THE 5-MINUTE CONSULT
Clinical Companion
TO WOMEN'S
HEALTH

Kelly A. McGarry, Iris L. Tong

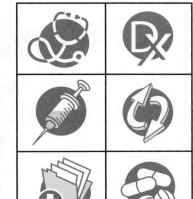

Wolters Kluwer | Lippincott Williams & Wilkins
Health

Philadelphia · Baltimore · New York · London
Buenos Aires · Hong Kong · Sydney · Tokyo

Acquisitions Editor: Sonya Seigafuse
Managing Editor: Lauren Aquino
Production Manager: David Murphy
Senior Manufacturing Manager: Benjamin Rivera
Marketing Manager: Kimberly Schonberger
Design Coordinator: Doug Smock
Production Services: Techbooks
Printer: Courier Westford

© 2007 by **LIPPINCOTT WILLIAMS & WILKINS**- a Wolters Kluwer business

**530 Walnut Street
Philadelphia, PA 19106 USA
LWW.com**

Printed in USA

Library of Congress Cataloging-in-Publication Data

McGarry, Kelly A.
    The 5-minute consult : clinical companion to women's health / Kelly A. McGarry, Iris L. Tong.
      p. ; cm.
    Includes bibliographical references.
    ISBN 0-7817-8338-0 (case)
    1. Women—Diseases—Handbooks, manuals, etc. 2. Women—Health and hygiene—Handbooks,
manuals, etc. I. McGarry, Kelly A. II. Tong, Iris L. III. Title. IV. Title: Five-minute consult
clinical companion to women's health.
    [DNLM: 1. Women's Health—Handbooks.   WA 39 M478z 2007]
  RC48.6.M44   2007
  613'. 04244—dc22   2006030778

PREFACE

It is with great pride that we present *The 5-Minute Consult Clinical Companion to Women's Health.* This book is a quick reference guide to the diagnosis and management of symptoms and disorders that commonly occur in women. Its main mission is to present concise, up-to-date information about disorders that are distinctive to women, occur disproportionately in women, or have different clinical presentations and/or prognoses in women. Written by primary care physicians, family practitioners, obstetrician-gynecologists, and specialists, the book presents evidence-based information in a format designed for quick and speedy consultation. Any healthcare provider who cares for women will find this book constructive and valuable. Students and residents preparing for oral and written in-service and certification exams will discover that this informative book is a useful study aid.

Providers have increasingly recognized that women have unique health needs and challenges. The field of women's health has undergone enormous advances in the last few decades. Research trials now are inclusive of women, whereas in the past treatment decisions for our female patients were based on data extrapolated from studies examining mostly men. Moreover, clinicians are constantly challenged with the unique physiological and sociological issues faced by women. This book is intended to be a handy reference that can be readily integrated into the practice of the busy clinician, providing highly relevant, clinically useful knowledge without the need for hours of reading, which is not practical in the office setting.

Therefore, we offer you this innovative book and ask you to make your own decision as to whether it is, in fact, all that we intended.

ACKNOWLEDGMENTS

We have enjoyed participating in this wonderful project. We have learned a great deal about the amount of work it takes to accomplish a task of this magnitude. We have had the opportunity to work with many wonderful people, from the individuals at Lippincott to all of our contributing authors.

This book has been an extraordinary opportunity for the two of us to grow professionally and personally, and we thank those working with us who have made it possible. We would like to thank Dr. Michele Cyr who gave us this incredible opportunity. We thank all our contributing authors for their hard work and dedication. Their efforts, knowledge, and expertise are the foundation of this book.

The Lippincott staff has been supportive and helpful from the first friendly and enthusiastic meeting at the Annual American College of Physicians (ACP) meeting to our subsequent lunch meeting at ACP two years later when the book was nearing its completion. We especially would like to thank Lauren Aquino, Mary Choi, and Sonya Seigafuse for all their guidance and efforts on our behalf.

We would also like to thank Gwen LaRiviere for all her organizational work and administrative support.

We have had an incredible experience in editing *The 5-Minute Consult Clinical Companion to Women's Health.* We hope that health care providers find this book useful and become as interested in the field of women's health as we are.

Kelly McGarry, M.D. and Iris Tong, M.D.

I would like to thank Dr. Karen Rosene-Montella, Chief of Medicine, Women and Infants' Hospital, Providence, Rhode Island, who has given me the support and time to dedicate to this project. Her mentorship has furthered my professional growth clinically and academically. And lastly, I would like to thank my partner, Michael, for his unconditional support and love in everything that I undertake.

Iris Tong, M.D.

CONTRIBUTORS

Purva Agarwal, M.D.
Resident Physician
Brown University
Providence, Rhode Island

Homayoon M. Akbari, M.D., Ph.D., F.R.C.S.(C).
Assistant Professor
Department of Surgery
Brown University Medical School
Rhode Island Hospital
Providence, Rhode Island

David Anthony, M.D., M.Sc.
Assistant Professor of Family Medicine
Assistant Director of Predoctoral Education
Brown University
Providence, Rhode Island

Michelle A. Stozek Anvar, M.D.
Assistant Professor of Medicine (Clinical)
Department of Medicine
Brown University
Providence, Rhode Island

Etsuko Aoki, M.D., Ph.D.
Fellow
M. D. Anderson Cancer Center
Houston, Texas

Sudeep K. Aulakh, M.D., C.M.
Attending Physician
Department of Medicine
Baystate Medical Center
Springfield, Massachusetts

John P. Bas, M.D., M.H.S.A.
Resident Physician
Department of Family Medicine
Memorial Hospital of Rhode Island
Pawtucket, Rhode Island
Brown University
Providence, Rhode Island

Anjali Basil, M.D.
Resident Physician
Department of Internal Medicine
Brown University Medical School
Providence, Rhode Island

Agnieszka K. Bialikiewicz, M.D.
Resident Physician
Department of Family Medicine
Memorial Hospital of Rhode Island
Pawtucket, Rhode Island
Brown University
Providence, Rhode Island

Amy Boardman, M.D.
Assistant Professor of Medicine
Division of Gastroenterology and Hepatology
Mayo Clinic College of Medicine
Rochester, Minnesota

Lori A. Boardman, M.D., Sc.M.
Associate Professor of Obstetrics/Gynecology
Department of Obstetrics and Gynecology
Brown University
Providence, Rhode Island

Alice E. Bonitati, M.D.
Associate Professor (Clinical)
Department of Medicine
Brown University
Providence, Rhode Island

Suzanne Bornschein, M.D.
Staff Physician
Department of Medicine
Rhode Island Hospital
Providence, Rhode Island

Kelly Bossenbroek, M.D.
Brown University
Providence, Rhode Island

Ghada Bourjeily, M.D.
Assistant Professor of Medicine
Pulmonary and Critical Care
Department of Medicine
Brown University
Director of Pulmonary Function Laboratory
Department of Medicine
Women and Infants' Hospital
Providence, Rhode Island

Maria Chiara Cantarini, M.D.
Dipartimento di Medicina Interna
Cardioangiologia
Epatologia
Bologna, Italy

Contributors

John P. Carvalho, M.B.A., L.R.E.P., C.M.P.E.
Dynamic Health Resources
Chesapeake, Virginia

Nadia Chammas, M.D.
Pulmonologist
Department of Pulmonary and Sleep Medicine
Minot, North Dakota

Sybil Cineas, M.D.
Clinical Assistant Professor of Medicine and
 Pediatrics
Department of Internal Medicine and
 Pediatrics
Brown University
Staff Physician
Department of Internal Medicine and
 Pediatrics
Rhode Island Hospital
Providence, Rhode Island

Courtney A. Clark, M.D.
Resident
Department of Medicine
Brown Medical School
Resident
Department of Medicine
Rhode Island Hospital
Providence, Rhode Island

Jennifer G. Clarke, M.D., M.P.H.
Assistant Professor
Department of Medicine
Brown University
Providence, Rhode Island
Director of Health Disparities Research
Department of Medicine
Memorial Hospital of Rhode Island
Pawtucket, Rhode Island

Michele G. Cyr, M.D., F.A.C.P.
Professor
Department of Medicine
Brown Medical School
Director
Division of General Internal Medicine
Rhode Island Hospital
Providence, Rhode Island

Silvia D. Degli-Esposti, M.D.
Associate Professor of Medicine (Clinical)
Department of Medicine
Brown Medical School
Director, Center for Women's Gastrointestinal
 Disorders
Department of Medicine
Women and Infants' Hospital
Providence, Rhode Island

Joseph A. Diaz, M.D.
Assistant Professor of Medicine
Division of General Internal Medicine
Brown Medical School
Providence, Rhode Island

Christy L. Dibble, D.O.
Clinical Assistant Professor
Department of Medicine
Brown University
Providence, Rhode Island

Christine Duffy, M.D., M.P.H.
Assistant Professor of Medicine
Department of Medicine
Brown University
Providence, Rhode Island

Staci A. Fischer, M.D., F.A.C.P.
Assistant Professor
Department of Medicine
Brown Medical School
Providence, Rhode Island

Jennifer S. Gass, M.D., F.A.C.S.
Clinical Assistant Professor
Department of Surgery
Brown University
Chief of Surgery
Women and Infants' Hospital—Breast Health
Providence, Rhode Island

Geetha Gopalakrishnan, M.D.
Assistant Professor
Department of Medicine
Brown University
Providence, Rhode Island

Amy S. Gottlieb, M.D.
Assistant Professor of Medicine and
 Obstetrics and Gynecology (Clinical)
Brown University
Providence, Rhode Island

Rebecca A. Griffith, M.D.
Medical Director Consult Service
Department of Medicine
Morristown Memorial Hospital
Morristown, New Jersey

Mina J. Guico, M.D.
House Staff
Department of Internal Medicine
North Florida Regional Medical Center
Gainesville, Florida

Fadlallah G. Habr, M.D.
Assistant Professor of Medicine
Department of Medicine
Brown University
Providence, Rhode Island

Megan Hebert, M.A.
Research Program Coordinator
Substance Abuse Research Unit
Department of Medicine
Brown University
Providence, Rhode Island

Mary H. Hohenhaus, M.D.
Clinical Instructor
Department of Medicine
Brown University
Providence, Rhode Island

Jennifer R. Hur, M.D.
Assistant Professor of Clinical Medicine
Indiana University School of Medicine
Indianapolis, Indiana

Lynn E. Iler, M.D.
Clinical Assistant Professor
Department of Dermatology
Brown University
Providence, Rhode Island

Neeta Jain, M.D.
Clinical Assistant Professor
Department of Psychiatry and
    Human Behavior
Brown University
Providence, Rhode Island

Jennifer Jeremiah, M.D.
Clinical Associate Professor
Department of Medicine
Brown University
Providence, Rhode Island

Elaine C. Jones, M.D.
Assistant Professor
Department of Medicine
Boston University
Boston, Massachusetts

Colleen R. Kelly, M.D.
Fellow
Department of Medicine
Brown University
Providence, Rhode Island

Jamie D. Kemp, M.D.
Resident Physician
Department of Medicine
Brown University
Providence, Rhode Island

Suzette M. LaRoche, M.D.
Assistant Professor
Department of Neurology
Emory University School of Medicine
Atlanta, Georgia

Lucia Larson, M.D.
Associate Professor
Department of Medicine and
    Obstetrics/Gynecology
Brown University
Providence, Rhode Island

Marco Lenzi, M.D.
Associate Professor
Dipartimento di Medicina Interna,
    Cardioangiologia, Epatologia
Università di Bologna
Bologna, Italy

Lori Lieberman-Maran, M.D.
Rheumatology Fellow
Department of Medicine
Boston University
Boston, Massachusetts

Mohsin K. Malik, M.D.
Assistant Clinical Instructor
Department of Medicine
Brown University
Providence, Rhode Island

Kelly A. McGarry, M.D.
Assistant Professor
Department of Medicine
Brown University
Providence, Rhode Island

Rohini McKee, M.D.
Resident Physician
Department of Surgery
Brown University
Providence, Rhode Island

Lynn McNicoll, M.D., F.R.C.P.C.
Assistant Professor of Medicine
Brown University
Providence, Rhode Island

Contributors

Niharika Mehta, M.D.
Assistant Clinical Professor
Department of Medicine
Brown University
Providence, Rhode Island

Margaret (Peg) A. Miller, M.D.
Assistant Professor
Department of Medicine
Brown University
Providence, Rhode Island

Bismruta Misra, M.D., M.P.H.
Clinical Instructor
Department of Medicine
Brown University
Providence, Rhode Island

Chad Morse, M.D.
Gastroenterology Fellow
Department of Medicine
Brown University
Providence, Rhode Island

Anne W. Moulton, M.D.
Associate Professor of Medicine
Department of Medicine
Brown University
Providence, Rhode Island

Rossana Moura, M.D.
Assistant Professor
Department of Medicine
Brown University
Providence, Rhode Island

Jill Newstead-Angel, M.D., F.R.C.P.(C).
Assistant Professor
Department of Medicine
University of Saskatchewan
Saskatoon, Saskatchewan, Canada

Melissa Nothnagle, M.D.
Assistant Professor of
  Family Medicine
Brown University
Providence, Rhode Island

Carolyn J. O'Connor, M.D.
Assistant Clinical Professor
Yale University School of Medicine
Department of Medicine
St. Mary's Hospital
Waterbury, Connecticut

Laura M. Ofstead, M.D.
Clinical Assistant Professor
Department of Medicine
Brown University
Providence, Rhode Island

Cristina Pacheco, M.D.
Assistant Clinical Instructor
Department of Family Medicine
Brown University
Providence, Rhode Island

Elvis Pagan, M.D.
Fellow
Department of Obstetric Medicine
Women and Infants' Hospital
Providence, Rhode Island

Michael P. Plevyak, M.D.
OB/GYN
Baystate Medical Center
Springfield, Massachusetts

Raymond O. Powrie, M.D.
Associate Professor
Department of Medicine and
  Obstetrics/Gynecology
Brown University
Providence, Rhode Island

Archana Pradhan, M.D., M.P.H.
Assistant Professor
Department of Obstetrics, Gynecology, and
  Reproductive Sciences
Robert Wood Johnson Medical School
New Brunswick, New Jersey

Ricardo Restrepo-Guzman, M.D.
Psychiatry
Providence, Rhode Island

Ramona L. Rhodes, M.D., M.P.H.
Fellow
Center for Gerontology and Health
  Care Research
Brown University
Providence, Rhode Island

Sumona Saha, M.D.
Fellow in Gastroenterology
Department of Medicine
Brown University
Providence, Rhode Island

Benjamin L. Sapers, M.D.
Assistant Professor (Clinical)
Department of Medicine
Brown University
Providence, Rhode Island

Eleanor Bimla Schwarz, M.D., M.S.
Assistant Professor of Medicine
Department of Medicine and Obstetrics,
    Gynecology and Reproductive Sciences
University of Pittsburgh
Pittsburgh, Pennsylvania

Catherine Malone Smitas, M.D.
Clinical Instructor
Department of Medicine
Brown University
Providence, Rhode Island

Sharon B. Stechna, M.D.
Assistant Professor
Department of Obstetrics and Gynecology
University of Medicine and Dentistry of
    New Jersey
New Brunswick, New Jersey

Vivian W. Sung, M.D., M.P.H.
Assistant Professor
Department of Obstetrics and Gynecology
Brown University
Providence, Rhode Island

Julie S. Taylor, M.D., M.Sc.
Assistant Professor
Department of Family Medicine
Brown University
Providence, Rhode Island

Iris L. Tong, M.D.
Assistant Professor (Clinical)
Department of Internal Medicine
Brown University
Providence, Rhode Island

Lidia Trejo, M.A.
Research Assistant
University of Rhode Island
Kingston, Rhode Island

Audrey R. Tyrka, M.D., Ph.D.
Assistant Professor
Department of Psychiatry and Human Behavior
Brown University
Providence, Rhode Island

Jody A. Underwood, M.D.
Clinical Assistant Professor
Department of Psychiatry and
    Human Behavior
Brown University
Providence, Rhode Island

Lauren M. Wier, B.S.
Research Assistant
Butler Hospital
Providence, Rhode Island

Susannah S. Wise, M.D., F.A.C.S.
Assistant Professor of Surgery
Department of General Surgery
Robert Wood Johnson Medical School
New Brunswick, New Jersey

Traci Wolbrink, M.D.
Resident Physician
Department of Internal Medicine/Pediatrics
Brown University
Providence, Rhode Island

Eric A. Wright, D.O.
Resident Physician
Brown University
Providence, Rhode Island

Margaret C. Wyche, B.S.
Research Assistant
Mood Disorders Research Program
Butler Hospital
Providence, Rhode Island

CONTENTS

Contents

THE 5-MINUTE CONSULT
Clinical Companion
TO WOMEN'S
HEALTH

Kelly A. McGarry, Iris L. Tong

ABNORMAL PAP SMEAR

Iris L. Tong, MD

KEY CLINICAL POINTS

- The papanicolaou (Pap) smear is an ideal screening test for cervical cancer, because it can identify the disease in its premalignant phase.
- Human Papilloma Virus (HPV) infection is strongly associated with cervical neoplasia.
  - Spontaneous clearance of HPV can occur.
  - Advocate safe sex practices.
- Cervical cancer is more likely in women who have not received screening within last 5 years.

 BASICS

DESCRIPTION

- Cervical cancer was the leading cause of cancer deaths in American women until widespread screening with the Pap smear began in 1941.
- The Pap smear, which is a sampling of cervical cells, is an ideal screening test because:
  - Cervical cancer has a premalignant phase of many years.
  - Screening on a regular basis is likely to identify the disease in its premalignant phase.
  - The test is inexpensive and can be performed in the outpatient setting.
- HPV is a sexually transmitted infection (STI) strongly associated with the development of cervical intraepithelial neoplasia (CIN) and cancer.
- Cervical cancer cell types:
  - Squamous cell cancer: 80%
  - Adenocarcinoma: 15%
  - Adenosquamous carcinoma: 5%

GENERAL PREVENTION

- Safe sex practices to prevent HPV transmission
- Regular screening with Pap smear
  - American College of Obstetricians & Gynecologists (ACOG):
    - Screening should begin 3 years after first sexual intercourse or by age 21
    - For women <30, annual Pap smear
    - For women >30,
      o Pap smear q2 to 3 years after 3 consecutive negative Pap smears OR
      o Pap smear with HPV testing. If both (−), screen with PAP and HPV testing q3 years.
    - Discontinue screening in:
      o Women who have had a hysterectomy for benign reasons and have no history of abnormal or cancerous cell growth
      o Women who have had hysterectomy for benign reasons and a history of CIN II or CIN III after 3 consecutive negative Pap smears
      o Older women on an individual basis
    - Annual pelvic exams should be performed regardless of frequency of Pap smears.
  - United States Preventative Services Task Force (USPSTF):
    - Screen q3 years
    - Discontinue at age 65
  - American Cancer Society (ACS):
    - Screen q3 years
    - Discontinue in women >70 years, unless high risk

- HPV vaccine against types 16 and 18
  - Effective against cervical infection and associated cytological abnormalities
  - However, vaccination is controversial as spontaneous clearance of HPV can occur (see Pathophysiology and Etiology).

EPIDEMIOLOGY

Incidence

- In the United States, 8 per 100,000 women.
- Estimated 10,000 new cases per year
  - Fifty percent of the cases are found in women who have never been screened.
  - Ten percent of the cases are found in women who have not been screened within the preceding 5 years.
- In the United States, peak incidence occurs in women 45 to 49 years of age.
  - Only 10% of the cases occur in women >75 years of age.

Prevalence

- In developed countries, cervical cancer is uncommon secondary to Pap smear screening.
  - In the United States, cervical cancer is the third most common gynecologic malignancy, but is associated with a low mortality rate.
  - Over past 50 years, there has been a 75% decrease in incidence and mortality of cervical cancer in developed countries
- Worldwide, cervical cancer is the most common cause of mortality from gynecologic malignancy
  - Second most common cancer among women
  - Third most common cause of cancer-related death

RISK FACTORS

- HPV infection
  - Unprotected intercourse
  - Multiple sexual partners
  - Early onset of sexual activity
- Tobacco use
- Immunocompromise
- Low socioeconomic status
- African American and Hispanic ethnicity
- History of STIs
- History of vulvar or vaginal squamous dysplasia
- Lack of Pap smear screening in last 5 years

PATHOPHYSIOLOGY

- Transmission of HPV via sexual contact leads to the malignant transformation of the vaginal and cervical epithelium.
- HPV DNA can be identified in at least 95% of dysplastic and malignant cervical lesions.
- HPV alone is not sufficient to cause cervical neoplasia.
  - Most HPV infections are transient.
    - Up to 50% of sexually active women have been exposed to HPV, but only a small number will develop high-grade CIN or invasive cervical cancer.
    - Seventy percent of CIN I, 50% of CIN II, and 30% of CIN III infections clear spontaneously.
  - Not all HPV types are oncogenic.

ETIOLOGY

- HPV subtypes 16 and 18
  - Responsible for up to 70% of cervical cancers

- Additional high-risk subtypes include 31, 33, 35, 39, 45, 51, 52, 56, 59, and 68

ASSOCIATED CONDITIONS
- Sexually Transmitted Infections (STIs)

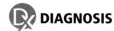

DIAGNOSIS

SIGNS AND SYMPTOMS
History
- Asymptomatic in early stages
- With more advance stages, symptoms may include:
  - Intermenstrual spotting
  - Postcoital bleeding
  - Postmenopausal bleeding
  - Vaginal discharge
    - Can be watery, mucoid, bloody, or purulent and malodorous
  - Severe back or pelvic pain
  - Alteration of bowel and bladder function
  - Enlarged lymph nodes
  - Obstructive uremia

Physical Exam
- Cervical exam
  - Can be grossly normal
  - If abnormal, can find
    - Superficial ulceration
    - Exophytic tumor
    - Endophytic tumor: enlarged, indurated cervix with smooth surface
- CVA tenderness if hydronephrosis present
- Inguinal lymphadenopathy

TESTS
Lab
- Consider screening for STIs: *Chlamydia Trachomatis, Neisseria Gonorrhea, Trichomonas Vaginalis,* Syphilis, Hepatitis B and C, HIV

Imaging
- CT or MRI of abdomen/pelvis for work-up of metastatic disease when indicated

Diagnostic Procedures/Surgery
- Pap Smear
  - Liquid medium system is slightly more sensitive than traditional slide system
  - Annual screening with liquid-based cytology may not be more cost effective
- Biopsy
  - Colposcopy with directed biopsy if abnormal cervical cytology without visible lesion
  - Cone biopsy is necessary for diagnosis of microinvasive disease
  - Punch biopsy and endocervical curettage for an unusually firm or expanded cervix

Pathologic Findings
According to the revised 2001 Bethesda System:
- Unsatisfactory specimen:
  - Repeat Pap smear
- Negative for intraepithelial lesion or malignancy:
  - Rescreen in 1 year if age <30
  - Rescreen in 3 years if age >30 and history of 3 consecutive negative Pap smears

- Atypical cells of unknown significance (ASCUS):
  - Rescreen q4 to 6 months × 2. If (−) × 2, then return to q year screening OR
  - Perform HPV polymerase-chain reaction DNA testing (only available with liquid-based cytology)
    - If positive for high-risk strains, refer to colposcopy
    - If negative for high-risk strains, rescreen in 1 year
    - Can be ordered as "reflex" such that if result of Pap smear is ASCUS, sample will be automatically sent for HPV testing
- Refer to colposcopy for
  - Atypical cells of unknown significance, cannot rule out high-grade lesion (ASC-H):
  - Low-grade squamous intraepithelial lesion (LGSIL)
    - Consistent with mild dysplasia (CIN I)
  - High-grade squamous intraepithelial lesion (HGSIL), which has two categories:
    - Moderate dysplasia (CIN II)
    - Severe dysplasia (CIN III or carcinoma in situ)
  - Atypical glandular cells of unknown significance (AGUS):
    - May also need endometrial biopsy

ALERT
- No endocervical cells, excessive blood, inflammation, reactive changes:
  - Repeat in 4–6 months if
    - History of abnormal Pap smears
    - HPV infection
    - Immunosuppression
    - HIV-positive
  - Rescreen in 1 year if no high-risk factors
- HIV(+) women
  - Repeat Pap smear q6 months until (−) × 2, then screen q year
- Postmenopausal women:
  - No endocervical cells: rescreen in 1 year
  - ASCUS: estrogen cream × 7 days, then repeat PAP smear
  - AGUS: colposcopy and endometrial biopsy

DIFFERENTIAL DIAGNOSIS
- Cervicitis
- Vaginitis
- Uterine cancer
- Nabothian cysts
- Endometriosis

TREATMENT

GENERAL MEASURES
- For LGSIL (CIN I), observation and close follow-up is appropriate
- Cervical cancer is staged from 0 to IVb
- Surgery is mainstay of treatment for lower stage tumors
- Radiation is mainstay of treatment for higher stage tumors
- Chemotherapy often used as adjuvant therapy

Activity
- Safe sex practices to prevent STI transmission

Radiotherapy
- Mainstay of treatment for higher stage tumors
  - Large, bulky tumors at Stage Ib or greater:
    - Radiation therapy with chemotherapy
  - Stage IIb, III and IVa Tumors: extension to local organs
    - Radiation therapy with chemotherapy
  - Stage IVb: distant metastases
    - Chemotherapy with or without radiation

MEDICATION (DRUGS)

- Chemotherapy: Cisplatin
  - Used as adjuvant therapy
    - Bulky and higher stage tumors
    - Postoperatively in patients considered to be at high risk for recurrent disease

SURGERY

- Mainstay of treatment for lower stage tumors
  - CIN II: cryotherapy OR laser vaporization
  - CIN III: loop excision
  - Stage Ia: invasive cancer identified only microscopically
    - Hysterectomy without pelvic lymph node dissection OR
    - Cone biopsy with close follow-up
  - Stage Ib/IIa: lesions confined to the cervix and/or upper vagina
    - Radical hysterectomy and dissection of pelvic lymph nodes OR
    - Radiation therapy

FOLLOW-UP

Issues for Referral

- Refer to gynecology for colposcopy
- Refer to gynecology/oncology for lesion consistent with cancer

PROGNOSIS

- Five-year survival rate of cervical cancer
  - Stage Ia: >95%
  - Stage IIa/Ib: 80% to 90%
  - Stage IIb, III and IVa Tumors: 20% to 65%
  - Stage IVb: 25%

COMPLICATIONS

- Metastatic disease
  - Direct extension to uterus, vagina, parametria, peritoneal cavity, bladder, and/or rectum
  - Lymphatic dissemination: external iliac, common iliac, paraaortic, and/or parametrial
  - Hematogenous dissemination

PATIENT MONITORING

- For cervical cancer, Pap smear q3 months × first 2 years after treatment then q6 months

Pregnancy Considerations

- Pregnancy does not increase the risk or change the course of cervical cancer.
- Diagnosis (with biopsy via colposcopy and confirmatory cone biopsy) carries increased risk of hemorrhage and poor perinatal outcome
- <20 weeks of gestation: radical hysterectomy can be performed with fetus in situ

- >20 weeks gestation: evacuation of fetus recommended before surgery
  - In stage I disease, can delay therapy until fetal survival is assured
  - In more advanced disease, delay of therapy is not recommended
- Delivery should be performed as soon as fetal lungs are mature
- Route of delivery is controversial
  - Cesarean delivery
    - Route advocated by most experts
  - Vaginal delivery
    - Recurrence at site of episiotomy possible
    - Increased risk of hemorrhage, obstructed labor, and infection with advanced disease

REFERENCES

1. Baer A, Kiviat NB, Kulasingam S, et al. ACOG Practice Bulletin. *Obstet Gynecol*. 2003;102:417–427.
2. Baer A, Kiviat NB, Kulasingam S, et al. ACOG Practice Bulletin. *Obstet Gynecol*. 2005;105:905–918.
3. Baer A, Kiviat NB, Kulasingam S, et al. Liquid-based papanicolaou smears without a transformation zone component: Should clinicians worry? *Obstet Gynecol*. 2002;99:1053–1059.
4. Canavan TP, Doshi NR. Cervical cancer. *Am Fam Physician*. 2000;61:1369–1376.
5. Harper DM, Fransco EL, Wheeler C, et al. Efficacy of a bivalent L1 virus-like particle vaccine in prevention of infection with human papillomavirus types 16 and 18 in young women: A randomized controlled trial. *Lancet*. 2004;362:1757–1765.

CODES
ICD-9-CM

- 795.0 Abnormal Pap smear of cervix
- 795.00 Nonspecific abnormal Pap smear of cervix, unspecified (Abnormal glandular cells)
- 795.09 Other nonspecific abnormal Pap (unsatisfactory smear, benign cellular changes)
- 622.1 Dysplasia of cervix (CIN I, II, LGSIL, HGSIL)
- 233.1 Carcinoma in-situ of cervix (CIN III)
- V76.2 Routine cervical Pap smear
- V72.3 General gynecological examination
- V72.32 Pap smear to confirm findings of recent normal smear following initial abnormal smear

KEY WORDS

- Abnormal Pap Smear
- Atypical Cells of Unknown Significance
- LGSIL
- HGSIL
- Atypical Glandular Cells
- Cervical Dysplasia
- Carcinoma in Situ
- Cervical Cancer

ABNORMAL UTERINE BLEEDING

Jamie D. Kemp, MD
Amy Boardman, MD

KEY CLINICAL POINTS

- AUB is a broad spectrum of menstrual cycle irregularities.
- Establishing a diagnosis depends on the patient's history, age, and exam findings.
- Treating AUB depends on whether or not the patient ovulates.
- Failure to effectively treat certain causes of AUB can lead to significant morbidity.

 BASICS

DESCRIPTION
Abnormal uterine bleeding can be divided into one or more of the following groups:
- Menorrhagia—heavy or prolonged menstrual bleeding
- Metrorrhagia—intermenstrual bleeding
- Hypomenorrhea—unusually light menses
- Menstrual bleeding with irregular cyclicity
  - Oligomenorrhea (periods that are more than 35 days apart)
  - Polymenorrhea (periods that are too frequent)
- Postcoital bleeding
- Postmenopausal bleeding

EPIDEMIOLOGY
- One-third of ambulatory gynecologic visits are due to abnormal uterine bleeding.
- The true frequency of AUB is difficult to assess.
  - Many women will experience AUB, although it may be sporadic.
  - Any one woman may experience different types of AUB.
  - Many women will not complain of AUB to their practitioners.
- AUB accounted for almost 4 million outpatient visits in the United States in 1996.
- Menorrhagia and uterine fibroids account for up to 75% of all hysterectomies worldwide.

Prevalence
Prevalence increases with age and peaks prior to menopause.

RISK FACTORS
Risk factors for AUB depend on the entity responsible. Important factors to consider include:
- Vaginal, pelvic, or abdominal trauma
- Personal or family history of AUB
- Personal or family history of bleeding diathesis
- Family history of premature ovarian failure or early menopause
- Associated symptoms of acne, weight gain, or hirsutism
- History of endocrinologic disease
- Medication use
- Eating disorders or excessive exercise
- Severe physical or emotional stress, including medical and psychiatric illness

PATHOPHYSIOLOGY
See Etiology.

ETIOLOGY
The causes of AUB depend upon age.
- Premenopausal women
  - Pregnancy
  - Malignancy
    - Cervix

- Vagina
    - Endometrium
  - Anatomic/Structural Abnormalities
    - Adenomyosis
    - Fibroids
    - Polyps
  - Anovulation
  - Bleeding Disorders
  - Trauma
  - Endocrine Disease
    - Thyroid
    - Pituitary
    - Adrenal
- Perimenopausal women
  - Includes the causes listed above for premenopausal women, but the incidences of anovulation and malignancy increase
  - Bleeding from sites other than the reproductive tract
- Postmenopausal women
  - Malignancy
  - Atrophy of the vaginal epithelium or endometrium
  - Bleeding from sites other than the reproductive tract

ASSOCIATED CONDITIONS
See causes of AUB above.

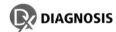 **DIAGNOSIS**

PRE-HOSPITAL
Generally, the workup for AUB is performed in an outpatient setting.

SIGNS AND SYMPTOMS
- Unusually heavy menstrual bleeding
- Irregularities in the amount of menstrual flow or the timing of menses
- Bleeding after intercourse or defecation
- Symptoms of anemia, including fatigue, dyspnea, lightheadedness

History
- Is the patient sexually active?
- Does she have a history of prior menstrual irregularities?
- When did menarche begin?
- When was her last period?
- Does she have a history of STD's?
- Does she have bleeding from other sites, such as the nose, gums, or rectum?
- Does the patient take medications, including oral contraceptives?

Physical Exam
All patients who complain of AUB should have a thorough physical exam, including speculum examination, bimanual examination, rectal examination, Papanicolou testing, STD testing, and examination of the vaginal discharge.
- Look for acne, hirsutism, or other signs of virilization. Examine the thyroid for abnormalities.
- Pelvic examination may allow direct visualization of a bleeding source.
- Abnormalities on bimanual exam may indicate uterine cancer or fibroids.

- Wet-prep may reveal evidence of vaginitis; STD testing is indicated to rule out cervicitis or PID.
- Pap smears can evaluate for cervical cancer, a common cause of intermittent and postcoital bleeding.
- Rectal examination assists in the diagnosis of hemorrhoids and fecal occult blood testing evaluates for GI bleeding.

TESTS
The first steps in evaluating AUB are to rule out pregnancy and to determine ovulatory status.
- Patients may complain of hypomenorrhea, metrorrhagia, or amenorrhea during pregnancy, which can be ruled out with urine or serum beta-hCG testing.
- Since the evaluation of AUB associated with ovulation differs from that of anovulatory cycles, attention must be paid to whether or not the patient ovulates regularly.
  - Cyclic menses occurring at regular intervals are most likely ovulatory. Cycle charting and basal body temperature testing are helpful in this regard.
  - A serum progesterone concentration greater than 2 ng/mL during the luteal phase is consistent with ovulation.

Lab
Chronic medical illness may cause AUB directly (as is the case with bleeding disorders), or can induce anovulation. Laboratory testing may be helpful in the workup of AUB, but should be guided by the history and physical.
- Liver, thyroid, or renal function testing may reveal another medical diagnosis.
- PTT, PT/INR, platelet count may be indicated; if there is suspicion for a bleeding disorder, one can check factor VIII or von Willebrand antigen levels.
- In a nonpregnant woman with amenorrhea or hypomenorrhea, obtaining a prolactin level may be helpful.
- Hirsutism or signs of hyperandrogenism may suggest PCOS; checking total testosterone, 17-hydroxyprogesterone and DHEA-S are indicated.
- Rarely, FSH may be helpful if premature ovarian failure is suspected; levels greater than 30 mIU/mL suggest menopause.

Imaging
Transvaginal ultrasound can sensitively detect structural lesions such as leiomyomata and can measure the thickness and regularity of the endometrial stripe.
- Uterine fibroids less than 5 mm may not be detected.
- Myometrial lesions cannot be accurately characterized as benign or malignant by TVUS.
- Endoluminal lesions, such as polyps, may not be readily visible unless sonohysterography is performed.
- Sonography is operator-dependent and is associated with significant cost.

Diagnostic Procedures/Surgery
Endometrial biopsy is indicated in women over age 35 to rule out malignancy or endometrial hyperplasia. Biopsy may be warranted in younger women with significant risk factors for malignancy, including anovulation, a history of unopposed estrogen use, obesity, or a family history of breast, uterine, or ovarian cancer.

DIFFERENTIAL DIAGNOSIS
The practitioner should rule out bleeding that does not come from the reproductive tract. Additionally, oral, transdermal, and intravaginal contraceptives, as well as the IUD, commonly cause abnormal uterine bleeding that is not harmful.
- Combined estrogen-progestin contraceptives regularly cause AUB during the first three cycles. If bleeding continues for more than 3 months, assess for compliance, concomitant pregnancy, or the use of other medications (anticonvulsants, antibiotics).
- Progestin-only medications, including depot contraception and the levonorgestrel-containing IUD, frequently induce amenorrhea during the first 6 to 12 months of use.

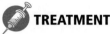 TREATMENT

PRE-HOSPITAL
Most cases of AUB can be treated in the outpatient setting.

INITIAL STABILIZATION
Ensure that there is no actively bleeding lesion visible on exam. Evaluate for anemia, hypotension or orthostatic hypotension.

GENERAL MEASURES
Proper treatment depends upon accurate diagnosis of the cause of AUB.

IV Fluids
Normal saline or lactated ringer's can be used for volume support if the patient is hypotensive.

 MEDICATION (DRUGS)

- Ovulatory bleeding and anovulatory bleeding that cannot be attributed to a particular cause can be treated similarly.

First Line
- Oral contraceptives induce withdrawal bleeding in anovulatory women, reduce menstrual flow, and improve cycle regularity in ovulatory women.
- Cyclic progestins induce bleeding in anovulatory women with adequate estrogen.
- The levonorgestrel IUD significantly reduces the amount of menstrual blood loss.
- In women with PCOS, OCP's have been shown to be helpful.

Second Line
- NSAIDS reduce menstrual blood flow and dysmenorrhea significantly, but have no effect on frequency or cyclicity.
- In severe cases, GnRH agonists (leuprolide, buserelin) may be used to induce a hypogonadotropic state.

SURGERY
Surgery is infrequently necessary, but can be used in severe cases.
- Endometrial ablation
- Hysterectomy
- Uterine artery embolization

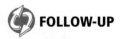 FOLLOW-UP

DISPOSITION
Admission Criteria
If the patient is dangerously anemic or hypotensive, or if she has an actively bleeding lesion that cannot be stopped by conservative measures in the office, admission may be warranted.

Issues for Referral
Most cases of AUB can be managed by the patient's primary health care provider; some situations require referral to specialists.
- Malignancy should be referred to a gynecologic oncologist.
- Multi-system endocrine disease or disease that fails to respond to usual management may warrant referral to an endocrinologist.

- Bleeding diatheses should be followed by a hematologist.

PROGNOSIS

When appropriately diagnosed and treated, most women with AUB will experience resolution or relief of their symptoms.

COMPLICATIONS

- Frequent or prolonged menstrual bleeding can cause iron-deficiency anemia.
- Unopposed estrogen exposure from chronic anovulation is a risk factor for endometrial cancer.
- Infrequent or irregular periods, perimenopause, and anovulation can result in infertility.

REFERENCES

1. Wren BG. Dysfunctional uterine bleeding. *Australian Family Physician*. 1998;54:61.
2. Bayer SR, DeCherney A. Clinical manifestations and treatment of dysfunctional uterine bleeding. *JAMA*. 1993;269:1823.
3. Dilley A, Drews C, Miller C, et al. von Willebrand's disease and other inherited bleeding disorders in women diagnosed with menorrhagia. *Obstetrics and Gynecology*. 2001;97:630–636.
4. Farquhar CM, Lethaby A, Sowter J, et al. An evaluation for risk factors for endometrial hyperplasia in premenopausal women with abnormal menstrual bleeding. *American Journal of Obstetrics and Gynecology*. 1999;181:525.

ADDITIONAL READING

Current Obstetrics and Gynecologic Diagnosis and Treatment. 9th ed. Alan H. DeCherney, Lauren Nathan: McGraw-Hill; 2003.

CODES
ICD9-CM

- 626.2 Excessive or frequent menstruation (includes menorrhagia, menometrorrhagia, polymenorrhea)
- 626.6 Metrorrhagia
- 627.1 Postmenopausal bleeding

KEY WORDS

- Heavy Menstrual Bleeding
- Irregular Menstrual Bleeding
- Hirsutism
- Bleeding after Intercourse
- Mucosal Bleeding

ABORTION, SPONTANEOUS

Jamie D. Kemp, MD
Archana Pradhan, MD, MPH

KEY CLINICAL POINTS

- Spontaneous abortion (SAB) is the most frequent complication of pregnancy.
- Advanced maternal age and previous miscarriage are the two strongest factors that predict future miscarriage.
- Most spontaneous abortions are associated with congenital or chromosomal abnormalities.

 BASICS

DESCRIPTION

Spontaneous abortion, or miscarriage, is the spontaneous loss of a pregnancy prior to 20 weeks gestation.
- Fifteen percent of clinically recognized pregnancies end in miscarriage.
- Up to 30% to 45% of unrecognized pregnancies end in miscarriage.
- Most SABs (80%) occur in the first trimester with the incidence decreasing with increasing gestational age.

RISK FACTORS

There are many recognized risk factors for spontaneous abortion.
- Advancing maternal age
  - The prevalence of miscarriage in women under 20 is 12% compared to greater than 25% in women over 40 years of age.
- Prior miscarriage
  - The risk of another miscarriage is 20% after one spontaneous abortion, 28% after two, and 43% after three.
- Alcohol
  - Moderate alcohol consumption (greater than 3 drinks per week) increases the risk of spontaneous abortion, especially in the first 10 weeks of pregnancy.
- Cocaine
- Cigarette smoking
- Caffeine
  - There is a modest increase in the rate of spontaneous abortion in women who drink more than 4 cups of coffee (or other caffeine-containing beverages) per day.
- NSAID use
  - If used at or around conception, NSAID use increases the incidence of miscarriage.

PATHOPHYSIOLOGY

- Threatened abortion is uterine bleeding from a gestation of less than 20 weeks without any cervical dilatation or effacement.
- Incomplete abortion is the passage of some but not all placental tissue through the cervix before 20 weeks gestation.
- Inevitable abortion is uterine bleeding from a gestation of less than 20 weeks accompanied by cervical dilatation, but without expulsion of any placental or fetal tissue through the cervix.
- Completed abortion occurs when all products of conception have been expelled before 20 weeks gestation.
- Missed abortion occurs when fetal expulsion does not occur despite intrauterine fetal demise less than 20 weeks gestation.
- Septic abortion is any type of abortion associated with fever, chills, pain, and purulent uterine discharge.

ETIOLOGY

There are numerous causes of spontaneous abortion.
FETAL:
- Chromosomal abnormalities
  - Half of spontaneous abortions are caused by karyotype abnormalities.
  - Most of these abnormalities occur de novo and are not inherited.
MATERNAL:
- Endocrinopathies
  - Hyperandrogenism
  - Hyperprolactinemia
  - Poorly controlled diabetes
- Hypercoagulable disorders
  - Systemic lupus erythematosus
  - Antiphospholipid syndrome
  - Factor V Leiden
- Trauma
- Infection
  - Rubella
  - Primary herpes simplex infection
  - Toxoplasmosis
  - Listeria monocytogenes
  - CMV
  - Anatomic
  - Leiomyomas
  - Cervical insufficiency
  - Intrauterine adhesions

ASSOCIATED CONDITIONS

- Recurrent spontaneous abortion—three or more consecutive miscarriages

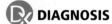 **DIAGNOSIS**

SIGNS AND SYMPTOMS

- Vaginal bleeding is the most common symptom reported in women with spontaneous abortion.
  - Occurs in up to 40% of all pregnant women and half of these will end up being spontaneous abortions
  - May be painful or painless
- There may be abdominal or pelvic pain.
- There may be fever or chills.
- The prior symptoms of pregnancy (nausea, vomiting, breast tenderness, fatigue) may disappear.

History

- Is there a history of previous miscarriage?
- What is the gestational age?
- Has the patient passed any blood clots or recognizable products of conception?
- Has she recently been ill?
- Has she been taking any medications or using any illicit substances?
- Has there been any trauma to the abdomen or pelvis?

Physical Exam

- Temperature, heart rate, blood pressure
- A speculum exam should be performed to locate the source of bleeding.

- On bimanual exam, assess if the cervix is open/closed, if the uterus is boggy or tender

TESTS
Lab
- Serum human chorionic gonadotropin level may be inappropriately low. This value is not diagnostic, however, unless a quantitative level was previously checked
- Maternal hemoglobin to assess for potentially harmful blood loss
- Type and Screen to determine 1) maternal blood type and Rh status, 2) also necessary if there has been significant bleeding and there is a likelihood of transfusion
- Blood cultures and cervical cultures if septic abortion is suspected

Imaging
Ultrasonography is the most helpful imaging tool in diagnosing spontaneous abortion.
- Absence of fetal heart activity
- Assessment of the presence/absence/size of the gestational sac, fetal pole and yolk sac

DIFFERENTIAL DIAGNOSIS
Because vaginal bleeding occurs frequently in the first trimester of pregnancy, this symptom does not always signal miscarriage.
- Implantation bleeding
- Bleeding from other sites in the gynecologic tract
- Ectopic pregnancy

 ## TREATMENT

INITIAL STABILIZATION
- Assess the patient for hemodynamic stability.
- If the patient is unstable, large bore IVs should be placed and IV fluids should be started.

GENERAL MEASURES
- Complete abortion does not require further medical therapy, but care should be made to support the patient psychologically.
- Septic abortion requires antibiotics and prompts surgical evacuation.
- Incomplete, inevitable, or missed abortion may be treated expectantly, medically, or surgically, depending on the patient's clinical status.

SPECIAL THERAPY
- Medical therapy with misoprostol
- Expectant management—waiting for the products of conception to pass on their own
- Dilation and curettage

IV Fluids
Lactated ringers and normal saline are appropriate for fluid resuscitation if necessary.

 ## MEDICATION (DRUGS)

- Rh negative women should be given Rh immune globulin.

SURGERY
Dilation and curettage with suction curettage is recommended in certain situations, including:
- Septic abortion
- Unsuccessful treatment with misoprostol

- When expectant management has not resulted in expulsion
- In concordance with the patient's wishes
- Heavy bleeding

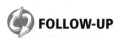 ## FOLLOW-UP

DISPOSITION
- Pelvic rest for 2 to 4 weeks

Admission Criteria
- Septic abortion
- Heavy bleeding
- Hemodynamic instability

Discharge Criteria
- All products of conception have been expulsed
- Psychologic issues have been addressed

Issues for Referral
- Patients with recurrent abortion may benefit from referral to a genetic specialist.
- Grief counseling may be appropriate.
- A diagnostic evaluation should be initiated in a patient with one second trimester SAB or two first trimester SABs.

PROGNOSIS
- There is an increased risk of spontaneous abortion in future pregnancies.

COMPLICATIONS
- When managed properly, spontaneous abortion is not generally associated with medical complications.
- There may be significant depression associated with the loss of a pregnancy.
- Infection rate of SABs: 1–2%

PATIENT MONITORING
- Monitor for prolonged vaginal bleeding
- Monitor psychological state

REFERENCES
1. Danforth's Obstetrics and Gynecology. 9th ed. Lippincott, Williams, and Wilkins.
2. Regan L, Braude PR, Trembath PL. Influence of past reproductive performance on risk of spontaneous abortion. *British Medical Journal*. 1989;299:541.
3. Regan L, Rai R. Epidemiology and the medical causes of miscarriage. *Bailliere's Clinical Obstetrics and Gynaecology*. 2000;14:839.
4. Bagratee JS, Khullar V, Regan L, et al. A randomized controlled trial comparing medical and expectant management of first trimester miscarriage. *Human Reproduction*. 2004;19:266.

CODES
ICD9-CM
- 634.1 Incomplete spontaneous abortion
- 634.2 Complete spontaneous abortion
- 632 Missed abortion

KEY WORDS
- Miscarriage
- Abortion
- Vaginal Bleeding

ACNE

Mohsin K. Malik, MD
Lynn E. Iler, MD

KEY CLINICAL POINTS

- Acne can cause permanent scarring as well as psychosocial distress.
- Therapeutic modalities should be chosen based on the morphology of lesions and the individual patient's response to, tolerance of, and desire for treatment.
- Patients with menstrual irregularity, hirsutism, or other signs of virilization should receive a hormonal evaluation to rule out:
  - Polycystic ovarian disease
  - Androgen-secreting tumors

BASICS

DESCRIPTION
Acne vulgaris is a disease of pilosebaceous units causing facial and truncal comedones, papules, pustules, and/or cysts.

EPIDEMIOLOGY
- Can affect any age from newborns onward
- Onset typically at menarche (onset of menses) or, less frequently, at adrenarche (increased adrenal gland activity associated with formation of secondary sex changes).

Prevalence
- Affects about 17 million persons in the United States
- Prevalence peaks at age 16–18 when 75–98% of the population is affected

RISK FACTORS
- Use of comedogenic facial and hair products
- Hormonal changes (flares 2–7 days before menses or during pregnancy)
- Excessive face washing and picking
- Stress
- Medications such as lithium, androgens (depo-provera), corticosteroids, and azathioprine
- Seasonal flares in some
- NOT caused by chocolate, soda, poor hygiene

PATHOPHYSIOLOGY
- Hyperproliferation of the follicular epithelium causes follicular plugging.
- Excess sebum production in the plugged follicle leads to inflammation, producing a favorable environment for *Propionibacterium acnes* colonization.
- Occlusion of follicles by cosmetics, hair products, or clothing can also be contributory.

ETIOLOGY
- Acne is caused by abnormal keratinization and sebum production associated with the pilosebaceous follicle.
- Hormonal influences also play a role.

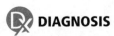

DIAGNOSIS

SIGNS AND SYMPTOMS
- Acne can present with:
  - Closed comedones (whiteheads)
  - Open comedones (blackheads)
  - Erythematous papules
  - Pustules
  - Nodules
  - Cysts
  - Postinflammatory hyperpigmentation
  - Scarring
- The face, neck, chest, upper back, and upper arms are most commonly affected.
- The trunk and buttocks may also be affected.
- Lesions (especially nodular ones) can be painful.
- Other systemic signs and symptoms should be absent.

History
- Evaluate for:
  - Time of onset of acne
  - Flare of acne around menses
  - Family history of acne
- Irregular menses, hirsutism or other virilization, or rapid onset of menses may signal an endocrinopathy.
- Polycystic ovarian syndrome must be considered in females with hirsutism, irregular menses, and/or obesity.
- An androgen-secreting ovarian or adrenal tumor should be considered in women with rapid onset of acne and virilization.

Physical Exam
- General appearance: Assess for signs of virilization and obesity
- Face and trunk: Comedones, papules, pustules, nodules, and/or cysts distributed on areas with the greatest number of sebaceous glands
- Presence of telengectasias makes diagnosis of rosacea more likely
- Lesions should be in various clinical stages; monomorphic comedones or pustules may signal exposure to halogenated hydrocarbons or topical or oral glucocorticoids.

DIFFERENTIAL DIAGNOSIS
- Polycystic ovarian disease
- Virilization by adrenal/ovarian tumor or androgens
- Rosacea
- Perioral dermatitis
- Folliculitis
- Abscess
- Furuncle/carbuncle

TREATMENT

GENERAL MEASURES
- Microcomedones take 8 weeks to mature so treatment must continue beyond this duration before evaluating the efficacy.
- Surface sebum and dirt are not pathogenic, and excessive washing or scrubbing can compromise the barrier function of skin and promote inflammation.
- Face washing should be limited to twice daily with a nonsoap cleanser or acne wash (benzoyl peroxide or salicylic acid).
- Patients should avoid rubbing their faces or picking at the skin.
- Washes, moisturizers, sunscreens, cosmetics, hair products, and any other products used on acne-prone skin should be labeled as "noncomedogenic" and preferably also "oil-free."
- Oil-free sunscreen should be used daily, because of increased photosensitivity with many topical and oral treatments.

MEDICATION (DRUGS)

First Line

For mild to moderate acne (comedonal, small inflamed papules and pustules), topical therapy is indicated. Topical therapy generally includes a topical retinoid and benzoyl peroxide/clindamycin combination.

- Topical retinoids (tretinon, adapalene, tazarotene) normalize rate of follicular keratinization
  - Minimal amounts should be applied to minimize irritation.
  - A "pea-sized" amount sufficient for entire face
  - Microsphere gels are least irritating, creams are intermediate, and gels are most irritating.
  - Should not be applied immediately after washing skin
  - Apply 2–3 times per week and increase as tolerated
  - Select concentration and vehicle based on skin type, for example:
    - For oily skin: Tazarotene cream 0.1% plus benzoyl peroxide/clindamycin gel
    - Dry skin: Tretinoin microsphere (Retin-A micro) gel 0.04%
  - Studies on relative efficacy of topical retinoids are incomplete, but tazarotene appears more effective and adapalene less irritating.
- Benzoyl peroxide gels are antimicrobial.
  - Warn patients of the risk of bleaching clothing, etc.
- Topical antibiotics are antibacterial and antiinflammatory.
  - Because of high resistance to erythromycin, clindamycin is first-line

Second Line

For moderate to severe acne (larger inflamed papules, pustules, cysts, +/– scarring), start with topical treatment with retinoids, +/– benzoyl peroxide/clindamycin as above. In addition, add:

- Systemic antibiotics (First line: Tetracycline, doxycycline, minocycline) are antibacterial, antiinflammatory, and immunomodulatory
  - Tetracycline (500 mg every day to b.i.d.)
    - Efficacious and relatively inexpensive
    - Must be taken on an empty stomach
  - Doxycycline (50–100 mg every day to b.i.d.)
    - Can be taken with food
  - Minocycline (50–100 mg every day to b.i.d.)
    - Does not cause photosensitivity like tetracycline and doxycycline
    - Potential adverse reactions are more serious (pseudotumor cerebri, hypersensitivity reaction, urticaria, elevated LFTs, exacerbation of systemic lupus erythematosus)
  - Women on antibiotic therapy are at increased risk for vaginal yeast infections.
  - These antibiotics do not reduce the efficacy of oral contraceptives
  - Course length varies; taper according to response
- Hormonal therapy is appropriate for female patients only.
  - Oral contraceptives (OC)
    - OCs can be used with any of the other treatment modalities.
    - Improvement of 40–70% has been reported with OCs alone
    - Ethinyl estradiol/norgestimate (Ortho Tri-Cyclen®)
    - Ethinyl estradiol/norethindrone (Estrostep®)
    - Ethinyl estradiol/drospirenone (Yasmin®)

- Androgen-receptor blockers are not FDA approved for use in acne. Agents that are effective and well-tolerated alone or with other treatment modalities include:
  - Spironolactone (50–150 mg daily): Serum potassium levels must be monitored.
  - Flutamide (250 mg daily): Liver function tests must be monitored with flutamide.

Third Line

For severe nodular acne or acne recalcitrant to other treatment, isotretinoin is indicated:

- Isotretinoin reduces sebum production and normalizes follicular keratinization.
- Physicians must receive FDA authorization before prescribing.
- Isotretinoin is teratogenic and females must use 2 forms of birth control.
- A single course of isotretinoin (0.5–1 gm/kg daily for 4–6 months) leads to a remission in about 75% of patients treated.
- About 25% require a 2nd course of isotretinoin, and a smaller subset requires further treatment.
- Systemic corticosteroids may additionally be required to achieve control in very severe cases of acne.

Pregnancy Considerations

Category B acne treatments are:

- Erythromycin or clindamycin, topically or orally
- Topical metronidazole
- Topical azelaic acid

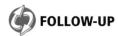 FOLLOW-UP

Issues for Referral

Scarring or cystic acne that is not responsive to second-line therapy should be referred to a dermatologist to evaluate for treatment with isotretinoin.

PROGNOSIS

- Prevalence of acne decreases after teenage years.
- The course and duration of disease cannot be predicted in a given individual.
- Acne often resolves during the early 20s.
- A subset of women has acne persisting into their 20s or beyond.
- Another subset of women does not have the onset of acne until their 20s.
- Seasonal variation in some
- Possible causes of flares:
  - Days just prior to menses
  - Excessive face washing
  - Use of comedogenic facial products
  - Stress: Not consistently proven
  - Diet: Role controversial

REFERENCES

1. Archer JS, Archer DF. Oral contraceptive efficacy and antibiotic interaction: A myth debunked. *J Am Acad Dermatol.* 2002;46:917–923.
2. Chan JJ, Rohr JB. Acne vulgaris: Yesterday, today and tomorrow. *Australas J Dermatol.* 2000;41:69–72.
3. Chiu A, Chon SY, Kimball AB. The response of skin disease to stress: Changes in the severity of acne vulgaris as affected by examination stress. *Arch Dermatol.* 2003;139:897–900.
4. Dreno B. Topical antibacterial therapy for acne vulgaris. *Drugs.* 2004;64:2389–2397.

5. Haider A, Shaw JC. Treatment of acne vulgaris. *JAMA*. 2004;292:726–735

6. Kaminer MS, Gilchrest BA. The many faces of acne. *J Am Acad Dermatol*. 1995;32:6–14.

CODES
ICD9-CM
706.1

KEY WORDS

- Acne Vulgaris
- Cyst
- Comedone
- Isotretinoin

ALCOHOL USE AND ABUSE

Ricardo Restrepo-Guzman, MD

KEY CLINICAL POINTS

- Clinical interview should include substance abuse history.
- Always maximize resources to treat substance abuse including different therapy modalities and different psychopharmacological approaches.
- Alcohol and other substance abuse is a chronic illness and should be treated as such.

 BASICS

DESCRIPTION

- The American Psychiatry Association (APA) definitions of Alcohol Use Disorders according to the Diagnosis Criteria For Mental Disorders (DSM –IV-TR):
  - Alcohol abuse (≥1 criteria for over 1 year):
    - Role impairment (failed work or home obligations)
    - Hazardous use (driving while intoxicated)
    - Legal problems related to alcohol use
    - Social or interpersonal problems due to alcohol
  - Alcohol Dependence (3 criteria for >1 year)
    - Tolerance (increase drinking to achieve same effect)
    - Alcohol withdrawal signs or symptoms
    - Drinking more than intended
    - Unsuccessful attempts to cut down on use
    - Excessive time related to alcohol (e.g., obtaining, hangover)
    - Impaired social/work activities due to alcohol
    - Use despite physical or psychological consequences

EPIDEMIOLOGY

- In 2003, an estimated 5.9% of women ≥ age 18 met criteria for abuse of or dependence on alcohol or an illicit drug in the past year.
- American Indian or Alaska native women >18 had higher rates of alcohol or illicit drug abuse or dependence than other racial or ethnic groups.
- Married women aged 18 to 49 had lower rate of alcohol or illicit drug abuse or dependence than women of any other marital status.
- Women with substance use disorders suffer greater secondary medical morbidity from substance abuse and higher mortality rate by all causes (including suicide).
- Female alcohol abusers start later than men, progress to abuse faster, abuse less total alcohol, and have higher rates of comorbid psychopathology.
- One in three college women now binge drink.
- In the United States, >40% of fatal car crashes are the result of driving under the influence.
  - Most of the drivers are men.
  - Almost 15,000 women drivers were involved in crashes in 2002, which is a number that has been increasing yearly.

RISK FACTORS

- Genetic influences
- Early initiation of drinking
- Victimization

Genetics

- Family, twin, and adoption studies have shown that alcohol related disorders have a genetic component.

PATHOPHYSIOLOGY

- Physiology/Metabolism
  - Sex differences in response to alcohol
    - Differential weight/body mass
    - Chemical absorption rates
    - Stomach enzymes
    - Ratios of body fat to water (Plant, 1997)
    - Higher peak blood alcohol concentrations in response to dose corrected by body
    - Higher body fat; lower body water-alcohol distributed in total body water, so is less dilute in women
    - Absorption of oral alcohol increased in women
    - Lower quantities of the enzyme ADH in the gastric mucosa
    - Higher levels of ADH in males (greater initial metabolism)
    - ETOH neurotoxic effects may be greater in women than in men.
- Comorbid Psychopathology
  - Anxiety disorders (PTSD), mood disorders, and eating disorders
  - Women are more likely to have a significant other who is also a substance abuser.
  - Women tend to have a history of trauma and to date the onset of their substance use disorder to a stressful event.

ASSOCIATED CONDITIONS

- For women in particular, the health related aspects of alcohol consumption include:
  - Different degree of impact on organ systems (e.g., liver, cognitive function)
  - Risks to fetal development
  - Compromised parenting capabilities
  - HIV/AIDS risk
- Fetal alcohol syndrome (FAS)
  - Prenatal drinking increases an infant's risk of dying during the first year by more than 50% and puts babies at risk for FAS.
  - FAS is one of most severe effects of drinking during pregnancy.
  - FAS is a lifelong condition that causes physical and mental disabilities, which are characterized by abnormal facial features, growth deficiencies, and central nervous system (CNS) problems.
  - People with FAS may have problems with learning, memory, attention span, communication, vision, hearing, or a combination of these.
  - FAS often leads to difficulties in school and problems getting along with others.
  - FAS is a permanent condition.
  - The amount of alcohol needed to develop FAS is unclear.
- Birth defects
- Mental retardation
- Neuro-developmental disorders (possibly ADHD)
- Heavy alcohol consumption affects:
  - CNS: mental function
  - Cardiac: cardiomyopathy
  - Liver: cirrhosis
  - GI system: ulcers, pancreatitis
  - Risk of cancers: throat, bladder, breast
    - Women alcohol abusers have higher risk of breast cancer than nonabusers.
  - Weight, nutrition, absorption
  - Reproductive health
  - Injury: falls, accidents

ALERT

- Alcohol is one of the leading known preventable causes of mental retardation and birth defects.
- The CDC recommends that women not drink any amount of alcohol during pregnancy or while trying to become pregnant.

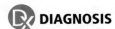 **DIAGNOSIS**

SIGNS AND SYMPTOMS

- Alcohol Intoxication

Blood Alcohol Level (mg/dL)	Signs of Intoxication
20–99	Incoordination, changes in mood, behavior, and personality Impairment of sensory functions
100–199	Slurred speech, marked incoordination/ataxia, impairment in cognitive functioning, reaction time prolonged
200–299	Nausea and vomiting, diplopia, marked ataxia
300–399	Hypothermia, severe dysarthria, amnesia
400–700	Coma, respiratory failure, death

- Remember BAL of 0 does not mean 0 risk for seizures, withdrawal, and delirium.
- Screening
  - CAGE Questionnaire:
    - Have you ever felt you should *Cut down* on your drinking?
    - Have people *Annoyed* you by criticizing your drinking?
    - Have you ever felt bad or *Guilty* about your drinking?
    - Have you ever had a drink first thing in the morning to steady your nerves or to get rid of a hangover (*Eye opener*)?
  - Scoring:
    - Item responses on CAGE are scored 0 or 1
    - Higher score indicates alcohol problem
    - Score ≥ 2 is considered clinically significant.

TESTS
Lab
- No one test is diagnostic.
- γ-Glutamyltransferase (GGT) is the most sensitive indicator of alcoholism.
- GGT level >30 units/L is induced by alcohol (4 or + drinks/day × 2 weeks).
- MCV ≥ 100 μm^3 in females
- Elevation of AST, ALT, and alkaline phosphate

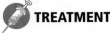 **TREATMENT**

- Coordination of care
  - Routinely ask patients about their alcohol and illicit drug use.
  - Inform patients of reproductive age about hazardous of alcohol or illicit drug use during and after pregnancy.
  - Offer help, written materials, and referrals.
  - Refer women patients to treatment programs and clinicians especially sensitive to women's needs.

- Educate patient with audiovisual and reading materials.
- Prepare and inform patients about the chronic nature of the illness and how to cope with relapses.
- Models of treatment
  - Harm reduction:
    - Recognizes that most people regularly use drugs of some type, such as alcohol.
    - Rather than aiming exclusively for abstinence, the goal is to reduce drug use or change drug use behavior so it is less harmful to the drug user.
  - Motivational interview
    - Patient encouraged to reduce drug use by exploring consequences of addiction and benefits of behavior change
  - Relapse prevention therapy:
    - Behavioral self-control program designed to teach individuals who are trying to maintain changes in their behavior how to anticipate and cope with relapse
  - Self help groups: AA meetings
  - Women groups
  - Therapeutic communities: women attend these programs for months or years
    - Half way house
    - Residential programs

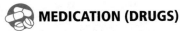 **MEDICATION (DRUGS)**

- **Benzodiazepines:**
  - Medication of choice for detoxification
  - Conflicting data about teratogenicity
  - Risks of withdrawal far more serious than risks of medications
  - Clinical Institute Withdrawal Assessment for Alcohol (CIWA)
    - Symptom-triggered dosing
    - Need to monitor patient frequently
  - Long acting benzodiazepines (Chlordiazepoxide and diazepam)
  - Short acting benzodiazepine (lorazepam)
- **Disulfiram:**
  - Blocks alcohol oxidation at acetaldehyde stage
  - Accumulation of acetaldehyde in blood produces highly unpleasant symptoms referred to as disulfiram-alcohol reaction.
  - Patient should not take disulfiram for at least 12 hours after drinking.
  - Reaction may occur for up to 2 weeks after disulfiram has been stopped.
  - Dosage: 125–500 mg a day.
  - Indicated in selected chronic alcoholic patients who want to remain in state of enforced sobriety so that supportive and psychotherapeutic treatment may be applied to the best advantage.
  - Do not prescribe when the patient is using alcohol-containing foods or products. The same rule applies with metronidazole.
  - Disulfiram inhibits enzyme induction and may interfere with drug metabolism. It enhances the effect of warfarin and phenytoin.
  - Monitor LFTs, CBC, and Chem 7 periodically.
- **Naltrexone:**
  - Opioid antagonist that blocks the pleasurable effects of alcohol and reduces cravings.
  - First dose may be 25 mg (one-half tablet), then 50 mg (one tablet) every day
  - Causes withdrawal symptoms in people who are using narcotics

– Avoid if opioids have been ingested during the prior 7–10 days
– Monitor liver enzymes.

- **Acamprosate**:
  – Recent evidence suggests the main interaction is with the glutamate system, inhibiting excitatory NMDA receptor.
  – Indicated for maintenance of abstinence in patients with dependence who are abstinent at treatment initiation
  – Begin treatment as soon as possible after the period of alcohol withdrawal and after the patient has achieved abstinence.
  – Two tablets (666 mg per dose) PO tid
  – It should be used as part of the treatment program that includes counseling and support.
  – Can continue drug even in event of relapse
  – Renal insufficiency is a contraindication.

Complementary and Alternative Medicine
- Thiamine, Folic acid, multi-vitamins
- Replace nutrional deficiencies
- Encourage PO hydration
- IV fluids if severe vomiting and diarrhea
- Correct electrolyte deficiencies (Ca, Mg, K)

Pregnancy Considerations
- In pregnant women, detoxification is the same as with nonpregnant women, although it is usually done in a medical setting with fetal monitoring (especially if the fetus is viable 23 to 24 weeks of gestation).
- Medications
  – Disulfiram
    - Not studied in pregnant women
    - Few reports of birth defects in infants
  – Naltrexone
    - Not studied in pregnant women
    - Causes unwanted effects when given in very large doses in animal studies
    - Category C
  – Acamprosate
    - Not studied in pregnant women
    - Causes birth defects or other problems in animal studies
- Breast-feeding
  – Disulfiram
    - Not known whether excreted in human milk
    - Advisable to discontinue nursing before administering disulfiram to mother
  – Naltrexone and Acamprosate
    - Not known whether passes into breast milk

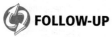 **FOLLOW-UP**

Issues for Referral
- Referral criteria for inpatient detoxification:
  – Outpatient detoxification failure or multiple relapses

– Suicidal ideation or acute psychosis
– History of Delirium Tremens
– Comorbid medical problems requiring frequent daily monitoring
- Referral criteria for specialized long-term alcoholism treatment
  – History of multiple treatment failures
  – Serious comorbid psychiatric conditions
  – Abuse of others substances
  – Unstable socioeconomical conditions

ADDITIONAL READING
- Web references:
  – http://www.nida.nih.gov
  – http://www.samhsa.gov
  – http://www.niaaa.nih.gov

 MISCELLANEOUS

- Always monitor for alcohol withdrawal, Delirium Tremens, and withdrawal seizures.
- Always ask about other substances.

CODES
ICD-9
- 303.90 Alcohol dependence
- 305.00 Alcohol abuse

REFERENCES
1. Romans SE, Seeman Mary V. *Women's Mental Health: A Life Cycle Approach. Substance Use and Abuse in Women*. 1st ed. Philadelphia: Lippincott Williams and Wilkins; 2006: 179–190.
2. Zweben JE. *Principles in Addiction Medicine: Special Issues in Treatment: Women*. 3rd ed. Chevy Chase, MD: Graham A, Schultz P; ASAM. 2003:569–578.
3. American Psychiatric Association. DSM-IV-TR. Washington, DC: American Psychiatric Press; 2000.
4. Bradley KA, Boyd-Wickizer J, Powell SH, et al. Alcohol screening question-naires in women. *JAMA*. 1998;280:166–171.
5. Galanter M, Kleber H. *The American Publishing Textbook of Substance Abuse Treatment. Addiction in Women*. 3rd ed. Washington: American Psychiatric Publishing Inc; 2004: 539–546.

KEY WORDS
- Alcoholism
- Alcohol Use
- Alcohol Withdrawal

ALOPECIA

Mohsin K. Malik, MD
Lynn E. Iler, MD

KEY CLINICAL POINTS

- Early hair loss may not be clinically apparent to the physician, but the patient may notice hair shedding or a decrease from baseline.
- Common causes of hair loss are present at similar frequency in men and women.
- The presence of alopecia in a woman does not require a hormonal work-up unless other signs or symptoms of androgen excess are present.

 ## BASICS

DESCRIPTION

- While rates of more common types of alopecia are similar in males and females, women may be more aware of hair loss and may experience more distress by hair loss for social reasons.
- Female pattern hair loss (androgenic alopecia)
  - Most common form of hair loss in women
  - Generally presents as thinning of the hair in women rather than as complete hair loss
  - Analogous to male pattern baldness
- Telogen effluvium
  - Diffuse hair thinning that is usually precipitated by a stressful life event
- Alopecia areata
  - Immune-mediated form of hair loss
  - Presents with focal patches of hair loss or, less frequently, complete hair loss
- Traumatic causes of hair loss
  - May present secondary to grooming practices or because of psychiatric causes genetic

EPIDEMIOLOGY

Female pattern hair loss
- Usually begins between 12 to 40 years of age
- About half of the population has some degree of involvement by age 50
- Peak onset in women in third and fifth decades

Telogen effluvium
- More frequent in postmenopausal women
- Common cause of alopecia, but exact incidence or prevalence unknown

Other forms of alopecia are less common.

Incidence
- Alopecia areata:
  - Rate: 20 per 100,000 population
  - Similar rates in both genders
  - More than half present before age 20

PATHOPHYSIOLOGY

- Normal growth in an individual hair follicle progressively cycles through 3 stages:
  - Anagen, the growth phase
    - Lasts 2 to 6 years
    - Approximately 90% to 95% of scalp hair is in anagen at any given time
  - Catogen, the degenerative phase
  - Anagen, the growth phase
    - Lasts 2 to 4 weeks
    - Approximately 1% to 3% of scalp hair is in catogen
  - Telogen, the resting phase
    - Lasts 2 to 4 months
    - Approximately 5% to 10% of scalp hair is in telogen
    - Hair becomes loosely attached during telogen
    - Generally shed at the end of telogen or when new hair growth begins in the subsequent anagen phase
    - Approximately 75 to 100 telogen hairs shed daily, and about the same number enter the anagen phase.
- Female pattern hair loss
  - Dihydrotestosterone binds to the androgen receptor of hair follicles and regulates gene expression.
  - With each successive growth cycle, large, terminal follicles become progressively miniaturized.
  - Local or overall increases in androgen levels may play a role, but most women have normal androgen levels.
  - Different areas of the scalp have varying sensitivity to androgens, which partially explains why hair is preferentially lost from some areas and not others.
- Telogen effluvium
  - Stressors cause increased numbers of hair to enter telogen phase prematurely.
  - The telogen hairs are shed 2 to 5 months after the stressor.

ETIOLOGY

- Female pattern hair loss
  - Genetic component with polygenic pattern of inheritance
  - Elevated androgen levels, either locally or systemically, also appear to play a role
- Telogen effluvium
  - Usually precipitated by life stressors
  - Caused by a disruption in the normal hair growth cycle
  - Less common causes of alopecia include hypothyroidism, iron deficiency, and drugs.
- Alopecia areata has genetic and immune-mediated components, but the exact etiology is unknown.
  - Genetic: 10% to 40% have family history
  - Immune: hair follicle dysfunction mediated by activated T cells; autoimmune etiology likely but target antigen not identified
- Traumatic causes of hair loss are purely mechanical. Common causes in women include:
  - Traction alopecia (hairstyles such as tightly pulled ponytails or tightly braided hair)
  - Cosmetic products and instruments (dyes, pomades, oils, curling irons, rollers)
  - Trichotillomania (hair pulling), which is an impulse-control disorder, can cause alopecia.

ASSOCIATED CONDITIONS

Alopecia areata
- Association with other autoimmune diseases including systemic lupus erythematosus, rheumatoid arthritis, and myasthenia gravis
- Increased prevalence of antinuclear, antismooth muscle, and antithyroid antibodies
- About 4-fold increased risk of vitiligo
- About 10% incidence of thyroid disease

DIAGNOSIS

SIGNS AND SYMPTOMS
History
A history of the onset of alopecia several months after starting a drug can be elicited in some cases
- Female pattern hair loss: gradual hair thinning
- Telogen effluvium
  - Rapid hair thinning, often following stressful life events
    - Pregnancy
    - Major illness, surgery
    - Significant weight loss
    - Other psychosocial stressors
  - A history of the onset of alopecia several months after starting a drug can be elicited in some cases.
  - No inciting factor can be found in about 1/3 of cases.
- Alopecia areata
  - Abrupt loss or graying of hair
  - May also be precipitated by stressful life events in some patients

Specific complaints
- Female pattern hair loss
  - Able to see scalp
  - Increased width of hair part on frontal scalp
- Telogen effluvium and alopecia areata
  - Hair may come out in handfuls, especially at the onset of a disease.
  - Hair clogging shower/sink drain
  - Women may bring bags of shed hair to the physician.

Evaluate for other causes of hair loss
- Androgen excess: menstrual irregularities, infertility, hirsutism, severe cystic acne virilization, galactorrhea
- Weight loss, malnutrition

Physical Exam
Pattern of hair loss
- Female pattern hair loss
  - Thinning hair classically occurs on the vertex or midscalp (area anterior to vertex).
  - There may also be in a bitemporal pattern.
  - The frontal hairline is usually maintained.
  - Large areas of balding are rare.
  - The remaining hair may be of uneven lengths and texture.
- Telogen effluvium
  - Thinning hair over entire scalp
  - Often worst over temporal scalp
  - Complete balding does not occur
  - "Pull test"
    - Grasp and pull as much hair as fits between two fingers and a thumb
    - Up to 3 to 5 hairs pulled normally ("negative pull test")
    - A greater number of pulled hairs is abnormal, especially if it is pulled telogen (club) hair.
    - Negative test does not rule out
- Alopecia areata
  - Scalp involvement is most common, but may involve any area of hair
  - Round/oval areas of complete balding
  - Smooth surface of skin in areas of hair loss
  - Short, broken hairs at margins between alopecia and remaining hair
  - Diffuse hair loss over the entire scalp is less common.

- The pull test may be positive, often with hypopigmented roots of pulled hair.
- Proximal nail pitting may be present.
- Traumatic hair loss
  - Pattern of hair loss depends on method of injury.
  - Traction alopecia due to ponytails or braiding is usually at the hair margins.
  - Trichotillomania: "pull test" tends to be negative, because hair that is easily pulled out has already been removed.

TESTS
Lab
- Alopecia areata: CBC, TSH
- All other causes, also check: iron, ferritin, TIBC, ANA, RPR
- If clinical suspicion of androgen excess, check:
  - DHEA-S
  - Testosterone (free and total)
- Suspicion of dietary deficiency, check:
  - Zinc
  - Biotin

Diagnostic Procedures/Surgery
- A biopsy may be required to differentiate between the forms of alopecia.
  - Two 4-mm punch biopsies in active areas of alopecia
  - Specimens should be processed horizontally and vertically by special request.

DIFFERENTIAL DIAGNOSIS
- Tinea capitis
- Folliculitis or other infection (may be scarring)
- Thyroid disease
- Anagen effluvium, loose anagen syndrome, and other abnormalities of hair cycling
- Discoid lupus erythematosus (usually scarring)
- Other connective tissue disease
- Secondary syphilis
- Zinc or biotin deficiency
- Hypervitaminosis A

TREATMENT

GENERAL MEASURES
- Nonmedical approaches to alopecia include wigs or hairstyles that cover the areas of hair loss.
- For traumatic alopecia or drug-induced telogen effluvium, the inciting agent should be identified and withdrawn.
- For trichotillomania, behavioral therapy and/or antidepressant drugs are used.

MEDICATION (DRUGS)

- Female pattern hair loss
  - Minoxidil is the mainstay of therapy.
    - A 2–5% solution applied twice daily
    - Several months are required for clinically apparent hair re-growth.
    - Re-growth is lost with discontinuation of the treatment.
  - Spirinolactone 50–200 mg daily can be added if response to minoxidil is poor.
- Telogen effluvium: efficacy of treatment not well described, but options include:

- Minoxidil solution 2–5% applied twice daily
- Spirinolactone 50–200 mg daily
- Alopecia areata
  - Intralesional corticosteroid injection is first-line therapy with limited involvement
  - Use of topical corticosteroid monotherapy is less effective than other methods, but clobetasol propionate 0.05% applied nightly under plastic film occlusion may be effective.
  - Minoxidil and anthralin, alone or in combination, are the second lines of therapy.
    - Minoxidil solution 5% applied twice daily can be used for partial scalp involvement.
    - Anthralin 0.25–1% can be applied nightly or for 10–30 minutes and washed off. Irritation occurs with the application, but tolerance can develop.
  - Topical immunomodulators are reserved for widespread disease and require an experienced practitioner (dinitrochlorobenzene, squaric acid dibutyl ester, or diphenylcyclopropenone).
  - Oral corticosteroids are effective for hair re-growth, but systemic side effects limit their use. A relapse is common upon discontinuation.

SURGERY
- Surgical options for alopecia include follicular unit transplantation, plug grafts, flaps, and scalp reduction.

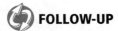 **FOLLOW-UP**

Issues for Referral
- Scarring alopecia should be referred to a dermatologist.

PROGNOSIS
- Female pattern hair loss
  - Women do not tend to have the same degree of hair loss as men and generally do not become bald.
- Telogen effluvium
  - Usually self-limited
  - Shedding of hair ceases in 3–6 months and normal hair begins to grow thereafter.
  - Minority of cases progress to chronic telogen effluvium, defined as persistence >6 months.
- Alopecia areata
  - Unpredictable course
  - Patients usually have several episodes over a lifetime.
  - Involvement ranges from limited areas of hair loss to diffuse alopecia involving scalp, eyebrows, and other areas (alopecia totalis/universalis).
  - There may be complete, partial, or no re-growth of hair.
  - Predictors of poor prognosis include extensive involvement, other autoimmune disease, atopy, family history of alopecia areata, and young age at onset.

- Traumatic alopecia
  - The prognosis depends on the success of identifying and withdrawing the traumatic agent.
  - Chronic or long-standing trauma may result in scarring which destroys hair follicles.

REFERENCES
1. Bernstein RM, Rassman WR. Follicular unit transplantation: 2005. *Dermatol Clin*. 2005;23:393–414.
2. Chartier MB, Hoss DM, Grant-Kels JM. Approach to the adult female patient with diffuse nonscarring alopecia. *J Am Acad Dermatol*. 2002;47:809–818; quiz 818–820.
3. Harrison S, Sinclair R. Telogen effluvium. *Clin Exp Dermatol*. 2002;27:389–395.
4. Madani S, Shapiro J. Alopecia areata update. *J Am Acad Dermatol*. Apr 2000;42(4):549–566; quiz 567–570.
5. Olsen EA. Female pattern hair loss. *J Am Acad Dermatol*. Sep 2001;45(suppl):70–80.
6. Price VH. Treatment of hair loss. *N Engl J Med*. 1999;341:964–973.
7. Safavi KH, Muller SA, Suman VJ, et al. Incidence of alopecia areata in Olmsted County, Minnesota, 1975 through 1989. *Mayo Clin Proc*. 1995;70:628–633.
8. Sawaya ME, Price VH. Different levels of 5alpha-reductase type I and II, aromatase, and androgen receptor in hair follicles of women and men with androgenetic alopecia. *J Invest Dermatol*. 1997;109:296–300.
9. Thiedke CC. Alopecia in women. *Am Fam Physician*. 2003;67:1007–1014.
10. Whiting DA. Chronic telogen effluvium: increased scalp hair shedding in middle-aged women. *J Am Acad Dermatol*. 1996;35:899–906.
11. Whiting DA. Traumatic alopecia. *Int J Dermatol*. 1999;38(suppl):34–44.

CODES
ICD9-CM
- 704.01 Alopecia areata
- 704.02 Telogen effluvium
- 312.39 Trichotillomania (Disorders of impulse control, not elsewhere classified)
- 704.00 Other causes of alopecia: (Alopecia, unspecified)

KEY WORDS
- Alopecia
- Alopecia Areata
- Telogen Effluvium
- Female Pattern Hair Loss
- Androgenic Alopecia

ALZHEIMER'S DISEASE

Elaine C. Jones, MD

KEY CLINICAL POINTS

- Alzheimer's disease is a slowly progressive disorder associated with aging and characterized by memory loss and other cognitive problems.
- As the population over age 65 expands in the coming years, there will be a significant increase in the frequency of Alzheimer's disease.
- Disease specific treatments are now available. These slow the progression of the disease and have proven impact on quality of life and delay time to nursing home placement.

BASICS

DESCRIPTION
- Dementia is a slow, gradual process characterized by changes in memory, behavior, and even physical decline.
- Patterns of brain involvement will determine what symptoms are experienced and what type of dementia the person has.
- Alzheimer's disease is the most common form of dementia, followed by vascular dementia (caused by ischemia). Other less common forms of dementia include frontotemporal dementia, and dementia with Lewy Bodies.
- Delirium differs from dementia:
  - Shorter duration
  - More fluctuation in symptoms during the day
  - More delusions or hallucinations, and
  - Often the patient is aware of the problem.

GENERAL PREVENTION
- Currently there are no known preventive measures for Alzheimer's disease.
- Antiinflammatory medications have been suggested to decrease the risk of Alzheimer's disease but this has not been proven at this time.

EPIDEMIOLOGY
- The biggest factor is age. Before age 65, the prevalence is less than 1%.
- Women seem to be more affected than men, even when correcting for greater longevity in women.
- All races and socioeconomic groups are affected.

Incidence
- 1% per year before age 65.
- Increases to 6% per year after age 65.

Prevalence
- Not well established but estimated at 4 million people in the US.
- The projected increase is to 7 million people by the early 21st century.
- From age 65–85, prevalence doubles every 5 years.
- Over age 85, prevalence is 35–40% currently.

RISK FACTORS
- 4–fold increase in risk with history of AD in 1st-degree relative
- Women more affected than men
- Lower level of education
- Single severe head injury or repeated injuries
- Estrogen replacement therapy was thought to offer a protective effect; however, a recent study demonstrated increased risk for other diseases that outweighed any benefits.

Genetics
- Familial forms have been identified
  - Younger onset
  - Associated with chromosomes 1, 14, and 21.
- Apolipoprotein E
  - Increased susceptibility in those homozygous for E4 alleles
  - Genes are located on chromosome 19.

PATHOPHYSIOLOGY
- Grossly:
  - Marked brain atrophy in all areas but with relative sparing of occipital lobes
- Microscopically:
  - Loss of neurons, neuritic plaques (NP) and neurofibrillary tangles (NFT)
    - NP = central core of fibrous protein (amyloid) the result of abnormal processing of amyloid precursor proteins
    - NFT = found inside neurons and made up of tau proteins
- Chemically:
  - Reduction of the enzyme, choline acetyltransferase, which produces acetylcholine: 50–90%
  - Glutaminergic neurons are also lost in large numbers.

ETIOLOGY
Not currently known.

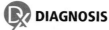

DIAGNOSIS

SIGNS AND SYMPTOMS
- Insidious onset with gradual, persistent worsening over time, usually years
- Memory loss is the cardinal feature and often the presenting complaint.
  - Recent information recall is affected first, and then older information gradually becomes involved.
- Language
  - Initially problems with naming and loss of fluency
- Visuospatial
  - Getting lost, misplacing things, drawing figures affected, driving may become affected
- Behavioral
  - Agitation, wandering in some, depression

History
- Patients may be unaware of the problems they are having.
- Therefore, it is very important to obtain history from families or other individuals.
- Specific questions targeting memory are most helpful:
  - Trouble recognizing familiar people
  - Remembering appointments
  - Doing household chores
  - Cooking
  - Shopping
  - Driving
  - Wandering
  - Getting lost, etc.
- It is important to assess mood as depression can mimic dementia.

Physical Exam
- An important part of the physical exam is doing the mini-mental status test (MMSE). This 30-point test is a very basic test of areas affected by dementia.
  - Normal: 26–30
  - Mild dementia: 20–26

- Moderate dementia: 10–20
- Severe dementia: <10
- Clock-drawing task is very sensitive as well.
  - Investigator draws a circle
  - Ask the patient to put in the numbers.
  - Ask the patient to place the hands at 2:25.
- Focal physical exam findings may suggest other diagnoses than Alzheimer's disease, at least early on in the disease.
  - Later Parkinsonian findings (rigidity, bradykinesia, gait disturbances, tremor) may become present.

TESTS

Neuropsychological testing can be very helpful in diagnosing Alzheimer's disease and distinguishing other forms of dementia.

Lab

The primary goal is to rule out reversible causes of cognitive complaints.

- CBC, chemistry panels, thyroid function tests, B12 levels
- When appropriate, ESR, urinalysis, syphilis, HIV, heavy metal screens

Imaging

It is appropriate to rule out other causes of cognitive complaints.

- CT brain is usually sufficient to rule out extensive ischemia (vascular dementia).
- MRI may be useful if there are significant focal physical exam findings.

DIFFERENTIAL DIAGNOSIS

- Vascular dementia
  - Characterized by sudden, step-wise deterioration
  - Can be associated with more focal neurologic exam findings
- Lewy Body Dementia
  - Memory impairment can be less prominent
  - Visual hallucinations/illusions/delusions prominent
  - Parkinsonian symptoms also prominent.
- Frontotemporal dementia (Pick's disease)
  - Early and severe behavioral features
  - Early aphasia

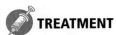 **TREATMENT**

GENERAL MEASURES

- Patients with memory problems usually benefit from writing things down, making lists, and gentle reminders by family.
- Routine is very important. Many patients become more agitated and confused when their environment is changed or if the routine is disrupted.
- Current treatments are proven to slow the progression of the dementia.
  - There is no cure.
  - Slowing the progression can allow a patient to continue to function in work, participate in activities, and stay in their home longer.

Diet

- No specific diet issues have been identified.
- In the past, it was thought that exposure to aluminum through cookware was a cause for Alzheimer's disease, but this has been disproven.

Activity

- Patients who remain active tend to do better longer.
- Cognitive task (puzzles, crosswords, card games) can help maintain function longer.

- Social interactions are also important. This can decrease depression and help maintain function.

Physical Therapy

- Patients who have gait problems may benefit from physical therapy.
- In general, however, physical therapy has little to offer.

Complementary and Alternative Medicine

- Vitamin E 400 international units (IU) daily have been shown to help with cognitive decline.
- Vitamin E at high doses (>600 IU/day) have been associated with increased risk for heart disease but lower doses may slow the development of atherosclerosis.
- Ginkgo biloba has been studied in limited trials and has not shown any benefits.
- Antiinflammatory medications have been suggested to decrease the risk of Alzheimer's disease but this has not been proven at this time.

 MEDICATION (DRUGS)

- Acetylcholinesterase inhibitors: Approved for mild to moderate dementia.
  - Donepezil (Aricept): 5 mg daily for 1 month then 10 mg daily
    - Common side effects include nausea, diarrhea, and syncope.
  - Galantamine (Razadyne): 4–12 mg b.i.d.
    - Common side effects include nausea, vomiting, diarrhea, bradycardia, and weight loss.
    - GI side effects can be minimized by taking on a full stomach.
  - Rivastigmine (Exelon): 3–6 mg b.i.d.
    - Common side effects include nausea, vomiting, diarrhea, bradycardia, and weight loss.
    - It also affects butyrylcholinesterase, which may play role, although it has not been proven.
- NMDA-receptor antagonist: Approved for moderate to severe dementia.
  - Memantine (Namenda): 5 mg daily, increase by 5 mg weekly to max 10 mg b.i.d.
    - Common side effects include dizziness, confusion, and headache.
- Behavioral management
  - Neuroleptics
    - Haloperidol: May cause Parkinsonism or tardive dyskinesia.
  - Atypical neuroleptics: Recently shown to be associated with increased mortality, but etiology is unclear
    - Risperidone (Risperdal): May cause orthostatic hypotension, nausea
    - Olanzapine (Zyprexa): Can cause weight gain, elevated liver enzymes
    - Quetiapine (Seroquel): Can cause sedation
  - Benzodiazepines
    - Lorazepam (Ativan): Can cause confusion, sedation, dependence

SURGERY

- Patients with dementia do not always do well with surgery.
- They are more susceptible to delirium at the time of surgery and some have a decline in functioning from their presurgical levels.
- This should be taken into account when surgery is being considered.

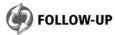 **FOLLOW-UP**

DISPOSITION
- With good outpatient services, families are often able to take patients home.
- For patients who have behavioral issues including wandering, nursing home placement may be necessary.

Admission Criteria
Patients with Alzheimer's disease are very susceptible to developing delirium.
- May present as sudden decline in functioning, increased confusion, and agitation
- May result in a need for admission.
- Common causes for delirium include:
  - Simple urinary tract infections
  - Changes in medications
  - Metabolic derangements (hyponatremia, etc.)

Issues for Referral
- When declining faster than 2 points on MMSE exam in 6 months
- When significant behavioral issues are present
- When memory loss is a minor part of the syndrome

PROGNOSIS
- This is a chronic, progressive disease that currently has no cure.
- The average duration from diagnosis to death is 10 years with a range of 4–16 years.

COMPLICATIONS
- The greatest risk in Alzheimer's patients is with wandering.
  - Not all patients will wander.
  - If they do, there is significant risk of injury and even death.
- Additional problems have arisen when Alzheimer's patients have left the stove on.
- Driving can be a big risk, but it is difficult to take away because of the impact on independence.
  - Most states have laws and guidelines regarding driving.
  - These should be reviewed by health care providers.

PATIENT MONITORING
- Because this is a slowly progressive disease, frequent monitoring is not necessary.
- Depending on the patient, a 3- to 6-month follow-up is generally sufficient.
- Patients can be monitored by using MMSE.
  - A decline of more than 2 points a year may suggest nonresponsiveness to medication.
  - Switching to a different agent or addition of another agent may be indicated.

 MISCELLANEOUS

- Caregivers of Alzheimer's patients have been shown to have increased health problems, probably from the stress of care giving.
- Respite care is available in many cities and allows for the caregiver to get some time away for themselves.
- The Alzheimer's Association and Department of Elderly Affairs can be great resources for patients and families.
- Currently significant research is directed at diagnosing dementia earlier in the course of the disease.
  - The term mild cognitive impairment (MCI) is used to identify this phase.
  - Subtypes of MCI are being identified so those who will go onto develop dementia can be treated earlier.

REFERENCES
1. Corey-Bloom J. Alzheimer's disease. *Continuum: Lifelong Learning in Neurology*. 2004;10:29–57.
2. Manly JJ, Bell-McGinty S, Tang MX, et al. Implementing diagnostic criteria and estimating frequency of mild cognitive impairment in an urban community. *Arch of Neurol*. 2005;62:1739–1746.
3. Mayeux R, Saunders AM, Shea S, et al. Utility of the apolipoprotein E genotype in the diagnosis of Alzheimer's disease. *N Engl J Med*. 1998;338:506–511.
4. Small SA, Mayeux R. Alzheimer disease and related dementia. In: Rowland LP, ed. *Merritt's Neurology*. 11th ed. Philadelphia: Lippincott Williams & Wilkins; 2005:771–776.

ADDITIONAL READING
Mace NL, Rabins PV. The 36-Hour Day: A Family Guide to Caring for Persons with Alzheimer's Disease. New York: Warner Books; 1999.

CODES
ICD9-CM
- 331.0 Alzheimer's disease
- 780.93 Memory loss
- 290.40 Vascular dementia
- 331.82 Lewy Body dementia

KEY WORDS
- Dementia
- Delirium
- Vascular Dementia
- Memory Loss
- Senility

AMENORRHEA

Traci Wolbrink, MD
Sybil Cineas, MD

KEY CLINICAL POINTS

- Amenorrhea can be divided into primary and secondary amenorrhea.
- Pregnancy is the most common cause of amenorrhea and must be excluded in both primary and secondary amenorrhea.
- Amenorrhea can be caused by many different disease mechanisms and therapy should be directed at treating the specific underlying illness.

 BASICS

DESCRIPTION

- Amenorrhea is the absence of menses. It may be divided into primary and secondary amenorrhea.
- Primary amenorrhea refers to the absence of menses by age 14 in the absence of secondary sexual characteristics or by age 16 in the setting of normal secondary sexual development.
- Secondary amenorrhea is the absence of menses for more than three cycles or 6 months in women who previously menstruated.

GENERAL PREVENTION

- Several causes of amenorrhea may be prevented by:
  - Treating underlying illness
  - Maintaining an appropriate caloric intake and expenditure balance
  - Avoidance of excessive stress

EPIDEMIOLOGY

- Amenorrhea affects only women during their reproductive years.

Incidence

- The incidence is approximately 3% in the United States for both primary and secondary amenorrhea.

Prevalence

- In the United States, 3–4% of women will have amenorrhea not related to pregnancy, lactation, or menopause.

RISK FACTORS

- Obesity
- Weight loss
- Exercise
- Stress
- Uterine instrumentation

PATHOPHYSIOLOGY

- Normal menstrual function requires an intact complex pathway that is under the regulation of many hormones and factors.
- Normally, the hypothalamus releases pulsatile GnRH, which causes the pituitary to release LH and FSH.
- These gonadotropins act on the ovaries to produce follicular development, ovulation, and function of the corpus luteum.
- The ovaries secrete estrogen and progesterone, which act on the uterus to cause proliferation and maturation of the endometrium.
- In the absence of fertilization, bleeding occurs. Menstrual blood exits through a normal female anatomical genital tract, which includes uterus, cervix, vagina, and vaginal orifice.
- Any alterations in this pathway can lead to amenorrhea.

ETIOLOGY

- The four most common causes of primary amenorrhea:
  - Ovarian failure (49%)
  - Congenital absence of uterus and vagina (16%)
  - GnRH deficiency (8%)
  - Constitutional delay of puberty (6%)
- Causes of secondary amenorrhea after exclusion of pregnancy and lactation:
  - Ovarian disease
    - Polycystic ovarian syndrome (PCOS)
    - Premature ovarian failure
    - Ovarian tumors
  - Hypothalamic dysfunction
    - Eating disorders
    - Exercise
    - Stress
    - Severe systemic illness
    - Infiltrative diseases
  - Pituitary disease
    - Prolactinoma and hyperprolactinemia of other etiologies (i.e., medications)
    - Postpartum hemorrhage of the pituitary (Sheehan's syndrome)
  - Uterine disease
    - Intrauterine synechiae (Asherman's syndrome) from uterine instrumentation
  - Endocrine disorders
    - Thyroid disease
    - Adrenal disorders
- The causes of secondary amenorrhea may also lead to primary amenorrhea, if they occur before menarche.

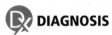 **DIAGNOSIS**

- Evaluation of amenorrhea should start with a history and physical exam and urine or serum βHCG to rule out pregnancy.

SIGNS AND SYMPTOMS

- Absence of menses

History

The patient should be questioned regarding:

- Presence of menarche
- Sexual activity
- Eating and exercise habits
- Galactorrhea, headaches, visual field defects, polyuria, polydipsia
- Signs and symptoms of endocrinological disorders
- Recent stress or illness
- Signs of androgen excess
- Medication use
- Symptoms of estrogen deficiency such as hot flashes, vaginal dryness, decreased libido
- History of uterine instrumentation
- Recent pregnancy
- Risk factors for tuberculosis or HIV

Physical Exam

The patient should be examined with close attention to:

- Height and weight (BMI)
- Secondary sexual characteristics
- External and internal genitalia
- Breast exam, especially looking for galactorrhea
- Signs of androgen excess, such as acne and hirsuitism

TESTS
- Pregnancy is the most common cause of amenorrhea and must be ruled out in both primary and secondary amenorrhea.

Lab
- If genital exam normal:
  - Urine or serum βHCG
  - FSH, prolactin
  - TSH
- If signs of hyperandrogenism:
  - Serum DHEAS and testosterone
- If symptoms of hypoestrogenism:
  - FSH
  - Estradiol
  - TSH, thyroid antibodies
  - Chemistry profile
- If low BMI:
  - LH
  - FSH
  - βHCG
  - TSH
- If symptoms/physical findings suggestive of genetic disorder:
  - Karyotype to evaluate for genetic defects, such as Turner Syndrome

Imaging
- If abnormal genital exam:
  - Abdominal ultrasound to confirm presence of normal structures
- If abnormal gonadal structures on ultrasound:
  - Karyotype to rule out genetic defect, such as Turner Syndrome
- If elevated prolactin levels:
  - MRI of brain to rule out pituitary tumor (i.e. prolactinoma)
- If history of uterine instrumentation:
  - Hysteroscopy to rule out uterine synechiae, which may also be therapeutic if synechiae are lysed with laser therapy

Diagnostic Procedures/Surgery
- A progesterone challenge may be performed to evaluate ovarian production of estrogen indirectly.
  - Medroxyprogesterone acetate (10 mg orally for 5–10 days) or intramuscular progesterone (100–200 mg once) is given.
  - If the ovaries are producing estrogen, withdrawal bleeding will follow administration of progesterone.
- A failed progesterone challenge may suggest:
  - Uterine cause (i.e. Asherman's syndrome)
  - Hypothalamic dysfunction
  - Ovarian dysfunction
- Asherman's syndrome can be ruled out by the lack of bleeding following administration of conjugated estrogen (2.5 mg orally for 25 days), then medroxyprogesterone acetate (10 mg orally on days 16–25).

DIFFERENTIAL DIAGNOSIS
- Pregnancy
- Anatomical defect
- Turner Syndrome
- Muellerian agenesis
- Complete androgen resistance
- Hypothyroidism
- Polycystic ovarian syndrome (PCOS)
- Prolactinoma
- Premature ovarian failure
- Hypothalamic amenorrhea
- Stress
- Weight loss

- Excessive exercise
- Chronic disease
- Androgen producing tumors
- Congenital adrenal hyperplasia

 ## TREATMENT

GENERAL MEASURES
- Reduce stress when possible
- Weight loss for patients with obesity +/− hyperandrogenism
- Normalization of BMI and appropriate exercise behaviors for patients with malnourishment, excessive exercise, and eating disorders

Diet
- Healthy, well-balanced to achieve normal BMI

Activity
- Competitive athletes must try to maintain a caloric intake equal to the exercise expenditure.

 ## MEDICATION (DRUGS)

- Cyclical estrogen-progesterone may be offered to the following as there may be cardiovascular and bone density benefits:
  - Patients with hypoestrogenic states (i.e., premature ovarian failure)
  - Functional disorders of the hypothalamus
- Patients with functional disorders of the hypothalamus that desire pregnancy may be offered the following to induce ovulation:
  - Clomiphene citrate
  - Exogenous gonadotropins
  - Pulsatile GnRH

SURGERY
- Hymenectomy if imperforate hymen
- Resection if tumor
- Lysis of synechiae if Asherman's syndrome
- If gonadal dysgenesis and XY karyotype, gonads should be removed to prevent malignant transformation (may occur in up to 25% if not removed)

 ## FOLLOW-UP

DISPOSITION
The evaluation and treatment for amenorrhea is usually done in the outpatient setting.

Issues for Referral
- Many causes of amenorrhea can be managed by the primary care provider.
- Causes that require the help of a specialist include:
  - Anorexia nervosa: psychiatrist or eating disorder specialist
  - PCOS: endocrinologist
  - Pituitary tumors: neurosurgeon and endocrinologist
  - Other types of tumors: oncologist, gynecologist, and/or general surgeon
  - Asherman's syndrome: gynecologist

PROGNOSIS
- Prognosis is based upon the underlying etiology, but is generally good.
- Many patients will recover from amenorrhea following therapy for the underlying condition, especially in cases of endocrine diseases, functional hypothalamic dysfunction, and PCOS.

- Most tumors can be treated.
- Many women can undergo induction of ovulation with medications such as clomiphene citrate.

COMPLICATIONS

- Hypoestrogenic states can lead to bone mineral density loss and possible increase in cardiovascular complications.
- Many causes of amenorrhea result in anovulation and infertility if patients remain undiagnosed and untreated.
- Women with PCOS may also have insulin resistance and should be screened for diabetes.

REFERENCES

1. Laughlin D, Thorneycroft IH. Amenorrhea. In: DeCherney AH, Nathan LI, eds. *Current Obstetrics & Gynecologic Diagnosis & Treatment*. 9th ed. New York: McGraw-Hill; 2003.
2. The Practice Committee of the American Society for Reproductive Medicine. Current evaluation of amenorrhea. *Fertility & Sterility*. 2004;82(suppl):33–39.
3. Timmreck LS, Reindollar RH. Contemporary issues in primary amenorrhea. *Obstet & Gynecol Clin North Am*. 2003;30:287–302.
4. Warren MP. Evaluation of secondary amenorrhea. *J Clin Endocrinol and Metab*. 1996;81:437–442.
5. Kalantaridou SN, Makrigiannakis A, Zoumakis E, et al. Stress and the female reproductive system. *J Reprod Immunol*. 2004;62:61–68.
6. Mitan LAP. Menstrual dysfunction in anorexia nervosa. *J Pediatric & Adolesc Gynecol*. 2004;17:81–85.

 MISCELLANEOUS

Internet resources:
- UpToDate Online 13.3: Welt CK, Barbieri RL. Etiology, diagnosis, and treatment of primary amenorrhea. 2005
- UpToDate Online 13.3: Welt CK, Barbieri RL. Etiology, diagnosis, and treatment of secondary amenorrhea. 2005

CODES

ICD9-CM

- 626.0 Amenorrhea (primary or secondary)
- 256.8 Amenorrhea (due to ovarian dysfunction)
- 256.8 Amenorrhea (hyperhormonal)

KEY WORDS

- Menarche
- Ovarian Failure
- Eating Disorders
- Polycystic Ovarian Syndrome
- Thyroid Disease
- Prolactinoma
- Turner Syndrome

ANXIETY DISORDERS

Audrey R. Tyrka, MD, PhD
Margaret C. Wyche, BS

KEY CLINICAL POINTS

- Individuals diagnosed with an anxiety disorder have a suicide risk that is at least ten times greater than the general population.
- The natural response is to avoid anxiety-provoking stimuli but this worsens anxiety disorders.
- Treatment options include antidepressants or anxiolytics and psychotherapy, especially CBT.

BASICS

DESCRIPTION

Anxiety disorders are a cluster of diagnoses sharing anxiety as a common theme.

- **Panic Disorder** is characterized by recurrent, unexpected panic attacks followed by a month or more of worry or avoidant behavior. Panic disorder can occur with or without agoraphobia.
- **Agoraphobia** involves anxiety about being in a situation from which escape would be difficult.
- **Specific phobia** is characterized by an excessive fear of a particular object or situation that is avoided or endured with marked distress.
- **Social phobia (Social Anxiety Disorder)** is an irrational fear of negative social evaluation, such as scrutiny by unfamiliar people or performance in unfamiliar situations.
- **Obsessive Compulsive Disorder (OCD)** is characterized by obsessions (intrusive, uncontrollable, anxiety provoking thoughts) that are alleviated by the performance of compulsions.
- **Posttraumatic Stress Disorder (PTSD)** is a reaction to a traumatic experience that involves reexperiencing of the trauma through nightmares and flashbacks. The reaction includes increased arousal and emotional numbing and efforts to avoid reminders of the event.
- **Generalized Anxiety Disorder (GAD)** involves persistent and excessive worry pertaining to multiple events or domains that continues for 6 months or more. Physical symptoms of GAD include feelings of restlessness, tiring easily, muscle tension, and sleep disturbance.

EPIDEMIOLOGY

- Anxiety disorders are the most common cluster of mental disorders.
- Anxiety disorders are more common in women.
- Phobic disorders are the most common mental disorder among women in the United States.

Prevalence

- Lifetime prevalence of any anxiety disorder in the United States is estimated at 30 million individuals.
- Lifetime prevalence of individual anxiety disorders range from 2–3% (OCD) to estimates as high as 25% for specific phobia.

RISK FACTORS

- Family history of anxiety disorders
- Temperamental factors such as behavioral inhibition
- Environmental stressors, including emotional and physical abuse

Genetics

- There is evidence for genes involved in serotonin neurotransmission, including:
  - The serotonin transporter gene (5HTTLPR)
  - The tryptophan hydroxylase gene (TPH)
  - The serotonin 2A receptor gene (HTR2A)
- Corticotropin-releasing hormone gene is associated with behavioral inhibition (i.e., avoidance of novel situations) in children at risk for anxiety disorders.

ETIOLOGY

- Implicated neurotransmitters include norepinephrine, serotonin, dopamine, gamma-aminobutyric acid (GABA), and glutamate
- Dysregulation of the hypothalamic-pituitary-adrenal axis in PTSD
- Misinterpretation of somatic sensations in panic disorder

ASSOCIATED CONDITIONS

- In a primary care setting, anxiety and depressive disorders present more commonly together than in isolation.
  - Panic Disorder and GAD are the anxiety disorders most commonly associated with depression.

ALERT

- Individuals diagnosed with an anxiety disorder have a suicide risk that is at least ten times greater than the general population.

DIAGNOSIS

- See description
- Specific criteria are listed in *The Diagnostic and Statistical Manual of Mental Disorders*, 4th ed., Text Revision
- Rule out substance use disorders
- Rule out general medical conditions that cause anxiety

SIGNS AND SYMPTOMS

- Hypervigilance
- Frequent worry
- Panic attacks
  - Discrete periods of intense physical symptoms that peak and resolve within a short time
  - Patients will often present to emergency care settings during or following panic attacks.
- Social withdrawal
- Physical symptoms of anxiety and panic including increased heart rate, muscle tension, difficulty sleeping, nausea, chest pain, and difficulty breathing
- Common obsessions include cleanliness, order, completeness, and fear of aggression
- Common compulsions include handwashing, ordering, and checking, particularly for safety
  - Examples include door locks and stoves

History

- A thorough psychiatric evaluation and family history will influence treatment decisions.
  - Specifically evaluate for history of substance use disorders.

TESTS

- Screen for drugs of abuse
- Check TSH

DIFFERENTIAL DIAGNOSIS

- Medical conditions associated with anxiety include disorders of the following systems:
  - Cardiovascular
  - Pulmonary
  - Neurologic
  - Endocrine
  - Gastrointestinal
- Other psychiatric disorders associated with anxiety
  - Substance intoxication and withdrawal
  - Tourette's disorder
    - Up to two-thirds of individuals with Tourette's have comorbid OCD.
  - Other mental disorders including mood disorders, Body Dysmorphic Disorder, hypochrondriasis, and personality disorders

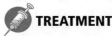 **TREATMENT**

INITIAL STABILIZATION

- Benzodiazepines and psychotherapeutic techniques can be used to decrease anxiety while awaiting the full effects of treatment with antidepressant medications or psychotherapy.

GENERAL MEASURES

- Cognitive Behavioral Therapy (CBT)
  - Relaxation techniques
  - Desensitization
  - Exposure and response prevention
  - Cognitive restructuring
  - Patient education
- Group or individual psychodynamic therapy
  - Particularly useful with PTSD

 MEDICATION (DRUGS)

- Antidepressants treat anxiety disorders even in the absence of depressive symptoms.
- Medication generally does not play a role in the treatment of specific phobia.

First Line

- Selective Serotonin Reuptake Inhibitors (SSRIs): first-line treatments for all anxiety disorders except specific phobia
  - Fluoxetine (OCD, Panic: start 20 mg PO q am, usual dose 20–60 mg/day)
  - Paroxetine (GAD, OCD, Panic, PTSD, Social Phobia: start 20 mg PO q am, usual dose 20–50 mg/day)
  - Sertraline (OCD, Panic, PTSD, Social Phobia; start 50 mg PO qd, usual dose 50–200 mg/day)
  - Citalopram (start 20 mg PO qd, usual dose 20–60 mg/day)
  - Escitalopram (GAD: start 10 mg/day, usual dose 10–20 mg/day)
  - Fluvoxamine (OCD: start 50 mg PO qhs, usual dose 100–300 mg/day divided bid)
    - Short term side effects of SSRIs include headache, anxiety or agitation, gastrointestinal distress, and fatigue.
    - Sexual dysfunction is a common and persisting side effect of SSRIs.
  - For each disorder, some SSRIs but not others have FDA indications.
  - There are indications for each drug listed above in parentheses, but off-label prescribing is common as other SSRIs are also effective.

- Serotonin norepinephrine reuptake inhibitor
  - Venlafaxine (GAD, Social Phobia; start 37.5–75 mg PO qd; usual dose 75–150 mg/day)
  - In addition to the side effects associated with SSRIs, venlafaxine has a small dose-related risk of inducing hypertension.
- To avoid discontinuation syndromes (headache, dizziness, nausea for SSRIs and venlafaxine), medication should be tapered when discontinued.

Second Line

- Buspirone (GAD: Initial dose 5–10 mg PO b.i.d., usual dose range 15–40 mg in divided doses)
- Tricyclic antidepressants and monoamine oxidase inhibitors: generally considered second- or third-line drugs due to a greater side-effect burden and concerns regarding toxicity
- Other drugs including mirtazapine, anticonvulsants, and atypical antipsychotics have some initial evidence of efficacy for some of the anxiety disorders.
- Benzodiazepines: effective for most anxiety disorders, but long-term treatment is usually restricted to cases that are resistant to other treatments due to concerns regarding tolerance, withdrawal, and abuse and dependence.

Pregnancy Considerations

Pregnancy and the postpartum period are particularly vulnerable times for the development and worsening of anxiety symptoms.

- Pregnancy concerns
  - Panic symptoms often improve during pregnancy.
  - In vulnerable women, OCD can develop or worsen during pregnancy.
  - Pharmacotherapy during pregnancy:
    - It is best to avoid medication during the first twelve weeks of gestation and near delivery if possible.
    - The smallest effective doses should be used.
    - SSRIs and TCAs have generally been thought to be safe during pregnancy, but recent data indicate a modest but significant increase in risk for adverse fetal outcomes such as prematurity, low birth weight, persistant pulmonary hypertension, and congenital malformations.
    - Prescribe TCAs generally with greater risk than SSRIs
    - A recent FDA MedWatch warning reports that paroxetine exposure during the first trimester has been associated with an increased risk of birth defects.
    - Benzodiazepines should be avoided in the first trimester.
    - MAOIs should not be used during pregnancy.
- Postpartum concerns
  - GAD more common in postpartum women
  - Subclinical symptoms of generalized and social anxiety frequently occur during the postpartum period.
  - Postpartum women are vulnerable to the development of OCD.
    - One particularly common type of obsession centers on the fear of harming the baby.
  - Pharmacotherapy in breast-feeding mothers:
    - All antidepressants have been shown to be present in breast milk.
    - Sertraline, paroxetine, and nortryptyline are preferred antidepressant treatments in breast-feeding mothers as they result in undetectable drug levels in infants.

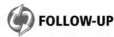 **FOLLOW-UP**

Issues for Referral

- Refer to a psychiatrist for complex, comorbid, severe, or treatment-refractory cases.

- Consider hospitalization for patients with suicidality or extreme difficulty functioning.
- Refer to psychotherapist (psychologist, psychiatrist, social worker or other licensed psychotherapist) according to patient preference and ability to participate in therapy.

PROGNOSIS
- With the exception of specific childhood phobias, which often remit spontaneously with age, untreated anxiety disorders are chronic and often worsen with time.
- Treatment of OCD complicated both by potential relapse and incomplete response
- PTSD is often chronic. Up to one-third of patients are still symptomatic 10 years after diagnosis.
- Despite this, prognosis for most anxiety disorders with appropriate treatment and follow up care is good.
  – A combination of psychotherapy and pharmacotherapy may be more effective than either treatment alone.
  – Supportive psychotherapy may prevent relapse. This is particularly important given the chronic course associated with most anxiety disorders.
- Length of treatment
  – Treatment response is comparable for both psychotherapy and pharmacotherapy and may take 6 to 12 weeks
  – Maintenance therapy recommended for 12 to 18 months, in some cases longer

COMPLICATIONS
- Frequent comorbidity with other psychiatric disorders, especially with other anxiety disorders
  – Comorbid depressive symptoms are particularly common in the postpartum period.
- Insomnia
- Suicidality
  – Suicidality must be carefully assessed and is more common when there is a comorbid depressive disorder.

REFERENCES

1. American Psychiatric Association. *Diagnostic and Statistical Manual of Mental Disorders*. 4th ed. Text Revision. Washington, DC: American Psychiatric Association; 2000.
2. Bladwin DS, Anderson IM, Nutt DJ, et al. Evidence-based guidelines for the pharmacological treatment of anxiety disorders: Recommendations from the British Association for Psychopharmacology. *J Psychopharmacology*. 2005;19:567–596.
3. Kallen B. Neonate characteristics after maternal use of antidepressants in late pregnancy. *Arch Pediatr Adolesc Med*. 2004;158:312–316.
4. Maron E, Nikopensius T, Kõks S, et al. Association study of 90 candidate gene polymorphisms in panic disorder. *Psychiatr Genetics*. 2005;15:17–24.
5. Smoller, JW, Yamaki LH, Fagerness JA, et al. The corticotropin-releasing hormone gene and behavioral inhibition in children at risk for panic disorder. *J Biol Psychiatry*. 2005;57:1485–1492.
6. Weissman AM, Levy BT, Hartz AJ, et al. Pooled analysis of antidepressant levels in lactating mothers, breast milk, and nursing infants. *Am J Psychiatry*. 2004;161: 1066–1078.
7. Wenzel A, Haugen EN, Jackson LC, et al. Anxiety symptoms and disorders at eight weeks postpartum. *Anxiety Disord*. 2005;19:295–311.

CODES
ICD9-CM
- 300.01 Panic Disoder without Agoraphobia
- 300.21 Panic Disorder with Agoraphobia
- 300.22 Agoraphobia
- 300.29 Specific phobia
- 300.23 Social anxiety disorder or social phobia
- 300.3 Obsessive Compulsive Disorder (OCD)
- 309.81 Posttraumatic Stress Disorder (PTSD)
- 300.02 Generalized Anxiety Disorder (GAD)

KEY WORDS

- Anxiety
- Panic Disorder
- Agoraphobia
- Specific Phobia
- Social Phobia
- Obsessive Compulsive Disorder
- Posttraumatic Stress Disorder
- Generalized Anxiety Disorder

ASTHMA

Ghada Bourjeily, MD
Nadia Chammas, MD

KEY CLINICAL POINTS

- A history of intermittent wheezing with peak flow variability suggest asthma.
- A diagnosis of asthma is established by the documentation of reversible airway obstruction or airway hyperresponsiveness to challenges.
- Asthma teaching and patient self-monitoring are crucial steps in the management of the condition.
- Eliminate known triggers and stimuli. Emphasize the importance of smoking cessation.
- Follow a step-wise approach in the long-term management of asthmatics.
- Poor technique and noncompliance are major factors contributing to suboptimal control.
- Early treatment is crucial in acute exacerbations.

 BASICS

DESCRIPTION
Asthma is a chronic inflammatory disease of the airways characterized by:
- Airway obstruction that is reversible either spontaneously or with medications
- Airway hyperresponsiveness to various allergens and triggers

EPIDEMIOLOGY
- The incidence and prevalence of asthma are uncertain due to the difficulty identifying the cases.
- Seems to vary significantly worldwide.
- The annual age-adjusted prevalence rate of self-reported asthma increased between 1982 and 1992 by about 42%.
- Mortality and the rate of hospitalizations related to asthma are increasing in the United States and are higher in African Americans.
- During childhood (age <10), asthma is more prevalent in boys. At puberty, (age 10–14), asthma prevalence is about the same in both sexes. After puberty (age 15–44), the risk of asthma is significantly higher in females.
- There is a significant increase in the prevalence of asthma in women of childbearing age. There is no clear explanation for this.

RISK FACTORS
Multiple factors have been shown to increase the risk of asthma. These include:
- Low birth weight
- Prematurity
- Personal or family history of allergic disease
- Various environmental exposures, such as tobacco smoke, organic volatile compounds, and house-dust mites
- Prolonged breast-feeding may have a protective effect against asthma in infants.

PATHOPHYSIOLOGY
- Asthma is characterized by eosinophilic and mononuclear cell infiltration, airway remodeling, and mucous metaplasia, leading to reversible airway obstruction and bronchial hyperresponsiveness.

- Th-2 dominated tissue inflammation is the underlying mechanism with elevated levels of interleukin (IL) 4, IL-5, IL-9 and IL-13.
- Widespread, but variable, airway obstruction ensues, which is often reversible spontaneously or with bronchodilators.
- The inflammation is also associated with an increase in airway hyperresponsiveness.
- In some patients, subbasement membrane fibrosis occurs, accounting for the persistent abnormalities in lung function.
- Premenstrual asthma has been reported in multiple studies.
  - Cutaneous response to histamine and specific allergens show a marked menstrual variability in the general population
  - In asthmatic women, there is a decrease in the density of the beta-2 adrenoreceptors in the luteal phase and exogenous administration of progesterone in the follicular phase is associated with a downregulation of the beta-2 adrenoreceptor density. The opposite response to exogenous progesterone occurs in nonasthmatics.
  - There is a significant airway hyperreactivity among premenstrual susceptible asthmatic women around the midluteal phase with significant drops in FEV1 and peak flows in late luteal phase.
  - In most studies, airway responsiveness to methacholine over the menstrual cycle does not show significant changes.
- Among smokers, women have more airway hyperreactivity than men do.

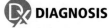 DIAGNOSIS

History
A history of intermittent wheezing or dyspnea after certain triggers (extreme temperatures, allergens, exercise). At times symptoms may start without any obvious triggers. Patients are typically asymptomatic between attacks.

SYMPTOMS
- Wheezing and chest tightness are common symptoms.
- May manifest with chronic cough only
- May also present with dyspnea

SIGNS
- The physical exam may be normal between attacks.
- Monophonic wheezing is a common sign.
- During exacerbations, use of accessory muscles and flaring of the nostrils are signs of severity.
- Asthma severity is classified by the National Asthma Education and Prevention Program (NAEPP) Expert Panel Report II to help simplify the therapeutic approach in adults and children older than 5 years. It has been divided into mild intermittent asthma and persistent asthma (Table 1).

DIFFERENTIAL DIAGNOSIS
Asthma may mimic a variety of pulmonary diseases, such as COPD, pulmonary emboli, upper airway obstruction, and vocal cord dysfunction.

TESTS
- Peak flow variability of more than 20% is a common finding in symptomatic, sub-optimally controlled asthmatics.
- Spirometry; when patients are symptomatic, the spirometry frequently shows an obstructive physiology (FEV1/FVC <70, with normal or variable degrees of reduction in FEV1). Once the

Table 1 Classification of Asthma Severity (Clinical Features Before Treatment)*

	Symptoms†	Nighttime symptoms	Lung function
STEP 4 **Severe** **Persistent**	Continual symptoms Limited physical activity Frequent exacerbations	Frequent	FEV1 or PEF ≤60% pred PEF variability >30%
STEP 3 **Moderate** **persistent**	Daily symptoms Daily use of short-acting beta 2-agonist Excerbations affect activity Excerbations >2 times/week	>1 time a week	FEV1 or PEF 60–80% pred PEF variability >30%
STEP 2 **Mild** **persistent**	Symptoms >twice/week, but <once/day Exacerbations may affect activity	>2 times a month	FEV1 or PEF ≥80% pred PEF variability 20–30%

STEP 1
Mild
intermittent
	Symptoms ≤2 times a week
	Asymptomatic and normal PEF
	    between exacerbations
	Exacerbations brief (from a few
	    hours to a few days); intensity
	    may vary
		≤2 times a month	FEV1 or PEF ≥80% pred
			PEF variability <20%

*The presence of one of the features of severity is sufficient to place a patient in that category. An individual should be assigned to the most severe grade in which any feature occurs. The characteristics noted in this figure are general and may overlap because asthma is highly variable. Furthermore, an individual's classification may change over time.

† Patients at any level of severity can have mild, moderate, or severe exacerbations. Some patients with intermittent asthma can experience severe and life-threatening exacerbations separated by long periods of normal lung function and no symptoms.

symptoms resolve, either with medications or spontaneously, spirometry should normalize, unless airway remodeling and loss of lung function have occurred. Documentation of an obstructive physiology on the spirometry is neither sensitive nor specific for the diagnosis of asthma and should be coupled with findings on the medical history and the pattern of symptoms.

• Documentation of bronchial hyperresponsiveness is needed if the diagnosis is not established based on the above. Methacholine is the most commonly used agent in airway challenge. Other challenges include hypertonic saline, allergens, and cold air, but those are used less frequently.

Lab
Hypoxemia is rare in pure asthma outside of exacerbations. Mild hypoxemia is a common finding in acute exacerbations. Hypocapnia, normocapnia, and hypercapnia can be seen in acute exacerbations depending on the severity of the attacks.

Imaging
• Chest radiographs may show evidence of hyperinflation and may be helpful in exacerbations to rule out pneumonia as a precipitating cause for the exacerbation as well as rule out potential complications of asthma exacerbations such as pneumothorax and pneumomediastinum.
• Other imaging modalities are not needed unless alternative diagnoses are being contemplated.

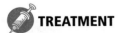 **TREATMENT**

PRE-HOSPITAL
• Long term management of asthma
  – Patient education is crucial in the long-term management of asthma given the fact that early intervention and treatment may prevent serious complications.
  – Compliance with medications is a major issue in asthma care. Simplifying the regimen and using combination drugs and less frequent dosing when appropriate may aid in compliance.
  – Inhaler technique should be reviewed on multiple visits with newly diagnosed patients and reviewed periodically.
  – Written instructions and asthma action plans detailing specific interventions for different symptoms and various peak flow levels are very helpful to patients in directing their care even prior to reaching their health care provider.
  – A small supply of steroids such as prednisone may be given to patients with a history of severe asthma who are reliable and understand how and when to use them in case their symptoms are severe.
  – Treatment of the inflammatory response in asthma is the mainstay of therapy.
  – A stepwise approach for the long-term management of asthma has been suggested by the NAEPP Expert Panel Report II (Table 2).
  – Omalizumab, a recombinant, humanized anti-IgE antibody reduces circulating free IgE, improves methacholine responsiveness, and reduces exacerbation rates. Its use is recommended in patients with a major allergic component to their asthma who are not controlled on usual therapy or who require steroid therapy chronically. It is supplied as a powder for subcutaneous injections every 2–4 weeks.
  – In a large managed care organization, women generated more cost for health care use and required more prescription medications, such as inhaled corticosteroids.
• Management of acute exacerbations
  – Exacerbations of asthma are acute or subacute episodes of worsening dyspnea, wheezing, chest tightness, or cough associated with significant reductions in peak expiratory flow (PEF) or FEV1.
  – A written action plan outlining what action to take based on peak flow numbers and symptoms helps guide the patient through exacerbations.

Table 2 Stepwise Approach for Managing Asthma in Adults and Children Older Than Five years of Age: Treatment-Preferred treatments are in bold print

	Long-term control	Quick relief	Education

STEP 4
Severe
persistent
	Daily medications
	Preferred treatment:
	   High–dose inhaled corticosteroids
	AND
	   Long-acting inhaled beta 2-agonists
	AND, if needed
	   Corticosteroid tables or syrup long term
	   (2 mg/kg/day, generally do not exceed
	   60 mg per day). (Make repeat attempts to
	   reduce systemic corticosteroids and
	   maintain control with high-dose inhaled
	   corticosteroids).
		Short–acting bronchodilator:
		inhaled beta 2–agoinsts as
		needed for symptoms. Intensity of
		treatment will depend on severity
		of exacerbation; see component
		3-Managing
		Exacerbations. Use of short-acting
		inhaled beta 2-agonists on a daily
		basis, or increasing use, indicates
		the need for additional
		long-term-control therapy.
			Steps 2 and 3 actions plus:
			Refer to individual
			education/counselling

STEP 3
Moderate
persistent
	Daily medications:
	Preferred treatment:
	   Low–to–medium dose inhaled
	   corticosteroids and long-acting inhaled
	   beta 2-agonists.
	Alternative treatment (listed alphabetically):
	   Increase inhaled corticosteroids within
	   medium–dose range
	OR
	   Low–to–medium dose inhaled
	   corticosteroids and either leukoriene
	   modifier or theophylline.
	If needed (particularly in patients with
	recurring severe exacerbations):
	Preferred treatment:
	   Increase inhaled corticosteroids within
	   medium–dose range and add long-acting
	   inhaled beta 2-agonists
	Alternative treatment:
	   Increase inhaled corticosteroids within
	   medium–dose range and add either
	   leukotriene modifier or theophylline.
		Short–acting bronchodilator:
		inhaled beta 2–agoinsts as
		needed for symptoms. Intensity of
		treatment will depend on severity
		of exacerbation; see component
		3-Managing
		Exacerbations. Use of short-acting
		inhaled beta 2-agonists on a daily
		basis, or increasing use, indicates
		the need for additional
		long-term-control therapy.
			Step 1 actions plus:
			Teach self-monitoring
			Refer to group education if
			available
			Review and update
			self-management plan

STEP 2
Mild
persistent
	Preferred treatment:
	   Low-dose inhaled corticosteroids
	Alternative treatment (listed alphabetically):
	   Cromolyn, leukotriene modifier,
	   nedocromil,
	OR sustaind release theophylline to serum
	   concentration of 5–15 mcg/mL.
		Short–acting bronchodilator:
		inhaled beta 2–agoinsts as
		needed for symptoms. Intensity of
		treatment will depend on severity
		of exacerbation; see component
		3-Managing
		Exacerbations. Use of short-acting
		inhaled beta 2-agonists on a daily
		basis, or increasing use, indicates
		the need for additional
		long-term-control therapy.
			Step 1 actions plus:
			Teach self-monitoring
			Refer to group education if
			available
			Review and update
			self-management plan

STEP 1 Mild persistent	No daily medication needed. Severe exacerbations may occur, separated by long periods of normal lung function and no symptoms. A course of systemic corticosteroids is recommended.	Short–acting bronchodilator: **inhaled beta 2–agoinsts** as needed for symptoms. Intensity of treatment will depend on severity of exacerbation; see component 3-Managing Exacerbations.	Teach basic facts about asthma Teach inhaler/spacer/holding chamber technique Discuss roles of medications Develop self-management plan

Table 2 Stepwise Approach for Managing Asthma in Adults and Children Older Than Five years of Age: Treatment-Preferred treatments are in bold print (Continued...)

Long-term control	Quick relief	Education
	Use of short-acting inhaled beta 2-agonists more than two times a week may indicate the need to initiate long-term-control therapy	Develop action plan for when and how to take rescue actions, especially for patients with a history of svere exacerbations Discuss appropriate environmental control measures to avoid exposure to known allergens and irritants

Step down
Review treatment every one to six months; a gradual stepwise reduction in treatment may be possible.

Step up
If control is not maintained, consider step up. First, review patient medication technique, adherence, and environmental control (avoidance of allergens or other factors that contribute to asthma severity).

NOTE:

The stepwise approach presents general guidelines to assist clinical decisionmaking; it is not intended to be a specific prescription. Asthma is highly variable; clinicians should tailor specific medication plans to the needs and circumstances of individual patients.

Gain control is quickly as possible; then decrease treatment to the least medication necessary to maintain control. Gaining control may be accomplished by either starting treatment at the step most appropriate to the initial severity of the condition or starting at a higher level of therapy (e.g., a course of systemic corticosteroids or higher dose of inhaled corticosteroids).

A rescue course of systemic corticosteroids may be needed at any time and at any step. Some patients with intermittent asthma experience severe and life-threatening exacerbations separated by long periods of normal lung function and no symptoms. This may be especially common with exacerbations provoked by respiratory infections. A short course of systemic corticosteroids is recommended.

At each step, patients should control their environment to avoid or control factors that make their asthma worse (e.g., allergens, irritants); this requires specific diagnosis and education. Referral to an asthma specialist for consultation or comanagement is recommended if there are difficulties achieving or maintaining control of asthma or if the patient requires step 4 care. Referral may be considered if the patient requires step 3 care (see also component 1-initial Assessment and Diagnosis).

- Treatment should be started as soon as possible to avoid unnecessary hospitalizations.
- Rapid reversal of airflow obstruction is attempted using inhaled short acting beta-2 agonists, either repetitively or continuously.
- Administration of a short acting anticholinergic has been shown to result in additional bronchodilation when used in acute exacerbations.
- Administration of systemic corticosteroids may be needed if PEF is <80% of predicted or of personal best after 3 treatments.
- Heliox may help in the early treatment of acute exacerbations and respiratory failure secondary to asthma. Heliox has been shown to improve the degree of respiratory acidosis as well as decrease pulsus paradoxus and peak flows. The improvements are seen in the first 20 minutes but treated groups and control groups showed no difference in peak flow numbers or dyspnea scores 6 hours after the treatment.
- Methylxanthines do not add to the benefit of beta-2 agonists and may cause increased side effects.
- Magnesium sulfate and intravenous albuterol are of uncertain benefit.
- Intubation and mechanical ventilation are at times necessary in cases of apnea, depressed mental status or worsening hypercapnia. Care should be taken in mechanically ventilated patients to prevent hyperinflation and elevated airway

pressures in order to avoid complications. Ventilator management should be done by experienced health care providers.

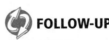 **FOLLOW-UP**

DISPOSITION
Admission Criteria
Patients requiring hospital admission include:
- Those who are hypoxemic or acidemic.
- Those with peak flow less than 50% after initial treatment. Decision for admission in patients with a peak flow of 50–70% should be individualized.
- One should have a low threshold to admit patients with moderately severe exacerbations who are newly diagnosed, have little knowledge about their disease, or are not comfortable managing exacerbations at home.
- Patients on systemic steroids at the time of presentation
- Patients with a history of frequent hospitalizations or emergency room visits

Discharge Criteria
- Patients can usually be discharged when their symptoms have improved and their peak flows are 70% or above.

- Discharge decisions on patients with peak flows of 40–70% should be individualized. For example, more knowledgeable patients with a long standing history of mild asthma who are compliant enough to have short term follow up may be discharged.

Issues for Referral

Guidelines set forth by the National expert Panel Report II on patients requiring specialist referral include: Those with a life-threatening asthma exacerbation, those not meeting the goals of asthma therapy after 3–6 months of treatment, those with atypical symptoms, those with the presence of complicating conditions (such as COPD, GERD, sinusitis, severe rhinitis), or patients with a question of occupational influence on symptoms, patients that need additional help with education and compliance, those with moderate to severe persistent asthma, or patients requiring immunotherapy or high dose inhaled steroids or oral steroids.

COMPLICATIONS

- Poor asthma control may lead to irreversible airway disease and airway remodeling.
- Patients requiring repeat or prolonged steroid therapy should be monitored for possible complications that may include hyperglycemia, hypertension, glaucoma, osteoporosis, and depression.

REFERENCES

1. De Marco R, Locatelli F, Sunyer J, et al. Differences in incidence of reported asthma related to age in men and women. A retrospective analysis of the data of the European Respiratory Health Survey. *Am J Respir Crit Care Med*. 2000;162:68–74.
2. Elias JA, Lee CG, Zheng T, et al. New insights into the pathogenesis of asthma. *J Clin Invest*. 2003;111:291–297.
3. National Health Lung and Blood Institute expert panel report 2. NIH publication. No. 97-4051, 1997.
4. Ten Hacken NH, Postma DS, Timens W. Airway remodeling and long term decline in lung function in asthma. *Curr Opin Pulm Med*. 2003;9:9–14.

ADDITIONAL READING

Cabana MD, Le TT. Challenges in asthma patient education. *J Allergy Clin Immunol*. 2005;115:1225–1227.

Mapp CE, Boschetto P, Maestrelli P, et al. Occupational asthma. *Am J Respir Crit Care Med*. 2005;172:280–305.

CODES

ICD9-CM

- 493.00 Asthma

KEY WORDS

- Asthma
- Peak Flows
- Spirometry
- Management

ATROPHIC VAGINITIS

Mary H. Hohenhaus, MD

KEY CLINICAL POINTS

- Common diagnosis in menopausal women, but can occur with any prolonged low estrogen state
- Many women are asymptomatic.
- Estrogen therapy is effective, but the risks and benefits for the individual woman should be weighed carefully.

 ## BASICS

DESCRIPTION

- Atrophic vaginitis is the thinning of the vaginal epithelium with associated inflammatory changes in response to decreased endogenous estrogen.
- Can also affect urinary epithelium
- Usually requires prolonged estrogen deficiency
- Most women with mild to moderate vaginal atrophy are asymptomatic.

GENERAL PREVENTION

- Regular sexual intercourse

EPIDEMIOLOGY

- The true incidence and prevalence are unknown, because many women are asymptomatic and up to 25% of symptomatic women do not seek treatment.

Prevalence

- Symptomatic in up to 50% of postmenopausal women

RISK FACTORS

Menopause is the most common risk factor, but there is an increased risk with any low estrogen state including prolonged breastfeeding.

- Cigarette smoking
- Decreased frequency of sexual intercourse

PATHOPHYSIOLOGY

Lack of estrogen alters the normal vaginal environment

- Atrophy of vaginal epithelium
- Decreased glycogen levels
- Loss of normal population of lactobacilli
  - Decreased lactic acid production
  - Increased vaginal pH
  - Overgrowth of gram negative rods
- Decreased blood flow
  - Decline in normal vaginal secretions

ETIOLOGY

Any condition causing significant decrease in circulating estrogen levels

- Menopause
- Oophorectomy
- Anti-estrogenic medications
  - Danazol
  - Gonadotropin-releasing hormone (GnRH) agonists (such as goserelin, leuprolide, nafarelin)
  - Progestins (such as medroxyprogesterone acetate)
  - Tamoxifen
- Prolonged breastfeeding (elevated prolactin level)
- Ovarian failure
  - Radiation therapy
  - Chemotherapy
  - Immune disorders

ASSOCIATED CONDITIONS

- Urinary incontinence
- Urinary tract infection
- Pelvic organ prolapse

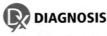 ## DIAGNOSIS

SIGNS AND SYMPTOMS

- Vaginal
  - Dryness, itching
  - Occasional spotting
  - Pain during intercourse
  - Burning sensation or spotting after intercourse
  - Leukorrhea
  - Yellow, malodorous discharge
- Urinary
  - Frequency, urgency
  - Painful urination
  - Hematuria
  - Stress incontinence

History

- Use of sanitary pads, soaps, lubricants, feminine hygiene products, spermicides, or other potential irritants
- Medication use
- Recent or recurrent urinary tract infection
- Sexual history, including risks for sexually transmitted infections
- Menstrual history, including date of last menstrual period
- Reproductive history, including recent or current breastfeeding

Physical Exam

ALERT

To avoid vaginal trauma, evaluate width and depth of introitus before attempting to insert a speculum

- External genitalia
  - Thinning of pubic hair
  - Decreased turgor and elasticity
  - Vulvar atrophy
  - Vulvar lesions
  - Fusion of labia minora
- Vagina
  - Narrowed introitus
  - Pale, smooth, shiny mucosa, may be friable
  - Loss of folds
  - Dryness
  - Fissures
  - Diffuse or patchy erythema
  - Petechiae or ecchymoses
  - Watery or serosanguinous discharge
  - Cystocele, rectocele, uterine prolapse
- Urinary
  - Urethral polyp or caruncle
  - Eversion of urethral mucosa

TESTS
Lab
- Urinalysis, urine culture, and sensitivity to evaluate for urinary tract infection
- Serum estrogen level

Imaging
- Transvaginal ultrasonography: thinning of endometrial stripe (4–5 mm) supports estrogen deficiency

Diagnostic Procedures/Surgery
- Vaginal pH taken from upper third of side wall: elevated (5.0–7.0)
- Microscopy of saline and potassium hydroxide wet mounts taken from upper third of vaginal side wall
  - Increased numbers of polymorphonuclear leukocytes
  - Decreased numbers of lactobacilli
  - May show evidence of coexisting infection
- Papanicollaou smear to assess for estrogen effect: take specimen from upper third of vaginal side wall and request maturation index to distinguish from smear taken for cervical cytology
  - Increased number of immature squamous epithelial cells
  - Inflammatory exudates
- Cervical cultures for sexually transmitted infections if indicated

DIFFERENTIAL DIAGNOSIS
- Bacterial vaginosis
- Trichomoniasis
- Vaginal candidiasis
- Vulvar dermatitis
- Contact irritation

 ## TREATMENT

INITIAL STABILIZATION
- Treat any coexisting infectious cause of vulvovaginitis

GENERAL MEASURES
- Avoid tight-fitting clothing and synthetic undergarments.
- Avoid potential irritants, such as soaps, sanitary pads, and feminine hygiene products.
- Discontinue offending medication if possible.
- Weigh the severity of the symptoms against benefits of prolonged breastfeeding.
- The use of water-based personal lubricant can help relieve vaginal itching and irritation as well as intercourse-related pain.
  - Polycarbophil-based vaginal moisturizers may promote maturation of vaginal epithelium and a more acidic pH.

Complementary and Alternative Therapies
Many agents, including phytoestrogens, black cohosh, dong quai, ginseng, and red clover have been used to treat menopausal symptoms, but information on their effectiveness is limited.

 ## MEDICATION (DRUGS)

- Need for treatment in asymptomatic women is unknown
- Estrogen most effective treatment
  - Estrogen contraindicated in known or suspected breast or estrogen-dependent cancers, undiagnosed vaginal bleeding, history of thromboembolism, active thrombophlebitis, or pregnancy
  - Estrogen use controversial in breastfeeding.
    - Secreted in breast milk, decreased quantity and quality
    - Unopposed estrogen may induce fertility
    - The benefits of local estrogen therapy or combination oral contraceptives in women more than 6 months postpartum may outweigh the risks.
  - Local estrogen therapy is preferred for isolated atrophic vaginitis given the concerns about long-term risks of malignancy and cardiovascular disease with systemic therapy.

- Few well-designed trials of local therapy
- All forms appear effective for vaginal symptoms, effect on urinary symptoms unclear
- The safety of local therapy beyond 1 year is unknown.
- Use the lowest effective dose for the shortest duration possible.
- Although estrogen exposure is assumed to be minimized with local therapy, systemic absorption occurs; consider addition of cyclic or daily progestin to prevent endometrial hyperplasia in women with an intact uterus, especially with long-term treatment.
- The cream may be less acceptable to women than vaginal tablet or ring, which may affect adherence.
- Conjugated estrogens vaginal cream (0.625 mg/gram)
  - 0.5–2 grams vaginally daily given cyclically (3 weeks on, 1 week off)
- Estradiol 0.01% vaginal cream
  - 2–4 grams vaginally daily for 1–2 weeks, then taper to half the starting dose over 1–2 weeks; administer 1–3 times weekly for maintenance
- Estradiol 0.025 mg vaginal tablet
  - One tablet vaginally daily for 2 weeks, then twice weekly for maintenance
- Estradiol vaginal ring (0.0075 mg per day)
  - Silicone ring placed vaginally every 3 months
  - It may not be appropriate for women with narrow, short, or stenosed vagina.
  - Expulsion may be more common in women with prior hysterectomy.
- Systemic estrogen therapy may be indicated in postmenopausal women with atrophic vaginitis in addition to moderate to severe vasomotor symptoms or in women taking long-term GnRH agonists.
  - Women with an intact uterus require cyclic or continuous progestin to prevent endometrial hyperplasia.

 ## FOLLOW-UP

PROGNOSIS
- Many women remain asymptomatic.
- Symptoms usually improve markedly within 2 weeks of local estrogen therapy, but may recur after treatment is stopped.

COMPLICATIONS
- Uterine bleeding, breast pain, perineal pain secondary to estrogen use
- Vaginal irritation secondary to local estrogen therapy

PATIENT MONITORING
- Review use of estrogen every 3–6 months and attempt to taper or discontinue its use.
- An annual clinical breast exam and mammography is recommended for women on estrogen therapy.
- Endometrial biopsy to evaluate postmenopausal bleeding, especially in women on estrogen therapy
- Consider transvaginal ultrasound to evaluate endometrium in women on prolonged estrogen therapy.

REFERENCES

1. Bachmann GA, Nevadunsky NS. Diagnosis and treatment of atrophic vaginitis. *Am Fam Physician*. 2000;61: 3090–3096.

2. Crandall C. Vaginal estrogen preparations: A review of safety and efficacy for vaginal atrophy. *J Womens Health*. 2002;11:857–877.
3. Davila GW, Singh A, Karapenagioten I, et al. Are women with urogenital atrophy symptomatic? *Am J Obstet Gynecol*. 2003;188:383–388.
4. Palmer AR, Likis FE. Lactational atrophic vaginitis. *J Midwifery Women's Health*. 2003;48:282–284.
5. Suckling J, Lethaby A, Kennedy R. Local oestrogen for vaginal atrophy in postmenopausal women. Cochrane Database of Systematic Reviews. 2003, Issue 4. Art. No.: CD001500. DOI: 10.1002/14651858.CD001500.
6. Van der Laak JAWM, de Biel MT, de Leen WH, et al. The effect of Replens on vaginal cytology in the treatment of postmenopausal atrophy: Cytomorphology versus computerized cytometry. *J Clin Pathol*. 2002;55:446–451.

CODES
ICD9-CM
616.10 Vaginitis and vulvovaginitis, unspecified

KEY WORDS

- Dyspareunia
- Menopause
- Urinary Incontinence
- Urogenital Atrophy
- Vaginitis

AUTOIMMUNE HEPATITIS

Silvia D. Degli-Esposti, MD
Marco Lenzi, MD

KEY CLINICAL POINTS

- Presents as acute or chronic hepatitis
- More frequent in women
- It is associated with other autoimmune diseases.
- Active disease progresses to end-stage liver disease without treatment.
- Prognosis with treatment is generally good.
- Rare asymptomatic patients with minimal hepatitis on the liver biopsy may not require therapy.

 BASICS

DESCRIPTION
Autoimmune hepatitis (AIH) is a chronic inflammatory disease of unknown cause, which leads to the progressive destruction of the liver parenchyma.

- The presence of a variety of serum auto antibodies is common, which leads to the classification of the disease into 3 groups (I–III).
  - Type I + antinuclear antibodies (ANA) and/or l anti-smooth muscle antibodies (SMA)
  - Type II + antiliver/kidney/microsomal antibodies (LKM/LC-1)
    - Group 1 typical features of Type I
    - Group 2 associated with hepatitis C in Europe
  - Type III + antimitochondrial antibodies (AMA) and +/– antisoluble liver antigen/liver pancreas antigen (SLA/LP)
- Overlapping syndromes
  - AIH has features in common (10%) with primary sclerosis cholangitis (PSC), primary biliary cirrhosis (PBC), and autoimmune cholangitis.

GENERAL PREVENTION
Early diagnosis and appropriate therapy will prevent progression to end stage liver disease.

EPIDEMIOLOGY
- AIH affects predominantly women of all ages, all ethnic origins.
- 1/2 of the patients with type I classic AIH are women under age of 40.
- Gender ratio: 3.6:1
- The clinical course is more aggressive in children.
- Elderly may have milder disease.
- AIH accounts for 5.6% of all liver transplants in the United States.

Incidence
1.9/100,000 white North European population

Prevalence
16.9/100,000 white North European population

RISK FACTORS
High index of suspicion for patients with autoimmune phenotype and elevated aminotransferases

Genetics
AHI is strongly associated with HLA class II phenotype DR 3 and DR 4 in Caucasian and North American patients. HLA phenotype influences disease expression and clinical behavior as well as susceptibility.
- AIH Type I DRB1*0301: Younger patients, aggressive disease, less response to therapy

- AIH Type I DRB1*0401: Older patients, better response to therapy
- AHI Type II DRB1*0701: More common in Southern Europe

PATHOPHYSIOLOGY
The pathogenesis of the disease is only partially understood.
- External factors interacting with host genetic susceptibility trigger immunoreactions targeted to hepatic cells.
- Antibody-dependent and cellular mediated hepatocyte cytotoxicity
- Targeted antigens in the liver are not known.
- Serum autoantibodies are not involved in the direct damage. They are useful in the diagnosis and to monitor the disease.
- Inflammation causes necrosis and fibrosis deposition in the liver parenchyma.

ETIOLOGY
Agent(s) triggering the autoimmune process in classical AIH are unknown (idiopathic)
- Can be caused by specific drugs
  - Clinically similar, responds to drug withdrawal
  - Methyldopa, Minocylline, Isoniazide, Nitrofuradantoin, Hydralazine
- Can be associated with viral hepatitis (EBV, A, C)

ASSOCIATED CONDITIONS
AIH is associated with full spectrum of autoimmune disorders:
- Diabetes mellitus type1
- Rheumatoid artritis
- Polyglandular syndrome (AIH type 2)
- Antiphospolipid antibody
- Autoimmune thyroiditis
- Ulcerative colitis
- Vasculitis
- Autoimmune hemolysis
- Alopecia
- Polyendocrinophaty-candidiasis-ectodermal dystrophy (APS-1)

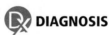 **DIAGNOSIS**

PRE-HOSPITAL
Diagnosis is reached using clinical, laboratory, and histological data.
- Easy diagnosis in typical cases
- No pathognomonic features
- Diagnostic criteria have been codified and updated by an international panel (IAIHG) and require the presence of characteristic features and exclusion of other known causes of liver disease.
- A scoring system that attributes negative and positive points to clinical and laboratory features is useful in difficult diagnoses.

ALERT
AIH is a treatable cause of end stage liver disease; any effort should be made to achieve diagnosis

SIGNS AND SYMPTOMS
- Malaise
- Fever
- Artralgia
- Fatigue
- RUQ discomfort

- Jaundice
- Acute hepatitis: 30–40% of all cases, usually symptomatic
- Chronic hepatitis: Usually asymptomatic, discovered during routine work up for abnormal LFTs
- Cirrhosis: Patients with cirrhosis at time of initial presentation; asymptomatic or with signs and symptoms of end stage liver disease
    - 1/2 of the children with AIH will present with cirrhosis.

History
- Personal or family history of autoimmune diseases
- History of medications known to cause chronic hepatitis
- Personal history of other liver diseases
- Inquire about alcohol use

Physical Exam
Signs of chronic liver disease may be present:
- Jaundice, muscular wasting, spider angioma
- Hepatoslenomegaly, ascites
- Peripheral edema
- Hyperreflexia, asterixis

TESTS
Required to confirm AIH and exclude other liver diseases

Lab
- AST and ALT >5 × normal
- Polyclonal hyperglobulinemia Yglobulin ≥1.5 × normal
- ANA, SMA, LKM1 ≥1:80
- Absent marker of viral infection (B, C, A)
- Normal a1 antitripsin phenotype, ceruloplasmin, iron, and ferritin levels

Imaging
Abdominal ultrasound with Doppler and CT scan with contrast can be useful in ruling out other causes of abnormal LFTs (Budd-Chiari, fatty liver, space occupying lesions), but are not critical for the diagnosis.

Diagnostic Procedures/Surgery
A liver biopsy is required for the diagnosis.

Pathologic Findings
- Periportal hepatitis (interface hepatitis)
- Predominant lymphocytes, plasma cells often present
- Variable degree of fibrosis
- Absence of biliary changes and granulomas

DIFFERENTIAL DIAGNOSIS
Other causes of acute or chronic hepatitis must be excluded to make a diagnosis.
- Overlapping syndromes pose a challenge
    - Primary biliary cirrhosis (PBC): Autoimmune chronic hepatitis with destruction of biliary epithelia leading to cirrhosis may present with AIH feature
        - Cholestatic syndrome
        - AMA often present (rarely in AIH)
        - Biliary epithelia infiltration, granulomas in liver biopsy
    - Primary sclerosis cholangitis (PSC), Autoimmune cholangitis: Autoimmune chronic hepatitis with destruction of small intrahepatic biliary ducts and /or large extra hepatic ducts, auto antibodies may be present
        - Predominantly cholestatic picture
        - Abnormal ERCP
- In overlapping syndromes and atypical presentation
    - Order additional antibodies (pANCA, anti-LC-1,anti-SLA/LP, anti-ASGPR)
    - HLA type
    - Use score system

Pregnancy Considerations
- Autoimmune hepatitis may occur de novo in pregnancy.
- Pregnant women with AIH have higher frequency of prematurity, low birth weight infants, and fetal losses.
- Liver biopsy must be performed if suspected and therapy started.
- Corticosteroid and azathioprine are probably safe in pregnancy.

 ## TREATMENT

PRE-HOSPITAL
Once the diagnosis is confirmed, treatment should be initiated as soon as possible.

INITIAL STABILIZATION
- Outpatient treatment is the norm.
- Acute hepatitis may require hospitalization if severe.
    - Acute liver failure has been described (rare).
    - Monitor coagulopathy and mental status
    - A liver transplant is indicated for acute liver failure.

GENERAL MEASURES
Avoid hepatotoxic drugs and alcohol.

Diet
- Nonrestrictive
- Decompensated liver disease requires dietary modification (salt, water, and animal protein restriction).

Activity
As tolerated

Complementary and Alternative Medicine
- None have been demonstrated effective.
- Consider possible hepatotoxicity of herbal preparations.

 ## MEDICATION (DRUGS)

Goal of therapy is to achieve remission:
- In the 1st 3 years of therapy, 80% of the patients will achieve biochemical and histological remission.
- Long-term remission: 15%
- Approximately 85% will relapse after discontinuation of the therapy and require long-term treatment.
- Nonresponders: 20%
    - Prompts reevaluation of diagnosis
    - Consider an increased dose or change in regimen
- Acute severe hepatitis not responding to therapy should be referred for liver transplant.
- Absolute indication for therapy: AST >10 × normal; AST >5 × upper limit of normal and gamma globulin level >2 × normal; bridging or multilobular necrosis in biopsy
- The benefit of therapy in mild, asymptomatic disease has not been established.

First Line
- Prednisone alone 60 mg/day or Prednisone 30 mg/day + azathioprine 50 mg/day
- Use a prednisone tapering schedule to reach the maintenance dose of 10–20 mg/day in 4–6 weeks.
- Clinical and biochemical normalization occurs in first 3–6 months. Histology lags behind.
- The duration of therapy has not been established; however, after initial tapering, maintenance doses should be continued at least for 1 year.

Second Line

New immunosuppressants have been used in nonresponders.

- Butesonide, cyclosporin A, tacrolimus, and mycophenolate mofetil

SURGERY

Acute liver failure and decompensated cirrhosis benefit from liver transplant.

- The disease recurs, but is generally mild and doesn't affect graft survival.

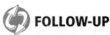 **FOLLOW-UP**

DISPOSITION

The length of therapy is individualized.

- Follow aminotransferases and gamma globulin to normalization
- Long-term therapy with immunosuppressants may be required if remission is not achieved.
- Liver biopsy at 1 year of therapy is required for the diagnosis of sustained remission and the discontinuation of therapy.

Admission Criteria

Patients may require hospitalization for complications of decompensated liver disease.

Discharge Criteria

When stabilization is achieved

Issues for Referral

- Refer to a hepatologist for liver biopsy and initial diagnosis and treatment
- Refer to transplantation center for decompensated liver disease

PROGNOSIS

Untreated AIH has a poor prognosis.

- Survival at 10 years: 10%
- Improves to 80–93% with corticosteroid treatment

COMPLICATIONS

- Cirrhosis
- Hepatocellular carcinoma is rare.

PATIENT MONITORING

Patients need to be followed biannually given the potential of recurrence.

REFERENCES

1. Alvarez F, Berg PA, Bianchi FB, et al. International Autoimmune Hepatitis Group Report: Review of criteria for diagnosis of autoimmune hepatitis. *J Hepatol*. 1999;31:929–938.
2. Czaja AJ, Freese DK. Diagnosis and treatment of autoimmune hepatitis. *Hepatol*. 2002:36:479–497.
3. Donaldson PT. Genetics of autoimmune and viral liver disease; understanding the issues. *J Hepatol*. 2004;41:327–332.
4. Kogan J, Safadi R, Ashur Y, et al. Prognosis of symptomatic versus asymptomatic autoimmune hepatitis: A study of 68 patients. *J Clin Gastroenterol*. 2002;35:75–81.
5. Talwalxar JA, Keach JC, Anqulo P, et al. Overlap of autoimmune hepatitis and primary biliary cirrhosis: An evaluation of modified scoring system. *Am J Gastroenterol*. 2002;97:1191–1197.

CODES

ICD9-CM

- 570.0 Acute-subacute necrosis of liver
- 571.4 Chronic hepatitis nonalcoholic
- 571.9 Unspecified disease of the liver

KEY WORDS

- Autoimmune Liver Diseases
- Acute Hepatitis
- Primary Biliary Cirrhosis

BACTERIAL VAGINOSIS

Iris L. Tong, MD

KEY CLINICAL POINTS

- Bacterial Vaginosis (BV) is caused by an imbalance of vaginal flora.
  - Overgrowth of *Gardnerella vaginalis* (*G. vaginalis*) is most common.
- Treatment of women with asymptomatic BV is not always necessary.
- However, BV is associated with higher transmission rates of HIV and complications in pregnancy.

 ## BASICS

DESCRIPTION

- Vaginitis is inflammation of the vagina resulting in discharge with or without pain.
- BV is the most common cause of vaginitis.
  - Accounts for up to 50% of vaginitis in women of childbearing age
- Other common causes of vaginitis include
  - Candidal vulvovaginitis
  - Trichomoniasis
- Bacterial Vaginosis is caused by an imbalance of the normal flora in the vaginal milieu, leading to the presence of vaginal discharge.

GENERAL PREVENTION

- Avoiding douching
- Safe sex practices as higher number of sexual partners associated with higher rates of BV

EPIDEMIOLOGY

Prevalence

- Prevalence of 5% to 60% worldwide
- Difficult to estimate exact prevalence as many women are asymptomatic
- Can occur in heterosexual and lesbian women
  - High prevalence among women who partner with women
- Prevalence among pregnant women in the United States: 10% to 35%

RISK FACTORS

- Vaginal douching
- Use of intrauterine device
- Younger age of first sexual intercourse
- Multiple sexual partners
- History of STDs
- Pregnancy
- Tobacco use

PATHOPHYSIOLOGY

- Caused by imbalance of normal flora
  - Decrease in lactobacilli and proliferation of
    - *G. vaginalis*, most commonly
    - *Mycoplasma hominis*
    - Anerobes such as *Mobiluncus*, *Bacteroides* and *Peptostreptococcus* species
- It remains unclear whether the initial pathogenic event is the overgrowth of anaerobes or the decrease in lactobacilli.
- The role of sexual transmission is controversial.
  - Higher-risk sex practices (higher number of sexual partners) have been associated with higher rates of BV in both heterosexual and lesbian women.

- However:
  - Treating male partners of women with BV is not beneficial.
  - Women who are not sexually active can develop BV.

ETIOLOGY

- Proliferation of the following organisms in the vaginal milieu:
  - *G. vaginalis*, most commonly
  - *Mycoplasma hominis*
  - Anerobes such as *Mobiluncus*, *Bacteroides* and *Peptostreptococcus* species

ASSOCIATED CONDITIONS

- Increases susceptibility to HIV and other sexually transmitted infections (STIs)
- Complications in pregnancy
  - Preterm labor and delivery
  - Premature rupture of membranes
  - Spontaneous abortion

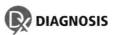 ## DIAGNOSIS

- Diagnosis is made by the presence of 3 of the 4 criteria, known as Amsel's criteria:
  - Thin, white, homogenous discharge
  - Vaginal pH >4.5
  - Positive Whiff test (amine odor when KOH added)
  - Presence of clue cells on light microscopy
    - Squamous cells with irregular borders secondary to studding of bacteria to cell membrane
  - Sensitivity = 69%, specificity = 93%
- A recent prospective, observational study demonstrated that the presence of any two of Amsel's criteria is associated with similar sensitivity and specificity.
  - Vaginal pH highest sensitivity
  - Presence of amine odor has highest specificity

SIGNS AND SYMPTOMS

- Many women are asymptomatic.

History

- +/− Vaginal douching or heavy soap use
- Thin, white, homogenous discharge
- Malodorous, "fishy" discharge

Physical Exam

- Inspection and speculum exam reveals normal vulva, vaginal mucosa, and cervix.
- Signs of mucosal erythema and irritation are typically absent.
- Thin, white, homogenous discharge is present in the vaginal vault.

TESTS

Lab

- pH >4.5 (normal = 4.5)
- Light Microscopy (see below)
- 10% Potassium Hydroxide (KOH) preparation for Whiff test
  - Small amount of vaginal discharge is placed on glass slide
  - A drop of KOH is added to slide
  - Production of an amine (or "fishy") odor indicates a positive Whiff test
- Gram stain
  - Often considered the gold standard

- Presence of small gram-negative rods or gram-variable rods and the absence of longer lactobacilli is highly predictive of BV
  - Less convenient for establishing diagnosis in office
- DNA probe
  - Commercially available probe that simultaneously detects presence of *Candida* species, *G. vaginalis*, and *Trichomonas vaginalis* from single vaginal swab
  - Results within hours
  - Must be performed in the laboratory
  - Sensitivity 73–89%, specificity 88–97%
  - Does not detect BV that is caused by organisms other than *G. vaginalis*
- Colorimetric pH and amine card
  - Detection of pH >4.7 and presence of vaginal fluid amines
  - Rapid diagnosis in office setting
  - Sensitivity, 40–89% and specificity, 61–95%
- Screen for STIs if indicated:
  - HIV
  - Chlamydia
  - Gonorrhea
  - Trichomonas
  - Syphilis
  - Hepatitis B and C

ALERT
- Samples for pH, microscopy, DNA probe, and culture should be obtained from the posterior fornix or vaginal wall.
- Obtaining a sample from cervical os may reveal normal cervical mucous.

Diagnostic Procedures/Surgery
- Light microscopy
  - Normal saline wet preparation slide
    - Place thin layer of discharge on glass slide
    - Add one drop of normal saline to slide
  - Findings
    - Presence of clue cells
    - Absence of lactobacilli
    - Few white blood cells

DIFFERENTIAL DIAGNOSIS
- Atrophic vaginitis
- Trichomoniasis
- Candidal vulvovaginitis

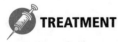 # TREATMENT

ALERT
- Treatment of asymptomatic women is not always necessary.
- However, complications can occur in patients with untreated BV, particularly
  - Pregnant women
  - Women undergoing gynecologic procedures and/or surgeries
  - Women at risk for sexually transmitted infections (STIs)

GENERAL MEASURES
Activity
- Avoid douching/heavy soap use

Complementary and Alternative Therapies
- Lactobacillus suppositories and oral lactobacillus may resolve symptoms briefly, but are associated with high rates of recurrence.

- A small crossover study of 46 women demonstrated that oral yogurt with live *lactobacillus acidophilus* cultures was associated with a reduction of episodes of BV.
- Twice daily yogurt douches × 7 days has been shown to be an effective treatment in a study of 84 pregnant women.

 # MEDICATION (DRUGS)

First Line
- Metronidazole 500 mg PO b.i.d. × 7 days
  - Avoid in the first trimester of pregnancy as possible teratogenicity

Second Line
- Metronidazole gel 0.75%
  - 5 g intravaginally per day × 5 days
- Clindamycin cream 2%
  - 5 g intravaginally q.h.s. × 7 days
- Clindamycin PO 300 mg PO b.i.d. × 7 days
- Metronidazole 2 g PO × 1 dose
  - Higher rate of recurrence associated with single dose regimen versus 7-day regimen
- Clindamycin ovules
  - 100 g intravaginally q.h.s. × 3 days

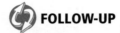 # FOLLOW-UP

DISPOSITION
- Cure rate with first line medication ranges from 84–96% versus 75–94% with second line regimens

Admission Criteria
- Treatment is primarily outpatient

Issues for Referral
- Consider referral to obstetrician/gynecologist if no resolution of symptoms after treatment

COMPLICATIONS
- Untreated BV is associated with higher risks of the following:
  - Transmission of HIV and other STIs
  - Complications in pregnancy (see below)
  - Complications in patients undergoing gynecologic procedures or surgeries
    - Vaginal cuff cellulitis
    - Pelvic inflammatory disease
    - Endometritis
- Recurrence
  - Occurs in approximately 30% within first 3 months after treatment
  - More common with single dose Metronidazole
  - Unclear if recurrence occurs secondary to
    - Failure to restore balance of normal flora because of organisms resistant to current antibiotic regimens
    - Failure to treat an unidentified pathogen
    - Reinfection from untreated partners
    - Hygiene practices that disrupt the balance of normal flora
    - OR a combination of these factors
  - Regimens
    - Treatment with metronidazole 500 mg PO b.i.d. × 10–14 days
    - Consider suppression with metronidazole 0.75% vaginal gel × 10 days then biweekly × 4–6 months

Pregnancy Considerations
- In pregnancy, BV has been associated with the following:
  - Preterm delivery

– Preterm labor
– Premature rupture of membranes
– Spontaneous abortion
• The U.S. Preventive Services Task Force (USPSTF) Recommendations:
  – Treatment of symptomatic pregnant women is appropriate.
    • Avoid oral metronidazole treatment in the first trimester of pregnancy.
    • Topical or single-dose oral antibiotic regimens are not recommended as they may not reduce the risk of pregnancy complications.
  – Treatment of asymptomatic pregnant women
    • May not improve pregnancy outcomes
    • Therefore, USPSTF recommends against routine screening of average-risk asymptomatic pregnant women.
  – High-risk pregnant women
    • High-risk usually defined as prior preterm delivery
    • Screening is an option, but USPSTF does not recommend for or against routine screening given insufficient evidence.

PATIENT MONITORING
Consider screening for STIs.

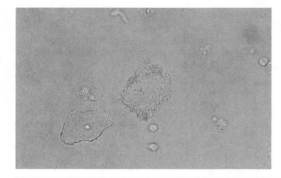

Figure 1 Absence of lactobacilli and clue cells:obliteration of sharp borders of squamous cells secondary to studding of bacteria to cell membrane.

REFERENCES

1. Bradshaw CS, Morton AN, Garland SM, et al. Higher-risk behavioral practices associated with bacterial vaginosis compared with vaginal candidiasis. *Obstet Gynecol*. 2005;106:105–114.
2. Gutman R, Peipert JF, Weitzen S, et al. Evaluation of clinical methods for diagnosing bacterial vaginosis. *Obstet Gynecol*. 2005;105:551–556.
3. Owen MK, Clenney TL. Management of vaginitis. *Am Fam Physician*. 2004;70:2125–2132.
4. US Preventive Task Forces. Screening for bacterial vaginosis: recommendations and rationale. *Am J Prev Med*. 2001;20:59–61.
5. Van Kessel K, Assefi N, Marrazzo J, et al. Common complementary and alternative therapies for yeast vaginitis and bacterial vaginosis: a systematic review. *Obstetrical and Gynecological Survey* 2003;58:351–358.

ADDITIONAL READING

Alfonsi GA, Shlay JC, Parker S. What is the best approach for managing recurrent bacterial vaginosis? *J Fam Pract*. 2004;53:650–652.
Neri A, Sabah G, Samra Z. Bacterial vaginosis in pregnancy treated with yoghurt. *Acta Obstet Gynecol Scand*. 1993;72(1):17–19.
Shalev E, Battino S, Weiner E, et al. Ingestion of yogurt containing Lactobacillus acidophilus compared with pasteurized yogurt as prophylaxis for recurrent candidal vagintis and bacterial vaginosis. *Arch Fam Med*. 1996;5:593–596.

CODES
ICD9-CM
• Bacterial Vaginosis
• 616.1 Vaginitis and vulvovaginitis
• 623.5 Vaginal discharge NOS

KEY WORDS
• Vaginal Discharge
• Vaginal Itching
• Bacterial Vaginosis
• Gardnerella Vaginalis

BARTHOLIN'S CYST

Sudeep K. Aulakh, MD
Michael P. Plevyak, MD

KEY CLINICAL POINTS

- Common problem in women of reproductive age
- Symptomatic cysts should be treated with surgical intervention.
  - Infection of a cyst can cause a gland abscess.
  - An abscess should be considered in a painful, rapidly growing cyst.
- A vulvar mass in peri- or postmenopausal women should be evaluated for malignancy.

 BASICS

DESCRIPTION

- Bartholin glands (0.5 cm size) are located bilaterally in the base of the labia minora and drain through 2.5 cm long ducts into the vestibule at approximately the 4 o'clock and 8 o'clock positions. They provide moisture for the vestibule but are not required for sexual lubrication.
- Occlusion of the duct opening can lead to cyst formation.
  - Most cysts are small (1–3 cm) and asymptomatic.
- Infection of a cyst can lead to abscess formation.
  - Most abscesses will rupture spontaneously in 3–5 days.

EPIDEMIOLOGY

- About 2% of women develop a cyst or abscess.
- Most common in women 20–29 years of age

RISK FACTORS

- Prior history of cysts or abscesses
- Sexually transmitted diseases (STD)
- Trauma
- Nulliparity
- White and black women are at higher risk for cyst formation than Hispanic women.

PATHOPHYSIOLOGY

- Inflammation (infection and trauma) may cause occlusion of the distal duct.
  - Congenital narrowing of the duct and thick mucous may contribute to ductal obstruction.
- The obstruction results in retention of secretions leading to dilatation of the duct and formation of a cyst.
- Cysts can get infected, resulting in a gland abscess. The infection is usually polymicrobial, but STDs (Neisseria gonorrhoeae, Chlamydia trachomatis) should always be considered.

ASSOCIATED CONDITIONS

- STD (Neisseria gonorrhoeae, Chlamydia trachomatis) possible

 DIAGNOSIS

SIGNS AND SYMPTOMS

- Cyst
  - Asymptomatic or vulvar discomfort in the medial labia majora or lower vestibule
  - Discomfort aggravated by sitting, walking and sexual intercourse
- Abscess
  - Painful vulvar mass
  - Often rapid growth

  - Pain aggravated by sitting, walking and sexual intercourse
  - Fever is rare

History

- Age
- Prior history of STD
- Prior history of Bartholin's cyst or abscess

Physical Exam

Cyst
- Soft, painless mass in the medial labia majora or lower vestibule

Abscess
- Tender mass in medial labia majora or lower vestibule
- Edema and erythema may be present.
- May have surrounding cellulitis
- Fever is rare

TESTS

- Cysts are usually sterile.
- Abscesses are often polymicrobial.

Lab

Abscess secretions should be cultured for:
- Neisseria gonorrhoeae, Chlamydia trachomatis
- Anaerobes and aerobes

DIFFERENTIAL DIAGNOSIS

- Epidermal inclusion or sebaceous cyst
- Vestibular mucous cyst
- Gartner's duct cyst
- Skene's duct cyst
- Cyst of the canal of Nuck
- Fibroma
- Lipoma
- Hernia
- Neurofibroma
- Leiomyoma
- Hidradenoma
- Bartholin's gland malignancy (rare)

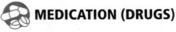 **TREATMENT**

- Asymptomatic cyst
  - <40 years old do not require therapy
  - Peri- and postmenopausal women require biopsy to rule out cancer.
- Symptomatic cysts require drainage.
- All solid nodules should be biopsied to rule out malignancy.

GENERAL MEASURES

Sitz baths (warm water soaks) if:
- Early abscess to help the abscess form a point
- Spontaneous rupture of a cyst or abscess to provide relief and promote drainage

MEDICATION (DRUGS)

- Pain control
- Broad spectrum antibiotics if cellulitis is present
  - Cefriaxone 125 mg IM or cefixime 400 mg PO (one dose) and clindamycin 300 mg q.i.d. (7 days)

– If cultures are positive for Chlamydia trachomatis, add azithromycin 1 g (one dose).

ALERT

Diabetic patients should be followed closely due to the risk of necrotizing infections.

SURGERY

- Indicated for all symptomatic lesions
- Establishing a drainage path is essential to prevent recurrence.

Office Based Procedures

- Incision and drainage alone (not recommended due to high recurrence)
- Word catheter (inflatable bulb tipped catheter) placement
  – Put it into the cyst after incision and drainage. The bulb is inflated and left in place for 2–4 weeks to allow formation of an epithelialized tract for drainage of glandular secretions.
- Marsupialization should be delayed if infection is present.
  – Elliptical incision with removal of 1–2 cm oval portion of the vulvar roof
  – The cyst wall is everted and sewn with interrupted sutures to the vestibular mucosa.
  – Usually used after Word catheter has failed
- Silver nitrate
  – After incision and drainage, a crystalloid silver nitrate stick is put in cyst. After 48 hours, necrotized tissue and remaining silver nitrate particles are removed.
  – Mild burning may occur.

ALERT

- Biopsy all solid nodules and all lesions in women >40 years old.

Day Surgery

- Excisional biopsy of the gland (often a difficult procedure with high morbidity):
  – If conservative therapy repeatedly fails
  – In perimenopausal and menopausal women to rule out cancer if biopsy not definitive
- CO_2 laser
  – Incision and drainage followed by vaporization of glandular capsule

FOLLOW-UP

Issues for Referral

- Gland excision required
- Biopsy suggestive of cancer

PROGNOSIS

- Recurrent infections resulting in cystic dilatation of the duct are likely unless a permanent opening for drainage is established
  – Ductal cysts recurrence rate after marsupialization: 5–10%
  – Failure rate with incision and drainage: 13%

COMPLICATIONS

- Hemorrhage and hematoma
- Infection
- Scarring
- Dyspareunia

REFERENCES

1. Omole F, Simmons BJ, Hacker Y. Management of Bartholin's duct cyst and gland abscess. *Am Fam Physician.* 2003;68:135–140.
2. Kaufman RK. Cystic tumors. In: Kaufman RK, Faro S, Brown D, eds. *Benign Diseases of the Vulva and Vagina.* 5th ed. Philadelphia: Elsevier Mosby; 2005:216–256.
3. Droegemueller W. Infections of the lower genital tract. In: Stenchever MA, Droegemueller W, Herbst AL, Mishell DR, eds. *Comprehensive Gynecology.* 4th ed. St. Louis: Mosby; 2001:641–706.
4. Eilber KS, Raz S. Benign cystic lesions of the vagina: a literature review. *J Urology.* 2003;170:717–722.
5. Penna C, Fambrini M, Fallani MG. CO(2) Laser Treatment for Bartholin's Gland Cyst. *Int J Gynaecol Obstet.* 2002;76:79–80.

CODES

ICD9-CM

- 616.2 Bartholin's gland or duct cyst
- 616.3 Bartholin's gland abscess

KEY WORDS

- Vulvar Mass
- Vulvar Pain
- Dysparenuia
- Bartholin's Gland

BREAST CANCER

Jennifer S. Gass, MD, FACS

KEY CLINICAL POINTS

- Annual mammographic screening of women over 40 is the single most effective tool in reducing breast cancer mortality.
- Patients who are appropriate candidates for Breast Conserving Therapy (BCT) do not compromise their survival.
- Sentinel node biopsy is an effective tool for staging the axilla.
- Neoadjuvant chemotherapy can enhance chances for BCT and lend insight to prognosis.

 BASICS

DESCRIPTION
- Most common noncutaneous cancer in women.
- Leading cause of death in women between the ages of 30–70.
- Invasive ductal carcinoma is the most common histologic type.

GENERAL PREVENTION
- Tamoxifen reduced the incidence of breast cancer by 49% in a NSABP P-1 Trial.
- Prophylactic mastectomy effectively reduces the risk of breast cancer by >90%.

EPIDEMIOLOGY
- Average age: 61
- Most common in North American females
- Asian immigrant's risk approaches American counterparts in two generations

Incidence
- Lifetime risk is 1 in 8.
- Caucasian American women rate per year: 115/100,000
- Native American < Hispanic < Asian< African American; 50 to 101/100,000 in racial subgroups

RISK FACTORS
Mild RR <3.0
- Early onset menarche <12
- Late menopause >55
- Nulliparity
- Delayed first pregnancy after 30
- Excessive alcohol consumption, >20 g/day particularly in postmenopausal women on HRT
- Prolonged use of HRT, especially combined estrogen and progestin
- Smoking, particularly premenopausal
- Increased bone mineral density

Moderate RR 3 to 10
- Family history, particularly 2 first degree relatives
- Personal history of breast cancer
- History of mantle irradiation for Hodgkin's disease
- History of Atypical Hyperplasia, or LCIS

High RR >10
- BRCA1/2 mutation
- Atypical Ductal Hyperplasia (ADH)/Atypical Lobular Hyperplasia (ALH) or Lobular Carcinoma In Situ (LCIS) and family history

No demonstrated risk
- Breast implants
- AIDS
- Environmental exposures to PCB/organotoxins
- Electromagnetic fields
- Abortion

- Low dose OCP

Protective
- Breast feeding >12 months
- Increased parity
- Preeclampsia
- Physical activity

Genetics
- Genetic syndromes account for 5–10% of breast cancer
- BRCA1 and 2 mutations (80% of genetic breast cancer) confer a lifetime risk of 44–78% and 31–56%, respectively. This mutation also carries a 25–49% lifetime risk for ovarian cancer.

  – While the prevalence of BRCA1 in the general population is 0.06%, in the Ashkenazi Jewish (AJ) population, the prevalence is 1–2%.
  – Early onset breast cancer in all women has a risk of 3–13% of BRCA1/2 positivity. And 30% for those of AJ heritage
  – Among mutation carriers, only 45% have family history of breast cancer.

- Cowden's Syndrome, Li-Fraumeni Syndrome, Ataxia-telangiectasia, and Peutz-Jeghers syndrome, CHEK2 mutation account for the remaining 20%
- A family history of bilateral breast, breast and ovary, lymphoma, prostate, melanoma, colon, pancreatic, and stomach cancer suggests the risk of a genetic mutation.
- Families with small sib ships or mutations passed through the paternal lineage can mask significant family histories.

PATHOPHYSIOLOGY
- A proposed paradigm describes proliferatory stimuli inciting progressive changes from normalcy to ductal hyperplasia to atypical hyperplasia to ductal carcinoma in situ and then to invasive carcinoma.
- The exact determinants of the timing and progression remain undefined.

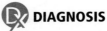 **DIAGNOSIS**

SIGNS AND SYMPTOMS
Major differences between screen-detected cancer and an interval cancer, one detected between screening, or one detected before screening begins

Cancers detected on screening are by definition asymptomatic. Interval cancers are detected in between screenings and, therefore, symptomatic almost a priori.

History
- Painless persistent breast mass
- Unilateral new nipple inversion, rash, discharge
- Nonresolving breast cellulitis
- Screen for signs of systemic disease
- Family history of breast and ovary cancer
- Ethnicity: Ashkenazi Jewish, Icelandic, Norwegian, Swedish

Physical Exam
- Painless breast mass
- Fixation relative to skin/chest wall
- Peri-areolar rash, spontaneous nipple discharge, nipple inversion
- Regional nodal adenopathy
- Altered breath sounds, dullness to percussion
- Hepatomegaly, advanced disease

TESTS
- CBC, liver function tests

Imaging
- Mammogram and Ultrasound for palpable masses
  - Spiculated density on mammography
  - Irregular hypoechoic lesion on ultrasound
- Microcalcifications: clustered, pleomorphic or casting
- Breast MRI in the face of a negative mammogram/ultrasound especially when index of suspicion is high (i.e., pathologic nipple inversion or nonresolving cellulites).

Diagnostic Procedures/Surgery
- Core needle biopsy
- Rarely needle localization surgical biopsy is indicated for lesions unapproachable by stereotaxis.
- Skin punch biopsy for cellulitic changes, or rash

Pathological Findings
- Infiltrating ductal carcinoma 80% to 90%, which is characterized by a sclerotic mass forming lesion
- Other subtypes of invasive cancer: Lobular, tubular, medullary, mucinous squamous
- Infiltrating lobular can be radiographically occult.
- Malignant cystsarcoma phyllodes represents a sarcomatous form of breast malignancy
- Pure ductal carcinoma in situ is noninvasive.
- Lobular carcinoma in situ is a histologic finding indicating increased risk of cancer in either breast more than a true precursor lesion.

DIFFERENTIAL DIAGNOSIS
- Radial scar
- Sclerosing adenosis
- Fibroadenoma
- Lymphoma

 TREATMENT

Radiotherapy
- Whole breast external beam radiotherapy delivered over 5–6 weeks reduces the risk of local recurrence when paired with BCT for invasive and in situ disease.
- Lower risk patients may be eligible for partial breast radiation delivered in shorter intervals or for close observation without radiotherapy.
- Postmastectomy radiotherapy reduces local recurrence in high-risk patients (multiple nodes or larger sized lesions).

Physical Therapy
A combination of massage and compression garments is effective is controlling lymphedema.

Complementary and Alternative Therapies
Support groups have been the mainstay of complementary therapy. The role of acupuncture, Reiki therapy, and other avenues enhancing the mind-body connection continue to be explored. **Particular interest in the ramifications of postchemotherapy cognitive disorders as well as sexuality issues.**

 MEDICATION (DRUGS)

Neoadjuvant chemo
- Skin/chest wall fixation, satellitosis, cellulitis, or tumor size prohibiting BCT

- No survival advantage but tumor response to chemo segregates subgroups in terms of survival, (NSABP 18, 27)

First Line
- Adriamycin and Cytoxan (A/C) are the mainstay of therapy. Node + and high-risk node negative may also receive taxane therapy to reduce risk of distant recurrence.
- CALGB 49909 showed the value of Herceptin for Her 2 neu positive cancers.
- Five years of endocrine therapy is recommended for all ER+ cancers.
  - Premenopausal: tamoxifen
  - Post: aromatase inhibitor or tamoxifen

Second Line
Adjuvant
- CMF remains reasonable therapy in node negative, Her 2 neucancers

SURGERY
Breast Conservation Therapy
- A lumpectomy, quandrantectomy, partial mastectomy, or wide local excision describes a technique of achieving a tumor free margin around the index lesion.
- Multicentric disease is a nearly certain contraindication to BCT.
- Multifocal disease requires a greater volume of tissue removal, but still may afford BCT.
Axillary surgery
- Sentinel node biopsy, a technique of labeling the "gatekeeper" node has virtually replaced axillary dissection in the clinically negative axilla.
- The technique involves injection of either/or both technetium 99 and a blue vital dye injection. These agents are then tracked to the axilla using direct visualization or a hand held gamma probe.
- At excision, when the sentinel node is suspicious, an intraoperative touch prep is performed and, if positive, axillary dissection is completed.
- If the sentinel node is negative, the chance that there is a residual positive node in the axilla is <5%.
- When the sentinel node is positive, it is the only positive node in 50% of patients.
- Completion axillary dissection is the standard of care for all node positive patients.

Mastectomy
- Mastectomy is indicated for large primary tumors that are ineligible for neoadjuvant chemo therapy and also for multicentric disease, or for patients ineligible for post lumpectomy radiotherapy.
- Skin sparing mastectomy has been shown to be safe, effective and with low risk of local recurrence. This technique affords particularly extraordinary cosmetic results.
- Immediate reconstruction can be offered to all mastectomy candidates. However, patients clearly needing postmastectomy radiotherapy should considered delayed reconstruction to achieve most secure cosmetic results.
- Mastectomy can be paired with either sentinel node biopsy or axillary dissection.

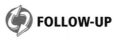 **FOLLOW-UP**

Once patients have completed their therapy, they should be seen every 3 months for the first year as long as they remain asymptomatic. A new baseline mammogram is obtained at 6 months postoperatively in the affected breast, and then annual mammography resumes.

There is no data suggesting a survival advantage for follow up screening with any other modalities such as bone scan, CT scan, or tumor markers in the absence of prior documented lesions or new patient symptoms.

DISPOSITION

Admission Criteria

- BCT can be performed as outpatient surgery.
- BCT and axillary dissection may require overnight observation.
- Mastectomy and nodal surgery is federally mandated to have access to 2 postoperative hospital days.
- Complications of chemotherapy can cause admission—most commonly febrile neutropenia.

PROGNOSIS

- The prognosis is best determined by the stage. Patients with maximally treated Stage I cancers have a 90% survival rate.
- Patients achieving a pathologic complete response to neoadjuvant chemotherapy have an improved survival beyond that indicated by their stage at diagnosis.

COMPLICATIONS

- The majority of local recurrences will occur within the first 2 years.
- Most systemic recurrences occur within the first 5 years; however, now with extended endocrine therapy further late recurrences may occur.

REFERENCES

1. Cady B, Chung M. Mammographic screening: No longer controversial. *Am J Clin Oncol*. 2005;28:1–4.
2. Malone KE, Daling JR, Thompson JD, et al. BRCA1 mutations and breast cancer in the general population: Analyses in women before age 35 years and in women before age 45 years with first-degree family history. *JAMA*. 1998;279:922–929.
3. Hartmann LC, Schaid DJ, Woods JE, et al. Efficacy of bilateral prophylactic mastectomy in women with a family history of breast cancer. *N Engl J Med*. 1999;340:77–84.
4. Fisher B, Costantino JP, Wickerham DL, et al. Tamoxifen for prevention of breast cancer: Report of the National Surgical Adjuvant Breast and Bowel Project P-1 Study. *J Natl Cancer Inst*. 1998;90:1371–1388.
5. Hughes KS, Schnaper LA, Berry D, et al. Lumpectomy plus tamoxifen with or without radiation in women 70 years of age or older with early breast cancer. *N Engl J Med*. 2004;3;351:963–970.

ADDITIONAL READING

Singletary SE, Robb GL, Hortobagyi GH, eds. *Advanced Therapy of Breast Disease*. 2nd ed. Ontario: BC Decker Inc; 2004.

CODES

ICD9-CM

- 174.9 Breast cancer
- 233.0 DCIS
- 793.0 Abnormal mammogram
- V16.3 Family history breast cancer
- V10.3 Personal history breast cancer

KEY WORDS

- Breast Mass
- BRCA 1/2
- Ovarian Cancer

BREAST DISCHARGE

Courtney A. Clark, MD
Susannah S. Wise, MD, FACS

KEY CLINICAL POINTS
- Rarely associated with malignancy
- High index of suspicion if:
  - Unilateral, unprovoked, from a single duct
  - Serous, serosanguinous, bloody
- Galactorrhea is always bilateral.

BASICS

DESCRIPTION
- There are many variations of breast discharge including:
  - Color of discharge: clear, white, gray, brown, yellow, green, red
  - Provoked (i.e., with nipple stimulation) vs. spontaneous
  - Unilateral vs. bilateral
- Rarely a sign of malignancy
- Concern regarding malignancy if discharge occurs without provocation, is persistent, and unilateral
- Consider a malignancy when the colors of the discharge are serous, serosanguinous, and bloody.
- The older the woman, the greater the likelihood that the breast discharge may be related to a malignancy.
- Intraductal papilloma, which has no risk for developing into an invasive cancer, is the most common cause of bloody nipple discharge.
- Malignancies may be associated with breast discharge, most commonly, ductal carcinoma in situ.
- Galactorrhea is bilateral milk production occurring in a nonlactating woman.

EPIDEMIOLOGY
Incidence
- Discharge is a common complaint from women of all ages; 10–15% of the women with benign breast disease experience breast discharge.
- Only 5–15% of patients with breast discharge have cancer.

RISK FACTORS
- Smoking
- Genetics

PATHOPHYSIOLOGY
Varies depending on etiology of the breast discharge
- A trigger to the pituitary gland (i.e., from nipple stimulation or certain medications) causes the release of prolactin, which may induce nipple discharge.
- Malignant invasion of the duct lining can cause bloody discharge, as can an intraductal papilloma.
- Most bilateral discharge from multiple ducts that comes only with manipulation is a normal physiologic response.

ETIOLOGY
- Causes of galactorrhea include pituitary tumor, thyroid dysfunction, and chronic renal failure.
- Several medications can cause galactorrhea.
  - Tranquilizers (i.e., thorazine)
  - Birth control pills
  - Antihypertensives (i.e., Methyldopate HCl)
  - Illicit drugs (i.e., marijuana)

ASSOCIATED CONDITIONS
- Pregnancy
- Prolactinoma
- Thyroid disease
- Renal failure

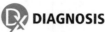

DIAGNOSIS

SIGNS AND SYMPTOMS
History
- Practitioners should obtain a through history including, timing and quality of the breast discharge and if occurring from one or both breasts. History regarding the location of the draining duct or ducts should be obtained.
- Relationship to menstrual cycle, menopause, or of starting a new medication
- Symptoms of thyroid disease

Physical Exam
- Clinical breast exam
- Evaluation of the breast discharge
- Increased suspicion for malignancy if breast discharge is associated with a mass or lump

TESTS
Lab
- Pregnancy test
- Lab tests to check for galactorrhea include prolactin level and thyroid function tests.
- Evaluation of breast discharge includes cytology, immunology (i.e., carcinoembryonic antigen-CEA), and occult blood testing (likely to be done by a breast specialist after referral).

Imaging
- Mammography and ultrasound should be done initially as the first radiological studies.
- Galactography: to visualize a space occupying lesion by inserting dye into a single breast duct
- MR Galactography
- Fiber-ductoscopy
- Duct injection mammography

Diagnostic Procedures/Surgery
- Duct lavage for cytology
- Exploration and/or removal of breast ducts
- Breast biopsy
- Excision of a prolactinoma if there is a pituitary adenoma

Pathologic Findings
- Cytological findings of atypia or malignancy
- Occult Blood (via Hemoccult Testing)

DIFFERENTIAL DIAGNOSIS
- Thrombophlebitis
- Infection
- Fat necrosis

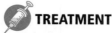

TREATMENT

GENERAL MEASURES
- The majority of patients with breast discharge require no further treatment outside of reassurance.

- Anyone with possible pathologic discharge (unilateral, single duct, spontaneous, and persistent discharge) should have a complete evaluation and likely will need a central duct excision and biopsy of the region of concern.
- Treatment of the underlying condition (i.e., prolactinoma) when indicated

 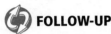

MEDICATION (DRUGS)

Medication for galactorrhea caused by a hyperprolactin state is the dopamine agonist, bromocriptine.

FOLLOW-UP

DISPOSITION
Issues for Referral
Refer all patients with discharge suspicious for malignancy (i.e., unilateral and spontaneous) to a breast surgeon.

PROGNOSIS
- Excellent if not related to malignancy
- Removal of an intraductal papilloma is curative.

REFERENCES

1. Cabioglu N, Hunt K, Singletary SE, et al. Surgical decision making and factors determining a diagnosis of breast carcinoma in women presenting with nipple discharge. *J Am Coll Surg*. 2003;196:354–364.
2. Orel S, Dougherty C, Reynolds C, et al. MR imaging in patients with nipple discharge: Initial experience. *Radiology*. 2000;216:248–254.
3. Hou M, Tsai K, Ou-Yang F, et al. Is a one-step operation for breast cancer patients presenting nipple discharge without palpable mass feasible. *The Breast*. 2002;11:402–407.
4. Leung A, Pacaud D. Diagnosis and management of galactorrhea. *Am Fam Physician*. 2004;70:543–550, 553–554.
5. Love S. *Dr. Susan Love's Breast Book*. 3rd ed. Cambridge: Perseus Publishing; 2000.
6. Okazaki A, Hirata K, Okazaki M, et al. Nipple discharge disorders: Current diagnostic management and the role of fiber-ductoscopy. *Eur Radiol*. 1999;9:583–590.
7. Santen R, Mansel R. Current concepts: Benign breast disorders. *N Engl J Med*. 2005;353:275–285.
8. Stoppard M. *The Breast Book*. New York: DK Publishing; 1996.

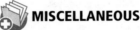

MISCELLANEOUS

CODES
ICD9-CM
- 611.79 Nipple Discharge
- 676.6 Galactorrhea

KEY WORDS

- Nipple Discharge
- Galactorrhea
- Galactography

BREAST MASS

Jennifer S. Gass, MD, FACS

KEY CLINICAL POINTS

- A dominant breast mass requires an ultrasound and a mammogram.
- A solid breast mass can be diagnosed definitively by ultrasound guided core biopsy.
- Cystic lesions must resolve completely with aspiration or further diagnostic intervention is required.

 ## BASICS

DESCRIPTION

- Breast masses are delineated into four categories: acute abscesses, benign physiologic masses, benign tumors, and cancer.
- Benign masses include cysts, galactoceles, papillomas, fibroadenomas, phyllodes tumor, and fibrocystic nodules.
- Cancerous masses are painless dominant masses that persist.

RISK FACTORS

- Breast abscess
  - Breast-feeding
  - Smoking
- Galactoceles
  - Pregnancy and postpartum
- Fibroadenoma, papilloma, phylodes tumor, and fibrocystic nodules
  - No defined risk factors
- Cancer
  - See Breast Cancer chapter

PATHOPHYSIOLOGY

- Breast Abscess
  - Peripartum
    - Milk stasis
    - Staphylococcus aureus
  - Nonperipartum
    - Squamous metaplasia and chronic fibrosis
- Galactocele
  - Termination of lactation

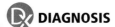 ## DIAGNOSIS

SIGNS AND SYMPTOMS

- Breast Abscess
  - Painful mass
  - Fever
  - Swelling
- Galactocele
  - Mass during or after lactation
- Fibroadenoma and benign tumors
  - Usually noncyclic painless mass
- Fibrocystic Nodules
  - Tender nodules that wax and wane with menstrual cycle
  - Pruritic pain radiating to axilla
- Papilloma
  - Bloody nipple discharge

History

- Last menstrual cycle
- Relationship to menses
- Tenderness
- Response to NSAIDs
- Termination of lactation
- Smoking
- Family history of cancer

Physical Exam

- An erythema, edema, and a tender dominant mass favor breast abscess.
- A tender mass without erythema and edema favors a fibrocystic nodule or cyst.
- A discreet mobile nontender nodule favors a benign tumor (i.e., fibroadenoma).

TESTS

Imaging

- Ultrasound for all ages
- Mammogram for patients over 30 or at an age 10 years younger than the age at which a first degree relative developed breast cancer
- MRI for dense breasts where the clinical suspicion for cancer is high

Diagnostic Procedures/Surgery

- Ultrasound guided core needle biopsy for solid masses
- Ultrasound guided aspiration for fluid filled masses if not a simple cyst
- Incision and drainage for breast abscesses

Pathologic Findings

- Pathologic evaluation of a core needle biopsy effectively diagnoses the underlying lesion.
- Cytologic evaluation of an FNA for a solid mass is less accurate, and cytologic evaluation of benign cyst contents is often misleading.

ALERT

If pathologic findings and imaging or physical exam are nonconcordant, then a definitive biopsy is needed.

DIFFERENTIAL DIAGNOSIS

The diagnoses discussed represent the most common differential diagnosis.

GENERAL MEASURES

The most important intervention is an accurate diagnosis.

Diet

Cysts: Avoidance of products with methylxanthines has been shown to decrease mastalgia and the fibrocystic masses and gross cysts associated with the process.

Nursing

For galactoceles and postpartum breast abscess maintenance of nursing is recommended.

Complementary and Alternative Therapies

- Use of evening primrose oil (gamma linolenic acid) has been shown to have a clinically useful response rate of 58% at 3 g/day per package recommendations for cyclic mastalgia.
- Adverse symptoms of mild GI upset in <2% of patients

 ## MEDICATION (DRUGS)

Tamoxifen at 10 mg per day has been used in refractory mastalgia.

SURGERY

Indications for surgery

- Cystosarcoma phyllodes
  - Surgical excision required to define benignity
- Fibroadenoma, papilloma, hamartoma, lipoma
  - Surgical excision for symptoms or enlargement
- Breast Abscess
  - Surgical I&D for treatment
- Fibrocystic nodules and galactoceles
  - Surgical excision not recommended unless there is a concern for missed malignancy
- Lack of concordance between exam and core biopsy

 FOLLOW-UP

Fibroadenomas, papillomas, and hamartomas require 6-month follow up imaging with mammogram and ultrasound to document stability at a 6 month interval for 1–2 years.

Admission Criteria

Nonresolving breast cellulitis may require inpatient therapy with IV antibiotics.

Issues for Referral

- Nonresolving breast cellulitis
- Persistent mass
- Lack of concordance between core biopsy and exam
- Any mass with chest wall/skin fixation
- Recurrent breast abscess

PROGNOSIS

- Fibroadenoma
  - The risk of a recurrence is minimal with adequate excision.
  - For nonexcised lesion
    - About 50% will disappear in 5 years
    - In postmenopausal women, they should be stable or diminish in size.

ALERT

- If a fibroadenoma in a postmenopausal woman enlarges, it should be removed.
- Hamartoma, lipomas, and papillomas have an excellent prognosis with or without excision.
- A breast abscess definitively treated is unlikely to recur.
- Galactoceles usually resolve without surgical intervention.
- Cysts seen on mammography will regress, more than one-half by the first year and more than two-thirds by the second year, leaving only 12% after 5 years.

COMPLICATIONS

Error in diagnosis is the major complication and can be avoided by a core biopsy and concordance evaluation.

REFERENCES

1. Hindle WH, Arais RD, Florentine B, et al. Lack of utility in clinical practice of cytologic examination of nonbloody cyst fluid from palpable breast cysts. *Am J Obstet Gynecol*. 2000;182:1300–1305.
2. Cowen PN, Benson EA. Cytological study of fluid from breast cysts. *Br J Surg*. 1979;66:209–211.
3. Santeen RJ, Mansel R. Benign breast disorders. *N Engl J Med*. 2005;353:275–285.
4. Brenner RJ, Bein ME, Sarti DA, et al. Spontaneous regression of interval benign cysts of the breast. *Radiology*. 1994;193:365–368.
5. Cant PJ, Madden MV, Coleman MG, et al. Non-operative management of breast masses diagnosed as fibroadenoma. *Br J Surg*. 1995;82:792–794.

ADDITIONAL READING

Singletary SE, Robb GL, Hortobagyi GH, eds. *Advanced Therapy of Breast Disease*. 2nd ed. Ontario: BC Decker Inc; 2004.

CODES

ICD9-CM

- 611.72 Breast mass
- 611.79 Nipple inversion,discharge
- 217 Benign neoplasm of breast
- 238.3 Neoplasm of breast, uncertain
- 611.0 Breast abscess
- 610.0 Breast cyst
- 611.5 Galactocele
- 217 Fibroadenoma
- 214 Lipoma

KEY WORDS

- Breast Mass
- Fibroadenoma
- Breast Cyst
- Hamartoma
- Papilloma
- Galactoceles
- Breast Abscess

BREAST-FEEDING

Julie S. Taylor, MD, MSc

KEY CLINICAL POINTS

- Breast-feeding has numerous short- and long-term benefits for both mothers and children.
- Current recommendations are exclusive breast-feeding for 6 months followed by breast milk for at least 1 year as solid foods are gradually introduced.
- Physician counseling to promote breast-feeding as the optimal form of infant nutrition should begin early in prenatal care, if not before, and occur frequently.

 BASICS

DESCRIPTION
- Feeding a child human milk either directly from a lactating breast or milk that has been expressed.
- Exclusive breast-feeding means that a child receives nothing other than breast milk for nutrition.

EPIDEMIOLOGY
- Nadir in 1971: 25% of women initiated breast-feeding.
- Peak in 2002: 70% of women initiated breast-feeding.
- In 2003,
  - 66% of women initiated breast-feeding
  - 33% were breast-feeding at 6 months
  - 19% were breast-feeding at 1 year

FACTORS ASSOCIATED WITH AN INCREASED LIKELIHOOD OF BREAST-FEEDING
- Caucasian ≥ Hispanic > African-American
- Older age
- Being married
- Higher socioeconomic status
- More years of education
- Intended pregnancy
- Vaginal delivery
- Healthy mother (e.g., no diabetes)
- Healthy baby (e.g., not premature)
- Support from the father of the baby and the family
- Support from the medical community
- Support from the employer

PHYSIOLOGY
- Based primarily on supply and demand. Initial feed should be within the first 1 hour of life followed by feeds on demand 8–12 times every 24 hours.
- Initially colostrum is produced. Milk comes in after 2–5 days. Often it takes a full month to get a milk supply well established.

MATERNAL BENEFITS*
Immediate
- Faster return to prepregnancy weight
- Less postpartum bleeding
Long-term
- Lower rates of premenopausal breast cancer, ovarian cancer, and endometrial cancer
- Improved bone density/lower fracture rates
General
- Bonding
- Cost (savings of up to $4,000/year in formula, fewer doctors visits, less time away from work for parents)
- Ease (no bottles to wash or warm unless pumping)

PEDIATRIC BENEFITS*
- Immunity
  - Lower rates of multiple different infections, especially colds, ear infections, and gastroenteritis
- Lower rates of chronic diseases
  - Type I diabetes
  - Allergies
  - Eczema
  - Obesity
- Increased IQ scores later in life
- Lower rates of sudden infant death syndrome (SIDS)
  *Many benefits are dose-related.

 TREATMENT

COMPLICATIONS
- Especially important to monitor in the first few days to weeks postpartum.

ALERT
None of these conditions are reasons to stop breast-feeding!
- **Latch/Sore Nipples**
  - Normally breast-feeding does NOT hurt.
  - If it does, something is not right.
  - Observe a feed. Watch for the following:
    - Position of the baby
    - Size and shape and condition of the mother's nipples (? flat or inverted, ? cracks or raw areas)
    - How baby's mouth attaches (are lips flanged, does the baby have most of the nipple in its mouth?)
    - Sucking and swallowing
  - There are multiple safe over-the-counter preparations that can soothe sore nipples:
    - Lansinoh®
    - Soothies®
  - Avoid "nipple confusion": getting milk out of a bottle is initially easier than getting it out of a breast.
    - Do not use pacifiers or bottles in the first month of life.
  - Prevention is the key.
- **Concerns about inadequate milk supply**
  - Although a very common concern, most women produce more than adequate amounts of milk.
  - Frequent visits and monitoring by trained health care professionals are extremely helpful.
  - Adequate output = adequate intake.
    - Number of wet diapers per day (one for each day of life then usually 6–8 per day)
    - Number of stools per day (several per day, sometimes as often as after every feed)
    - Weight checks
      - Babies often lose up to 8% of their birth weight in the first week.
      - Breast-fed babies typically return to their birth weight by 10–14 days of life.
  - Try to avoid supplementation if at all possible as it interferes with the supply and demand mechanism.
  - May require pumping
- **Other common complications**
  - Jaundice
    - Treated the same in a breast or a bottle-fed infant
  - Mastitis

- A local infection as a result of milk stasis that often requires antibiotics
  - Candida infection
    - Should be considered when a woman develops burning nipple pain with feeding
    - Diagnosis can be difficult and is usually made clinically
    - Antifungal treatment is necessary for both mother and baby.

Pregnancy Considerations
A subsequent pregnancy is **not** a contraindication to breastfeeding.

MEDICATIONS (DRUGS)

- Vitamin D Supplementation
  - Vitamin D 200 IU/day beginning during the first 2 months of life
    - New recommendation in 2003 by the American Academy of Pediatrics for exclusively breast-fed infants to prevent rickets and Vitamin D deficiency:
  - Breast milk is not itself Vitamin D deficient, but many children are sunlight deficient.
  - Important resource for information on the safety of medications for lactating mothers:
    - Hale T. *Thomas Hale's Medications and Mother's Milk: A Manual of Lactational Pharmacology.* 11th ed. Texas: Pharmasoft Medical Publishing; 2004.

FOLLOW-UP

- Prolonged Breast-Feeding (Returning to school or work)
  - Manual breast pumps
    - Relatively inexpensive unilateral device typically good for infrequent or short-term use
    - Medical equipment that can be prescribed by physicians and is often covered by insurance
  - Electric breast pumps
    - More expensive, but virtually essential for women who will be separated from their children for prolonged periods of time
    - Bilateral device that often comes in a discreet pack with a place for storage of cold milk
    - Rarely covered by insurance companies
  - Storage of pumped milk. Storage bags are available in local pharmacies and on the internet. Milk can be kept:
    - At room temperature for 4 hours.
    - In the refrigerator for 5–7 days.
    - In a self-contained refrigerator freezer unit for 3 months.
    - In deep freeze for 6–12 months.

ALERT
- Never refreeze thawed breast milk.
  - Support from the school/employer
    - Time to feed or pump—typically 30 minutes every 3–4 hours
    - Privacy and sanitary conditions
    - NB: Several states in the United States have legislation that protects the rights of working lactating mothers.

Issues for Referral
- Consider referral to breastfeeding specialist (lactation consultant) if:
  - Difficulty with latching on
  - Nipple trauma
  - Jaundiced infant

- Pain throughout feeding
- Infant weight loss $\geq 8\%$
- Inadequate urine/stool output
- No audible swallowing after 24 hours of age
- History of unsuccessful breastfeeding
- History of breast surgery
- Abnormal infant oral anatomy
- Infant in critical care nursery
- Jaundiced infant
- Multiple births
- Premature infant

MISCELLANEOUS

- GENERAL SOURCES OF BREAST-FEEDING SUPPORT
  - "Warm lines" at individual hospitals
    - Warm line is a phone service designed to solve relatively minor problems or to prevent those problems from becoming serious.
  - Women, Infants, and Children (WIC) breastfeeding support peer counselors
  - Private physicians and lactation consultants in the community (MDs, CLCs, IBCLCs)
  - La Leche League International (LLLI): www.lalecheleague.org
  - The Academy of Breast-feeding Medicine: www.bfmed.org
  - Worldwide organization of physicians dedicated to the promotion, protection, and support of breast-feeding and human lactation

REFERENCES
1. Breast-feeding Trends 2003. Appendices 1 and 2. Mothers' Survey, Ross Products Division of Abbott.
2. American Academy of Pediatrics. Section on breast-feeding. Breast-feeding and the use of human milk. *Pediatr.* 2005;115:496–506.
3. Breast-feeding Pocket Guide to Help You Help Your Patients, Breast-feeding Support Services. TI Breastfeeding Coalition, Rhode Island Department of Health, Rhode Island, Division of Family Health, 12/04.
4. Satcher DS. DHHS blueprint for action on breastfeeding. *Public Health Rep.* 2001;116:72-73.
5. Prevention of rickets and vitamin D deficiency: New guidelines for vitamin D intake. *Pediatr.* 2003;111:908–910. Retrieved April, 2005 from http://aappolicy.aappublications.org/cgi/reprint/pediatrics; 111/4/908.
6. Sinusas K, Gagliardi A. Initial management of breast-feeding. *Am Fam Physician.* 2001;64:981–988.

CODES
ICD9-CM
- 783.3 Feeding difficulty (infant)
- 779.3 Feeding difficulty (newborn)

KEY WORDS
- Breast-feeding
- Lactation
- Neonatal
- Pediatrics
- Postpartum
- Pregnancy

CANDIDIASIS, VULVOVAGINAL

Iris L. Tong, MD

KEY CLINICAL POINTS

- Self-diagnosis of vulvovaginal candidiasis by patients is accurate in only 34% of cases.
- Patients who self-diagnose often have more than one type of vaginitis.
- Patients who have symptoms of vaginal discharge should be encouraged to be seen by a health care provider.

 BASICS

DESCRIPTION

- Vulvovaginal candidiasis is the second most common cause of vaginitis, after bacterial vaginosis (BV).
- *Candida albicans* is the most common organism and is responsible for 90% of cases.
- Recurrent vulvovaginal candidiasis (RVVC)
  - Can occur in up to 5%
  - Defined as more than 4 episodes in a 1-year period

GENERAL PREVENTION

- Avoid douching
- Optimal control of blood sugar in diabetic patients

EPIDEMIOLOGY

Prevalence

- It is estimated that 75% of women will have 1 episode of vulvovaginal candidiasis during their lifetime.
- Approximately 5% will have recurrent episodes.

RISK FACTORS

- Recent antibiotic use
- Diabetes mellitus
- HIV
- Steroid use
- Pregnancy
- Contraceptive use
  - Oral contraceptive pills
  - Diaphragm and spermicide
  - Intrauterine device (IUD)
- Douching
- Receptive anal and oral sex practices

PATHOPHYSIOLOGY

- Not sexually transmitted
- Changes in the vaginal milieu, such as increase in glycogen production from pregnancy or oral contraceptive pill use, lead to increased adherence of C. albicans to vaginal epithelium and germination of yeast.
- In recurrent vulvovaginal candidiasis
  - Some women may remain colonized with small numbers of yeast even after treatment.
  - When yeast increase in number, a recurrence of the symptoms occurs.

ETIOLOGY

- In the general population: 15–20% colonized with yeast
- Routine cultures will also identify asymptomatic women.
- Most common organisms
  - *Candida albicans*
    - Cause in 90% of cases
  - *Candida glabrata*
  - *Candida tropicalis*
  - *Candida parapsilosis*
  - *Saccharomyces cerevisiae*
- Recurrent vulvovaginal candidiasis
- *Candida glabrata, Candida parapsilosis,* and *Saccharomyces cerevisiae* are responsible for up to 33% of the cases.

ASSOCIATED CONDITIONS

Other types of vaginitis

- Bacterial vaginosis
- Trichomoniasis

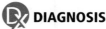 **DIAGNOSIS**

SIGNS AND SYMPTOMS

- Thick, white vaginal discharge
- Vaginal itching
- Vaginal irritation
- Dysuria
- Vulvovaginal swelling

History

- Recent antibiotic use
- Contraceptive use
- Diabetes
- Pregnancy
- Self-diagnosis by patients is only accurate in 34% of the cases.

Physical Exam

- Thick, white, "cottage cheese"-like discharge
- Vulvar and vaginal erythema and/or ulcerations

TESTS

Lab

- Vaginal pH
  - Normal in vulvovaginal candidiasis (<4.5)
- Light microscopy (see below)
- Negative in up to 50% of confirmed cases
- DNA probe
  - Commercially available probe that simultaneously detects the presence of *Candida* species, *G. vaginalis*, and *Trichomonas vaginalis* from a single vaginal swab
  - Results within 24 hours
  - Performed in laboratory
  - Sensitivity 82%, specificity 98.5%
- Culture
  - Fungal culture
    - Indicated in recurrent vulvovaginal as identifying causative organism helpful in guiding treatment
  - Viral Culture
    - In patients with ulcerations, a culture for the herpes simplex virus should be performed.
    - Gram stain
  - Less convenient for making diagnosis in outpatient setting
- Screening for sexually transmitted infections (STIs), if clinically indicated
  - Chlamydia
  - Gonorrhea
  - Trichomonas
  - Syphilis
  - Hepatitis B and C
  - HIV

CANDIDIASIS, VULVOVAGINAL

ALERT
- Samples for pH, microscopy, DNA probe, and culture should be obtained from the posterior fornix or vaginal wall.
- Obtaining a sample from the cervical os may reveal normal cervical mucous.

Diagnostic Procedures/Surgery
- Light microscopy
  - Normal saline or potassium hydroxide (KOH) preparation slide can be used.
    - A thin layer of discharge is placed on the slide.
    - A drop of normal saline or 10% KOH solution is added.
    - KOH causes lysis of epithelial cells, increasing the ability to identify the yeast forms.
    - KOH slides are associated with 50% sensitivity.
  - Presence of hyphae, pseudohyphae, and budding yeast cells (see image)
  - Lactobacilli should be present.
    - Lack of lactobacilli is suggestive of concomitant bacterial vaginosis
  - Few or no white blood cells (WBCs)
    - Ratio of WBCs to epithelial cells of >1:1 is suggestive of underlying infection, such as trichomonas or gonorrhea/chlamydia
- Biopsy
  - If ulcerations or chronic skin changes exist, consider vulvar biopsy to rule out lichen sclerosus, other vulvar dermatoses, or malignancy

DIFFERENTIAL DIAGNOSIS
- BV
- Trichomonas vaginalis
- Atrophic vaginitis
- Cervicitis

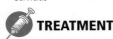 TREATMENT

GENERAL MEASURES
Diet
Dietary changes, such as yeast-free diets, have been frequently recommended for recurrent vulvovaginal candidiasis, but there is no evidence to support this approach.

SPECIAL THERAPY
- Cotton underwear
- Avoid tight-fitting pants

Complementary and Alternative Therapies
Most complementary and alternative therapies are recommended for patients with recurrent vulvovaginal candidiasis.
- Lactobacillus acidophilus containing yogurt
  - Small crossover study of 33 women with recurrent infection demonstrated that oral yogurt daily for 6 months decreased the rate of recurrent infection 3-fold.
- Boric Acid
  - For recurrent yeast infection caused by nonalbicans species
  - Often prepared as a powder in a gelatin capsule
  - Vulvovaginal burning can occur
  - Treatment dose: 600 mg intravaginally before bed for 14 days
  - Maintenance dose: 600 mg intravaginally twice weekly
- Tea tree oil
  - Multiple observation studies support antifungal activity of tea tree oil
  - 1–2 capsules intravaginally before bed for 6 days
  - Potential side effects: Allergic contact dermatitis

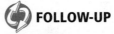 MEDICATION (DRUGS)

First Line
- Topical antifungal agents
  - Clotrimazole 1% cream: 5 g intravaginally every day for 7–14 days
  - Clotrimazole 100 mg tablet: intravaginally every day for 7 days OR intravaginally b.i.d. for 3 days
  - Miconazole 2% cream: 5 g intravaginally every day for 7 days
  - Miconazole: 100 mg vaginal suppository intravaginally every day for 7 days OR 200 mg every day for 3 days
- Oral antifungal agents
  - Fluconazole: 150 mg PO × 1 dose
    - Has been shown to be as effective as a 7-day treatment with topical clotrimazole.

Pregnancy Considerations
Oral azoles are not recommended in pregnancy.

FOLLOW-UP

DISPOSITION
Good response to topical or oral therapy but up to 5% will have recurrent vulvovaginal candidiasis.

Admission Criteria
Treatment is primarily in outpatient setting.

Issues for Referral
- To obstetrician/gynecologist if symptoms do not resolve after treatment
- To endocrinologist if poorly controlled diabetes is the cause of recurrent vulvovaginal candidiasis

COMPLICATIONS
- Complicated vulvovaginal candidiasis
  - Defined as:
    - Severe or repeat infections
    - Infection with Candida species other than C. Albicans
    - Infections in immunosuppressed, diabetic, or pregnant women
  - Topical therapy has been shown to be more effective than single-dose oral therapy.
  - Regimens
    - Extend topical therapy to 10–14 days
    - Fluconazole: 150 mg PO every three days × 2 doses can also be given
- For patients with severe discomfort, a low-potency steroid cream can be added to topical therapy.
- Recurrence
  - Fungal culture to identify organism
  - Identify possible precipitating factors
    - Poorly controlled diabetes
    - Underlying immunodeficiency
    - Oral contraceptive pill
    - Antibiotic therapy
  - Treatment regimens include initial and maintenance dosages:
    - Clotrimazole: 100 mg vaginal tablet intravaginally every day for 7days, then 500 mg intravaginally every week for 6 months
    - Fluconazole: 150 mg PO every day for 3 days, then 150 mg PO every week for 6 months
  - For albicans species, resistance to azoles rare
  - For nonalbicans species, resistance to azoles more common

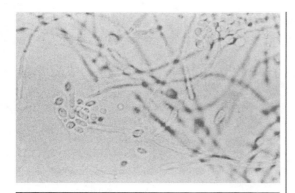

Figure 1 Blastospores, hyphae, and pseudohyphae

- In patients who failed standard azole therapy, can attempt trial of
  - Boric acid vaginal suppositories 600 mg every day for 14 days with topical flucytosine cream
- Severe complications are very rare.
  - Chorioamnionitis in pregnancy and vulvar vestibulitis syndrome have been reported.

PATIENT MONITORING
- Routine glucose monitoring for patients with diabetes
- Patients receiving weekly fluconazole suppressive therapy should have periodic liver function tests.
- For recurrent vulvovaginal candidiasis, a repeat fungal culture is helpful to confirm treatment success.
  - Positive culture with negative culture on follow-up associated with resolution of symptoms in 90% cases

REFERENCES

1. Ferris DG, Nyirjesy P, Sobel JD, et al. Over-the-counter antifungal drug misuse associated with patient-diagnosed vulvovaginal candidiasis. *Obstet Gynecol*. 2002;99:419–425.
2. Nyirjesy P. Chronic vulvovaginal candidiasis. *Am Fam Physician*. 2001;63:697–702.
3. Owen MK, Clenney TL. Management of vaginitis. *Am Fam Physician*. 2004;70:2125–2132.
4. Sobel JD, Wiesenfeld HC, Martens M, et al. Maintenance fluconazole therapy for recurrent vulvovaginal candidiasis. *N Engl J Med*. 2004;351:876–883.
5. Van Kessel K, Assefi N, Marrazzo J, et al. Common complementary and alternative therapies for yeast vaginitis and bacterial vaginosis: a systematic review. *Obstet Gynecol Survey*. 2003;58:351–358.

ADDITIONAL READING

Egan ME, Lipsky MS. Diagnosis of vaginitis. *Am Fam Physician*. 2000;62:1095–1104.

Hilton E, Isenberg HD, Alperstein P, et al. Ingestion of yogurt containing Lactobacillus acidophilus as prophylaxis for candidal vaginitis. *Arch Fam Med*. 1996;116:353–357.

CODES
ICD9-CM
- 112.1 Candidal vulvovaginitis
- 616.1 Vaginitis and vulvovaginitis
- 623.5 Vaginal discharge NOS

KEY WORDS
- Vaginal Discharge
- Vaginal Itching
- Yeast Infection
- Yeast Vaginitis
- Vulvovaginal Candidiasis

C

CELIAC DISEASE

Sumona Saha, MD
Silvia D. Degli-Esposti, MD

KEY CLINICAL POINTS

- Disease is immune-mediated, requires genetic and environmental factors
- Prevalence in United States greater than previously estimated
- Diagnosis commonly delayed due to the wide range of clinical presentations
- Lifelong surveillance for the development of complications

 BASICS

DESCRIPTION
- Disease is systemic
- Wide spectrum of clinical presentation
- Natural history
  - Latent disease
    - Symptoms absent
    - Biopsy normal
    - Autoantibodies positive
  - Silent disease
    - Symptoms minimal
    - Biopsy positive
    - Autoantibodies positive
  - Active disease
    - Symptoms present
    - Biopsy positive
    - Autoantibodies positive

GENERAL PREVENTION
Elimination of gluten and related proteins in genetically susceptible individuals with silent and latent disease

EPIDEMIOLOGY
- Female > male predominance (2.9:1)
- Diagnosis frequent in 4th to 6th decades of life.

Incidence
Estimates vary from 2 to 13/100,000 per year
- True incidence unknown, "new" cases are adults with 20 to 60 years of untreated disease
- Recent increase in incidence reflects increased use of serologic screening and diagnosis of asymptomatic disease

Prevalence
- Now estimated to affect 3 million Americans (approximately 1% of the U.S. population)
- Rare in East Asian and African populations (with the exception of Saharavi in North Africa)

RISK FACTORS
- Human leukocyte antigen (HLA) class II antigens DQ2 and DQ8 (necessary but not sufficient for disease development)
  - HLA-DQ2 is expressed in 85% to 95% of the patients.
  - HLA-DQ8 is expressed in the majority of the remainder of the patients.
- Early and massive gluten exposure
- Other autoimmune diseases

Genetics
Autosomal dominant transmission with incomplete penetrance
- Disease prevalence is 15% in first-degree relatives
- Concordance is 75% in monozygotic twins

PATHOPHYSIOLOGY
- HLA-DQ2 (DQ8) present modified gluten peptides to gluten-reactive T cells activating an abnormal mucosal response and inducing tissue damage
- The ubiquitous enzyme, tissue transglutaminase (tTG), modifies gluten molecules, allowing them to bind to HLA-DQ2 (DQ8) and launch an inflammatory response

ETIOLOGY
Dietary gluten in genetically susceptible individuals triggers T-cell response

ASSOCIATED CONDITIONS
- Type I diabetes
- Autoimmune thyroid disorders
- Addison's disease
- Reproductive disorders
- Alopecia areata
- Cerebellar ataxia
- Neuropathy
- Epilepsy
- Migraine
- Autoimmune myocarditis
- Anemia
- Osteoporosis
- Selective IgA deficiency
- Sjögrens syndrome
- Juvenile chronic arthritis
- Ulcerative colitis

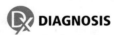 **DIAGNOSIS**

SIGNS AND SYMPTOMS
- Be aware that the presentation of celiac disease varies greatly.
- Clinical subtypes
  - Symptomatic or classic
    - Gastrointestinal symptoms predominate
  - Atypical
    - Gastrointestinal symptoms absent or less pronounced
    - Extraintestinal symptoms predominate
  - Asymptomatic
    - Positive biopsy found incidentally or positive serologic tests found on screening

History
- Gastrointestinal symptoms commonly include dyspepsia, upper abdominal pain, increased frequency of bowel movements, steatorrhea, and weight loss.
- Symptoms are often atypical (e.g., osteoporosis in men or premenopausal women, iron deficiency)
- Coexistent autoimmune disorders
- Obtain family history
- Previous diagnosis of irritable bowel syndrome (IBS) as 5% of individuals with IBS have celiac disease

Physical Exam
Physical findings range from absent to severe
- General exam
  - Short stature
  - Weight loss

- Abdominal exam
  - Distention
  - Tenderness
- Musculoskeletal exam
  - Fractures
  - Arthritis
- Neurological exam
  - Ataxia
  - Peripheral neuropathy
  - Depression
- Skin and mucosa exam
  - Dermatitis herpetiformis-pruritic, symmetric papulovesicular lesions
  - Apthous stomatitis
  - Hair loss

TESTS
- Screening usually done by serologic testing
- Small bowel biopsy while patient consumes gluten still necessary for diagnosis
- Gluten challenge only in patients on gluten-free diet despite not being diagnosed with celiac disease

Lab
- Serologic tests are used to screen patients and to monitor the response.
- The best available tests are the Riga tissue transglutaminase and IgA endomysial antibody (EMA).
- High sensitivity and specificity (>95%), false negative in IGA deficiency
- Screen for IGA deficiency with total IGA.
- Antigliadin antibody (AGA) is testing no longer recommended.
- When results are indeterminate can test for HLA haplotypes
  - Greater than 97% of those with celiac disease are DQ2 and/or DQ8 positive, compared with 40% of the general population

Imaging
CT findings
- Intestinal fold pattern abnormalities (most specific finding) quantified by intestinal fold count
- Mild to moderate bowel dilation with fluid excess
- Benign mesenteric lymphadenopathy
  - Can resolve with gluten-free diet

Diagnostic Procedures
- Upper endoscopy
  - An intestinal biopsy is necessary for the diagnosis.
  - Disease may be patchy
    - Obtain 4 to 6 biopsies from the descending duodenum
  - Endoscopic findings
    - Loss of intestinal folds
    - Scalloping of folds
- Wireless capsule endoscopy (WCE)
  - Can identify complications of celiac disease not identifiable by conventional imaging

Pathologic Findings
- Characteristic histologic features
  - Villous atrophy
  - Crypt hyperplasia
  - Increased intraepithelial lymphocyte count
- Marsh criteria are used to grade the disease (from 0 to 4).

DIFFERENTIAL DIAGNOSIS
- Infective gastroenteritis
- Bacterial overgrowth
- Lactose intolerance
- Anorexia nervosa
- Ischemic enteritis
- Tuberculosis
- Crohn's disease
- Hypogammaglobulinemia
- Tropical sprue
- Whipple's disease
- Zollinger-Ellison syndrome
- Intestinal lymphoma
- HIV enteropathy

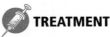 TREATMENT

INITIAL STABILIZATION
- Newly diagnosed patients should be screened for vitamin and mineral deficiencies.
  - Fat soluble vitamins (A, D, E, and K)
  - Water soluble vitamins (folate and B12)
  - Iron, Calcium, Phosphorus, Zinc
- Screen for osteoporosis.
- Screen for other autoimmune disorders.

GENERAL MEASURES
- Only begin the treatment after a complete diagnostic evaluation, which should include serology and a biopsy.
- Patients should be referred for consultation with a dietitian and to celiac disease advocacy groups shortly after diagnosis.
- Screen first- and second-degree relatives.

Diet
Management of celiac disease is a gluten-free diet for life.
- A gluten-free diet excludes wheat, rye, and barley; oats in a minimal quantity may be safe.
- Even small quantities of gluten can be harmful.
- Potential for cross-contamination with gluten during processing
- Use products labeled gluten-free.
- There are many barriers to compliance including poor palatability of foods, cost, limited availability of gluten-free foods, and confusing food labels.
- A gluten-free diet improves the quality of life even in patients without gastrointestinal symptoms.

Activity
As tolerated

Nursing
- Monitor weight
- Web resources
  - www.gluten.net
  - www.celiac.org

Complementary and Alternative Medicine
None advocated by the NIH consensus panel

MEDICATION (DRUGS)

- Gluten-free diet usually sufficient to produce disease remission
- Vitamin and mineral supplementation required in most patients

First Line
- Multivitamin
- Calcium supplementation
  - 1000–1500 mg/day
- Iron supplementation if needed

C

Second Line
Medication is used in refractory cases.
- Refractory sprue type I
  - Responsive to steroids and immunosuppressant (e.g., infliximab)
- Refractory sprue type II
  - Evolves into T-cell lymphoma
  - Novel therapies include IL-15 antagonists

SURGERY
In cases of celiac disease associated cancer, approximately 50% require laparotomy.
- Surgical complications: Hemorrhage, perforation, obstruction

Pregnancy Considerations
- Associated with reduced fertility
- Also associated with increased risk of adverse pregnancy-related events
  - Intrauterine growth retardation
  - Low birth weight

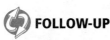

FOLLOW-UP

DISPOSITION
- First follow up visit 1–2 weeks after endoscopy with gastroenterologist
  - Refer to dietician and support group at this time
- Follow up 3–6 months then yearly
  - Discuss dietary compliance
  - Monitor for complications
  - No need to repeat endoscopy
  - Recheck autoantibodies (should clear within 1 year if responding to gluten free diet)

Issues for Referral
- Persistent symptoms despite gluten-free diet
  - Refer to dietician to evaluate for intentional or nonintentional gluten ingestion
  - Refer to gastroenterologist to evaluate for complications
    - May need repeat upper endoscopy, push enteroscopy, or WCE to make diagnosis
- Poor family support or limited literacy
  - Refer to social services

PROGNOSIS
Some studies report two-fold to four-fold excess in all-cause mortality compared with the general population.

COMPLICATIONS
- Nutritional deficiencies
- Osteoporosis

- Gastrointestinal tract malignancies
  - Enteropathy-associated T-cell lymphoma (EATL)
    - High grade Non-Hodgkin's lymphoma
    - Derived from clonal proliferation of intraepithelial lymphocytes
    - Strict adherence to gluten free diet helps to prevent lymphoma development.
  - Adenocarcinoma of the small bowel, pharynx, and esophgus
- Other malignancies
  - Primary hepatocellular carcinoma
  - Melanoma

PATIENT MONITORING
- Monitor for diet compliance
- Screen for nutritional deficiencies
- Monitor for complications

REFERENCES

1. Catassi C, Bearzi I, Holmes GK. Association of celiac disease and intestinal lymphomas and other cancers. *Gastroenterol*. 2005;128:79–86.
2. Dewar DH, Ciclitira PJ. Clinical features and diagnosis of celiac disease. *Gastroenterol*. 2005:128:19–24.
3. Rewers M. Epidemiology of celiac disease: what are the prevalence, incidence, and progression of celiac disease? *Gastroenterol*. 2005;128:47–51.
4. Green PHR. The many faces of celiac disease: Clinical presentation of celiac disease in the adult population. *Gastroenterol*. 2005;128:74–78.
5. National Institutes of Health. Consensus development conference statement on celiac disease, June 28–30, 2004. *Gastroenterol*. 2005;128:1–9.

CODES
ICD9-CM
- 579.0 Celiac disease
- 783.2 Abnormal loss of weight
- 789.0 Abdominal pain

KEY WORDS

- Abdominal Pain
- Malabsorption
- Diarrhea

CHRONIC FATIGUE SYNDROME

John P. Bas, MD, MHSA
David Anthony, MD, MSc

KEY CLINICAL POINTS

- No clear etiology has been identified.
- Less than 10% of patients with lasting fatigue have chronic fatigue syndrome (CFS).
- CFS is a disabling and frustrating illness in which close follow-up and trust-building are essential elements of therapy.
- Graded exercise programs and cognitive behavioral therapy (CBT) have each been shown to be effective in multiple RCTs.

 BASICS

DESCRIPTION
CFS is a debilitating illness with components of neurological, affective, and cognitive disorders. It is characterized by the acute onset of fatigue severe enough to lead to substantial reductions in activities of daily living (i.e., occupation, social, personal). Patients report no relief with rest. Symptoms must last greater than 6 months for CFS to be considered.

GENERAL PREVENTION
None

EPIDEMIOLOGY
- CFS is associated primarily with young to middle age adults, but cases have been discovered in children. Cases have also been discovered in the elderly, although coexisting medical conditions usually preclude considering this diagnosis in this population.
- CFS is twice as common among women. It is less commonly diagnosed among minorities and lower socioeconomic groups, but may be underestimated secondary to the lack of equivalent access to health care institutions in which CFS is studied.

Incidence
180 cases per 100,000 persons over 1 year.

Prevalence
- Estimates have ranged from 75–267 cases per 100,000 persons.
- The CDC estimates that up to a half a million people in the United States have undiagnosed CFS.
- The Chronic Fatigue and Immune-Dysfunction Syndrome (CFIDS) Association of America (www.cfids.org) states that 90% of the people with CFS have not been diagnosed and are not receiving care.

RISK FACTORS
Female sex

Genetics
No specific genetic abnormality has been identified.

PATHOPHYSIOLOGY
Unknown

ETIOLOGY
No clear etiologic agent has been identified. Studied causes include:
- Infection: EBV, retroviruses, HHV-6, Enteroviruses, Coxsackie B virus, Ross river virus, Borna disease virus. None have been consistently identified.
- Immune dysfunction: Chronic inflammation with low NK cell levels; findings inconsistent
- Neuroendocrine disorder: Low cortisol levels and high serotonin activity

- Neurally-mediated hypotension: Higher than expected rate of positive tilt table tests
- Depression: Clearly associated, but not clear if it causes or is caused by CFS

ASSOCIATED CONDITIONS
Fibromyalgia shares many of the symptoms and may be on a spectrum of illness with CFS.

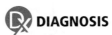 DIAGNOSIS

PRE-HOSPITAL
- No specific tests; diagnosis is one of exclusion
- Each case must have:
  - New onset of fatigue lasting >6 months; with severe reduction in ADLs (<50% of patient's premorbid condition)
  - Fatigue not relieved by rest
  - The exclusion of other conditions that can produce fatigue
  - Any 4 of the asterisked (*) symptoms below during and not predating the 6 months of illness

SIGNS AND SYMPTOMS
- Fatigue
- Sore throat*
- Arthralgias without arthritis*
- Impairment in memory*
- Impairment in concentration*
- Myalgias*
- Tender cervical or axillary nodes*
- Headache*
- Unrefreshing sleep*
- Postexertional malaise lasting >24 hours*
- Feverishness without true fever
- Emotional lability
- Decreased libido
- Mood swings
- Irritability
- Depression
- Allergies
- Vertigo
- Shortness of breath
- Chest pain
- Nausea
- Hot flashes
- Palpitations
- Abdominal cramps
- Night sweats
- Weight gain or loss
- Rash

History
A complete history is essential in order to rule out and exclude other underlying pathology.

Physical Exam
- Perform a complete exam to rule out other diagnoses.
- Painful lymph nodes without enlargement
- Mild nonexudative pharyngitis
- No evidence of joint inflammation

CHRONIC FATIGUE SYNDROME

TESTS
Lab
- Standard:
  - CBC w/ diff
  - ESR
  - Serum chemistries
  - Thyroid function tests
- Other tests only if clinically indicated:
  - Serum cortisol
  - Rheumatoid factor
  - Immunoglobulin levels
  - Lyme titers
  - HIV

Imaging
Although brain MR abnormalities are more common among people with CFS, there is no clear pattern and imaging is generally not useful in the diagnosis.

DIFFERENTIAL DIAGNOSIS
- Malignancy
- Autoimmune disease (i.e., Addison's disease shares 42 clinical features with that of CFS)
- Localized infection
- Chronic versus subacute bacterial disease (e.g., endocarditis, Lyme disease)
- Fungal disease (e.g., histoplasmosis, coccidiomycosis)
- Parasitic disease (e.g., giardiasis)
- HIV
- Psychiatric illness (e.g., depression, anxiety)
- Drug dependence
- Somatization
- Altered physiological states (i.e., pregnancy, over-exertion)
- Lifestyle derangements
- More controversial entities (e.g., chronic candidiasis, food allergies, environmental illnesses)

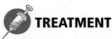 TREATMENT

GENERAL MEASURES
- Given the debilitating nature of CFS and the absence of a clear treatable etiologic agent, therapy should be supportive and focused on the patient's ability to function.
- Treat underlying conditions including psychiatric disorders.

Diet
No specific dietary recommendations

Activity
- Multiple RCTs have demonstrated the benefits of graded exercise. This involves 1–10 minutes of aerobic exercise (e.g., running) every other day. The duration of exercise is adjusted biweekly depending on symptoms with a goal of gradually increasing to 30 minutes. The effects can be lasting.
- Patients should be warned that sudden increases in activity may worsen symptoms.

SPECIAL THERAPY
RCTs have shown that cognitive behavioral therapy (CBT) is effective. As in graded exercise, beneficial effects may be lasting.

Complementary and Alternative Therapies
Many therapies have been studied (e.g., acupuncture and homeopathy); however, none have shown significant benefits.

 MEDICATION (DRUGS)

Multiple medications have been studied, including fluoxetine, fludrocortisone, and galantamine hydrobromide; however, none have shown consistent benefits.

Pregnancy Considerations
- No evidence suggests that CFS can be transmitted to an unborn child or that the condition will affect baby.
- Pregnancy does not consistently worsen or improve the symptoms of CFS.
- One study demonstrated increased spontaneous abortion and developmental delay of offspring in pregnancies complicated by CFS compared to pregnancies which occurred before the onset of illness. These increases, however, may be explained by increased maternal age and parity and likely are unrelated to CFS.

PATIENT MONITORING
Close and frequent follow-up is recommended. Patient-doctor rapport and trust is essential to illness management and care. Many patients feel their symptoms are ignored by physicians.

REFERENCES
1. Chronic Fatigue and Immune Dysfunction Syndrome. Statistics for CFIDS. Available at: www.cfids.org.
2. Bates DW, Schmitt W, Buchwald D, et al. Prevalence of fatigue and chronic fatigue syndrome in a primary care practice. Arch Intern Med. 1993;153:2759–2765.
3. Deale A, Husain K, Chalder T, et al. Long-term outcome of cognitive behavior therapy versus relaxation therapy for chronic fatigue syndrome: A 5-year follow-up study. Am J Psychiatry. 2001;158:2038–2042.
4. Mihrshahi R, Bierman R. Aetiolgy and pathogenesis of chronic fatigue syndrome: a review. N Z Med J. 2005;118:1780.
5. Powell P, Bentall RP, Nye FJ, et al. Patient education to encourage graded exercise in chronic fatigue syndrome: 2-year follow-up of randomized controlled trial. Br J Psych. 2004;184:142–146.
6. Schacterle RS, Komaroff AL. A comparison of pregnancies that occur before and after the onset of chronic fatigue syndrome. Arch Intern Med. 2004;164:401–404.
7. Wallman KE, Morton AR, Goodman C, et al. Exercise prescription for individuals with chronic fatigue syndrome. Med J Australia. 2005;183:142–143.

CODES
ICD9-CM
- 780.71 Chronic Fatigue Syndrome

KEY WORDS
- Chronic Fatigue
- Immune Dysfunction
- Fibromyalgia
- Graded Exercise
- Cognitive Behavioral Therapy

CHRONIC PELVIC PAIN (CPP)

Sharon B. Stechna, MD

KEY CLINICAL POINTS

CPP is a syndrome whose etiology remains unknown; however, uncovering a definitive diagnosis improves prognosis and treatment.

- Evaluate all organ systems in the pelvis-gynecologic, urologic, gastrointestinal, neurologic, and musculoskeletal.
- Screen for concomitant psychological disorders.
- A team approach between the specialists and the primary provider improves patient care and outcome.
- Establishing a supportive relationship is essential to care of the patient with CPP.
- Even in the patient with depression, chronic pelvic pain is not "all in her head." A combined approach of mind and body will provide optimal results.

 BASICS

DESCRIPTION

- CPP is any non-menstrual pain lasting more than 6 months.
- CPP is often vague and difficult to assess.
- The degree of pain is often out of proportion to the clinical findings.
- CPP is extremely distressing to women.
- CPP is extremely frustrating for physicians.
- Over 60% of patients never receive a diagnosis.

Incidence
- As high as 20% of women of reproductive age
- Accounts for 20% of laparoscopies
- Accounts for 12–16% of hysterectomies
- Associated medical costs total nearly $3 billion annually

ETIOLOGY
- CPP is a syndrome. Its etiology remains unknown.
- In patients without a clear source of pain, one theory is that an acute event triggers the pain, but the pain continues even after the trigger is gone.

ASSOCIATED CONDITIONS
- Interstitial cystitis
- Irritable bowel syndrome
- Depression/anxiety
- Dyspareunia
- Vulvar dystrophy

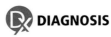 **DIAGNOSIS**

- CPP often remains undiagnosed.
- The identification of the source of CPP is elusive.
- Patient complaints can too often be ignored by the provider.

SIGNS AND SYMPTOMS
To help assess possible etiology:
- Vague pain is associated with a visceral/intra-abdominal process.
- Localized pain is associated with a musculoskeletal origin.
- Constipation/flatulence/bloating are associated with a gastrointestinal origin.
- Urinary frequency or burning is associated with a urinary origin.

History
- Obtaining a complete history is the key to the diagnosis.
- Assess the nature of the pain, intensity, distribution, associated symptoms, and temporal relations.
- Identify prior surgeries, infections, infertility, and birth complications.
- Evaluate the patient's bleeding patterns.
- Evaluate the patient for associated psychiatric symptoms, such as depression or anxiety.
- Evaluate the patient for current or prior sexual abuse.
- Determine the role pain plays in the patient's life.
- A 3-month pain diary may be helpful.

Physical Exam
- Evaluate each anatomic area individually:
  - Anterior abdominal wall/hernias
  - Pelvic bones/symphysis
  - Pelvic floor musculature/levator ani
  - Vulva/vestibule
  - Vagina
  - Urethra
  - Cervix
  - Viscera-uterus, adnexa, bladder
  - Rectum
  - Rectovaginal septum
  - Coccyx
  - Posture and gait
- Perform the exam standing, sitting, supine, and lithotomy.
- A bimanual exam alone is insufficient as it cannot differentiate between anterior abdominal wall, cervix, and intraabdominal organs.

TESTS
- **Basic Testing**:
  - Pap smear
  - Gonorrhea and chlamydia cultures
  - Wet mount if associated discharge or odor
  - Urinalysis
  - Urine culture
  - Pregnancy test
  - CBC with differential
  - Erythrocyte sedimentation rate (nonspecific for inflammatory process)
  - Pelvic ultrasound, which could possibly lead to MRI or CT
- **Specialized Testing** (as directed by findings of H & P):
  - Potassium sensitivity testing—interstitial cystitis (IC) requires evaluation by urology or urogynecology.
  - Cystoscopy/urethroscopy—IC, urethral diverticulum, neoplasia
  - Urodynamics—detrusor instability
  - Electrophysiologic studies—nerve compression, muscular spasm
  - X-ray—fracture
  - Laparoscopy—endometriosis, adhesions, hernia
  - Specialists may consider "awake laparoscopy" for pain mapping.

DIFFERENTIAL DIAGNOSIS
- The differential diagnosis for CPP is extensive.
- If the pain seems gynecologic in origin, the differential includes:
  - Adenomyosis
  - Adhesions

- Chronic ectopic
- Chronic Infection
- Endometriosis
- Ovarian carcinoma
- Ovarian cysts
- Ovulatory pain (Mittelschmerz)
- Pelvic congestion syndrome
- Pelvic organ prolapse
- Tuberculous salpingitis
- Uterine fibroids

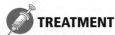 TREATMENT

A multidisciplinary approach to Chronic Pelvic Pain has been shown to be most effective

GENERAL MEASURES
- Identify the most likely organ system causing CPP and treat or refer appropriately.
- Recommend therapy for pain management techniques and emotional support.
- If the pain is gynecologic in origin:
  - Trial of NSAID's
  - Suppress the menstrual cycle with oral contraceptive or GNRH agonist for a 3-month trial.
  - If suppression fails, perform diagnostic laparoscopy.
  - A negative pelvic sonogram and diagnostic laparoscopy can be very reassuring to the patient.
  - A positive laparoscopy can be curative.
  - If muscular "trigger" points are identified, lidocaine injections may be considered.

Diet
- Identify triggers associated with food, such as lactose intolerance, celiac sprue, and acid reflux.
- Recommend a diet high in complex carbohydrates and fiber for general health and regular bowel movements.
- Avoid constipating food or foods that cause gaseous distension.

Activity
- Regular exercise has been shown to increase endorphins and, thus, pain tolerance is increased.
- Exercise has also been shown to improve symptomatic depression.
- Unless there is a specific indication (i.e., fracture), bed rest should be avoided.

 MEDICATION (DRUGS)

- Oral contraceptive
- GNRH agonist
- Progesterone
- NSAIDs
- Antidepressants for depression, but not pain
- Narcotic analgesics should be used under a "drug contract" for refractory pain.

SURGERY
- Laparoscopic fulgaration of endometriosis
- Lysis of adhesions has shown some benefit for thin adhesions where movement could cause tension on the band.

- Lysis of adhesions for dense adhesions has shown little benefit.
- Hysterectomy should be reserved for refractory cases where the etiology of the pain is thought to be gynecologic in origin.
- LUNA (laparoscopic uterine nerve ablation) has not been shown to be helpful.
- Hernia repair if hernia present

Physical Therapy
- For patients where the pain originates from muscular spasms, physical therapy can be helpful.
- Transcutaneous Electrical Nerve Stimulation (TENS) units may be of benefit.

Complementary and Alternative Medicine
- Results of clinical trials are limited.
- Acupressure and acupuncture have demonstrated efficacy equal to ibuprofen.
- Chiropractic and Osteopathic spinal manipulations may be of benefit.
- Meditation and breathing improve symptoms and relieve anxiety.
- Journaling may be of benefit.
- Saw Palmetto has insufficient information to support its use.

 FOLLOW-UP

DISPOSITION
- Establishing a supportive relationship is essential to care of the patient with CPP.
- It is very important to schedule regular visits to establish trust.
- Scheduled visits also eliminate the patient's need to have pain in order to have an office visit (eliminate secondary gain).
- A team approach with specialists improves patient care and outcome.

REFERENCES

1. ACOG. Pelvic Pain Practice Bulletin. No. 51 (March) 2004: 364–374.
2. Carter JE. Chronic pelvic pain: diagnosis and management [International Pelvic Pain Society Web site]. Available at: www.pelvicpain.org. Accessed 2005.
3. Wenof M, Perry CP. Chronic pelvic pain: A patient education booklet [International Pelvic Pain Society Web site]. Available at: www.pelvicpain.org. Accessed 1998.
4. Stones W, Cheong YC, Howard FM. Interventions for treating chronic pelvic pain in women In: The Cochrane Collaboration. Vol. 4, 2005.

CODES
ICD9-CM
- 625.9 Pelvic pain
- 625.0 Dyspareunia
- 617.1 Endometriosis

KEY WORDS

- Pelvic Pain
- Dyspareunia
- Endometriosis
- Abdominal Pain

CIRRHOSIS

Maria Chiara Cantarini, MD
Silvia D. Degli-Esposti, MD

KEY CLINICAL POINTS

- Progressive condition that represents the final common pathway for several chronic liver diseases
- The natural history includes a compensated stage and a decompensated stage; the latter is characterized by the onset of complications.
- Complications include: esophageal varices, ascites, encephalopathy, hepatocellular carcinoma, and liver failure.
- Treatment and prevention of complications and timely referral for liver transplant are crucial.

BASICS

DESCRIPTION

- Accumulation of scar tissue in the liver parenchyma with functional impairment of the organ: histologic features of fibrosis and regenerative nodules in the liver
- Liver cirrhosis results from sustained chronic liver injury over time regardless of the offending agents.
- It is a progressive condition leading to portal hypertension and liver failure.

GENERAL PREVENTION

- Primary prevention and treatment of underlying chronic liver diseases
- Obesity, excessive alcohol consumption, and other hepatoxins may accelerate the development of cirrhosis in all chronic liver diseases.
- Cirrhotic patients need to be vaccinated against hepatitis B and A, pneumococcal disease, and influenza.

EPIDEMIOLOGY

- Cirrhosis is the 12th leading cause of mortality among United State adults.
- It is the 5th leading cause of death for individuals aged 45–54.
- Predominant sex: Male > Female (0.15% prevalence)

RISK FACTORS

- Chronic B, C, and D hepatitis
- Alcoholic liver disease
- NASH (non-alcoholic steatohepatitis)
- Genetic disease (hemochromatosis, alpha 1 antitripsin deficiency, Wilson's disease, galactosemia, tyrosinemia)
- Autoimmune hepatitis
- Primary biliary cirrhosis
- Primary sclerosis cholangitis
- Childhood biliary diseases (Alagille, Byler, Indian childhood cirrhosis)
- Severe right-sided congestive heart failure
- Veno-occlusive disease
- Budd Chiari

Genetics

- Several liver diseases leading to cirrhosis are the result of genetic mutations (hemochromatosis, alpha 1 antitrypsin, gaclatosemia, tyrosinemia, and Wilson disease).
- Genetic predisposition for hepatic fibrosis may be linked to polymorphism of genes encoding profibrogenic cytokines.

PATHOPHYSIOLOGY

The substitution of liver parenchyma by scar tissue has a profound effect on organ function and eventually causes liver failure.

- Impaired protein synthesis
- Impaired detoxification and filtering function
- Structural and functional resistance to the portal flow through the liver with subsequent portal hypertension
- Hemodynamic alterations: systemic hypotension and fluid retention

ETIOLOGY

Multiple etiologies (see risk factors) result in common injury causing:

- Perisinusoidal satellite cell activation and proliferation
- Matrix deposition and remodeling in the liver. The process is orchestrated by a network of profibrogenic mediators.

ASSOCIATED CONDITIONS

Complications of cirrhosis:

- Ascites
- Gastrointestinal bleeding
- Hypo/hyperglycemia
- Encephalopathy
- Pantocytopenia
- Infertility

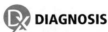 DIAGNOSIS

PRE-HOSPITAL

Diagnosis of cirrhosis requires clinical, laboratory, and histological evaluation.

SIGNS AND SYMPTOMS

Symptoms and signs correlate with the stage of the disease.

- Fatigue and weakness
- Fluid retention: ascites and edema
- Spider angiomas
- Bruising and bleeding
- Jaundice
- Itching
- Gastrointestinal bleeding (from esophageal or gastric varices, hypertensive gastritis, colic varices, hypertensive colitis)
- Hepatic encephalopathy: asterixis, disorientation, lethargy and coma
- Systemic hypotension

History

- Inquire about risk factors
- Family history of liver disease
- Travel history
- Hepatotoxic drugs or other toxic exposures

Physical Exam

- Decreased muscle mass
- Jaundice
- Ascites and edema
- Liver often a hard consistency with irregular borders
- Splenomegaly
- Superficial collateral circles (cava-cava, porto-cava)

CIRRHOSIS

- Spider angiomas
- Skin bruising
- Palmar erythema
- Flapping tremor

TESTS
Lab
- Thrombocytopenia
- Reduced albumin
- Prolonged prothrombin time
- Hypergammaglobulinemia
- Mild increase of ALT and AST, usually with AST/ALT >1
- Increased indices of cholestasis

Imaging
Abdominal ultrasound/Doppler and CT scan:
- The liver will be reduced in size; it will also have irregular borders and a granular texture.
- Ascites
- Portal vein: Increased diameter and reduced flow, reversal of flow direction
- Splenomegaly

Diagnostic Procedures/Surgery
- Endoscopy is recommended at time of diagnosis and every 3 years thereafter assessing:
  - Esophageal and gastric varices
  - Hypertensive gastritis
- Diagnostic paracentesis is recommended to rule out other causes of ascites

Pathologic Findings
- Liver biopsy is still necessary for definitive diagnosis
  - Fibrotic septa extending in the hepatic parenchyma surrounding regenerative nodules
  - Necroinflammation
  - Regeneration nodules
- Noninvasive methods to assess fibrosis are under evaluation at present (Fibrotest, Fibroscan)

DIFFERENTIAL DIAGNOSIS
- Ascites: Of all patients in the United States, 15% have a nonhepatic cause, such as peritoneal carcinomatosis, heart failure, tuberculosis, or nephrotic syndrome.
  - Perform paracentesis to narrow differential diagnosis.
- Hepatic encephalopathy: Consider other causes of confusion and coma in cirrhotic patients:
  - Hepatic encephalopathy does not present with focal neurological signs.
  - Encephalopathy is usually triggered by conditions, such as constipation, infection, intestinal bleeding, diuretics, and protein overload.
  - Obtain EEG, CT Scan, lumbar puncture if indicated
- Noncirrhotic causes of portal hypertension:
  - Traumatic/neoplastic arterioportal fistula
  - Tropical splenomegaly
  - Portal/splenic vein thrombosis
  - Acute fatty liver

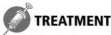 TREATMENT

PRE-HOSPITAL
Therapy aims to prevent and treat the complications of cirrhosis.
Diet
- Sodium restriction: 2,000 mg per day (88 mmol per day)

- Nutritious balanced diet
  - Restrict proteins only in the presence of hepatic encephalopathy: 1–1.5 g of protein/kg/day (vegetable or dietary proteins better than animal).
    - Oral branched amino acids are a better tolerated source of proteins.
    - Zinc supplementation

IV Fluids
- Fluid challenge is used for hepatorenal syndrome to correct intravascular depletion.
- IV fluids should be used with caution: rapid volume expansion may cause variceal bleeding and worsen ascites.

 MEDICATION (DRUGS)

- Ascites:
  - Oral diuretics: Antialdosterone diuretics (Spironoloactone or Potassium Canreonate) and loop diuretic (furosemide) beginning with 100 mg/day of the former and adding 40 mg/day of the latter to a maximum of 400 mg/day of spironolactone/canreonate and 160 mg/day of furosemide.
  - Monitor response by daily weight: 1 lb/day in patients without peripheral edema and 2 lb/day in patients with edema.
  - Paracentesis is indicated in patients with:
    - Tense or refractory ascites: Large volume ($\geq$4 L), consider albumin infusion of 8–10 g per L of fluid removed.
    - To rule out spontaneous bacterial peritonitis (SBP); on ascitic fluids perform: Cell count, total protein, serum-ascites albumin gradient (SAAG $\geq$1.1 g/dL in ascites is due to portal hypertension), fluid culture.
    - SBP diagnosis—PMN count $\geq$250 cells/mm^3 and/or positive fluid culture. Treat with appropriate antibiotics.
- Hepatic Encephalopathy
  - Remove precipitating conditions (gastrointestinal hemorrhage, infections, constipation, renal failure, and excessive dietary protein).
  - Catharsis
    - Nonabsorbable disaccharides (lactulose) administrated by mouth, enemas or naso-gastric tube)
  - Nonabsorbed oral antibiotics (rifaximine)
- Esophageal varices
  - Primary prevention of bleeding (indicated in presence of medium and large varices)
    - Nonselective beta-blockers (propranolol)
    - Endoscopic variceal ligation (EVL)
  - Secondary prevention (patient with previous history of variceal bleeding)
    - Eradicate varices with ELV (Endoscopic sclerotherapy if EVL is not available)
    - Beta-blockers
  - Acute bleeding:
    - Hemodynamic stabilization
    - Endoscopy with EVL or sclerotherapy
    - Drugs: Teripressin, Glypressin (both synthetic analogues of Vasopressin), Vasopressin associated with nitroglycerine, Octreotide.
    - Uncontrolled bleeding: Transjugular intrahepatic portosystemic shunt (TIPSS) or surgical shunt

SURGERY
- Liver transplantation is indicated for patients < age 70 with decompensated liver disease and absence of comorbidity.
- Sobriety for a period of 3–6 months is required.

- Allocation of organs is performed nation-wide according to a international score system (MELD), a severity index to predict short-term mortality.
- Transplantation is the only curative treatment.
- Shortage of cadaveric livers is a limiting factor. Currently many centers offer transplant from living donors and split organs technique.

Pregnancy Considerations
- Compensated cirrhosis is no longer a contraindication to pregnancy.
- Worsening of cholestasis may occur.
- Upper endoscopy should be performed in the first trimester to treat varices with EVL. There is a high risk of bleeding during the third stage of delivery.
- Cesarean section should be performed with caution, correct coagulopathy with fresh frozen plasma, and platelets.
- Antibiotic therapy is recommended to avoid bacterial peritonitis.
- Successful pregnancy has been reported after liver transplant.

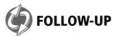 FOLLOW-UP

Admission Criteria
Refractory ascites, spontaneous bacterial peritonitis, encephalopathy, progressive liver failure

Discharge Criteria
Achieved stabilization and/ or liver transplant evaluation

Issues for Referral
- Refer the patients to a hepatologist for initial diagnosis and management
- Refer decompensated patients for liver transplant evaluation

PROGNOSIS
- Compensated cirrhosis: median survival 7 to 10 years from diagnosis
- Decompensated cirrhosis: 2 year survival rate is 50%. Death occurs from progressive liver failure, hepatocellular carcinoma, gastrointestinal bleeding, sepsis and renal failure.

COMPLICATIONS
Occurrence per year
- Ascites: 5% per year
- Hepatic encephalopathy: 6% per year

- Esophageal varices: 4–12% per year
- Hepatocelluar carcinoma: 1–6% per year

PATIENT MONITORING
- Monitor well compensated patient yearly for disease progression
- Monitor every 6 months for HCC: alpha-fetoprotein and liver ultrasound
- Endoscopy for gastroesophageal varices:
  – No gastroesophageal varices: re-endoscopy every 3 years
  – Varices Grade I: re-endoscopy after 1 year
  – Varices Grade II-III: prophylaxis (see above)
  – Monitor every 3 years for recurrence of treated varices

REFERENCES

1. Talwalkar JA, Kamath PS. Influence of recent advances in medical management on clinical outcomes of cirrhosis. *Mayo Clin Proc*. 2005;80:1501–1508.
2. Runyon BA. Practice Guidelines Committee, American Association for the Study of Liver Diseases (AASLD). Management of adult patients with ascites due to cirrhosis. *Hepatology*. 2004;39:841–856.
3. Blei AT, Cordoba J. Practice Parameters Committee of the American College of Gastroenterology. Hepatic encephalopathy. *Am J Gastroenterol*. 2001:96:1968–1976.
4. Bruix J, Sherman M. Practice Guidelines Committee, American Association for the Study of Liver Diseases. Management of hepatocellular carcinoma. *Hepatology*. 2005;42:1208–1236.
5. Jalan R, Hayes PC. UK guidelines on the management of varcieal haemorrhage in cirrhotic patients. British Society of Gastroenterology. *Gut*. 2000;46:1–II

CODES
ICD9-CM
- 571.5 Cirrhosis of the liver without mention alcohol
- 789.5 Ascites
- 456.0 Esophageal varices with bleeding

KEY WORDS
- Cirrhosis
- Chronic Liver Disease

C

COLON CANCER

Christy L. Dibble, DO

KEY CLINICAL POINTS

- Colorectal cancer (CRC) is the 3rd most commonly diagnosed cancer and the 2nd leading cause of cancer death in the United States.
- Colonoscopy is an excellent screening and diagnostic test for CRC.
- Routine colon cancer screening among women and minorities remains a challenge.

 BASICS

DESCRIPTION

- CRC is the 3rd most commonly diagnosed cancer in the United States.
- It is the second leading cause of cancer death in the United States.

GENERAL PREVENTION

- Dietary/environmental considerations for prevention.
  - Limit red meat, increase fiber and vegetables in diet.
  - Avoid excessive alcohol or tobacco use.
  - Avoid obesity and a sedentary lifestyle.
- Adherence to a CRC cancer screening program is a high priority clinical preventative service due to the aging of the American population and the increased incidence of CRC in patients aged over 50 years.
  - Early detection increases probability of cure and options of less invasive treatment, e.g., polypectomy.
  - Clinical trials, research, and technology advances constantly expand the evidence-base for national screening recommendations.
  - Translating national standards for CRC screening into actual high screening rates remains a challenge, particularly for women and minorities.
- CRC screening—determine risk stratification
  - Average risk (Absence of 1st-degree relative under 65 with colon cancer or adenomatous polyp): begin screening at age 50 with:
    - Fecal occult blood test (FOBT) annually, and /or sigmoidoscopy every 5 years *or*
    - Colonoscopy every 10 years *or*
    - Double contrast barium enema every 5–10 years
  - Increased risk:
    - Screening colonoscopy at 40 years or
    - 10 years younger than index case and repeat every 5 years
    - Groups at increased risk include:
      - Family history: 1 or more 1st degree relatives with CRC or adenomatous polyp < age 65
      - Personal history of inflammatory bowel disease
      - Personal history of prior colorectal cancer or adenomatous polyp
  - Family history suggestive of genetic syndrome (Familial adenomatous polyposis or hereditary nonpolyposis CRC)
    - Initiate screening pertinent to the particular syndrome.
  - Initiate CRC screening in African American's at 45 based upon increased risk of earlier CRC and increased CRC morbidity and mortality.
- Current concepts to facilitate CRC screening in women and minorities:

  - Shared decision making recognizes patient values and personal choices to promote motivation and greater satisfaction with cancer screening.
  - Consider cultural factors that may influence patient values.
  - Recognize role of socioeconomic factors affecting accessibility of screening to avoid disparities in screenings:
    - Recommend colonoscopy every 10 years rather than annual FOBT to increase adherence in groups with cultural barriers to care.
  - Women illustrate more pure right-sided polyps, lesions that would be missed on sigmoidoscopy.
  - Lack of female endoscopists result in barriers to screening.
  - Based on prospective study 90% of women illustrated gender preference for screening colonoscopy and were willing to wait until female endoscopist available—attitudes remained unchanged after procedure.
  - Colonoscopy completion rate lower in women than men—81.6% versus 88.9%, respectively.
  - Cecal intubation prolonged by female gender
    - Contributing factors
      - BMI <28
      - Constipation/laxative use
      - Prior abdominal-pelvic surgery
      - Lower annual endoscopist case volume

EPIDEMIOLOGY

Incidence

- CRC is a common disease.
- Approximately 145,290 new cases diagnosed yearly in the United States.
- In 2005, greater than 56,000 Americans died of CRC.
- Higher incidence and mortality of CRC in African Americans than in whites or any other racial or ethnic group.
- Among women, CRC screening rates are still relatively low (30–40%) and are comparable to mammography rates 20 years ago.
- Although good evidence-based screening technologies are available for CRC screening, decision making is complicated by the availability of more than one option.

RISK FACTORS

- Low fiber diet
- Alcohol
- Tobacco
- Obesity/sedentary lifestyle
- Family history of colon cancer or adenomatous polyp prior to age 65
- Personal history of prior colorectal cancer or adenomatous polyp
- Personal history of inflammatory bowel disease
- Family history of genetic syndrome
  - Familial adenomatous polyposis
  - Hereditary nonpolyposis

Genetics

- Sporadic CRC-adenomatous polyp to carcinoma paradigm.
- Hereditary nonpolyposis colorectal cancer-germ line mutations in MLH and MSH genes, usually associated with microsatellite instability (MSI)
- Familial adenomatous polyposis (FAP)-mutations in the adenomatous polyposis coli gene.

PATHOPHYSIOLOGY
- Progression of normal colon lining to an adenoma or polyp and eventually to carcinoma.
- Progression occurs at the genetic level with accumulation of DNA mutations in colonic cells.

ETIOLOGY
- Inherited mutations combined with environmental/lifestyle factors give rise to most cases of familial CRC.
- Some inherited mutations cause highly penetrant syndromes with extreme CRC risk, such as those associated with hereditary nonpolyposis colorectal cancer (HNPCC) and familial adenomatous polyposis.

ASSOCIATED CONDITION

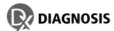 **DIAGNOSIS**

SIGNS AND SYMPTOMS
CRC may be asymptomatic and discovered during routine screening of average and high risk subjects.

History
- Abdominal pain
- Change in bowel habit
- Hematochezia or melena
- Weakness
- Anemia
- Weight loss
- Intestinal obstruction and/or perforation.
- Rare presentations include local invasion, contained perforation, abscess, or fistulization to surrounding organ.

Physical Exam
- Palpable mass on abdominal exam, infrequently.
- Presence of ascites
- Hepatomegaly
- Lymphaderypathy
- FOBT positive stool or palpable rectal mass or "shelf" on digital rectal exam.

TESTS
The fecal occult blood test can be used for screening in certain individuals.

Lab
- CBC
  - Iron deficient anemia may or may not be present.
- Serum CEA often used for staging (see below)

Imaging
- Imaging modalities are used for clinical stating once a diagnosis of CRC is established.
- Local and distant extent of disease needs to be determined.
  - CXR
  - CT scan of abdomen and pelvis

Diagnostic Procedures/Surgery
- Colonoscopy:
  - Majority of CRC are endoluminal adenocarcinomas that arise from a polyp in the mucosa.
  - Colonoscopy is the single best diagnostic test since it can localize lesions, biopsy mass lesions, detect synchronous neoplasms, and remove polyps.
- Barium enema:
  - Of patients with CRC, 5–10% may require the addition of a barium enema if colonoscopy cannot be completed.
  - Barium enema will rule out synchronous lesions in the colon.

- Tissue biopsy
  - A histologic examination of the resected specimen is required for the pathological staging of cancer.

Pathologic Findings
Most colon cancers arise from adenomatous polyps and will illustrate adenocarcinomas.

DIFFERENTIAL DIAGNOSIS
- Majority of CRC are adenocarcinomas.
- The differential diagnosis of a colon mass include:
  - Kaposi's sarcoma
  - Lymphoma
  - Carcinoid tumors
  - Metastases from other primary cancers, such as ovarian

 TREATMENT

GENERAL MEASURES
- Surgery is the mainstay of treatment
- Adjuvant chemotherapy is indicated in advanced or node-positive cases
- See the Prognosis Section for staging.

 MEDICATION (DRUGS)

Chemotherapy:
- 5 FU-Leucovorin or a FOLFOX-like regimen
  - Advanced lesions, T3 or above
  - Node positive CRC
- Combination regimens including irinotecan, oxaliplatin, and capecitabine may become standard adjuvant therapy.

SURGERY
Surgical resection is the primary treatment for CRC and the outcome is closely related to extent of disease at presentation.

 FOLLOW-UP

Issues for Referral
- To gastroenterology for routine screening colonoscopy or for diagnostic colonoscopy in individuals with signs and symptoms consistent with CRC
- To colorectal surgeon for patients with diagnosis of CRC

PROGNOSIS
- Pathologic stage at diagnosis remains best indicator for both colon and rectal cancer.
- Important characteristics:
  - presence of distant metastases
  - local tumor extent
  - nodal positivity
  - residual disease
- 5-year survival statistics
  - Dukes A or $T_1N_0M_0$ (Stage I)
    - If limited to submucosa: >90%
  - Dukes B or $T_2N_0M_0$ (Stage I)
    - If within bowel wall: 85%
  - Dukes B_2 or $T_{3-4}N_0M_0$ (Stage II)
    - If it extends through wall but no nodes: 70–75%
  - Dukes C, or $T_2N_1M_0$/Dukes C_2 or $T_3N_1M_0$ (Stage III)
    - If lymph nodes involved: 35–65%
  - Dukes D or $T_xN_xM_1$ (Stage IV)
    - If distant metastases (e.g. liver, lung): <5%

COMPLICATIONS
- Metastatic disease
  - Approximately 15% to 20% have distant metastatic disease at the time of the presentation.
  - Can spread by lymphatic, hematogenous, contiguous, or transperitoneal routes
  - Most common sites of metastasis:
    - Regional lymph nodes
    - Liver
    - Lungs
    - Peritoneum
- Intestinal obstruction

PATIENT MONITORING
- History and physical:
  - Every 3 months for 2 years then
  - Every 6 months for a total of 5 years, then
  - Annually for 5–10 years.
- CEA:
  - Every 3 months for 2 years then
  - Every 6 months for T2 or greater lesions for 5–10 years
- Colonoscopy:
  - After 1 year, repeat in 1 year if abnormal, or 3 years if normal
  - Repeat colonoscopy every 3–5 years

REFERENCES

1. Jenal A, Murray T, Ward W, et al. Cancer statistics, 2005. *CA Cancer Journal Clinic.* 2005;55:10.
2. Agrawal S, Bhupinderjil A, Bhutani MS, et al. Colorectal cancer in African Americans. *Am J Gastroenterol.* 2005;100:515–523.
3. Rise LAG, Eisner MP, Kosary CL, et al. Seer cancer statistics review, 1975–2000. Bethesda, MD: National Cancer Institute; 2003. Available at: http://seer.cancer.gov/cst1975–2000.
4. Morrin MM, Farrell RJ, Raptopulos V, et al. Role of virtual computed tomographic colonoscopy in patients with colorectal cancers and obstructing colorectal lesions. *Disease of Colon and Rectum.* 2000;43:303.

CODES
ICD9-CM
- 153.9 Malignant neosplasm of the colon, unspecified
- V12.72 Colonic polyps

KEY WORDS
- Colorectal Cancer
- Colon Cancer
- Colonic Polyp

CONSTIPATION

Rohini McKee, MD
Homayoon M. Akbari, MD, PhD, FRCS(C)

KEY CLINICAL POINTS

- Despite high prevalence, very few patients have life-altering constipation.
- It is important to rule out a structural cause, especially in the older population.
- The majority of patients can be managed with simple alterations in diet and medication.
- Surgical therapy is appropriate for carefully selected patients with slow transit constipation after correction of other contributory factors.

 BASICS

DESCRIPTION
Constipation is present when two or more of the following exist for at least 12 weeks in the past 12 months (Rome II criteria):
- <3 bowel movements a week
- Straining >25% of the time
- Incomplete evacuation or anorectal blockage >25% of the time
- Hard stools >25% of the time
- Manual maneuvers to facilitate defecation >25% of the time

GENERAL PREVENTION
- Increase dietary fiber and fluid intake
- Avoid delaying bowel movements when urge present
- Increase physical activity

EPIDEMIOLOGY
- More common in women and African-Americans
- More common in older individuals
- Constipation is responsible for up to 2 million physician visits per year in United States.

Prevalence
- Prevalence of 2% in the general population
- Prevalence of 25% in individuals >60 years

RISK FACTORS
- Low fiber diet
- Inadequate fluid intake/dehydration
- Lack of exercise/inactivity
- Endocrine/electrolyte abnormalities
- Laxative abuse
- Low socioeconomic status

PATHOPHYSIOLOGY
- Visceral neuropathy in patients with slow-transit constipation; degeneration of myenteric plexus
- Congenital or acquired colonic myopathy: Pseudo-obstruction/megacolon
- Congenital aganglionosis/hypoganglionosis: Hirschsprung disease
- Disorders of pelvic floor
  - Rectocele
  - Rectal prolapse/intrarectal mucosal prolapse
  - Descending perineum syndrome

ETIOLOGY
- Extracolonic:
  - Endocrine and metabolic disorders:
    - Diabetes mellitus
    - Hypercalcemeia, hypokalemia
    - Hypothyroidism
    - Pregnancy
    - Uremia
  - Neurologic disorders:
    - Cerebrovascular accident
    - Multiple sclerosis
    - Parkinsons disease
  - Collagen vascular and muscle disorders:
    - Scleroderma
    - Amyloidosis
    - Myotonic dystrophy
  - Drugs:
    - Anticonvulsants
    - Calcium channel blockers
    - Opiates
- Colonic
  - Structural
    - Stricture (diverticular, Crohn's, ischemic)
    - Carcinoma or large polyp
    - Hirschsprung's disease
    - Rectal prolapse or rectocele
    - Descending perineum syndrome
  - Colonic inertia:
    - Slow transit constipation
    - Intestinal pseudo-obstrustion (Ogilvie's syndrome)
    - Irritable bowel syndrome

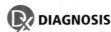 **DIAGNOSIS**

SIGNS AND SYMPTOMS
- Abdominal distention
- Bloating
- Abdominal pain
- Hard bowel movements

History
- Age of onset
  - Young age of onset more consistent with congenital abnormality
  - More recent age of onset may indicate colorectal structural pathology
- Laxative and enema use: Type, frequency
- Bowel diary of frequency, consistency of stool
- Abdominal pain, bloating between bowel movements
- History of straining with bowel movements
- Sensation of incomplete evacuation

Physical Exam
- The abdominal exam is usually normal.
  - A stool-filled colon may be palpated.
  - Diffuse abdominal tenderness may be present.
- The anorectal exam may reveal a rectal mass, rectocele, or stool-filled rectum.
- The anal exam may also reveal associated pathology: hemorrhoids, anal fissure.

TESTS
Lab
- Thyroid function tests
- Electrolytes, including calcium, BUN

Imaging
- Plain radiograph of abdomen
- Colonoscopy or barium enema
- Colonic transit marker study:
  - Ingestion of radioopaque markers on day 0
  - 80% should be eliminated by day 5
  - All should be passed by day 7
- Defecography to evaluate disorders of defecation and pelvic floor dysfunction
- Anorectal manometry to evaluate neurogenic causes, such as Hirschsprung's disease or obstructed defecation
- Small bowel transit study to exclude pan-intestinal dysmotility

Diagnostic Procedures/Surgery
Rectal biopsy if abnormal manometry/defecography indicates possible aganglionic segment

 TREATMENT
GENERAL MEASURES
- Limit constipating medications
- Increase physical activity
- Improve dietary habits, particularly in patients with suspected eating disorders

Diet
- Increase dietary fiber to 25–30 g per day.
- Increase fluid intake (at least 8 glasses of noncaffeinated beverage per day).

Activity
Increase activity/exercise:
- Many patients report improvement in bowel function with walking 20 minutes per day.

Complementary and Alternative Medicine
- Acupuncture in patients with irritable bowel symptoms (bloating, abdominal pain with constipation)
- Chinese herbal medicines

 MEDICATION (DRUGS)
First Line
Bulk laxatives:
- Psyllium
- Methylcellulose: Less bloating and flatulence than psyllium preparations

Second Line
- Stool softeners
  - Docusate
- Osmotic laxatives
  - Magnesium hydroxide
  - Magnesium citrate
  - Polyethylene glycol
  - Sodium biphosphate
  - Lactulose
- Stimulant laxatives
  - Bisacodyl
  - Cascara
  - Senna
  - Castor oil
- Prokinetics
  - Tegasorod
    - 5HT4 receptor agonist
    - Approved for constipation predominant irritable bowel syndrome

Pregnancy Considerations
Bisacodyl and senna are safe in pregnancy.

SURGERY
- Surgical repair of rectocele or pelvic organ prolapse (i.e., rectal prolapse, sigmoidocele, enterocele) if defecography consistent with obstructed defecation
- Total abdominal colectomy with either ileorectal or ileosigmoid anastamosis if radiographic and physiologic studies consistent with a diagnosis of slow transit constipation/colonic inertia

 FOLLOW-UP
Issues for Referral
- Gastroenterology to evaluate for structural cause with colonoscopy; initial evaluation of functional constipation
- Colorectal surgeon if surgically correctable cause found on testing

PROGNOSIS
- Most of the patients (80–90%) have improvement in the frequency of their bowel movements following total abdominal colectomy for colonic inertia.
- Abdominal bloating and distention may persist in many patients after total abdominal colectomy.

COMPLICATIONS
- Diarrhea and incontinence following total abdominal colectomy seen in 15–20% of patients.
- There is a high incidence of adhesive disease.
- Patients with pelvic outlet obstruction and colonic inertia may require an ileostomy for continued constipation following colectomy.

REFERENCES

1. Locke GR, Pemberton JH, Phillips SF. AGA Technical review on constipation. *Gastroenterol*. 2000;119:1161–1178.
2. Rao SC. Constipation: Evaluation and treatment. *Gastroenterology Clinics*. 2003;32:659–683.
3. Young-Fadok TM, Pemberton JH. Constipation. In: Fazio VW, ed. *Current Therapy in Colon and Rectal Surgery*. 2nd ed. Elsevier Mosby; 2005.

ADDITIONAL READING

Piccirillo MF, Reissman P, Wexner SD. Colectomy as treatment for constipation in selected patients. *Dis Colon Rectum*. 1997;40:273–279.
Thompson WG, Longstreth GF, Drossman DA, et al. Functional bowel disorders and functional abdominal pain. *Gut*. 1999;45:1143–1147.

CODES
ICD9-CM
- 564.00 Constipation, unspecified
- 564.01 Slow transit constipation
- 564.02 Outlet dysfunction constipation
- 564.1 Irritable bowel syndrome

KEY WORDS

- Constipation
- Laxatives

CHRONIC OBSTRUCTIVE PULMONARY DISEASE (COPD)

Ghada Bourjeily, MD
Nadia Chammas, MD

KEY CLINICAL POINTS

- Chronic obstructive pulmonary disease (COPD) is diagnosed by a postbronchodilator forced expiratory volume in 1 second/forced vital capacity <70%.
- Smoking cessation and long-term oxygen therapy in patients that qualify improves mortality.
- Bronchodilators improve dyspnea, exercise tolerance, and quality of life.
- Steroid inhalers reduce the rate of exacerbations and may improve lung function in a select patient population.
- Pulmonary rehabilitation should be considered in patients with moderate to severe COPD.

 ## BASICS

DESCRIPTION

- COPD is a chronic disorder characterized by irreversible or partially reversible airway obstruction.
- It is closely associated with smoking, which is an addiction and a relapsing disorder.

EPIDEMIOLOGY

- COPD is the fourth leading cause of mortality in the United States and Europe.
- Mortality has doubled in women in the last 20 years.
- In the United States, the estimated prevalence of mild COPD was 6.9% and of moderate COPD was 6.6%, according to the National Health and Nutrition Examination Survey (NHANES).

RISK FACTORS

The most common risk factor is smoking; other less common risk factors include:

- Environmental exposure to dusts and organic antigens
- Airway hyper-responsiveness and allergic phenotype
- Genetic predisposition
- Recurrent respiratory infections in childhood
- Antioxidant deficiencies and molecular risk factors

PATHOPHYSIOLOGY AND PHYSIOLOGY

- A Th-1 dominated response is prominent and leads to the production of interferon gamma and tumor necrosis factor, which are thought to contribute to the pathogenesis.
- Mucous hypersecretion and ciliary dysfunction are consequences of the inflammatory response described above.
- In addition to the spirometric changes described above, pulmonary function tests can show evidence of hyperinflation and gas trapping evidenced by an increase in total lung capacity (TLC), residual volume (RV), and the ratio of RV/TLC as well as a reduction in the inspiratory capacity (IC).
- An increase in airway resistance (Raw) can also be observed.
- Impairment in gas exchange is usually seen in the later stages of COPD and is seen as a reduction in DLCO and hypoxemia; in severe disease, hypercapnia ensues.

- Women may be more predisposed to the development of COPD, in part because of their smaller airway size and their increased susceptibility to tobacco smoke.

 ## DIAGNOSIS

History

- The diagnosis of COPD should be considered in any patient with a chronic cough, sputum production, or dyspnea, especially if there is a history of exposure to cigarette smoking or air pollutants.
- Dyspnea is a prominent symptom in women, whereas sputum production is more prominent in men.
- Women are often diagnosed later in life and only after more prominent symptoms develop compared with men.

SIGNS AND SYMPTOMS

The physical examination of patients with early COPD can be deceivingly normal.

- As the disease progresses, tachypnea with a prolonged expiratory phase, wheezing, and rhonchi are found on the lung exam.
- An increase in the antero-posterior diameter of the chest occurs, as well as diaphragmatic depression
- Auscultation can reveal a prominent S2 as well as neck vein distention, hepatojugular reflux, and lower extremity edema, all suggesting right ventricular dysfunction.
- During exacerbations, patients may use their accessory muscles and show flaring of the nostrils depending upon the severity of the attacks.
- Systemic manifestations of COPD include skeletal muscle dysfunction, weight loss, and anorexia. Patients with COPD are also thought to be at higher risk for osteoporosis and cardiovascular disease.

TESTS

The diagnosis is established by demonstrating an irreversible or partially reversible airway obstruction.

- This requires a spirometry showing a postbronchodilator forced expiratory volume in second (FEV1)/forced vital capacity (FVC) <70%. The lack of full reversibility is suggestive of COPD.

Lab

- Alpha-1 anti-trypsin deficiency should be considered in those patients that present with irreversible airway obstruction at an early age and especially if a family history of COPD is present.
- Arterial blood gases may range from normal in early stages of COPD to variable degrees of hypoxemia and hypercapnia as the disease progresses.

Imaging

- Chest radiographs may show evidence of hyperinflation or bullous disease but these findings are not diagnostic of COPD.

DIFFERENTIAL DIAGNOSIS

- Differential diagnosis of COPD includes:
  - Asthma, pulmonary embolism, bronchiectasis, recurrent aspiration

Table 1 Therapy at Each Stage of COPD						
Old	O: At Risk	I: Mild	II: Moderate		III: Severe	
			IIA	IIB		
New	O: At Risk	I: Mild	II: Moderate	III: Severe	IV: Very Severe	
Characteristics	• Chronic symptoms • Exposure to risk factors • Normal spirometry	• FEV_1/FVC <70% • FEV_1 ≤80% • With or without symptoms	• FEV_1/FVC <70% • 50% ≤FEV_1 <80% • With or without symptoms	• FEV_1/FVC <70% • 30% ≤ FEV_1 <60% • With or without symptoms	• FEV_1/FVC <70% • FEV_1 <30% or FEV_1 <50% • predicted plus chronic respiratory failure	
		Avoidance of risk factor(s); Influenza vaccination				
			Add Short-acting bronchodilator when needed			
				Add regular treatment with one or more long-acting bronchodilators *Add* rehabilitation		
					Add Inhaled glucorticosteroids if repeated exacerbations	
						Add long-term oxygen if chronic respiratory failure *Consider* surgical treatments

— Cardiac disease, such as angina and heart failure, should be considered in heavy smokers with dyspnea on exertion.

• Different stages of COPD have been elucidated. The classification set forth by the Global Initiative for Chronic Obstructive Pulmonary Disease helps in directing therapy and is shown in Table 1.

LONG TERM MANGEMENT OF COPD

SMOKING CESSATION

• It is the most important step in the management of symptomatic and asymptomatic patients with COPD.
• Cessation of smoking at any age is associated with a reduction in the rate of decline of lung function and prolongs survival.
• A stepwise approach has been suggested by the Global Initiative for Chronic Obstructive Pulmonary Disease and is shown in Table 1.
• This requires systematic identification of smoking habits at every visit and a strong personalized recommendation to quit.
• Willingness needs to be assessed on every patient periodically and help offered to assist in counseling, support, and in recommending appropriate pharmacotherapy.
• Women have a greater difficulty sustaining from tobacco than men.
• Women with COPD who became sustained quitters in the lung health study had a 2.5 times greater improvement in their FEV1 % predicted compared with men.

BRONCHODILATORS

• These include beta agonists, anticholinergics, and methylxanthines

• There is often a greater improvement in symptoms than one would expect given the minimal improvement in FEV1 with these medications. Bronchodilators also produce a reduction in residual volume and a delay in the onset of dynamic hyperinflation.
• Short-acting beta agonists help reduce symptoms and improve exercise tolerance acutely.
• Long-acting beta agonists reduce symptoms, reduce the need for rescue medications, and increase the time between exacerbations.
• Short-acting anticholinergics alleviate dyspnea, improve exercise tolerance, improve FEV1, and the quality of life.
• Combination beta agonists/anticholinergics produce a greater improvement than either agent alone.
• The 1 available long-acting anticholinergic in the United States, Tiotropium, reduces exacerbations and the rate of hospitalizations.
• Methylxanthines are weak bronchodilators, but have mild anti-inflammatory properties.

ANTI-INFLAMMATORIES

• Inhaled corticosteroids have been shown to reduce the number of exacerbations.
• They are recommended in patients with COPD with an FEV1 <50%.
• Inhaled steroids are also beneficial in patients with a significant bronchodilator response on spirometry.
• Oral corticosteroids have little proven benefit if used chronically in patients with COPD except in a very select patient population. There is no set criterion that predicts those who would benefit from chronic steroids; however, those that exacerbate every

time they are taken off steroids despite maximal therapy and those with a history of asthma prior to COPD might require long-term steroids.

- Corticosteroids are beneficial in the treatment of acute exacerbations.
- Combination inhalers improve compliance with medications, but have less dosing flexibility.

NONPHARMACOLOGIC THERAPY

- Long-term oxygen therapy
  - The need for long-term oxygen therapy should be assessed under stable conditions.
  - Has been shown to improve survival, exercise tolerance, sleep quality, and cognitive abilities
- Noninvasive mechanical ventilation
  - Can be used in the setting of acute hypercapnic respiratory failure
  - Has been shown to improve quality of life, slightly reduce daytime $PaCO_2$ in patients with severe COPD and chronic respiratory failure
  - It can be considered in select patients. Patients with hypercapneic and hypoxic failure as well as patients with a history of sleep apnea may benefit form bi-level positive pressure.
- Nutritional assessment and intervention should be periodically performed in every patient with COPD because low body mass index (BMI) is associated with increased mortality.
- Pulmonary rehabilitation, a multidisciplinary approach aimed at improving muscle performance of both the upper and lower extremities and increasing exercise tolerance
  - Has been shown to reduce the rate of hospitalizations
  - Adjuncts are now available for exercise training, such as transcutaneous electrical neuromuscular stimulation to the lower extremities, and were shown to improve exercise tolerance.

SURGICAL TREATMENT OF COPD

- Bullectomy, lung volume reduction surgery, and lung transplantation have been shown to improve symptoms, lung volumes, and exercise capacity in a highly selective patient population.
- Clinical trials are now being performed to attempt endoscopic lung volume reduction.
- End of life issues need to be addressed in patients with severe disease, preferably as an outpatient in a stable environment.

MANAGEMENT OF ACUTE EXACERBATIONS OF COPD

- The management of acute exacerbations of COPD involves the identification of and treatment of the underlying cause of the exacerbation, bronchodilation, adequate oxygenation, and avoiding intubation and mechanical ventilation.
- Definite criteria for hospitalization include acute respiratory acidemia and hypoxemia. Other criteria include significant comorbidities, failure to respond to initial treatment, diagnostic uncertainty, older age, marked intensity of symptoms, and severe background disease.

- Pharmacologic therapy should include:
  - Short-acting beta agonists, either by MDI or nebulizers. There is no benefit to continuous therapy or doubling the nebulizer dose.
  - Short-acting anticholinergic, Ipratropium, adds to the bronchodilator effects of Albuterol and may be administered vianebulizer or MDI every 2–4 hours.
  - Systemic corticosteroids, usually parenterally. Initial doses of 80 to 125 mg of methylprednisolone or equivalent are recommended 2–4 times daily. There have been studies showing that oral regimens have resulted in the same reduction in hospital stay as parenteral regimens.
  - If sputum is purulent or abundant, antibiotics help to accelerate the improvement in lung function.
  - Methylxanthines have no benefit in the treatment of acute exacerbations.
  - Oxygen therapy should be administered to ensure adequate oxygenation (oxygen saturation of 90% or above) even if it results in hypercapnia. Venturi masks are preferred given that FiO_2 is better controlled.
  - In the event of hypercapnic respiratory failure, noninvasive ventilation may be used prior to intubation and invasive mechanical ventilation.
  - Nutritional assessment should be done during acute exacerbations given that patients are in a negative nitrogen balance during exacerbations and high carbohydrate diets may increase the risk of hypercapnia.

Patients with chronic respiratory failure and COPD should certainly be seen by a pulmonologist. ATS recommends stage II and III be referred.

REFERENCES

1. Chapman KR. Chronic obstructive pulmonary disease: are women more susceptible than men? *Clin Chest Med*. 2004:25:331–341.
2. Agusti A. Systemic effects of chronic obstructive pulmonary disease. Proceedings of the American Thoracic Society. 2005;2:367–370.
3. Pauwels RA, Buist AS, Calverley PM, et al. Global strategy for the diagnosis, management, and prevention of chronic obstructive pulmonary disease. NHLBI/WHO Global Initiative for the Chronic Obstructive Lung Disease (GOLD) workshop summary. *AM J Respir Crit Care Med*. 2001;163:1256–1276.
4. ATS/ERS summary: Standards for the diagnosis and treatment of patients with COPD. *Eur Respir J*. 2004;23:932.
5. Scanlon PD, Connell JE, Waller LA, et al. Smoking cessation and lung function in mild to moderate chronic obstructive lung disease. *Am J Respir Crit Care Med*. 2000;161:381–390.
6. Bourjeily G, Rochester CL. Exercise training in chronic obstructive pulmonary disease. *Clinics in Chest Med*. 2000;21:763–781.
7. Bourjeily-Habr G, Rochester CL, Palermo F, et al. Randomized controlled trial of transcutaneous electrical muscle stimulation of the lower extremities in patients with chronic obstructive pulmonary disease. *Thorax*. 2002;57:1045–1049.

C

ADDITIONAL READING

Becklake MR, Kaufman F. Gender difference in airway behavior over the human lifespan. *Thorax*. 1999;54:1119–1138.

Proceedings of the American Thoracic Society. 2005;2:257–394.

KEY WORDS

- COPD
- Airway Obstruction
- Dyspnea

CORONARY DISEASE

Anne W. Moulton, MD

KEY CLINICAL POINTS

- Coronary heart disease (CHD) is the leading cause of death in women of all ages.
- CHD is a disease of older women.
- CHD is more common in certain racial and ethnic minorities (African Americans, Native Americans).
- Gender differences exist in presentation, evaluation, pathophysiology, and treatment.
- Women are still underrepresented in studies of the evaluation and treatment of CHD.

 BASICS

DESCRIPTION
- CHD is defined by the presence of atherosclerosis in the epicardial coronary arteries.
- Atherosclerosis forms plaque in coronary vessels, which progressively impairs myocardial blood flow.
  - Plaque in women more likely to be distributed diffusely without areas of critical stenosis
- The reduction in flow may be asymptomatic or symptomatic:
  - Angina: 70% to 80% stenosis.
  - Acute CHD (includes unstable angina, MI, sudden death) usually caused by rupture of plaque with less than 50% stenosis

EPIDEMIOLOGY
- Women develop CHD 10–15 years later than men, so they are at lower CHD risk until the 7th decade.
- Women with newly diagnosed CHD are more likely to present with angina, followed by MI, and least often, sudden death.
- Women are more likely to have silent MI.

Incidence
- The lifetime risk for women age 40 is 32% (49% in men).
- Even women free from disease at age 70 have a lifetime risk of 24% (35% in men).
- 250,000 CHD-related deaths in women/year

RISK FACTORS (RF)
- Individual risk factors are less predictive of CHD in women than men.
- Strongest predictors in women: Diabetes and low HDL cholesterol.

Strongest Risk/Well Established
- Diabetes:*
  - Stronger predictor of CHD risk and prognosis in women than men
- Smoking:
  - Associated with 50% of all coronary events in women
  - Risk elevated even with minimal use (1–4 cigs/day)
  - Increased risk in CHD with increasing levels of glucose intolerance
- Elevated cholesterol:
  - Low HDL more important than high LDL in women
  - Best estimate of risk in women: total to HDL cholesterol ratio
- Hypertension:
  - Most common risk factor for CHD in women
- Family history premature CHD (1st-degree male relative < the age of 55 or female relative < the age of 65)

- Peripheral vascular disease*
- Chronic kidney disease.*

Moderate Risk
- Hormones:
  - Low endogenous estrogen levels noted in premenopausal women presenting with signs and symptoms of CHD
  - Increase risk of CHD in post menopausal women (Women's Health Initiative)
  - Very small increased risk in young women on oral contraceptives
- Elevated triglycerides:
  - Significant risk factor in women only
- Obesity
- Sedentary lifestyle
- Metabolic syndrome: Consists of
  - Central obesity (waist >40 inches)
  - Glucose intolerance (FBS >110 mg/dL)
  - Elevated fasting triglycerides (>150 mg/dL)
  - Low serum HDL (<40 mg/dL)
  - Elevated blood pressure (>130/85)

Other Risk Factors/Less Data Available
- Psychosocial (stress, depression, anxiety)
- Markers of inflammation: CRP, WBC serum amyloid A
- Hemostatic factors: Fibrinogen, Factor V Leiden
- Homocysteine
- Microalbuminuria

Assessing Pre-Test Risk
Framingham Risk Score (FRS) most useful to date:
Incorporates age, gender, LDL-cholesterol, HDL-cholesterol, BP, and smoking to estimate risk of developing CHD within 10 years (diabetes = CHD equivalent)
Validated and works well in black and white women (and men)
May overestimate the risk of initial CHD events in other minority groups

PATHOPHYSIOLOGY
- Multiple factors contribute to the pathogenesis of atherosclerosis:
  - Abnormalities in lipid metabolism
  - Endothelial dysfunction—especially significant for women
  - Inflammatory and immunologic factors
  - Plaque rupture
  - Smoking
- Recent data suggest that there are gender differences in the relative contribution of each factor (probably mediated by hormone levels) to the process of atherosclerosis in women.

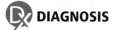 **DIAGNOSIS**

SIGNS AND SYMPTOMS
- Chest pain may occur with or without exertion, in stressful situations, and may even awaken someone from sleep.
- Chest pain may be absent: May have pain in neck, jaw, or back only.
- Shortness of breath is common.
- Atypical symptoms more likely:
  - Dizziness
  - Weakness
  - Fatigue

*Considered equivalent to having known CHD

History
Women delay presentation despite having symptoms of longer duration than men.

Physical Exam
- Vital signs:
  - BP and heart rate are variable.
- Cardiovascular exam—murmurs, extra heart sounds, point of maximum impulse (PMI)
- Lung exam—listen for crackles
- Abdominal exam—listen for bruits
- Peripheral vascular exam—assess for peripheral vascular disease

Differential Diagnosis for Noncardiac Chest Pain Varies by Age
- Young women: Costochondritis and GI causes predominate (GERD, gastritis, IBS).
- Middle aged women: Menopause, GI causes predominate.
- Older women: Aortic dissection, pulmonary, (PE, pneumonia, cancer). May also include costochondritis and GI causes.

TESTS
Lab
- BUN, creatinine, electrolytes, glucose, fasting lipid panel
- Troponin and MB-CPK in the acute setting
- CRP and homocysteine
- Urine microalbumin

EKG
- Women are more likely to have baseline EKG abnormalities due to heart size, axis, and estrogen levels.
  - Makes diagnosis of acute CHD more difficult
- Women are less likely to have a Q wave MI.

Noninvasive Testing: Test Characteristics Vary by Gender
- Exercise stress test: Sens 61%; spec 70%.
- Nuclear stress test: Sens 78%; spec 64%.
- Stress echocardiogram: Sens 86%; spec 79%.
- Coronary CT:
  - Measures coronary calcification: Increased amount is associated with increased cardiac mortality in women.
  - Role in evaluation of women with potential CHD needs further study.
- Coronary MRI:
  - Distinguishes endocardial from epicardial perfusion
  - Spectroscopy (with Phos-31) identifies changes in high-energy phosphates and, thus, provides a direct assessment of metabolic myocardial ischemia.
  - Particularly helpful in women with suspected impaired microvascular dysfunction

Cardiac Catheterization (CC)
- Women with a positive stress test are less likely than men to be referred for CC.
- Women have a significantly higher risk of death after CC (older age, higher comorbidity).
- Women are more likely to have single vessel disease and/or less significant stenoses, but may have ischemia in the setting of vascular dysfunction (see Noninvasive Functional Testing).

Noninvasive Functional Testing
- Up to 50% of women who present with chest pain and have a positive stress test necessitating CC have "nonsignificant" obstructive coronary disease.
- These women may have coronary microvascular dysfunction, which warrants referral to a cardiologist and additional testing (such as Cardiac MRI).

Pregnancy Considerations
- Acute MI 1/10,000 pregnancies:
  - Most in 3rd trimester
- Increased risk because of:
  - Hypercoagulable state
  - Increased myocardial oxygen demand
- Risk factors:
  - Age >33 years
  - Multigravid
- Causes:
  - Atherosclerosis with or without thrombosis: 43%
  - Coronary thrombosis without atherosclerosis: 21%
  - Coronary dissection: 16%; coronary aneurysm: 4%

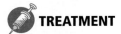 **TREATMENT**

INITIAL CARE FOR ACUTE CHD EVENT (ACE)
- Identify acute coronary syndrome and hospitalize for additional evaluation and stabilization:
  - No significant difference in acute presentation between women and men with ACE.
- Identify the extent of the coronary artery disease and the appropriate long-term treatment:
  - Women with a positive CC are equally likely to be referred for revascularization.
  - However, women have less favorable outcomes with revascularization (including percutaneous coronary intervention and bypass surgery).
- Address cardiovascular risk reduction (see Reduce Cardiovascular Risk).

OUTPATIENT MANAGEMENT OF CHD

 MEDICATIONS (DRUGS)

- Equal efficacy of beta blockers, ACE, nitrates in women post-MI or with active CHD
- Hormone therapy—no benefit and possible harm
- Aspirin is effective as a secondary prevention of CHD events; it may be effective as a primary prevention in high-risk women (those with multiple risk factors). Thus far, it has not been shown to be effective as primary prevention in low-risk women.

Reduce Cardiovascular Risk
- Smoking cessation:
  - Associated with rapid reduction in risk of MI
- Control of diabetes:
  - There are no clear data that tight diabetic control reduces macrovascular disease, i.e., CHD (although it does reduce microvascular disease).
  - Tight control of DM does improve other cardiac RF.
- Control of hypertension:
  - There is extensive evidence that the control of blood pressure reduces risk of CHD.
- Treatment of elevated cholesterol:
  - Primary prevention data support treatment in high-risk women with diabetes or chronic kidney disease or FRS >20% and elevated cholesterol.
- There is insufficient evidence to support cholesterol treatment in low risk women.
  - The secondary prevention benefit is well demonstrated.
- Weight loss:
  - Improves or prevents obesity related RF for CHD

- Weight loss associated with a 25% decrease in all-cause, CHD, and cancer mortality
- Diet:
  - Best diets include nonhydrogenated unsaturated fats (as predominant form of dietary fat), whole grains (for carbohydrates), lots of fruits and vegetables, and adequate omega-3 fatty acids
  - Reduces risk of development of CHD
- Exercise:
  - There is a strong inverse relationship between leisure time activity and a decreased risk of CHD.
  - Engage in 20 to 40 minutes of brisk exercise most days of week.

REFERENCES

1. Mieres JH, Shaw LJ, Arai A, et al. Role of noninvasive testing in the clinical evaluation of women with suspected coronary artery disease: consensus statement from the Cardiac Imaging Committee, Council on Clinical Cardiology, and the Cardiovascular Imaging and Intervention Committee, Council on Cardiovascular Radiology and Intervention, American Heart Association [AHA scientific statements]. *Circulation*. 2005;111:682–696.
2. Douglas PS, Poppas A. Determinants and management of cardiovascular risk in women. UpToDate Online 13.3 [serial online]. 2006;27 screens. Available from: URL: http://www.uptodate.com. Accessed January 22, 2006.
3. Bugiardini R, Merz CNB, Lauer MS. Angina with "normal" coronary arteries: A changing philosophy. *JAMA*. 2005;293:477–484.
4. Mosca L, Appel LJ, Benjamin EJ, et al. Evidence-based guidelines for cardiovascular disease prevention in women. *Arteriosclerosis, Thrombosis, and Vascular Biology*. 2004;24:29–50.
5. Walsh JME, Pignone M. Drug treatment of hyperlipidemia in women. *JAMA*. 2004;291:2243–2252.

USEFUL WEBSITES FOR PATIENTS

http://www.americanheart.org
http://www.womenshealth.gov

CODES
ICD9-CM
- 413 Angina pectoris
- 410 Acute myocardial infarction
- 414 Coronary atherosclerosis

KEY WORDS

Chest Pain
Acute Coronary Syndrome
Atherosclerosis

C

COSTOCHONDRITIS

Anjali Basil, MD
Joseph A. Diaz, MD

KEY CLINICAL POINTS

- Always rule out cardiac source of chest pain first.
- Angina and costochondritis can coexist.
- Consider costochondral infection in intravenous drug users. (The most common organisms in intravenous drug users are *Staphylococcus epidermidis* and *Candida albicans*.)

 ## BASICS

DESCRIPTION
Inflammation of any of the costochondral junctions

EPIDEMIOLOGY
- Accounts for 10% of chest pain complaints
- Women account for 70% of all cases of costochondritis
- Can occur at any age

RISK FACTORS
- Trauma
- Viral infections
- Strain from coughing
- Bacterial infection following intravenous drug use or upper chest surgery
- Association with seronegative spondyloarthropathies

PATHOPHYSIOLOGY
- Inflammatory process of costochondral or costosternal joints that causes localized pain and tenderness
- Any of the 7 costochondral junctions may be affected.
- More than 1 site is affected in 90% of the cases.

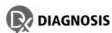 ## DIAGNOSIS

History
- History of repetitive or unaccustomed physical activity involving the upper trunk or arms
- Most chest wall pain is positional and lasts for hours to days.
- Localized to a specific area
- Sharp in character
- May radiate to back or abdomen or to left arm and neck

Physical Exam
- Chest wall tenderness over costochondral junctions
- Assess for areas of localized swelling over the the upper costochondral junctions
- The Crowing Rooster Maneuver is performed with the physician standing behind the patient and exerting traction on the upper arms by pulling them backward and slightly superiorly. This maneuver reproduces the pain.

TESTS
- No specific lab studies for costochondritis
- Rule out cardiac cause with EKG and other cardiac studies if necessary

- Rib and sternoclavicular joint radiographs to rule out other pathologies, such as localized tumors and fractures
- Gallium or technetium labelled radionuclide bone scintigraphy: Pattern of radionuclide uptake and Scintigraphic configuration is considered diagnostic of an inflammatory process especially in costochondritis of infectious etiology.
- Computed tomography is used to further evaluate other pulmonary or pleural causes of chest wall pain and also to evaluate lesions of the sternum or sternoclavicular joints.

DIFFERENTIAL DIAGNOSIS
- Coronary artery disease
- Teitze syndrome: Localized tender swelling of sternoclavicular, costochondral or costosternal joint
- Sternalis syndrome: Localized tenderness over body of sternum or overlying Sternalis muscle (Teitze syndrome and Sternalis syndrome are treated with analgesics, local heat and reassurance)
- Spontaneous sternoclavicular subluxation
- Neck, thoracic or shoulder pain with referral to chest
- Fibromyalgia
- Esophageal spasm
- Peptic ulcer disease
- Anxiety

 ## TREATMENT

- NSAIDS
- Cool compresses or heating pads
- Steroid injections, if no relief with conservative treatment
- Biofeedback
- Primary care follow-up for patients with persistent symptoms

 ## FOLLOW-UP

PROGNOSIS
- Course is generally self-limited
- Most cases of costochondritis resolve, although up to 1/2 of the patients may still have discomfort and 1/3 of the cases report persistent costochondral discomfort.

REFERENCES

1. Massie JD, Sebes JI, Cowles SJ. Bone ccintigraphy and costochondritis. *J Thoracic Imaging*. 1993;8:137–141.
2. Gilliland BC. Fibromyalgia, Arthritis Associated with Systemic Disease, and Other Arthritides. Kasper, et al, eds. 16th ed. Harrison's Principles of Internal Medicine. 2063.
3. Disla E, Rhim HR, Reddy A, et al. Costochondritis: A prospective analysis in an emergency department setting. *Arch Internal Med*. 1994;154:2466–2469.

CUSHING'S SYNDROME

Geetha Gopalakrishnan, MD

KEY CLINICAL POINTS

- Cushing syndrome can be characterized as ACTH dependent or independent glucocorticoid excess.
- Exogenous glucocorticoid is the most common cause of Cushing syndrome followed by pituitary, adrenal, and ectopic tumors, respectively.
- A 24-hour urine cortisol and a dexamethasone suppression test can confirm the diagnosis. ACTH levels, a high-dose dexamethasone suppression test, and imaging can help localize the lesion.
- Surgical resection of the ACTH or cortisol producing tumor is the first step. Radiation, adrenal enzyme inhibitors, and bilateral adrenalectomy can be considered for resistant tumors.
- Most symptoms of Cushing syndrome resolve once the source is removed.

 BASICS

DESCRIPTION
Cushing syndrome is a condition that results from excess glucocorticoids.

EPIDEMIOLOGY
- Affects about 3 times more women than men
- Exogenous glucocorticoids are the most common cause of Cushing syndrome followed by pituitary, adrenal, and ectopic tumors, respectively.

ETIOLOGY
- ACTH Dependent Cushing Syndromes: Excess ACTH causes bilateral adrenal hyperplasia and hypersecretion of cortisol.
  - Cushing disease: Hypersecretion of ACTH by the pituitary microadenomas (majority), macroadenoma (5%) or hyperplasia; associated with multiple endocrine neoplasia type 1 (MEN 1) syndrome
  - Ectopic ACTH syndrome: Hypersecretion of ACTH by nonpituitary tumors; tumors of the lung, pancreas, and thymus are commonly associated with ectopic ACTH production.
  - Excess corticotropin-releasing hormone (CRH) (rare): Hypothalamic or nonhypothalamic tumors producing CRH cause hyperplasia of pituitary corticotrophs and hypersecretion of ACTH, resulting in cortisol hypersecretion and bilateral adrenal hyperplasia.
  - Iatrogenic or factitious (rare): Due to administration of exogenous ACTH
- ACTH-independent Cushing Syndromes: Excess cortisol inhibits CRH and ACTH secretion.
  - Iatrogenic or factitious: Due to administration of exogenous glucocorticoids (most common cause of Cushing syndrome) or drugs that have glucocorticoid activity, such as megestrol acetate. Excess cortisol inhibits CRH and ACTH secretion resulting in bilateral adrenal atrophy.
  - Primary adrenocortical hyperfunction: Increase in cortisol production by benign or malignant adrenal tumors, micronodular dysplasia, or ACTH-independent macronodular hyperplasia can inhibit CRH and result in atrophy of the pituitary corticotrophs resulting in decreased ACTH secretion.
    - Benign or malignant adrenocortical tumor: Excess cortisol production by adrenal tumor inhibits CRH and ACTH

secretion resulting in atrophy of the normal adrenal zonae fasciculata and reticularis.
- Bilateral micronodular dysplasia (rare): Sporadic and familial (e.g., Carney complex) nodular hyperplasia of the adrenal gland resulting in cortisol excess
- Bilateral ACTH-independent macronodular hyperplasia (rare): Associated with stimulation of abberent receptors by hormones, such as gastric inhibitory polypeptide, vasopressin, serotonin, luteinizing hormone/chorionic gonadotropin, or leptin, resulting in adrenal hyperplasia and cortisol excess.

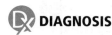 **DIAGNOSIS**

SIGNS AND SYMPTOMS
Cushing syndrome is associated with the following clinical features
- Progressive weight gain involving the face (moon faces), neck (supraclavicular fat pad), trunk, and abdomen; thin extremities
- Facial plethora, bruising, poor wound healing, striae (wide, reddish-purple streaks), hirsutism, acne, hyperpigmentation (induced by ACTH)
- Menstrual irregularities and infertility
- Proximal muscle weakness (e.g., difficult to get out of a chair or climb stairs)
- Bone loss increasing the risk for osteoporotic fracture
- Glucose intolerance that can progress to diabetes mellitus
- Hypertension
- Hyperlipidemia
- Emotional liability, depression, and psychosis
- Increased risk of infections

TESTS
Lab
Diagnosis of Cushing syndrome:
- Screening tests—consider 1 of the following screening tests to document elevated cortisol levels:
  - Midnight salivary cortisol: Normal or elevated (>7 μg/dL) in Cushing syndrome due to loss of circadian rhythm. In normal individuals, a nadir in the cortisol level is noted at midnight.
  - Overnight 1 mg dexamethasone suppression test: Give 1 mg of dexamethasone between 11 p.m. and midnight and check plasma cortisol level at 8 a.m. the following morning. Dexamethasone suppresses cortisol production to <5 mcg/dL in healthy individuals, but not in those with Cushing syndrome.
  - 24-hour urine cortisol: Elevated in Cushing syndrome (>300 μg/24 hours)
- Confirmatory—if screening cortisol levels are elevated, consider 1 of these confirmatory tests:
  - 24-hour urine cortisol: Elevated urine cortisol is more specific for Cushing syndrome.
  - Low dose dexamethasone suppression test: Dexamethasone 0.5 mg q6h for 2 days. Measure 24 hour urine for metabolites of cortisol. Urine hydroxysteroid is elevated with Cushing syndrome.
  - Low dose dexamethasone followed by CRH stimulation: Dexamethasone 0.5 mg q6h for 2 days followed by CRH stimulation. In PseudoCushing states the pituitary is responsive to CRH, but not with a pituitary tumor.

Localization:
- ACTH: Elevated in ACTH dependent Cushing Syndrome (e.g., pituitary and ectopic tumor) and low in ACTH independent Cushing Syndrome (e.g., adrenal tumors and exogenous glucocorticoids)
- Overnight 8 mg dexamethasone suppression test: Ectopic tumors are resistant to glucocorticoid negative feedback. Therefore, high-dose dexamethasone is more likely to suppress ACTH production by pituitary adenomas than an ectopic tumor. Give 8 mg of dexamethasone between 11 p.m. and midnight and check plasma cortisol level at 8 a.m. the following morning. Dexamethasone suppresses cortisol production by 50% in Cushing disease, but not in those with ectopic Cushing.
- High-dose dexamethasone suppression test: dexamethasone 2 mg q6h for 2 days. Check 24-hour urine free cortisol and 17-hydroxysteroid for 2 days. In Cushing disease, urine cortisol decreases by 90% and 17-hydroxysteroid by 64%.
- CRH stimulation: Pituitary adenoma (not ectopic or adrenal tumors) respond to CRH stimulation.

Imaging
- Computed tomography (CT) of adrenals: Primary adrenal tumor or hyperplasia
- CT of chest and abdomen: Ectopic tumor
- Magnetic resonance imaging (MRI) scan of the pituitary: Cushing disease

Diagnostic Procedures/Surgery
Petrosal sinus sampling: ACTH levels measured from the petrosal sinuses are compared with ACTH levels from the forearm vein. Higher ACTH in the petrosal sinuses indicates the presence of a pituitary adenoma and similar levels suggests an ectopic tumor. Consider this procedure if CT or MRI does not localize the tumor.

DIFFERENTIAL DIAGNOSIS
Pseudo-Cushing syndrome: Hypercortisolism associated with depression, stress, obesity, and alcohol

 ## TREATMENT

INITIAL STABILIZATION
Medication-associated Cushing syndrome: Discontinuation resolves symptoms. However, adrenal insufficiency is a complication of exogenous glucocorticoids and therefore, glucocorticoids needs to be tapered slowly to allow the pituitary and adrenal glands to resume normal function.

Treatment of Cushing disease: Transsphenoidal surgical removal of a pituitary adenoma has a cure rate of 60% to 70%. Hypopituitarism is a possible side effect requiring lifelong hormone replacement. Residual tumors can be treated with radiation. The effect of radiation on cortisol levels can be seen after 3–12 months. Therefore, adrenal enzyme inhibitors such as ketoconazole, metyrapone, and aminoglutethimide can be used to lower cortisol level in the interim. Surgical or medical adrenalectomy with mitotane (adrenocorticolytic drug that blocks adrenal hormone synthesis) is reserved for individuals who have failed pituitary surgery and radiation. After adrenalectomy, patients require lifelong glucocorticoids and mineralocorticoid replacement therapy. Persistent hypercortisolism can be treated with adrenal enzyme inhibitors.

Treatment of ectopic ACTH syndrome: Surgical removal of ectopic non-pituitary tumor resolves symptoms of Cushing in only 10% of individuals. Ketoconazole, metyrapone, and aminoglutethimide can be used to reduce adrenal cortisol level. Bilateral adrenalectomy is reserved for individuals who have failed surgery and medical management.

Treatment of hypothalamic or nonhypothalamic CRH tumor: Surgical removal of the CRH secreting tumor is the first step. Medications (e.g., ketoconazole metyrapone, and aminoglutethimide) and adrenalectomy are reserved for those who have failed initial surgery.
- Treatment of primary adrenocortical hyperfunction:
  - Adrenal adenoma: Surgical removal of the affected adrenal gland. Symptoms of Cushing usually resolve with surgery. Remaining adrenal gland resumes normal adrenal function.
  - Adrenal carcinomas: Require more aggressive management. Surgical removal of the affected adrenal gland, radiation, chemotherapy, and mitotane to lower cortisol levels. Poor prognosis. Adrenal insufficiency is a complication of treatment and requires glucocorticoids and mineralocorticoid replacement.
  - Nodular adrenal hyperplasia: Surgical removal of both adrenal glands. Can consider ketoconazole, metyrapone, or aminoglutethimide preoperatively to lower cortisol levels. Adrenal insufficiency is a complication of treatment and requires glucocorticoids and mineralocorticoid replacement

Pregnancy Considerations
Excess cortisol can cause preeclampsia, gestational diabetes, spontaneous abortion and premature delivery. Therefore, surgery to remove the adrenal or pituitary tumor is recommended to lower cortisol levels in the second trimester. If surgery is not an option, metyrapone can be used to treat hypercortisolism. Aminoglutethimide, Ketoconazole, and Mitotane should not be given to pregnant women.

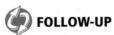 ## FOLLOW-UP

DISPOSITION
Most symptoms of Cushing syndrome resolve once the source is removed.

Issues for Referral
Endocrine consultation should be obtained for the evaluation and management of Cushing syndrome.

COMPLICATIONS
- Nelson syndrome: Characterized by an enlarging ACTH producing pituitary tumor in an individual who has undergone medical or surgical bilateral adrenalectomy for the treatment of Cushing disease. Pituitary irradiation prior to adrenalectomy can prevent this syndrome. A periodic MRI of the pituitary and plasma ACTH levels are recommended after adrenalectomy. Transsphenoidal surgery and irradiation recommended for Nelson's syndrome.
- Panhypopituitarism: Complication of transsphenoidal surgery and radiation treatment for Cushing disease. Lifelong pituitary hormone replacement is recommended including glucocorticoids and thyroid hormone replacement.
- Adrenal insufficiency: After medical or surgical bilateral adrenalectomy, patients require lifelong glucocorticoids and mineralocorticoid replacement therapy. Mitotane can increase the metabolism of dexamethasone and fludrocortisone, but not prednisone and hydrocortisone. Therefore, a higher replacement dose of dexamethasone and fludrocortisone is required with Mitotane.

REFERENCES

1. Newell-Price J, Trainer P, Besser M, et al. The diagnosis and differential diagnosis of Cushing's syndrome and pseudo-Cushing's states. *Endocr Rev.* 1998;19:647.

2. Orth DN. Medical progress: Cushing's syndrome. *N Engl J Med*. 1995;332:791.
3. Kemink SA, Smals AG, Hermus AR, et al. Nelson's syndrome: A review. *Endocrinologist*. 1997;7:5.

CODES
ICD9-CM
255.0 Cushing's disease or syndrome

KEY WORDS
Cushing's Syndrome
Cushing's Disease
Pituitary Tumor
Adrenal Tumor

C

DEPRESSION

Audrey R. Tyrka, MD, PhD
John P. Carvalho, BA

KEY CLINICAL POINTS

- Major depressive disorder (MDD) is a serious and debilitating mental illness with a defined set of physical and cognitive symptoms.
- The disorder is twice as common in women as in men and is the 2nd leading cause of medical disability for women in America.

 BASICS

DESCRIPTION

- MDD is a mood disorder characterized by depressed mood in conjunction with physical and cognitive symptoms which interfere with daily functioning.
- Can be classified as a single episode or recurrent (2 or more episodes)
- May present as mild, moderate, or severe depending on number and severity of symptoms
- Can be present with or without psychotic features
- Postpartum depression (PPD) is a major depressive episode occurring shortly after childbirth (see Postpartum Depression chapter).

ALERT

- MDD has a 15% suicide rate; suicidal intent of patients should be assessed.
- Rule out bipolar disorder before initiating treatment, because antidepressants can induce mania in bipolar disorder.

Prevalence

- Lifetime prevalence:
  - For females: 10–25%; for males: 5–12%
- Point prevalence:
  - For females: 4–9%; for males: 2–3%

RISK FACTORS

- Previous major depressive episode
- Family history of MDD
- Early-life stress
  - Loss of a parent
  - Abuse
  - Neglect
- Adult stressors
  - Loss of a spouse or child, etc.
- Poor social supports

ETIOLOGY

- Abnormalities of biogenic amines (serotonin, norepinephrine, dopamine) and other neurotransmitters
- Hypothalamic-pituitary-adrenal (HPA) axis dysfunction
- Personality/cognitive style
- Genetics
  - Family, twin, and adoption studies indicate that MDD is heritable.
  - Some candidate risk genes have been identified
    - A functional polymorphism of the serotonin transporter gene has been associated with depression among individuals with a history of stressful life events (e.g., Caspi et al., 2003).

ASSOCIATED CONDITIONS

- Depression often coexists with other psychiatric disorders, including:
  - Anxiety disorders
  - Dysthymic disorder
  - Substance abuse/dependence
  - Psychotic disorders
  - Somatoform disorders
  - Eating disorders
  - Attention deficit disorder
- Depression is also very common in patients with medical illness (see Differential Diagnosis).

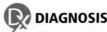 **DIAGNOSIS**

At least 5 of the following symptoms must occur most of the day nearly every day for at least a 2-week period.

- Depressed mood or anhedonia must be among the symptoms present.

SIGNS AND SYMPTOMS

- Depressed mood
- Loss of interest or pleasure in normally enjoyed activities (anhedonia)
- Decreased or increased appetite
- Insomnia or hypersomnia
- Loss of energy, fatigue
- Psychomotor agitation or psychomotor retardation
- Feelings of worthlessness or excessive, inappropriate guilt
- Trouble concentrating or making simple decisions
- Thoughts of death or suicidal ideation

History

- Determination of the number of previous episodes will inform treatment duration
- Rule out history of mania
  - Manic symptoms include:
    - Elevated, expansive, or irritable mood
    - Decreased need for sleep
    - Inflated self-esteem or grandiosity
    - Pressured speech
    - Racing thoughts
    - Distractibility
    - Increase in goal-oriented activity
    - Increase in pleasure-seeking activity
- Rule out substance-induced mood disorder
- Assess for history of suicide risk factors:
  - Age 15–24, or >65
  - Previous suicide attempts
  - Family history of suicide
  - Widowed or divorced
  - Unemployed
  - Chronic or terminal medical illness
  - Current risk factors:
    - Suicidal ideation
    - Specific plan
    - Availability of means/opportunity (e.g., firearm, medications)
    - Hopelessness
    - Impulsiveness

- Lack of social supports
- Substance abuse

TESTS
- Thyroid Stimulating Hormone (TSH)
- Complete Blood Count (CBC)
- Toxicology screen
- Other tests as appropriate to rule out medial conditions that may cause depressed mood and associated symptoms (see Differential Diagnosis).

DIFFERENTIAL DIAGNOSIS
- MDD shares symptoms and may co-occur with many other medical conditions, including disorders of the following systems:
  - Endocrine (e.g., hypothyroidism)
  - Neurologic (e.g., Parkinson's disease)
  - Cardiopulmonary
  - Infectious disease
  - Hematologic (e.g., anemia)
  - Autoimmune
  - Cancers (e.g., pancreatic)
- MDD also shares symptoms and may co-occur with other psychiatric disorders, including:
  - Bipolar disorder
  - Substance use disorders
  - Others
    - Dysthymic disorder
    - Adjustment disorder
    - Anxiety disorders
    - Schizophrenia
    - Eating disorders
    - Somatization disorders
    - Personality disorders

 TREATMENT

- Pharmacologic: Selective serotonin reuptake inhibitors (SSRIs), tricyclics (TCAs), monoamine oxidase inhibitors (MAOIs), and other antidepressants
- Psychotherapy: Supportive, cognitive-behavioral, interpersonal, family, and psychodynamic psychotherapy
- The combination of psychological and pharmacological treatments may be more effective than either treatment alone.
- Electroconvulsive therapy (ECT) is very effective but is limited by cognitive side effects and patient preference.
- Vagus Nerve Stimulation therapy has recently been FDA approved for treatment-resistant depression.

INITIAL STABILIZATION
- Initial treatment should begin with pharmacotherapy, psychotherapy, or a combination of the 2, depending on severity of disorder and patient's preference.
- Different antidepressants appear to have similar effectiveness for the treatment of MDD.
- Treatment choice should be based on patient characteristics.
- Psychotic features: Combined antidepressant and antipsychotic; consider hospitalization and psychiatric referral
- Suicidality: Avoid tricyclics and MAOIs, consider hospitalization and psychiatric referral.
- Anxious or insomnia: Benzodiazepines can be added during the acute stage while awaiting onset of antidepressant effect.
- Personal or family history of good response to a particular medication may warrant a trial with that medication.

- Personal preference and medical history influence the choice of the drug based on side effects and drug interaction profiles (see below).
- Medication costs may influence treatment choice.

 MEDICATION (DRUGS)

First Line
SSRIs and other newer antidepressants are generally better tolerated and safer than TCAs and MAOIs
- SSRIs include:
  - Fluoxetine: Start 20 mg PO in the a.m., usual effective dose 20–40 mg/day
  - Paroxetine: Start 20 mg PO in the a.m., usual effective dose 20–40 mg/day
  - Sertraline: Start 50 mg PO/day, usual effective dose 50–200 mg/day
  - Citalopram: Start 20 mg PO/day, usual effective dose 20–40 mg/day
  - Escitalopram: Start 10 mg/day, usual effective dose 10–20 mg/day
  - Short-term side effects of SSRIs include headache, agitation, gastrointestinal distress and fatigue; sexual dysfunction is a common persistent side effect.
- Other 1st-line antidepressants include:
  - Bupropion: Start 75 mg PO b.i.d, usual effective dose 150–300 mg/day
    - Not likely to cause sexual dysfunction or weight gain, but should be avoided by patients at risk for seizures
  - Mirtazapine: Start 15 mg PO q.h.s., usual effective dose 15–30 mg/day
    - Not likely to cause sexual side effects but may lead to weight gain and sedation
  - Venlafaxine: Start 37.5–75 mg PO/day; usual effective dose 75–225 mg/day
    - Dose-related risk of inducing hypertension in some patients
  - Duloxetine: start 20 mg PO b.i.d, usual effective dose 40–60 mg in single daily dose
    - May cause hepatic injury with preexisting liver disease or significant alcohol use.

Second Line
The following medication classes usually reserved as 2nd- or 3rd-line options due to greater side-effect burden and concerns regarding toxicity
- Tricyclics (TCAs): Amitriptyline, clomipramine, desipramine, imipramine, nortriptyline
- Monoamine Oxidase Inhibitors (MAOIs): Phenelzine, tranylcypromine, selegiline patch
- Combining antidepressants with complementary mechanisms of action
- Combining an antidepressant with an augmenting agent such as lithium, atypical antipsychotics, thyroid hormone, stimulant or lamotrigine

 FOLLOW-UP

- The response to the pharmacological treatment usually occurs within 2–6 weeks.
- If partial or no response after 4–6 weeks, dosage should be increased until maximum dose achieved or depression remits.
- After 2 trials within same antidepressant class, a new trial within a different class should be implemented.

- Periodically assess the patient for intolerable side effects, such as sexual dysfunction.
- Continue the medication for at least 6–9 months in patients with a 1st episode of MDD.
- For patients with numerous past episodes, treatment may be continued indefinitely.

PROGNOSIS

- The average duration of a major depressive episode without treatment is 6–9 months.
- The risk of relapse is high.
  - Of the patients with a single episode, 60% experience a 2nd episode.
  - Of the patients with a history of 2 episodes, 70% experience a 3rd.
  - Of the patients with a history of 3 episodes, 90% experience a 4th.
- 2/3 of depressive episodes end completely, whereas 1/3 remit only partially or not at all.

Pregnancy Considerations

- Between 10–20% of pregnant women experience major depression.
- Depression during pregnancy can lead to premature birth and can also negatively affect neonatal physiological, neurobiological, and behavioral development.
- Postpartum depression can interfere with bonding and parental care, which can hinder infant social, emotional, and behavioral development.
- Education, support and psychotherapy are important elements of treatment.
  - Cognitive-behavioral, interpersonal, group, family and marital, and supportive therapies
- Pharmacological treatment during pregnancy
  - Mild cases may be adequately treated with psychotherapy.
  - Moderate and severe cases may require antidepressant treatment.
  - Antidepressants are generally category C drugs (Bupropion is category B).
  - A recent study of women with a prior history of depression found that those who discontinued antidepressant treatment were 5 times more likely to relapse during pregnancy than those who continued treatment during pregnancy (Cohen, et al 2006)
  - Studies of antidepressant use during pregnancy have produced mixed results, with some finding no adverse effects and others showing small increases in adverse neonatal outcomes.
    - A recent large prospective study in Sweden revealed small but significant increases in hypoglycemia, premature birth, low birth weight, respiratory distress, low APGAR scores (odds ratio 1.62–2.33), and convulsions (odds ratio 4.70) in infants exposed to antidepressants in utero.
    - TCAs generally increased risk more than SSRIs (Kalra et al., 2005).
    - Paroxetine use in the 1st trimester has been significantly associated with birth defects (odds ratio 2.2; FDA Medwatch, 9/05).

- A recent study found that infants born to mothers who took SSRIs after the 20th week of pregnancy were 6 times more likely to have persistant pulmonary hypertension than those whose mothers did not take antidepressant (Chambers, et al, 2006).
  - Benzodiazepines should be avoided during the 1st trimester.
- When treating depression during pregnancy, it is important to compare potential benefits of treatment against potential risks.
- The risks of allowing a depressive episode to remain untreated may be far greater than those associated with antidepressants treatment.

Issues for Referral

- Referral to a psychiatrist should be considered for complex, treatment-resistant, or severe cases.
- Hospitalization is indicated for suicidal patients, some psychotic patients, and those who have severe impairments in functioning.
- Referral for psychotherapy should be considered according to patient-preference and ability to participate.

REFERENCES

1. American Psychiatric Association. Diagnostic and Statistical Manual of Mental Disorders. 4th ed. Washington, DC: American Psychiatric Association; 2000.
2. Caspi A, Sugden K, Moffitt TE, et al. Influence of life stress on depression: moderation by a polymorphism in the 5-HTT gene. *Science*. 2003;301:386–389.
3. Kalra S, Born L, Sarkar M, et al. The safety of antidepressant use in pregnancy. *Expert Opinion on Drug Safety*. 2005;4:273–283.
4. Mann JJ. The medical management of depression. *New Engl J Med*. 2005;353:1819–1834.
5. Weissman AM, Levy BT, Hartz AJ, et al. Pooled analysis of antidepressant levels in lactating mothers, breast milk, and nursing infants. *Am J Psychiatry*. 2004;161:1066–1078.
6. Cohen LS, Altshuler LL, Harlow BL, et al. Relapse of major depression during in women who maintain or discontinue antidepressant treatment. *JAMA*. 2006;295:499–507.
7. Chambers CD, Hernandez-Diaz S, van Marter LJ, et al. Selective serotonin-reuptake inhibitors and risk of persistant pulmonary hypertension of the newborn. *New Engl J Med*. 2006;354: 579–587.

CODES
ICD9-CM

- 296.2 Major depressive disorder, single episode
- 296.3 Major depressive disorder, recurrent episode

KEY WORDS

- Depression
- Antidepressant
- Suicide
- Depression and Pregnancy

DERMATOMYOSITIS

Mohsin K. Malik, MD
Lynn E. Iler, MD

KEY CLINICAL POINTS

- The mainstay of therapy for dermatomyositis is long-term steroids, with or without immunosuppressive agent.
- Pulmonary involvement is not universal, but is an important cause of morbidity and mortality.
- Patients with dermatomyositis have an increased risk of malignancy and should have an age-appropriate malignancy workup.

BASICS

DESCRIPTION

- Dermatomyositis is an idiopathic inflammatory myopathy which involves the muscles and skin.
- On laboratory testing, most patients have:
  - Antinuclear autoantibodies
  - Elevated muscle enzymes, notably creatine kinase
- A portion of patients also develop interstitial lung disease.
- Amyopathic dermatomyositis (dermatomyositis siné myositis) is a less common subset which lacks muscle involvement.
- Polymyositis is a closely related disease with similar, but not identical, muscle pathology, symptoms, treatment, and outcome, but lacks skin involvement.

EPIDEMIOLOGY

Incidence
Incidence varies by ethnic background and location of study:
- 0.8 per million population studied in Pennsylvania, United States.
- Female > Male (2:1)
- Higher incidence among African American women

RISK FACTORS

- Susceptibility genes (see genetics)
- Infectious agents may play a role in the development of dermatolmyositis, but have not been consistently implicated.

Genetics
Both HLA and TNF genes have been associated with dermatomyositis:
- HLA DRB1*03 in Caucasians, HLA DRB1*14 in Koreans
- TNF2 allele of TNFA gene

PATHOPHYSIOLOGY

- An autoimmune etiology is likely, but a target antigen has not yet been identified.
- Autoantibodies are thought to target the endothelium of endomysial capillaries.
  - Complement activation and deposition in the capillaries follows.
  - Complement deposition leads to capillary damage and eventually to muscle fiber ischemia and destruction.

ETIOLOGY

- An autoimmune etiology is supported by the findings of autoantibodies and by an association with histocompatibility genes.
- UV light can precipitate or exacerbate skin lesions.

ASSOCIATED CONDITIONS

- Increased risk of malignancy with reported incidence of cancer ranging from 7–30%.

- The risk is the highest in first 5 years after diagnosis.
  - Ovarian cancer may be over-represented.
  - Otherwise the distribution of the various types of cancers are roughly equal to the general population.
- Dermatomyositis can overlap with systemic scleroderma or mixed connective tissue disease.

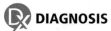

DIAGNOSIS

SIGNS AND SYMPTOMS

- The clinical picture is marked by:
  - Symmetric proximal muscle weakness of extremities
  - Characteristic skin lesions on the face, chest, and/or hand
- Universally accepted diagnostic criteria do not exist
- Diagnosis is made on a combination of the clinical picture and elevated muscle enzymes, with a muscle biopsy or MRI providing additional information when necessary.

History

- Muscle weakness
  - Often manifests as difficulty in daily activities such as rising from chair or bathtub, climbing stairs, combing hair
  - Pain/tenderness in affected muscle groups tends to be mild.
  - The facial and extraoccular muscles are NOT affected.
  - Less commonly dysphagia due to involvement of esophageal striated muscle
- Skin lesions (see below)
- Pulmonary involvement
  - Dyspnea
  - Nonproductive cough

Physical Exam

- Skin changes
  - Characterized by symmetric, confluent, often pruritic, violaceous erythema on:
    - Central face/forehead/scalp/periorbital areas (heliotrope rash: eyelid/periorbital involvement with edema)
    - Extensor fingers/hands/arms
    - Posterior neck/shoulders
    - "v" distribution (photodistribution) on anterior neck/upper chest ("shawl sign")
  - "Mechanic's hands": Thickening and cracking of lateral, and occasionally palmar, aspects of hands
  - Dilated capillary loops at base of fingernails may also be present.
  - Pathognomonic skin lesions:
    - Gottron's papules: Violaceous papules over dorsal/lateral interphalangeal/ metacarpophalangeal joints
    - Gottron sign: Symmetric, confluent, violaceous macules over interphalangeal/metacarpophalangeal joints, patellae, olecranon process, medial malleoli, with or without edema
- Muscle weakness
  - The spectrum ranges from mild weakness to quadraparesis.
  - The lower extremity is generally affected before the upper extremity.
- Pulmonary involvement
  - Up to 1/2 of patients develop interstitial pneumonitis
    - Bibasilar fine cracks/rales may be indicative of interstitial pulmonary disease

– Aspiration pneumonia and respiratory failure secondary to varying weakness of respiratory muscles
- Cardiac:
  – Conduction abnormalities
  – Myocarditis
- Joint contractures
- Subcutaneous calcifications

TESTS
Lab
- Muscle enzymes: Some, all, or none (rarely) may be elevated
  – Creatine kinase: Most sensitive for diagnosis, can be 50 times normal
  – Lactate dehydrogenase (LDH)
  – Aldolase
  – Aspartate aminotransferase (AST)
  – Alanine aminotransferase (ALT)
  – Normal troponin-I can rule out cardiac involvement
- Electromyography abnormal in 90%
- Autoantibodies
  – Anti–Jo–1 (anti–histidyl–tRNA synthetase)
    - Only present in about 20% but is the most specific antibody
    - Associated with interstitial lung disease, Raynaud phenomenon, arthritis, "mechanic's hands"
  – ANA positive in 60–80%
    - Not specific for dermatomyositis
    - High-titers suggest an overlap syndrome

Imaging
- MRI
  – Shows inflammation and edema
  – Fibrosis and calcification may also be present
  – Especially valuable because muscle pathology can be focal and biopsy sampling may miss disease process
- 31-P magnetic resonance spectroscopy
  – Highly sensitive, and especially useful for detecting subclinical myositis in patients with suggestive skin lesions
- Chest x-ray and/or high-resolution CT are indicated if there is suspicion for interstitial pneumonitis.
- Pulmonary function tests reveal a restrictive pattern with reduced diffusing capacity in patients with interstitial pneumonitis.

Diagnostic Procedures/Surgery
Muscle biopsy

Pathologic Findings
Muscle biopsy demonstrates:
- Decreased density of capillaries within muscle fibers
- Atrophy/necrosis of muscle fibers in groups, especially at edges of fascicles
- Degeneration and regeneration of muscle fibers
- Perifascicular or perivascular infiltrate consisting largely of B cells

DIFFERENTIAL DIAGNOSIS
- Polymyositis
- Inclusion body myositis
- Rhabdomyolysis
- Muscular dystrophy
- Myasthenia gravis
- Upper or lower motor neuron disease
- Hypothyroidism
- Connective tissue disease with myositis
- Systemic lupus erythematosus
- Mixed connective tissue disease
- HIV

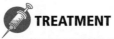

TREATMENT
INITIAL STABILIZATION
Disease onset is generally gradual.
- Life-threatening involvement of the esophagus or respiratory muscles should be ruled out at presentation.
- Supportive measures, high-dose systemic corticosteroids, and possibly intravenous immunoglobulin are indicated in these situations.

GENERAL MEASURES
- Malignancy workup
- UV protection
  – Sunscreen and avoidance of sun exposure should be employed to minimize exacerbation of the skin disease.
  – UV light also worsens muscle weakness in some patients.

Activity
Activity is as tolerated since exercise has not been shown to increase muscle inflammation.

SPECIAL THERAPY
Physical Therapy
Resistive muscular training and aerobic endurance training can reduce disability, but do not modify disease activity.

MEDICATION (DRUGS)
First Line
Systemic corticosteroids are the mainstay of treatment.
- Treatment protocol needs to be tailored to each patient's response and tolerance to therapy.
- Initial dose generally 0.5–1.5 g/kg oral prednisone daily.
  – Prednisone is tapered over weeks to months as the disease activity is controlled.
  – Patients may require a maintenance dose of corticosteroids, either in daily or alternate-day dosing.
  – Severe disease may require high-dose intravenous corticosteroids.

Second Line
- Azathioprine and methotrexate have a role in select patients including:
  – Patients with poor response to steroids
  – Serious or intolerable steroid side effects
  – Aggressive disease
  – Disease resistant to steroids
- Either azathioprine or methotrexate is generally given in combination with prednisone.
- Trials comparing the efficacy of azathioprine vs. methotrexate have not been conducted.
- Other therapies may also be effective and should be chosen based on the response to disease, the side effect profile, and comorbidities.
  – Cyclosporine
  – Mycophenolate mofetil
  – Tacrolimus
  – Cyclophosphamide/chlorambucil
  – Etanercept/infliximab
  – Rituximab
  – Intravenous immunoglobulin

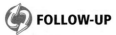
FOLLOW-UP

Issues for Referral
To dermatologist/rheumatologist to help with diagnosis and management

PROGNOSIS
Long-term outcomes are variable and range from remission to progressive disease and death.
- The disease typically has a relapsing and remitting course.
- On long-term follow-up, 15–40% of the patients achieve disease remission.
- Death occurs in about 10–20%, and tends to be due to cancer or pulmonary involvement.
- Older age is also associated with a relatively poor outcome.

COMPLICATIONS
Side effects of long-term steroids and immunosuppressive agents are additional, important causes of morbidity and mortality.

PATIENT MONITORING
- Age-appropriate cancer screening is warranted given the increased risk of malignancy.
- The benefit of searching for occult malignancy is unclear.

REFERENCES

1. Mastaglia FL, Phillips BA. Idiopathic inflammatory myopathies: epidemiology, classification, and diagnostic criteria. *Rheum Dis Clin North Am*. 2002;28:723–741.
2. Oddis CV, Conte CG, Steen VD, et al. Incidence of polymyositis-dermatomyositis: A 20-year study of hospital diagnosed cases in Allegheny County, PA 1963–1982. *J Rheumatol*. 1990;17:1329–1334.
3. Hassan AB, Nikitina-Zake L, Sanjeevi CB, et al. Association of the proinflammatory haplotype (MICA5.1/TNF2/TNFa2/DRB1*03) with polymyositis and dermatomyositis. *Arthritis Rheum*. 2004;50:1013–1015.
4. Plotz PH, Rider LG, Targoff IN, et al. NIH conference. Myositis: Immunologic contributions to understanding cause, pathogenesis, and therapy. *Ann Intern Med*. 1995;122:715–724.
5. Alexanderson H, Lundberg IE. The role of exercise in the rehabilitation of idiopathic inflammatory myopathies. *Curr Opin Rheumatol*. 2005;17:164–171.
6. Marie I, Hachulla E, Hatron PY, et al. Polymyositis and dermatomyositis: Short-term and long-term outcome, and predictive factors of prognosis. *J Rheumatol*. 2001;28:2230–2237.

CODES
ICD9-CM
710.3 Dermatomyositis

KEY WORDS
- Dermatomyositis
- Gottron Papules
- Heliotrope

D

DIABETES

Geetha Gopalakrishnan, MD

KEY CLINICAL POINTS

- Diabetes Mellitus (DM) results from an absolute or relative insulin deficiency.
- DM: Fasting plasma glucose (FPG) $\geq$126 mg/dL or postprandial plasma glucose (PPG) $\geq$200 mg/dL on 2 occasions.
- Absolute insulin deficiency (e.g., Type 1 DM or pancreatitis) requires insulin therapy. Oral agents and insulin can lower glucose in conditions associated with insulin resistance and relative deficiency (e.g., Type 2 DM).
- In pregnant women, diabetes needs to be treated aggressively with insulin.

 BASICS

DESCRIPTION
DM is a syndrome that results from an absolute or relative insulin deficiency

EPIDEMIOLOGY
- Prevalence of diabetes in the United States is 7.2% (80% Type 2, 10% Type 1, and 10% other)
- Gestational DM (GDM) affects 3% of pregnancies; 50% progress to Type 2 DM in 20 years.
- Increased risk of coronary artery disease (2- to 5-fold), stroke (2- to 3-fold), blindness (20-fold), kidney failure (25-fold), and amputation (40-fold). 5th leading cause of death in the United States.

ETIOLOGY
- Type 1 DM: Destruction of pancreatic beta cells leading to absolute insulin deficiency. Requires insulin therapy and can develop diabetic ketoacidosis (DKA). Genetic factors (HLA-D and 50% concordance in identical twins) and environmental inducers (mumps and rubella) have been associated with development of Type 1 DM.
  - Type 1A : Immune mediated destruction
  - Type 1B: Destruction without autoimmunity
- Type 2 DM: Combined insulin resistance and relative insulin deficiency results in Type 2 DM. Patients usually present with nonketotic hyperglycemia. Under certain circumstances such as infection, Type 2 DM can also develop DKA secondary to partial insulin deficiency. Genetic factors (e.g., 90–100% concordance in twins) and environmental inducers (e.g., obesity) have been associated with the development of Type 2 DM. Responsive to oral agents and insulin.
- Genetic defects
  - Maturity-onset diabetes of the young (MODY): 6 genetic abnormalities have been identified. Presents in childhood and is responsive to oral agents and insulin.
  - Other rare genetic defects including abnormalities in insulin action, mutation in the sulfonylurea receptor, Wolfram, and Prader-Willi can cause diabetes.
- Disease of the pancreas: Includes surgery, cystic fibrosis, hemochromatosis and pancreatitis. Associated with loss of both alpha and beta cells resulting in insulin and glucagon deficiency. These patients are prone to develop diabetes and hypoglycemia. Require insulin therapy.
- Endocrinopathies: Conditions such as Cushing syndrome, acromegaly, pheochromocytoma, and glucagonomas increase counter-regulatory hormones (hormones that antagonize the action of insulin) and lead to glucose intolerance and DM.

- Medications: Glucocorticoids, protease inhibitors, thiazides, niacin, beta blockers, calcium blockers, clonidine, anti-psychotics and alcohol can cause glucose intolerance.
- Viral infections: Cause both autoimmune and direct beta-cell destruction (e.g., hepatitis C, CMV)
- Immune mediated diabetes:
  - Stiff-man syndrome: Autoimmune (anti-GAD) disorder of the central nervous system characterized by progressive axial muscle stiffness leading to impaired ambulation.
  - Insulin receptor antibodies: Causes DM by blocking the binding of insulin to its receptor
- GDM: Insulin resistance and glucose intolerance develops in the 2nd or 3rd trimester secondary to increased dietary intake and counter-regulatory hormones such as human chorionic somatomammotropin secreted during pregnancy. Usually, GDM resolves after delivery.

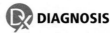 DIAGNOSIS

SIGNS AND SYMPTOMS
- High glucose levels: Asymptomatic, but can present with polyuria, polydipsia, weight loss, and blurred vision. Symptoms improve with treatment.
- Diabetic complications: Asymptomatic initially, but develop as diabetes progresses. Assess complication 3–5 years after initial presentation in Type 1 and at the time of presentation in Type 2.
- Diabetic eye complications:
  - Nonproliferative retinopathy: Microaneurysm, hemorrhages, hard exudates, macular edema, microinfarcts with cotton wool exudates and AV shunts
  - Proliferative retinopathy: Neovascularization, vitrious hemorrhage, fibrous scarring, and retinal detachment.
  - Cataract and glaucoma
- Diabetic nephropathy: Hypertension, pedal edema, uremic appearance
- Diabetic neuropathy:
  - Autonomic: Gastroparesis, constipation, diarrhea, neurogenic bladder, impotence, orthostatic hypotension, gustatory sweating
  - Peripheral:
    - Symmetrical polyneuropathy: Characterized by paresthesias, burning and gnawing pain sensation. Exam identifies decreased pinprick, light touch, pain, vibration, and DTR reflexes.
    - Asymmetric mononeuropathies: Cranial neuropathy, mononeuropathy, mononeuritis multiplex and entrapment neuropathy
    - Complications: Foot ulcers and Charcot's
- Macrovascular disease: Coronary artery, cerebrovascularor peripheral arterial disease
- Infections: Rhinocerebral mucormycosis, malignant otitis externa (pseudomonas), and emphysematous cholecystitis (clostridia)

ASSOCIATED CONDITIONS
Evaluation of other autoimmune conditions should be considered in Type 1 diabetes such as celiac disease, hypothyroidism, and pernicious anemia.

TESTS
Lab
- Diagnosis of diabetes: Abnormal blood glucose levels on 2 occasions.

- Random plasma glucose: Level 200 mg/dL or higher with symptoms of polyuria, polydipsia, and unexplained weight loss suggests diabetes.
- Fasting plasma glucose (8 hour fast): Level of 126 mg/dL or higher suggests diabetes.
- Oral glucose tolerance test: Plasma glucose is measured hourly for 3 hours after a glucose load. Level 200 mg/dL or higher 2 hours after a 75 gram glucose load suggests diabetes.
- Assess etiology of diabetes:
  - Islet-cell antibodies (ICA), antibodies to glutamic acid dehydrogenase (anti-GAD) and anti-insulin can confirm the diagnosis of type 1A.
  - Serum C-peptide reflects endogenous insulin secretion. Detectable levels rules out conditions associated with absolute insulin deficiency such as Type 1 diabetes.
  - Monitor diabetes and its complications:
    - Hemoglobin A1c (HgA1C): Correlates with mean blood glucose over the previous 8 to 12 weeks. HgA1C of 7% and 9% represent a mean blood glucose value of about 150 and 210 mg/dL, respectively. Normal values for hemoglobin A1c are usually lower than 6%. Treatment goals aim for HgA1C less than 7%.
    - Self-monitoring blood glucose and plasma glucose: Whole blood glucose measurements with a glucose meter vary by as much as 15% from plasma glucose measurement. Several glucose meters are now available with plasma readings.
    - Urine ketones: Test urine for ketones during periods of illness or stress.
    - Test creatinine and urine for microalbuminuria
      ○ Microalbuminuria: 30–300 mg albumin per 24 hours or 30–300 mg of albumin per gram of creatinine in spot urine sample.
      ○ Macroalbuminuria or nephropathy: >300 mg albumin per 24 hours or >300 mg of albumin per gram of creatinine.
    - Fasting lipids panel: Target goal for serum LDL cholesterol of <100 mg/dL, TG <150 mg/dL and HDL >40 mg/dL in men and >50 mg/dL in women.

Pregnancy Considerations
- At 24–28 weeks gestation, screening with 100 gram glucose tolerance test is recommended.
- Diagnosis of gestational diabetes requires more than 2 abnormal values: Fasting ≥95 mg/dL; 1 hour ≥180 mg/dL; 2 hours ≥155 mg/dL; and 3 hours ≥140 mg/dL.
- Earlier screening is recommended for high risk individuals. Fetal ultrasound surveillance is recommended for all diabetics.

DIFFERENTIAL DIAGNOSIS
Individual with impaired glucose intolerance (IGT) are at risk for developing diabetes and cardiovascular disease.
- Diagnostic Criteria:
  - Fasting Plasma Glucose: 100–126 mg/dL
  - 2 hour Postload Glucose: 140–200 mg/dL

TREATMENT

INITIAL STABILIZATION
Target goal: Hg A1C <7.0%, fasting glucose <130 mg/dL and postprandial glucose <180 mg/dL.

GENERAL MEASURES
- Exercise, diet and weight management are critical to blood glucose control.

- Recommend 30–45 minutes of moderate aerobic activity for 3–5 days/week and a balanced diet (40–50% carbohydrate, 20% protein, and 30–40% fat).
- Weight loss is achieved by reducing caloric intake and increasing physical activity. A decrease of 500 kcal/day results in a 1–2 lbs/week weight loss.

MEDICATION (DRUGS)

- Sulfonylureas: Lower blood glucose by increasing insulin secretion. Lowers HgA1C by 1–2%. Efficacy wanes over time due to beta cell exhaustion and failure. They are metabolized by the liver and cleared by the kidney. Side effects include hypoglycemia, weight gain and potential increase in CV mortality because of its effect of K^+ ATP channels. Dosed daily or b.i.d. in Type 2 DM.
  - 1st generation: Chlorpropamide, tolbutamide, acetohexamide, tolazamide
  - 2nd generation: Glipizide, glyburide, and glimepiride are the preferred agents.
- Meglitinides (Nateglinide and Repaglinide): Short-acting secretagogues given to lower postprandial blood glucose by increasing insulin secretion. Lower HgA1C by 1.0–1.5%. Metabolized by the liver and cleared by the kidney. Side effects include hypoglycemia and weight gain. Dosed t.i.d. with meals in Type 2 DM.
- Biguanides (Metformin): Lower blood glucose by decreasing hepatic glucose output and increasing insulin action. Metformin lowers HgA1C by 1.0–2.0%. Associated with modest weight reductions and decreased risk of all-cause mortality in obese individuals. Side effects include GI distress (diarrhea, nausea, and abdominal pain) and lactic acidosis (avoid in renal dysfunction, hepatic disease, cardiac disease, excess alcohol, IV iodinated contrast or surgical procedure.) Dosed b.i.d. or t.i.d. in Type 2 DM.
- Thiazolidinediones (Rosiglitazone and Pioglitazone): Lowers blood glucose concentrations by increasing insulin sensitivity. Lower A1C by 1.0–2.0%. Metabolized and cleared by the liver. Side effects include hepatotoxicity, fluid retention, CHF and weight gain. Dosed daily or b.i.d. in Type 2 DM.
- Alpha-glucosidase inhibitors (acarbose and miglitol): Interferes with digestion and absorption of complex carbohydrates. Lower HgA1C by 0.5–1.0%. Side effects include flatulence, diarrhea, and abdominal discomfort. Dosed t.i.d. with meals in Type 2 DM.
- Amylin analogs (pramlintide): Decrease gastric emptying and suppress glucagon secretion and hepatic glucose production. Side effects include nausea and hypoglycemia. Subcutaneous injections t.i.d. with meals for Type 1 and insulin-treated Type 2 DM.
- GLP-1 therapies (exenatide): Stimulates glucose-dependent insulin release from the pancreatic islets, slows gastric emptying, inhibits inappropriate postmeal glucagon release, and reduces food intake. Side effects include nausea and hypoglycemia when given with sulfonylureas. Subcutaneous injections within 1 hour of morning and evening meals in Type 2 DM on oral agents.
- Insulin: For all Type 1 and in Type 2 with inadequate blood glucose control on oral agents.
  - Rapid-acting (Lispro, Aspart, and Glulysine): Onset of action 30 minutes and duration of action 2–4 hours.
  - Short-acting (Regular): Peaks at 2–4 hours and duration of action 6–8 hours.
  - Intermediate-acting (NPH): Peak at 4–10 hours and duration of action 12–18 hours.

- Long-acting (Glargine): Onset 1–2 hours and duration of action up to 24 hours.
- Combine long acting insulin with short acting insulin to achieve glycemic control.
- Common regimens include Glargine at bedtime with Lispro/Aspart/Glulysine for meal time coverage or NPH/Regular before morning and evening meals. Insulin pump infuses continuous subcutaneous short or rapid acting insulin in Type 1 DM.
- In Type 2 DM, adding intermediate or long acting insulin to oral therapy is the first step before considering regimens with multiple injections.
- Side effects include hypoglycemia and weight gain.

Pregnancy Considerations

- GDM, Type 1 or Type 2 DM: Insulin (NPH, Regular and Lispro) is recommended for use in pregnancy.
- Target plasma glucose in pregnancy: fasting <95 mg/dL, 1 hour postprandial <140 mg/dL or 2 hours postprandial <120 mg/dL. During labor and delivery, insulin drip and glucose infusion is used to maintain maternal blood glucose concentration between 70 and 90 mg/dL.
- Insulin requirements decrease after delivery due to a drop in counter regulatory hormones.

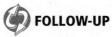 **FOLLOW-UP**

Admission Criteria

Diabetic ketoacidosis (hyperglycemia <800 mg/dL, ketone bodies, anion gap acidosis) and nonketotic hyperglycemia (hyperglycemia >800 mg/dL and plasma osmolality >320 mosmol/kg) require ICU admission for IV fluids, insulin drip, potassium replacement, and evaluation of precipitating event. Bicarbonate therapy reserved for severe acidosis.

COMPLICATIONS

- Glucose control decreases microvascular, not macrovascular, complications in Type 1 and Type 2 DM. However, strong trends in the reduction of macrovascular complications with glycemic control in two major trials.
- Other preventative measures include
  - Macrovascular disease:
    - Aspirin therapy: Recommended for individuals with CVD, >40 years of age, and 30–40 years with risk factors including smoking, HTN, dyslipidemia, and albuminuria.
    - Lipid management: Achieve target goals. Statin (30–50% LDL reduction) and fibrates (35–50% TG reduction) are 1st line.
    - Blood pressure control: Goal <130/80 mmHg. ACE Inhibitors and ARB are first line in DM.
    - Smoking cessation

- Neuropathy: Regular foot exam with referral to podiatry for foot care. Consider antidepressants (e.g., amitriptyline) and anticonvulsants (e.g., gabapentin) for pain control; metoclopramide for gastroparesis
- Retinopathy: Regular dilated eye exam by an ophthalmologist; consider photocoagulation and vitrectomy in symptomatic individuals
- Nephropathy: ACE Inhibitors and ARB decrease progression in individuals with microalbuminuria
- Vaccines: Flu vaccine every fall and pneumococcal vaccine

Pregnancy Considerations

- Hyperglycemia in pregnancy is associated with preeclampsia, polyhydramnios, macrosomia, intrauterine growth restriction, congenital anomalies, perinatal mortality, neonatal complications (e.g., hypoglycemia, hyperbilirubinemia) and childhood complications (e.g., DM, obesity). Normalizing glucose can reduce risk of complication.
- Several agents used in the treatment of diabetes and its complications are contraindicated during pregnancy including ACE inhibitors, ARBs, statins, and oral antidiabetic agents. Assessment of medications, glycemic control, and complication (e.g., blood pressure, retinopathy progression) is recommended prior to and during pregnancy.

REFERENCES

1. The Diabetes Control and Complications Trial Research Group. The effect of intensive treatment of diabetes on the development and progression of long-term complications in insulin-dependent diabetes mellitus. *N Engl J Med*. 1993;329:977.
2. Intensive blood-glucose control with sulphonylureas or insulin compared with conventional treatment and risk of complications in patients with type 2 diabetes. UK Prospective Diabetes Study Group. *Lancet*. 1998;352:837.
3. American Diabetes Association Position Statement. Diabetes Care. 2004;27.

CODES
ICD9-CM
250.0 Diabetes

KEY WORDS

- Diabetes
- Hyperglycemia
- Gestational Diabetes

DOMESTIC VIOLENCE

Amy S. Gottlieb, MD

KEY CLINICAL POINTS

- R: Remember to ask about domestic violence in the course of a routine patient encounter.
- A: Ask directly.
- D: Document findings in the medical record.
- A: Assess safety.
- R: Review options and refer as appropriate.

 BASICS

DESCRIPTION

- Domestic violence is characterized by a pattern of coercive behaviors that may include repeated battering and injury, psychological abuse, sexual assault, progressive social isolation, deprivation, and intimidation.
- These behaviors are perpetrated by someone who is or was involved in an intimate relationship with the victim.

EPIDEMIOLOGY

- United States incidence: 1.5 million women per year are physically assaulted or raped by a current or former husband, cohabitating partner, or date.
- Women are killed by intimate partners more often than by any other perpetrator.
- 25% of women will be physically assaulted or raped by an intimate in her lifetime.

Lifetime Prevalence by Clinical Setting

- Internal Medicine Clinics: 28% of women
- Prenatal Clinics: 23% of women
- Emergency Rooms: 37% of women
- Family Medicine Clinics: 39% of women

RISK FACTORS

Domestic violence occurs in all racial, socioeconomic, religious, and ethnic groups. Additional risk factors:

- Young age (<36 years of age)
- Single, separated, or divorced
- Coverage by medical assistance or uninsured

NATURAL HISTORY

Most domestic violence is characterized by ongoing, repetitive acts of relatively "minor" physical assaults accompanied by patterns of control, intimidation, and isolation.

- Control—over money, car, food—is used to instill dependence
- Intimidation—raised eyebrows, humiliation, open threats, stalking—creates a state of generalized anxiety for the battered woman
- Isolation—from family, friends, coworkers—prevents exposure of the violence and reinforces dependence on the abuser; deprives the battered woman of the support to escape

SCREENING

Most medical professional organizations recommend routine screening for domestic violence.

- Ask the patient questions in a safe, private setting.
- Ask directly:
  - "Have you been hit, kicked, punched, or otherwise hurt by someone in the past year? If so, by whom?"
  - "Do you feel safe in your current relationship?"
  - "Is there a partner from a previous relationship who is making you feel unsafe now?"
  - "Does your partner ever emotionally abuse you or force you to have sex?"

SIGNS AND SYMPTOMS

- Physical: Chest pain, dyspareunia, GI disturbances, headaches, palpitations, pelvic pain, trauma (sprains/fractures/cuts)
- Psychological: Anorexia/bulimia, depression, insomnia, irritability, lethargy, mood swings, suicidal ideation, suicide attempts

INTERVENTION

IF A WOMAN DISCLOSES ABUSE:
RECOGNITION & VALIDATION

Tell the patient she is not alone and no one deserves to be beaten.

SAFETY ASSESSMENT

The majority of domestic violence homicides involve physical abuse prior to the murder. Separation after cohabitation increases the risk of homicide.

- Establish the severity of the abuse:
  - Does the batterer have a weapon?
  - Has the batterer threatened to kill the patient?
  - Has the couple recently separated or stopped living together?
  - Does the patient feel she is in immediate danger?
- Establish the type(s) of abuse—physical, sexual, and/or emotional.
- Establish the pattern of abuse:
  - When was the first episode of abuse?
  - When was the most serious episode of abuse?
  - When was the most recent episode of abuse?
- Inquire about suicidal ideation.

SAFETY PLAN

- Provide the patient with information about available resources—e.g., local hotline & shelter phone numbers.
- Discuss a "quick escape" plan. Suggest that the patient keep copies of birth certificates, immunization records, driver's license, credit/bank card numbers, and (if possible) car keys in a safe, accessible place.

DOCUMENTATION

- Clearly document in the chart all physical findings, using a body map if possible.
- Document the patient's own words when describing abuse. For example, "He hit me with a hammer."
- If you suspect abuse but the patient does not disclose, document your suspicion in the chart.

MANDATORY REPORTING

Most states do NOT mandate reporting of partner abuse unless a weapon is involved. Contact your local domestic violence coalition for specific reporting requirements.

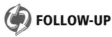 **FOLLOW-UP**

- Tell the patient that you are concerned about her home/personal life and possibly her safety and would like to check-in with her again.
- Bring the patient back for regular follow-up visits (e.g., every 3–4 months) to inquire about any violence in her life.

RESOURCES

- National Domestic Violence Hotline:1-800-799-SAFE (7233); 1-800-787-3224 (TTY)
- Family Violence Prevention Fund: http://endabuse.org
- American College of Obstetricians and Gynecologists: www.acog.org/from_home/departments/dept_web.cfm?recno=17
- American Medical Association: www.ama-assn.org/ama/pub/category/3242.html
- National Institutes of Health: www.nlm.nih.gov/medlineplus/domesticviolence.html
- World Health Organization: www.who.int/violence_injury_prevention/violence/global_campaign/en/

REFERENCES

1. Alpert EJ, Freund KM, Park CC, et al. Partner violence: How to recognize and treat victims of abuse. Massachusetts Medical Society. 1994;15.
2. Flitcraft AH, et al. AMA diagnostic and treatment guidelines on domestic violence. 1992;2.
3. Tjaden P, Thoennes N. Prevalence, incidence, and consequences of violence against women: findings from the national violence against women survey. National Institute of Justice-Centers for Disease Control and Prevention, Research in Brief. 1998;NCJ 172837:1–16.
4. Gin NE, Rucker L, Frayne S, et al. Prevalence of domestic violence among patients in three ambulatory care internal medicine clinics. *JGIM*. 1991;6:317–322.
5. Helton AS, McFarlane J, Anderson ET. Battered and pregnant: A prevalence study. *Am J Pub Health*. 1987;77:1337–1339.
6. Dearwater SR, Cohen JH, Campbell JC, et al. Prevalence of intimate partner abuse in women treated at community hospital emergency rooms. *JAMA*. 1998;280:433–438.
7. Hamberger LK, Saunders DG, Hovey M. Prevalence of domestic violence in community practice and rate of physician inquiry. *Family Med*. 1992;24:283–287.
8. McCauley J, Kern DE, Kolodner K, et al. The "battering syndrome": Prevalence and clinical characteristics of domestic violence in primary care internal medicine practices. *Ann Intern Med*. 1995;123:737–746.
9. Feldhaus KM, Koziol-McLain J, Amsbury HL, et al. Accuracy of 3 brief screening questions for detecting partner violence in the emergency department. *JAMA*. 1997;277:1357–1361.
10. Campbell JC. Health consequences of intimate partner violence. *Lancet*. 2002;359:1331–1336.
11. Campbell JC, Sharps PW, Gary FA, et al. Intimate partner violence and physical health consequences. *Arch Intern Med*. 2002;162:1157–1163.
12. Campbell JC, Webster D, Koziol-McLain J, et al. Risk factors for femicide in abusive relationships: Results from a multisite case control study. *Am J Pub Health*. 2003;93:1089–1097.
13. General mandatory reporting laws: When are health care practitioners required to report domestic violence victimization? Family Violence Prevention Fund. March 8, 2002.

CODES
ICD9-CM

- 995.81 Adult physical abuse
- 995.82 Adult emotional/psychological abuse
- 995.83 Adult sexual abuse
- V61.11 Domestic Violence counseling—victim

KEY WORDS

- Battered Woman
- Battered Wife
- Battering
- Domestic Violence
- Intimate Partner Violence
- Partner Abuse
- Sexual Abuse

DYSMENORRHEA

Jamie D. Kemp, MD
Suzanne Bornschein, MD

KEY CLINICAL POINTS

- Dysmenorrhea occurs in a large percentage of women and is a major cause of days missed at school or work.
- Most women with dysmenorrhea will have a normal physical exam; laboratory tests or diagnostic studies are generally not helpful unless a secondary cause is suspected.
- NSAIDS and hormonal therapy such as combined oral contraceptives are first line treatment.
- Dysmenorrhea may be associated with significant disability in some women; if severe symptoms persist in the absence of menses, other causes of pelvic pain must be considered.

 BASICS

DESCRIPTION
- Primary dysmenorrhea
  - Pain results from myometrial contraction and the production of prostaglandins.
  - There is no readily identifiable pelvic process.
  - Pain associated with menstruation that usually occurs within 1–2 years of onset of menarche
  - The pain usually begins on or the day before menses and lasts 1–3 days.
  - There is crampy, lower abdominal discomfort accompanied at times by nausea, vomiting, diarrhea, or headache.
- Secondary dysmenorrhea
  - Involves pelvic pathology such as infection, endometriosis, adhesions, ovarian cysts
  - Usually prompts a gynecologic referral

GENERAL PREVENTION
The general population should be screened for dysmenorrhea.

EPIDEMIOLOGY
Incidence
Decreases in incidence with increasing age, parity, and the use of oral contraceptives.

Prevalence
- Approximately 72% of adolescents experience dysmenorrhea, and 15% have severe symptoms.
- Among women in their 20s, 67% experience dysmenorrhea, whereas 10% have severe symptoms.

RISK FACTORS
- Nulliparity
- Young age
- Heavy menstrual flow
- Cigarette smoking
- High prostaglandin and vasopressin levels
- Depression/anxiety and sexual abuse are weaker risk factors

PATHOPHYSIOLOGY
- During the follicular phase of the menstrual cycle, hormonal stimulation of the endometrium results in the production of arachidonic acid.
- During menses, arachidonic acid is converted to leukotrienes and prostaglandins F2-α and E2.
- These chemical mediators as well as vasopressin cause strong uterine contractions that reduce blood flow to the myometrium by compressing small arterioles and capillaries.
- Muscular contractions and myometrial ischemia cause pain.

ETIOLOGY
- Secondary dysmenorrhea may occur in a number of pelvic diseases.
- Endometriosis, the presence of endometrial tissue outside the uterus
- Adenomyosis, the presence of endometrial tissue within the myometrium
- Uterine leiomyomas

ASSOCIATED CONDITIONS
Premenstrual mood dysphoric disorder (PMDD) may have overlap with dysmenorrhea; thus patients should be screened for PMDD.

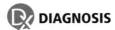 **DIAGNOSIS**

PRE-HOSPITAL
Dysmenorrhea is almost exclusively evaluated as an outpatient.

SIGNS AND SYMPTOMS
- Primary dysmenorrhea
  - Pain occurs shortly before or with the onset of menses, and may last for 1–4 days.
  - Cramping or colicky pain located in the lower abdomen.
  - There may be associated fatigue, nausea, vomiting, diarrhea, headaches, and malaise.
- Secondary dysmenorrhea
  - There may be pain in the absence of menses, as well as fever, dysuria, dyspareunia, menorrhagia, or metrorrhagia.

History
- When was menarche?
- Are menses regular and normal in flow?
- Does the patient smoke?
- Does the pain occur at times other than menstruation?

Physical Exam
- Women with primary dysmenorrhea have a normal physical exam.
- Women with secondary dysmenorrhea often have a normal exam, but the clinician may find:
  - An enlarged, irregularly shaped, or tender uterus or adnexae
  - Cervical displacement
  - Cervical stenosis

TESTS
- Most patients do not require extensive evaluation.
- As most women with dysmenorrhea do not have a secondary cause, a trial of NSAIDS may be helpful in diagnosis, as more worrisome causes of pelvic pain will not likely respond.

Imaging
Transvaginal ultrasound
- Aids in the characterization of physical exam abnormalities
- Allows the detection of uterine and adenexal lesions that may not be detectable on exam
- Highly sensitive for the detection of pelvic masses, but operator-dependent

Diagnostic Procedures/Surgery
- Exploratory laparascopy/laparatomy
- If the suspicion is high for a secondary cause of dysmenorrhea, and above studies unyielding, directly examining the uterus adnexae, and peritoneal cavity via laparoscopy or open surgical examination may be helpful.

Pathologic Findings
Described above.

DIFFERENTIAL DIAGNOSIS
- Endometriosis
- Adenomyosis
- Uterine leiomyomas
- Ovarian cyst

TREATMENT

PRE-HOSPITAL
Dysmenorrhea can almost always be treated as an outpatient.

GENERAL MEASURES
- Assess the patient's degree of symptoms.
- Many women will obtain relief with topical heat therapy.
  - Reduces pain by approximately 50% more than acetaminophen alone.
  - Similar to the relief obtained by low-dose ibuprofen

Diet
There is some evidence to suggest that low-fat and low-protein diets help some women, but the data are not strong enough to suggest dietary changes as a treatment.

Activity
Some women obtain relief with aerobic exercise, although other women see no benefit.

Complementary and Alternative Medicine
- There are promising early data supporting alternative treatments for dysmenorrhea, although more studies are needed before they can be recommended.
- Some data suggest that vitamins B1 and B6, and vitamin E, may be beneficial.
- 1 small study of 11 women revealed that 10 obtained significant pain relief with acupuncture.
- A meta-analysis from the Cochrane database reported no effectiveness with chiropractic manipulation.
- There is currently little more than empiric data supporting herbal therapy.

MEDICATION (DRUGS)

First Line
- NSAIDS and hormonal control are first-line therapy for dysmenorrhea.
- NSAIDS
  - Decrease prostaglandin production, thereby decreasing the discomfort of uterine contractions.
  - Partial or total pain relief is experienced by 72%, compared to 15% with placebo.
  - Must be used with caution in women who are trying to get pregnant, as well as in those with uncontrolled HTN, CAD, or a history of GI bleeding.
  - Mefenamic acid (Ponstel) is the best choice as its prevents:
    - Production of prostaglandins
    - Binding of prostaglandins to receptors

- Hormonal therapy
  - Combined oral contraceptives
  - Contraceptive patch: Intravaginal hormonal eluting devices (Nuvaring)
  - Levonorgestrel intrauterine system (Mirena)
  - Depo-medroxyprogesterone acetate (Depo-Provera)

Second Line
- COX-2 inhibitors can be considered for their easy dosing regimen, but may carry an increased incidence of cardiovascular events.
- Leuprolide acetate (Lupron)

SURGERY
- In women with disabling symptoms, hysterectomy is an option.
- In select women, lysis of adhesions or ablation therapy for endometriosis may be indicated.

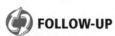

FOLLOW-UP

DISPOSITION
Admission Criteria
In extremely rare cases, women may need to be hospitalized for pain control.

Issues for Referral
If a secondary cause of dysmenorrhea or if another source of chronic pelvic pain is suspected, the patient may benefit from referral to a gynecologist with expertise in dealing with pelvic pain.

PROGNOSIS
- <20% of women with dysmenorrhea experience disabling symptoms.
- Symptoms improve with age and increasing parity.

COMPLICATIONS
- Some women experience significant psychological morbidity from dysmenorrhea.
- PMDD should be considered and treated if present.

PATIENT MONITORING
If the patient experiences depression or anxiety with dysmenorrhea, these symptoms must be reassessed during a pain-free period, as they may be independently present.

REFERENCES

1. Sundell G, Milsom I, Andersch B. Factors influencing the prevalence and severity of dysmenorrhoea in young women. *British J Obstet Gynaecol*. 1990;97:588.
2. Current Obstetrics and Gynecologic Diagnosis and Treatment. 9th ed. McGraw-Hill.
3. Novak's Gynecology. 13th ed. Philadelphia: Lippincott, Williams & Wilkins.
4. Akin M, Weingand KW, Hengehold DA, et al. Continuous, low-level topical heat in the treatment of primary dysmenorrhea. *Obstet & Gynecol*. 2001:97:343.
5. Proctor ML, Roberts H, Farquhar CM. Combined oral contraceptive pill (OCP) as treatment for primary dysmenorrhea. The Cochrane Database of Systematic Reviews, 2001.
6. Helms JM. Acupuncture for the management of primary dysmenorrhea. *Obstet Gynecol*. 1987;69:51.
7. Proctor ML, Hing W, Johnson TC, et al. Spinal manipulation for primary and secondary dysmenorrhea. The Cochrana Database of Systematic Reviews, 2001.

8. Daniels S, Torri S, Desjardins PJ. Valdecoxib for treatment of primary dysmenorrhea. *J General Intern Med*. 2005:20:62–67.
9. French L. Dysmenorrhea. American Family Physician. 2005;71:285.

CODES
ICD9-CM
- 625.3 Dysmenorrhea
- 625.9 Pelvic pain

KEY WORDS
- Abdominal Pain
- Pelvic Pain
- Premenstrual Mood Dysphoric Disorder
- Premenstrual Syndrome

D

EATING DISORDERS

Audrey R. Tyrka, MD, PhD
Lauren M. Wier, BS

KEY CLINICAL POINTS

- Eating disorders may have serious medical complications, which should be monitored during treatment and weight restoration.
- Early detection is associated with a better prognosis.
- Psychotherapy is mainstay of treatment and SSRIs appear to be helpful in the treatment of bulimia nervosa (BN) and binge-eating disorder (BED).

 BASICS

DESCRIPTION

- Eating disorders are characterized by severe disturbances in eating patterns and distortion of body image.
- BN
  - Repeated episodes of eating large amounts of food (binging) followed by inappropriate compensatory behaviors (purging)
- BED
  - Repeated episodes of binging, no purging
  - BED is not formally recognized as a diagnostic category; further study is necessary to determine its validity.
- Anorexia nervosa (AN)
  - Extreme dieting resulting in weight loss below 15% of ideal body weight
  - Individuals with AN may also engage in binging and purging.

EPIDEMIOLOGY

- Over 90% of people with eating disorders are female.
- In the United States, eating disorders are most common in Caucasian women, but occur across all ethnic groups and socioeconomic classes.

Prevalence

- Lifetime prevalence of AN
  - In women: 0.5–1%
- Lifetime prevalence of BN
  - In women: 1–3%
- Prevalence rates of BED
  - Vary greatly depending on sample populations
  - Rates of 0.7–4% have been reported in community samples
  - Occurring more often in females than males

RISK FACTORS

- Low self esteem
- Fear of losing control
- History of physical or sexual abuse
- Prior history of an eating disorder or multiple dieting attempts
- Age of onset most common in adolescence
- Female athletes (especially distance runners and gymnasts)
- Male athletes (especially body builders and wrestlers)
- Individuals with BED tend to be overweight and/or have a history of weight fluctuation

ETIOLOGY

- Genetics
  - Twin and family studies lend support to heritability of eating disorders.
  - The 5-HT$_{2A}$ receptor gene has recently been implicated in the etiology of Anorexia Nervosa.
  - Individuals with BN and BED have decreased 5-HT$_{2A}$ receptor binding and reduced 5-HT transporter binding, respectively.

- Cultural pressure
  - Particularly in Western society
- Psychosocial and environmental stressors
  - Physical or sexual abuse

ASSOCIATED CONDITIONS

- Conditions associated with AN:
  - Major depressive disorder
  - Obsessive compulsive disorder
  - Personality disorders (especially avoidant and obsessive compulsive)
- Conditions associated with BN:
  - Major depressive disorder
  - Anxiety disorders
  - Substance abuse disorders
  - Borderline and avoidant personality disorders

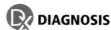 **DIAGNOSIS**

- AN
  - Characterized by self-starvation and excessive weight loss
  - Symptoms include:
    - Refusal to maintain appropriate body weight
      ○ Weight <85% of appropriate weight for height and age or BMI $\leq$17.5 kg/m^2
    - Intense fear of gaining weight
    - Distorted body image
    - Amenorrhea in postmenarcheal females
    - May involve purging with or without binge eating
- BN
  - Characterized by repeated episodes of secretive binge eating
  - In contrast to patients with AN who may also binge, patients with BN do not have excessive weight loss.
  - Symptoms include:
    - Lack of control during binges which occur at least twice weekly for 3 months
    - Eating beyond the point of comfortable fullness
    - Inappropriate compensatory behaviors after binges such as self-induced vomiting, excessive exercise, fasting, abuse of laxatives, diet pills and/or diuretics

SIGNS AND SYMPTOMS

- Starvation is associated with:
  - Excessive thinness, cachexia
  - Bradycardia
  - Hypothermia
  - Anemia
  - Leukopenia
  - Hypotension
  - Osteoporosis
  - Thyroid dysfunction
  - Electrolyte abnormalities
  - Cognitive impairment
  - Dry, scaly skin
  - Lanugo (baby fine hair covering the body)
- Purging is associated with
  - Dehydration
  - Erosion of tooth enamel
  - Enlarged parotid glands
  - Electrolyte abnormalities

History
- Assess for eating disorder symptoms
- Assess for comorbid psychiatric conditions including major depressive disorder, substance abuse, obsessive compulsive disorder and personality disorders
- Rule out medical conditions

Physical Exam
Physical examination to assess for signs of starvation and purging as above.

TESTS
- Laboratory tests to assess for signs of starvation and purging
  - CBC
  - Electrolytes
  - Urinalysis
  - EKG
- Test for medical conditions that may produce weight loss
  - TSH
  - Glucose
  - CBC
- Self report questionnaires may be helpful screening tools for eating disorders
  - The SCOFF questionnaire (Morgan, et al, 1999)
  - Eating Attitudes Test (Garner, 1997)

DIFFERENTIAL DIAGNOSIS
- Psychiatric disorders causing weight loss or decreased appetite:
  - Major depressive disorder
  - Anxiety disorders (e.g., obsessive compulsive disorder, fear of eating in public)
  - Psychotic disorders (e.g., schizophrenia)
- Medical conditions causing weight loss:
  - Hyperthyroidism
  - Cancer
  - Onset of diabetes mellitus
  - Gastrointestinal disorders

Pregnancy Considerations
- Women with a history of eating disorder may relapse during pregnancy.
- The lack of an increase in weight from one prenatal visit to the next during second trimester may be warning sign of eating disorder during pregnancy.
  - Purging should be distinguished from hyperemesis gravidarum.
- Pregnant women with current or past eating disorders are more likely to give birth to infants with low birth weight and smaller head circumferences.

ALERT
- There is >10% mortality rate in individuals with AN due to suicide or medical complications such as arrhythmia.
- Weight restoration in patients with eating disorders may worsen psychiatric and medical conditions, particularly if the weight gain is rapid.

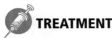

TREATMENT

INITIAL STABILIZATION
- If seriously underweight (<75% of ideal body weight) or other serious medical complications, consider hospitalization.
- Individuals with eating disorders may be resistant to treatment and deny disordered eating or being underweight.

- Family involvement and supportive environment may aid in treatment.

GENERAL MEASURES
- Treatment for AN or BN may be quite lengthy (5+ years) depending on severity of illness. Treatments include:
  - Individual psychotherapy
    - Cognitive-behavioral
    - Behavioral
    - Interpersonal
    - Psychoanalytic
    - Psychodynamic
  - Family psychotherapy
  - Support groups
    - With caution, because patients may compete to be the thinnest or most sickly in the group.
- Weight reduction programs, cognitive-behavioral therapy, and/or dialectical behavioral therapy may be helpful in the treatment of BED.

Diet
Nutritional rehabilitation and weight restoration
- May take place in an inpatient or outpatient setting, depending on severity and individual needs
- Ideal target body weight should be defined
  - Based on BMI or
  - Weight at which individual previously had normal menses
- Healthy rate of weight gain approximately
  - In an inpatient setting: 2–3 lb/week
  - In an outpatient setting: 0.5–2 lb/week
- Create and implement plan for weight restoration. May include:
  - Nutritional supplements
  - Structured diet
  - In extreme cases, nasogastric or parenteral feeding may be necessary
- Weight gain and decreased use of diuretics and/or laxatives may cause fluid retention, abdominal pain and, in rare cases, congestive heart failure.
- Weight gain may increase anxiety and depressive symptoms; suicidal ideation may also increase and should be monitored.

Activity
- Physical activity should be limited until sufficient weight has been gained.
- Emphasize that physical activity should be to maintain fitness and not to burn calories.
- Individuals who are physically restless and continually fidget may require higher caloric intake to stabilize weight.

MEDICATION (DRUGS)

Psychotropic medications, particularly SSRIs, can be helpful in treating comorbid psychiatric symptoms (e.g., depression, obsessive compulsive disorder) and in maintaining weight gain.
- AN
  - Psychotropic medications are not used as the primary treatment for AN.
- BN
  - Fluoxetine is the only FDA approved drug for treatment of BN.
  - Other SSRIs may also be effective.
    - MAOIs may be useful in curbing vomiting; their use requires stringent adherence to dietary restrictions and attention to drug interactions to avoid possibility of hypertensive crisis and serotonin syndrome.

E

- BED
  - Fluoxetine and other SSRIs may be effective in treating BED.
  - Some preliminary studies have found that:
    - Anticonvulsants may help control urges to binge.
    - Appetite suppressants may be helpful; however, more research is needed to determine their efficacy.

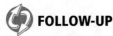

FOLLOW-UP

Issues for Referral
- Referral for nutritional counseling and psychotherapy generally indicated; long-term follow-up care including psychotherapy, support groups and/or medications may be necessary.
- Consider referral to a psychiatrist for management of comorbid conditions.
- Hospitalization may be necessary for severe malnutrition or other medical complications.

Discharge Criteria
- Before discharge from inpatient setting, weight and medical conditions should be stable.
- Individuals with higher discharge weights are less likely to relapse than individuals with lower discharge weights.

PROGNOSIS
A number of factors influence treatment outcome:
- Poorer prognosis is associated with
  - Failure to respond to previous treatment
  - Frequent vomiting
  - Poor quality of family relationships
  - Comorbid psychiatric illness
- Better prognosis is associated with:
  - Early detection
  - Higher initial body weight
  - Younger individuals

PATIENT MONITORING
During weight restoration:
- Vital signs, electrolytes, gastrointestinal symptoms, and cardiac function should be monitored.
- Individuals should be monitored for secretive binging and purging, and for feigning weight gain via excessive hydration.

REFERENCES

1. American Psychiatric Association. Diagnostic and Statistical Manual of Mental Disorders. 4th ed. Text Revision. Washington, DC: American Psychiatric Association; 2000.
2. Garner DM. Psychoeducational principals in the treatment of eating disorders. In: Garner DM, Garfinkel PE, eds. Handbook for Treatment of Eating Disorders. New York, NY: Guilford Press; 1997:145–177.
3. Husted DS, Shapira NA. Binge-eating disorder and new pharmacologic treatments. *Primary Psychiatry*. 2005;12:46–51.
4. Judge BS, Eisenga BH. Disorders of fuel metabolism: medical complications associated with starvation, eating disorders, dietary fads, and supplements. *Emerg Med Clin of North Am*. 2005;23:789–813.
5. Morgan JF, Reid F, Lacey JH. The SCOFF questionnaire: Assessment of a new screening tool for eating disorders. *Br Med J*. 1999;319:1467–1468.
6. Tyrka AR, Graber JA, Brooks-Gunn J. The development of disordered eating: Correlates and predictors of eating problems in the context of adolescence. In: Sameroff AJ, Lewis M, Miller SM, eds. Handbook of Developmental Psychopathology. 2nd ed. New York, NY: Kluwer Academic/Plenum Publishers; 2000: 607–624.
7. Yager J, Andersen A, Devlin M, et al. Practice guidelines for the treatment of patients with eating disorders. In: Practice Guidelines for the Treatment of Psychiatric Disorders. 2nd ed. Washington, DC: American Psychological Association compendium; 2002:697–766.

CODES
ICD9-CM
- 307.1 Anorexia nervosa
- 307.51 Bulimia nervosa

KEY WORDS

- Anorexia
- Bulimia
- Binge
- Body Image

ECTOPIC PREGNANCY

Iris L. Tong, MD
Archana Pradhan, MD, MPH

KEY CLINICAL POINTS

- High index of suspicion in
  - Women of child-bearing age presenting with lower abdominal pain
  - Absence of intrauterine gestational sac in women with β-HCG >2,000 IU/L
- A diagnosis can be confirmed with serial β-HCG levels and repeat transvaginal ultrasound.
- In appropriate candidates, treatment with methotrexate is comparable to surgical intervention.

 BASICS

DESCRIPTION

- An ectopic pregnancy results from the implantation of the blastocyst occurring at a site other than the uterine cavity.
- Can occur in the fallopian tube, cervix, ovary, broad ligament, and peritoneal cavity
- Approximately 98% of ectopic pregnancies occur in the fallopian tube

EPIDEMIOLOGY

- Leading cause of maternal death in the United States during the 1st trimester of pregnancy
- Accounts for approximately 10% of all pregnancy-related deaths

Prevalence
Occurs in 2% of all pregnancies

RISK FACTORS
High
- Prior tubal surgery
- Prior ectopic pregnancy
- Previous salpingitis
- Assisted reproduction
- In utero DES exposure

Moderate
- Previous pelvic infection
- Age <25
- Infertility

Slight
- Tobacco use
- Vaginal douching

PATHOPHYSIOLOGY

- 1/2 of cases result from impaired tubal function, particularly chronic salpingitis.
- Can result from factors inherent to the embryo, leading to premature implantation in fallopian tube.

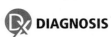 **DIAGNOSIS**

SYMPTOMS

- Symptoms occur 6–8 weeks after missed menstrual period
- Abdominal pain
- Amenorrhea
- Vaginal spotting/bleeding
- Dizziness
- Fainting
- Urge to defecate
- Pregnancy symptoms
- Passage of tissue
- Pain radiating to shoulder
- 50% asymptomatic

Physical Exam
- Adnexal tenderness
- Abdominal tenderness
- Palpable adnexal mass
- Uterine enlargement
- Hypotension, orthostatic changes
- Low grade fever
- Breast tenderness

TESTS
Lab
- Serial quantitative serum β-HCG: in normal pregnancy, β-HCG increases by 66% every 2 days up to 6–7 weeks gestation.
  - In ectopic pregnancy, impaired β-HCG production leads to prolonged doubling times.
  - An increase of $\leq$66% in a 48-hour period is associated with a nonviable pregnancy (either intrauterine or extrauterine).
- Serum progesterone: useful in excluding ectopic pregnancy
  - Levels >25 ng/mL associated with viable intrauterine pregnancies (98%)
  - Levels <5 ng/mL associated with nonviable pregnancies (99%)

Imaging
- Transvaginal ultrasound: In normal pregnancy, intrauterine pregnancy is seen when β-HCG >1,500 mLUm/L (5–6 wks gestation).
  - If the gestational sac is 10 mm, a yolk sac should be visualized.
  - If the yolk sac is 5 mm, a fetal pole should be visualized.
  - If the fetal pole is 5 mm, a fetal heart beat should be visualized.
  - Absence of intrauterine gestation with β-HCG >1,500 is suggestive of ectopic pregnancy.

Diagnostic Procedures/Surgery
Uterine curettage: The presence of chorionic villi excludes diagnosis of ectopic pregnancy as heterotopic pregnancies are rare (1/4,000 to 1/30,000).
- Limited diagnostic tool as false-negative rate of 20% of women undergoing elective termination
- After curettage, β-HCG level should fall $\geq$15% by 8–12 hours
- Failure to decline by 15% is diagnostic of ectopic pregnancy
- Useful management tool in patients hemodynamically stable patients with unclear diagnosis with undesired pregnancy

DIFFERENTIAL DIAGNOSIS
- Spontaneous abortion
- Early IUP
- Threatened abortion
- Ruptured ovarian cyst
- Ovarian torsion
- Pelvic inflammatory disease
- Appendicitis

- UTI/pyelonephritis
- Nephrolithiasis

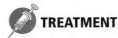

TREATMENT

GENERAL MEASURES
- The initial management is always based on the patient's stability.
- Rhogam should be given if the woman is Rh(D)– and the male partner is Rh(D)+ or unknown.
- Expectant Management:
  - 50–70% of ectopic pregnancies resolve spontaneously, but you do not know which 30–50% will rupture.
  - There is an 88% success rate with expectant management when the initial β-HCG is <200 mLU/mL.
  - Abandon this approach if there is any pain, β-HCG levels fail to decrease, or tubal rupture occurs with hemoperitoneum.

MEDICATION (DRUGS)

- Methotrexate is comparable to surgery in appropriate candidates with a success rate of $\cong$90%.
- Candidates for medical treatment:
  - Asymptomatic women
  - Ability/willingness of women to comply with post-treatment monitoring
  - β-HCG <15,000 mLU/mL prior to treatment (high levels strongly associated with Rx failure)
  - Unruptured mass <3.5 cm and no fetal cardiac activity on ultrasound
- Methotrexate 50 mg/m^2 of body surface area (BSA) IM × 1 dose
  - Evaluate candidate for contraindications, ensure that baseline renal, liver, bone marrow function is normal, check β-HCG
  - Check β-HCG levels, day 4
  - β-HCG levels may rise in the 72 hours following treatment.
  - β-HCG levels should decline 15% from day 4 to day 7.
  - Follow β-HCG levels until they are undetectable (<5 mLU/mL, usually reached in 5 weeks, but can take >3 months).
  - Common side effects include abdominal stomatitis, nausea, vomiting, diarrhea, and dizziness.
- A 2nd dose of methotrexate is given if the β-HCG level does not decrease by an appropriate percentage from day 4 to day 7.
  - A 2nd dose is required in 15–20% of the women
  - Women that require >2 doses: <1%
- Surgical intervention may be required for patients who do not respond to medical treatment or develop symptoms consistent with ruptured ectopic pregnancy.

SURGERY
- Candidates for surgical treatment:
  - Ruptured ectopic pregnancy, especially in hemodynamically unstable patients
  - Inability/unwillingness to comply with post-treatment monitoring with medical therapy
  - Lack of timely access to a medical facility if rupture occurs during conservative therapy
- Surgical options:
  - Laparoscopic vs. open
  - Salpingostomy vs. salpingectomy

- Type of surgery dependent on:
  - Hemodynamic stability of patient
  - Surgical skills of physician
  - Location of ectopic pregnancy

FOLLOW-UP

PROGNOSIS
- Spontaneous resolution:
  - May occur in up to 50–70% of cases
- Future fertility:
  - The subsequent fertility and tubal patency after medical treatment with methotrexate is comparable to surgical management.
  - The subsequent conception rate is approximately 60%, half of these are live births.

COMPLICATIONS
- Tubal rupture:
  - Leading cause of maternal death in 1st trimester
- Tubal abortion:
  - Expulsion of products of conception through fimbria into abdominal cavity
  - Can have minimal intra-abdominal bleeding or severe bleeding requiring surgery
- Recurrence:
  - Recurrence rate after 1 ectopic pregnancy: 15%
  - After 2 ectopic pregnancies: 30%

REFERENCES

1. Lemus J. Ectopic pregnancy: An update. *Curr Opinion in Obstet Gynecol.* 2000;12:369–375.
2. Lipscomb G, Stovall TG, Ling FW. Nonsurgical treatment of ectopic pregnancy. *New Engl J Med.* 2000;343:1325–1329.
3. Speroff L, Glass R, Kase, N. Ectopic pregnancy. In: Clinical Gynecologic Endocrinology and Infertility. Baltimore, MD: Lippincott Williams and Wilkins; 1999:1149–1167.
4. Tulandi T, Sammour A. Evidence-based management of ectopic pregnancy. *Curr Opinion in Obstet Gynecol.* 2000;12:289–292.

CODES
ICD9-CM
- 633.90 Unspecified ectopic pregnancy without intrauterine pregnancy
- 633.91 Unspecified ectopic pregnancy with intrauterine pregnancy
- 633.80 Other ectopic pregnancy without intrauterine pregnancy
- 633.81 Other ectopic pregnancy with intrauterine pregnancy
- 633.0 Abdominal pregnancy
- 633.1 Tubal pregnancy
- 633.2 Ovarian pregnancy

KEY WORDS

- Abdominal Pain
- Adnexal Pain
- Amenorrhea
- Vaginal Bleeding
- Miscarriage
- Pregnancy

ELDERLY FEMALE PATIENT

Ramona L. Rhodes, MD, MPH
Lynn McNicoll, MD, FRCPC

KEY CLINICAL POINTS

- Successful aging includes maintenance of cognitive and functional abilities.
- Cognitive decline is common in older women and results in reduced quality of life and dependence.
- Functional decline is a common marker of many illnesses or conditions. It is a marker of someone's ability to recover from illness and prognosis.

 BASICS

DESCRIPTION

- The keys to successful aging for the elderly female patient involve:
- Continuation of physical activity
- Maintenance of chronic medical conditions
- Prevention of cognitive impairment
- Prevention of morbidity in the form of falls, fractures, and preventable infections
- This chapter will focus on the prevention and management of cognitive and functional decline in the older woman.

GENERAL PREVENTION

- Cognitive decline
- Maintenance of social networks
- Mental exercises
- Proper nutrition
- Functional decline
- Physical exercise
- Diagnose and treat osteoporosis
- Pain management for osteoarthritis
- Evaluation and adjustment of environment (grab bars, raised toilet seats, removal of hazards)

EPIDEMIOLOGY

Women live an average of 6 years longer than men: Current life expectancy for women is 79.9 years.

- Older women spend more years and a larger percentage of their lives disabled.
- Nearly 80% of all older persons living alone are women.
- Studies have shown that among community dwelling adults age 65 and older, the prevalence of severe cognitive impairment in women was 4.7%.

RISK FACTORS

- Cognitive decline
- Family history of dementia
- Cerebrovascular disease
- Traumatic brain Injury
- Poor nutritional status
- Poor social networks
- Functional decline
- Poor social networks
- Widowhood

- Fractures/osteoarthritis
- Comorbid illnesses

ASSOCIATED CONDITIONS

- Cognitive decline
- Depression
- Hypothyroidism
- Vitamin B12 deficiency
- Folate deficiency
- Functional decline
- Osteoporosis
- Osteoarthritis
- Sarcopenia – the age-related loss of muscle mass and strength
- CAD/CHF

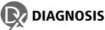 **DIAGNOSIS**

SIGNS AND SYMPTOMS

- Cognitive decline
- Problems with memory
- Difficulty performing instrumental activities of daily living (IADLs). See below.
- Depression
- Social isolation
- Functional decline
- Weight loss
- Decreased ambulation
- Difficulty performing activities of daily living (ADLs). See below.

History

History taking for cognitive and functional decline should include the following:

- Assessment of cognition
- When did the problem begin?
- Has it progressed, and if so, over how long a period of time?
- Assessment of ADLs (bathing, toileting, transferring, dressing, grooming, feeding, walking inside the home, getting in/out of bed)
- Is the patient disheveled?
- Can the patient walk around the home?
- Can the patient transfer into/out of bed?
- Can the patient feed herself?
- Review medications for drug interactions from polypharmacy and potential drug toxicities.
- Assessment of Instrumental ADLs (transportation, shopping, meal preparation, housework, finances, telephone use, medication management)
- Medication noncompliance
- Is the house disheveled?
- Do utilities (gas, electricity) get disconnected?
- Are the patient's finances in order?
- Is the patient missing appointments?
- Are there signs of abuse or neglect?
- Assessment of comorbid conditions

Physical Exam

The physical exam should be comprehensive, including a thorough neurological and musculoskeletal exam as well as a gait assessment for those with functional decline.

TESTS

- For cognitive decline
- The mini mental status exam (MMSE)
- Clock drawing
- The executive interview (EXIT) for: Those with suspected executive dysfunction
- The geriatric depression scale to assess for depression
- Neuropsychological testing if further differentiation is required for functional decline
- The "timed get-up-and go" test
- Katz activities of daily living scale
- Lawton instrumental activities of daily living scale
- Direct observation during exam

Lab

For cognitive decline:

- CBC: Megaloblastic anemia
- Electrolyte panel
  - Hyponatremia
  - Elevated glucose
  - Elevated BUN/CR signifying dehydration, acute renal failure, or uremia
  - Hypercalcemia
- Elevated liver function tests, if indicated
- Thyroid function tests
- Vitamin B12 /folate levels
  - For functional decline
- Albumin/pre-albumin to assess nutritional status
- VDRL or vitamin B12 level
- Thyroid function tests

Imaging

- For cognitive decline: CT scan of the brain, if focal deficit on neurological exam
- For functional decline
  - Plain film, if localized pain is causing decline in function (back, hip, knees, etc.)
  - DEXA to diagnose osteoporosis and initiate appropriate therapies to reduce fracture risk
  - Consider cancer workup (mammogram, CT abdomen/pelvis, colonoscopy, etc.)

Diagnostic Procedures/Surgery

For functional decline: Joint replacement/fixation if so indicated

DIFFERENTIAL DIAGNOSIS

- For cognitive decline
- Alzheimer's dementia
- Vascular dementia
- Dementia of lewy bodies
- Parkinson's disease
- Depression
- Hypothyroidism
- Pick's disease
- Normal pressure hydrocephalus
  - For functional decline
- Depression
- Malnutrition
- Osteoarthritis
- Stroke or other neurological condition
- Undiagnosed dementia

 TREATMENT

Physical Therapy

- For functional decline
- Home safety evaluation
- Gait assessment
- Ambulatory aids

 MEDICATION (DRUGS)

- Review current medications (including OTC/alternative medications) that may contribute to cognitive or functional decline.
- For cognitive decline
  - Cholinesterase inhibitors (for mild to moderate dementia)
    - Donepezil (Aricept™): Start with 5 mg PO q.h.s.; may increase to 10 mg PO q.h.s. in 4–6 weeks if tolerated
    - Rivastigmine (Exelon™): Start with 1.5 mg PO b.i.d. with food; may increase to 3 mg PO b.i.d. in ~2 weeks (max. dose 12 mg/day).
    - Galantamine (Reminyl™, Razadyne™): Start with 4 mg PO b.i.d. with meals; may increase to 8 mg PO b.i.d. after 4 weeks, then 12 mg PO b.i.d. after 4 weeks, if tolerated
  - NMDA receptor antagonists (for moderate to severe dementia)
    - Memantine (Namenda™): Has a titration schedule; increase by 5 mg/day at weekly intervals to a max. dose of 20 mg/day); dose >5 mg/day should be divided b.i.d.
- Vitamin B12 and/or folate, if indicated:
- For functional decline
  - Osteoporosis treatment and prevention
    - Bisphosphonates: Must be taken as directed to avoid GI side effects
      - Alendronate (Fosamax™):
        - Prevention: 35 mg PO a week
        - Treatment: 70 mg PO a week
      - Risedronate (Actonel™):
        - Prevention/treatment: 35 mg PO a week
      - Ibandronate (Boniva™):
        - Prevention/treatment: 150 mg PO a month (on same day of each month)
      - Raloxifene (Evista™):
        - Prevention/treatment: 60 mg PO a day
        - Increased risk of venous thrombosis and exacerbation of hot flushes
      - Calcitonin (Miacalcin™):
        - Treatment: 200 units nasal spray per day; 100 unit Sc/IM alternative is available
    - Parathyroid hormone/teriparatide (Forteo™)
      - Treatment: 20 μg daily SC injection
      - Anabolic agent for postmenopausal women at high risk for fracture
      - May cause leg cramps and dizziness
      - Avoid in patients with increased risk of osteosarcoma
    - Calcium: 1,200–1,500 mg/day
    - Vitamin D: 400–800 units/day
    - Multivitamins

 FOLLOW-UP

DISPOSITION

- An adjustment or change in environment may be beneficial.
- Home care companions or certified nursing assistants to assist in ADLs

- Involvement of family members in supervision of medications and physician visits
- Senior housing
- Adult day care
- Assisted living facilities
- Skilled nursing facilities for rehabilitation
- Hospitalization if acute changes in cognition or function raise concerns for delirium and an underlying acute medical condition

Issues for Referral
- For assessments of cognitive decline
  - Geriatrician for comprehensive geriatric assessment
  - Geriatric psychiatry
  - Neurology/dementia specialists
  - Neuropsychologist
  - Driving safety assessment
- For assessments of functional decline
  - Physical therapy
  - Occupational therapy
  - Visiting nursing
  - Social work

PROGNOSIS
The prognoses for cognitive and functional decline are variable depending on the reversibility of symptoms.

COMPLICATIONS
Complications for both conditions include:
- Higher risks of morbidity and mortality
- Nursing home placement
- Falls, fractures
- Accidents

PATIENT MONITORING
Outpatient assessment of cognitive and functional decline should include serial monitoring of each condition every 3 months.

REFERENCES
1. The Administration on Aging. http://www.aoa.gov. Accessed 10/21/05.
2. Hybels CF, Blazer DG. Epidemiology of late-life mental disorders. *Clin Geriatric Med*. 2003;19:663–696.

ADDITIONAL READING
The Centers for Disease Control and Prevention. The state of aging and health in America, 2004. http://www.cdc.gov/aging. Accessed 10/21/05.

Atkinson HH, Cesari M, Kritchevsky SB, et al. Predictors of combined cognitive and physical decline. *J Am Geriatrics Society*. 2005;53:1197–1202.

Singh MAF. Exercise and aging. *Clin Geriatric Med*. 2004;20:201–221.

CODES
ICD9-CM
- 290.0 Dementia
- 293.0 Delirium
- 783.7 Failure to thrive, adult
- 781.2 Gait disturbance

KEY WORDS
- Memory Loss
- Cognitive Impairment
- Functional Decline
- Disability
- Frailty

E

ELECTIVE BREAST SURGERY

Courtney A. Clark, MD
Susannah S. Wise, MD, FACS

KEY CLINICAL POINTS

- Augmentation mammoplasty: Enhances breast size
- Reduction mammoplasty: Reduces breast size
- Reduction surgery is a more complicated surgery than augmentation.
- Any breast surgery will change breast tissue and increase the challenge to examine and diagnose breast pathology in the future.
- Elective breast surgery may impair nipple sensation, affecting breast feeding and sexual pleasure.

 BASICS

DESCRIPTION

- How a woman views her breast size can have strong emotional and psychological impact on her self image.
- Common elective surgeries for women include: Augmentation mammoplasty to enhance breast size and reduction mammoplasty to reduce breast size.
- Breast enlargement is commonly a day surgery.
  - Surgery lasts an average of 1 ½–3 hours
  - Costs $4,000–$8,000
- Breast reduction is a more complicated surgery.
  - Surgery lasts an average of 3–4 hours
  - Typically it requires a 2- to 3-day hospital stay
  - Costs $6,000–$12,000
- Health insurance does not cover breast augmentation.
- Some health insurance covers breast reduction if considered medically necessary and if a minimum of 500 grams of breast tissue can be removed per breast.
- Patients undergoing reduction mammoplasty often find significant improvement in their quality of life with the reduction or elimination of preoperative complaints.

Pregnancy Considerations

- Pregnancy-associated breast changes will affect the look of both implanted and reduced breasts.
- Breast feeding is commonly affected by cosmetic breast surgery because of rearrangement of breast ducts and/or reduction of nipple sensation.
- Women may wish to undergo breast augmentation or reduction surgery after pregnancy and breast feeding is no longer desired.

RISKS

- There has never been shown an increased cancer risk with cosmetic breast surgery.
- Patients should be aware that any breast surgery will change breast tissue and increase the challenge to examine and diagnose pathology of the breast.

Surgical Risks

Includes reactions to anesthesia, bleeding, and infections

Other Risks

- Implants have never been proven to increase the risk of cancer, connective tissue, or autoimmune disease.
- An implant can last up to 20 years before there is deflation or leaking. Replacement requires additional surgery.
- All breast implants will have scar tissue formed around them called a capsule. The capsule can cause contracture, deformity, and pain.

- The Baker Scale is a descriptive measure of the severity of capsular formation around the breast implant.
  - Class I is minimal.
  - Class IV is severe and requires surgical correction.
- Implants do not typically feel nodular; therefore, if nodules are found on breast exam, they should be evaluated as per standard of care for suspicious breast masses.
- Implants may decrease visualization of breast tumors with mammography.
- Elective breast surgery may impair nipple sensation, affecting breast feeding and sexual pleasure.

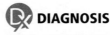 **DIAGNOSIS**

SIGNS AND SYMPTOMS

- Large breasts (macromastia, breast hypertrophy/hyperplasia) have numerous associated physical problems including:
  - Headache, neck pain, back pain, shoulder pain (including from bra strap grooves), skin irritation
- Women with large breasts may also face psychological and social stresses including inability to participate in exercise and other social functions.

History

- Prior to surgery, a woman should discuss with her primary care provider and surgeon the reasons why she wishes to have the surgery.
- Providers should explore how realistic are the woman's postoperative expectations.
- To assist a patient with her surgical options, surgeons should provide preoperative and postoperative photos of previous patients.

Physical Exam

- Basic preoperative exam including a thorough breast exam
- Any abnormality identified must be evaluated prior to elective breast surgery.

TESTS

Imaging

- Preoperative mammography is recommended for women ≥30 years to obtain a baseline.
- Any abnormality on mammogram must be evaluated prior to elective breast surgery.

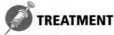 **TREATMENT**

Augmentation Surgery

- An implant is a silicone pouch filled with saline.
- Silicone filled implants are not approved for cosmetic use (only available in special cases including silicone implant replacement and reconstructive surgery for breast cancer or breast anomaly).
- An incision for the breast implant is made under the breast, around the areola, through the umbilicus, or in the axilla.
- The implant can be placed either submuscular (behind the pectoral muscle) or subglandular (between the breast tissue and the muscle). The submuscular approach is more common.

Reduction Surgery

There are a variety of surgical approaches for reduction surgery, typically preserving the nipple-areolar complex.

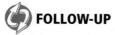 **FOLLOW-UP**

- The patient should expect some postoperative pain, swelling, and bruising.
- Reduction surgery typically requires the patient to have a drain in place for several days.
- Patients should avoid vigorous postoperative activity for 4–6 weeks.
- Over time the augmented breast will soften; however, it will never feel as soft as the natural breast.
- Patients may choose to massage the augmented breast to enhance softening and recover sensation.

REFERENCES

1. Chadbourne E, Zhang S, Gordon M, et al. Clinical outcomes in reduction mammoplasty: A systematic review and meta-analysis of published studies. *Mayo Clinic Proceedings*. 2001;76:503–510.
2. Freund R. *Cosmetic Breast Surgery*. New York, NY: Marlowe & Company; 2004.
3. Love S. *Dr. Susan Love's Breast Book*. 3rd ed. Cambridge, England: Perseus Publishing; 2000.
4. Ruot-Worley J. Augmentation mammoplasty: Implications for the primer care provider. *J of the Am Acad of Nurse Pract*. 2001;13:304–309.
5. Sarwer D, Nordmann J, Herbert J, et al. Cosmetic breast augmentation surgery: A critical review. *J Womens Health & Gender-Based Med*. 2000;9:843–855.
6. Smith M, Kent K. Breast concerns and lifestyles of women. *Clin Obstet Gynecol*. 2002;45:1129–1139.
7. Stoppard M. *The Breast Book*. New York, NY: DK Publishing; 1996.

CODES
ICD9-CM
- 85.31–85.32 Reduction mammoplasty
- 85.51–85.52 Augmentation of breast

KEY WORDS

- Mammoplasty
- Capsular Contracture
- Breast Hyperplasia
- Macromastia
- Reduction
- Augmentation
- Implants

E

ENDOMETRIAL CANCER

Etsuko Aoki, MD, PhD

KEY CLINICAL POINTS

- The most common gynecologic malignancy in the United States
- Primarily a disease of postmenopausal women presenting with abnormal uterine bleeding.
- There is an increased risk in women exposed to unopposed estrogen, those who have received tamoxifen therapy for breast cancer, and those who are at risk of hereditary nonpolyposis colorectal cancer (HNPCC).
- Most cases are diagnosed at an early stage when surgery alone may be curative.
- Diagnosis can be made with office-based endometrial biopsy, although a hysteroscopy with dilation and curettage (D&C) remains the gold standard.

 ## BASICS

DESCRIPTION

- Endometrial cancer is a malignancy of the epithelial lining of the uterine corpus.
  - Pathology: Adenocarcinoma (75–80%), serous carcinoma (<10%), clear-cell carcinoma, secretory adenocarcinoma
- Majority of cases are adenocarcinoma
- Serous carcinoma and clear-cell carcinoma are usually found in advanced stage in older women, whereas secretory adenocarcinoma tends to have good prognosis.

EPIDEMIOLOGY

- Usually seen in postmenopausal women, although 25% of cases occur in premenopausal women
- Higher incidence in Western countries; very low incidence in Eastern nations

Incidence

In 2005 in the United States: 40,880

RISK FACTORS

For endometrial cancer related to hormonal stimulation (type I endometrial carcinoma):

- Unopposed estrogen: Hormone replacement therapy
- Functional ovarian tumors
- Obesity
- High-fat diet
- Chronic anovulation: Polycystic ovary syndrome (PCOS)
- Nulliparity (infertility)
- Diabetes mellitus
- Hypertension (a small study showed HTN is independently associated with endometrial cancer)
- Endometrial hyperplasia
- Family history of endometrial, breast and/or colon cancer (HNPCC)
- Tamoxifen therapy

ETIOLOGY

Thought to be caused by a combination of genetic mutation and hormonal factors

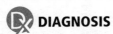 ## DIAGNOSIS

SIGNS AND SYMPTOMS

- Postmenopausal women:
  - Abnormal vaginal discharge (90%)
  - Abnormal vaginal bleeding (80%)

- Approximately 15% of women who present with abnormal bleeding will be found to have endometrial cancer
- Premenopausal women:
  - Diagnosis may be difficult
  - Should be suspected in women with prolonged, heavy menstruation, or mid-cycle bleeding

History

- History of tamoxifen use, unopposed estrogen use, nulliparous, diabetes, hypertension, HNPCC, and PCOS
- Protective factors in history include oral contraceptive use, high physical activity, and smoking

Physical Exam

- Most often pelvic exam will be normal
- May feel mass if advanced

TESTS

Lab

Serum CA-125 to predict extrauterine spread of the disease

Imaging

- Transvaginal ultrasonography to evaluate the endometrial thickness in postmenopausal women:
  - <5 mm; low risk
  - ≥20 mm; high risk
- Chest X-ray to evaluate for lung metastasis
- An abdominal CT scan is not routinely necessary unless extrapelvic disease is suspected.
- Enhanced MRI to evaluate myometrial invasion

Diagnostic Procedures/Surgery

- Endometrial biopsy for diagnosis; in 1 meta-analysis, the post-test probability of endometrial cancer was evaluated
  - After a positive test: 82%
  - After a negative test: 0.9%
- D&C with hysteroscopy: Gold standard, requires anesthesia
- Surgical staging (see Surgery in Treatment)

DIFFERENTIAL DIAGNOSIS

- Sarcoma of uterus
- Polyps
- Endometrial/vaginal atrophy
- Hormone replacement therapy
- Endometrial hyperplasia

 ## TREATMENT

SURGERY

Surgical staging includes hysterectomy with bilateral salpingo-oophorectomy, peritoneal cytology, and pelvic and paraaortic lymph nodes sampling or removal.

- Based on the results of surgical staging and pathological examination, the risk of recurrence is estimated by an experienced oncologist.
  - Low risk: Surgical staging alone is an adequate treatment
  - Intermediate risk: Surgical staging + adjuvant radiation
  - High risk: Surgical staging + extent of surgery + adjuvant radiation and/or chemotherapy ± progestin

Radiotherapy

- Adjuvant pelvic radiation after complete surgical staging in women with intermediate risk decreases the local recurrence, but does not prolong survival.

- For high-risk women, pelvic and whole abdominal irradiation reduce the risk of local recurrence and may prolong survival.

 ## MEDICATION (DRUGS)

Adjuvant chemotherapy should be considered in women with high risk disease.
- Anthracyclines, platinums, and taxanes (found to have antitumor activity)
- The most effective regimen and duration of therapy is unclear.

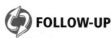 ## FOLLOW-UP

PROGNOSIS
The 5-year survival rates for localized, regional, and metastatic disease are 96%, 67%, and 26%, respectively.

COMPLICATIONS
Recurrence: 75–95% of recurrence occurs within the first 3 years of diagnosis
- Most local recurrence occurs in vagina; potentially curative surgery is often possible
- The major sites of metastasis are the abdominal cavity, liver, and lungs.

PATIENT MONITORING
Periodic evaluation by a gynecological oncologist including history, physical examination, and pelvic examination every 3–6 months for the 1st 5 years and yearly thereafter is recommended.

REFERENCES
1. Creasman WT, Odicino F, Maisonneuve P, et al. Carcinoma of the corpus uteri. *J Epidemiol Biostatistics*. 2001;6:47–86.
2. Jemal A, Murray T, Ward E, et al. Cancer statistics, 2005. *CA: A Cancer J Clinicians*. 2005;55:10–30.
3. Hale GE, Hughes CL, Cline JM, et al. Endometrial cancer: Hormonal factors, the perimenopausal "window risk," and isoflavones. *Journal of endoclinology and metabolism*. 2002;87:3–15.
4. Barakat RR, Hoskins WH, eds. Corpus: Epitherial tumors. In: Hoskins WH, et al., eds. *Principles and Practice of Gynecologic Oncology*. 2nd ed. Philadelphia, PA: Lippincott-Raven Publishers; 1997: 859.
5. Frumovits M, Singh DK, Meyer L, et al. Predictors of final histology in patients with endometrial cancer. *Gynecol Oncol*. 2004;95:463–468.

CODES
ICD9-CM
182.0 Endometrial cancer

KEY WORDS
- Vaginal Bleeding
- Postmenopausal Bleeding

E

ENDOMETRIOSIS

Mary H. Hohenhaus, MD

KEY CLINICAL POINTS

- Common diagnosis in women of reproductive age presenting with chronic pelvic pain
- Often asymptomatic, with lesions identified incidentally on laparoscopy
- Medical and surgical treatments are effective, but no single approach has been shown to be superior.
  - Individualize treatment based on patient age, preferences, and desire for pregnancy.

 ## BASICS

DESCRIPTION
- Endometriosis is the presence of endometrial tissue (glands and stroma) outside the uterus.
- Usually found at multiple sites
  - Dependent areas of pelvis, most commonly the ovaries
  - May occur at distant sites (bowel, bladder, lung, pleurae, skin)
- Classified by findings at laparoscopy
  - Minimal: Isolated implants without significant adhesions
  - Mild: Superficial implants of the peritoneum and ovaries measuring less than 5 cm in total without significant adhesions
  - Moderate: Multiple superficial and invasive implants, may involve adnexal adhesions
  - Severe: Multiple superficial and invasive implants, including endometriomas (cysts filled with menstrual tissue and fluid) with significant adhesions
- Often asymptomatic, but commonly associated with chronic pelvic pain
- The symptoms are not well correlated with the number or size of the implants, but may be related to peritoneal inflammation.
- The symptoms usually regress with pregnancy and menopause.
- Common indication for hysterectomy

EPIDEMIOLOGY
Endometriosis is typically diagnosed in women between 25 and 35 years. True incidence and prevalence are unknown because endometriosis is frequently found in asymptomatic women.

Prevalence
- Approximately 45% of the women of childbearing age undergoing laparoscopy for any indication.
- Approximately 30% of the women presenting with a primary complaint of chronic pelvic pain.

RISK FACTORS
- Caucasian race
- 1st-degree relative with endometriosis
- Congenital outflow tract obstruction

PATHOPHYSIOLOGY
- Not well understood
- Ovarian hormones may cause cyclic stimulation of endometrial implants, with bleeding into surrounding tissue, followed by inflammation and scarring

ETIOLOGY
- Multiple theories
  - Reflux of menstrual tissue into pelvis (retrograde menstruation)
  - Hematologic or lymphatic spread of menstrual tissue
  - Metaplasia of coelomic epithelium

- Implantation of endometrial tissue in surgical incisions
- Appears to require abnormal immune and inflammatory response to implanted tissue

ASSOCIATED CONDITIONS
- Increased risk of infertility
- Increased risk for epithelial ovarian cancer

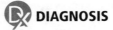 ## DIAGNOSIS

PRE-HOSPITAL
Clinical diagnosis appropriate if symptoms are mild to moderate and pelvic abnormality can be ruled out.

SIGNS AND SYMPTOMS
- Pelvic pain that increases 1–2 days before menstruation
- Pelvic heaviness
- Premenstrual spotting
- Dysmenorrhea
- Heavy menstrual bleeding
- Cyclic bleeding at distant sites (bowel, bladder, pleural cavity)
- Painful defecation during menstruation
- Deep pain with intercourse
- Difficulty conceiving
- Acute surgical abdomen (with rupture of a large ovarian endometrioma)

History
- Location, severity, timing of pain
- Prior diagnosis of endometriosis, response to treatment
- Menstrual, sexual, obstetrical histories

Physical Exam
May be normal; findings depend on location and size of implants; may be more pronounced during first few days of menses.
- Visible lesions on cervix or upper vaginal wall
- Tenderness of the posterior fornix, cul-de-sac, or uterosacral ligaments
- Tender nodules in the cul-de-sac, uterosacral ligaments, or rectovaginal septum
- Pain with uterine movement
- Tender adnexal masses
- Fixation of uterus (retroversion) or adnexa
- Rectal mass

TESTS
Lab
- Serum CA125 level may be elevated, but lacks sufficient sensitivity and specificity to be useful in diagnosis
- β-HCG to rule out pregnancy before treatment

Imaging
- Imaging studies lack sufficient resolution to detect endometrial implants.
  - Large endometriomas may appear as a mass.
- Pelvic ultrasonography useful to evaluate mass palpated on exam
- Pelvic ultrasonography, computed tomography, and magnetic resonance imaging are useful for ruling out other causes of pelvic pain.

Diagnostic Procedures/Surgery
Laparoscopy is the preferred method for diagnosis.
- Allows direct visualization of endometrial implants

- Visual identification alone without biopsy has positive predictive value <45%
- Permits evaluation for pelvic distortion that may contribute to infertility
- Allows treatment of lesions and adhesions

Pathologic Findings
- May be microscopic or macroscopic
- Wide variety in size, shape, and color of lesions
- Biopsy demonstrates endometrial glands and stroma mixed with fibrotic tissue, blood, and cysts

DIFFERENTIAL DIAGNOSIS
- Chronic pelvic pain
  - Chronic pelvic inflammatory disease
  - Ovarian cancer
  - Primary dysmenorrhea
  - Degeneration of uterine myoma
- Acute pelvic pain
  - Hemorrhage or torsion of ovarian cyst
  - Ectopic pregnancy
  - Appendicitis, diverticulitis
- Pelvic lesions
  - Endosalpingiosis, mesothelial hyperplasia, hemosiderin deposition, hemangioma
  - Metastatic breast or ovarian cancer
  - Adrenal rests, splenosis
  - Carbon deposition from prior ablative procedure, reaction to oil-based radiographic dye

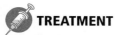 ## TREATMENT

PRE-HOSPITAL
Watchful waiting may be appropriate for women with mild symptoms or who are approaching menopause.

INITIAL STABILIZATION
Pain control with nonsteroidal antiinflammatory drugs as first-line agents

 ## MEDICATION (DRUGS)

- Indicated for mild to moderate symptoms
- Reduce pain by eliminating cyclic stimulation of endometrial implants.
- The selection of the agent depends on patient preferences, the side effect profile, and the cost.
- Not appropriate for women desiring pregnancy in near future as agents cause anovulation
- Not effective for treating adhesions or endometriomas
- Symptoms may recur within months after treatment is stopped.
- May be used in combination with surgery
  - Preoperative: May reduce size of endometrial implants and limit amount of surgical dissection required
  - Postoperative: Appears to prolong pain relief after ablation

First Line
Low-dose monophasic combination oral contraceptives (20 to 25 mcg ethinyl estradiol)
- Suppress ovulation and menstruation through hyperestrogenic effects
- May be administered cyclically or continuously
  - Consider continuous administration if only partial response to cyclic administration

- Schedule pill-free interval to allow for withdrawal bleeding every 3–4 months with continuous therapy
- Improvement in symptoms in up to 80%
- May be used indefinitely
- Up to 30% discontinue secondary to side effects (breast tenderness and weight gain most common)
- Not recommended for women >35 years who smoke or with history of thrombosis

Second Line
- Consider if symptoms do not improve with 1st-line agents or if patient has contraindication to or cannot tolerate them
- Progestins
  - Indicated for women who have contraindication to or cannot tolerate high estrogen regimen
  - Not recommended for women with history of thrombosis
  - Medroxyprogesterone acetate: 30–50 mg daily PO or 150 mg IM depot every 3 months
  - Improvement in symptoms in up to 80%
  - Associated with breakthrough bleeding, nausea, breast tenderness, fluid retention, weight gain, and depression
  - Depot formulation associated with prolonged return of ovulation
- Gonadotropin-releasing hormone (GnRH) agonists
  - Suppress ovulation and menstruation through hypoestrogenic effects
    - Leuprolide: 3.75 mg IM monthly or 11.25 mg IM depot every 3 months for up to 6 months
    - Nafarelin: 200 mcg intranasally twice daily (alternate nostrils) up to 800 mcg a day for up to 6 months
    - Goserelin: 3.6 mg implant SC every 28 days for up to 6 months
  - Improvement in symptoms in up to 90%
  - Side effects common: Hot flushes, vaginal dryness, insomnia, bone loss, irritability
  - Side effects may be largely eliminated and treatment extended to up to 12 months by the addition of estrogen and/or progestin at dosages used for menopausal symptoms.
- Danazol
  - Suppresses ovulation and menstruation through hypoestrogenic and hyperandrogenic effects
  - 400 to 800 mg daily PO in divided doses for 6 to 9 months
  - Improvement in approximately 75%, objective improvement on repeat laparoscopy in 90%
  - Barrier contraceptive for 1st month
  - Can inhibit hepatic clearance of multiple drugs, monitor for toxicity
  - Most patients (80%) experience side effects: Hot flushes, atrophic vaginitis, weight gain, fluid retention, decreased breast size, acne, hirsutism, deepening of voice, elevated liver enzymes, decreased high-density lipoprotein levels, and increased low-density lipoprotein levels.
  - Up to 30% recur 2 years after therapy stopped

SURGERY
- Indicated for moderate to severe symptoms, failure of medical management, presence of endometrioma or pelvic mass, distortion of pelvic organs, bowel or urinary tract obstruction, or when patient desires immediate pregnancy
- Allows treatment at time of diagnosis
- Improvement in pain in up to 70%
- Carries risk of bleeding, infection, injury to pelvic organs, and development of adhesions
- Laparoscopy
  - Indicated for conservative surgery where goal is preservation of the pelvic organs

- Endometrial implants and adhesions may be excised or destroyed by fulguration or laser vaporization; excision is recommended for endometriomas.
  - Shorter hospital stay and recovery compared with laparotomy
- Laparotomy
  - Indicated for radical surgery (hysterectomy with oophorectomy, removal of endometrial implants) when symptoms do not respond adequately to medical therapy or conservative surgery or when the patient has significant symptoms and does not desire future pregnancy
  - Ovaries may be preserved in young women; however, up to 30% have recurrent symptoms requiring later oophorectomy.
- Symptoms recur in 40–60% within 2 years after surgery.
- Adjunctive presacral neurectomy may improve pain, but is not well studied.

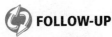 **FOLLOW-UP**

Issues for Referral
- Refer for laparoscopy if symptoms do not respond to medical treatment or if there are changes in symptom pattern or physical exam
- Refer to fertility specialist for management of infertility

PROGNOSIS
- Natural history poorly understood
- Recurrence common after medical and conservative surgical treatment, reported in up to 10% after radical surgery
- Pregnancy rates may improve after conservative surgery for moderate and severe disease
- May recur with postmenopausal hormone replacement

COMPLICATIONS
- Impaired fertility secondary to pelvic distortion
- Thromboembolism secondary to oral contraceptive use
- Osteoporosis secondary to hypoestrogenic effects of GnRH analogs

PATIENT MONITORING
- Regular assessment of symptoms; consider other causes of pelvic pain if symptoms do not improve with trial of therapy
- Role of repeat laparoscopy for monitoring is unknown

- Annual bone mineral density studies if GnRH agonists are continued >6 months; consider calcium and bisphosphonate therapy

REFERENCES

1. Gambone JC, Mittman BS, Munro MG, et al. Consensus statement for the management of chronic pelvic pain and endometriosis: Proceedings of an expert-panel consensus process. *Fertil Sterility*. 2002;78:961–972.
2. Olive DL, Pritts EA. The treatment of endometriosis: A review of the evidence. *Annals NY Academy of Sciences*. 2002;955: 360–372.
3. Rice VM. Conventional medical therapies for endometriosis. *Annals NY Academy of Sciences*. 2002;955:343–352.
4. Stenchever MA, Droegemueller W, Herpst AL, et al. Endometriosis. In: Stenchever MA, et al. *Comprehensive Gynecology*. 4th ed. Philadelphia, PA: Mosby, 2001;531–554.
5. Winkel CA. Evaluation and management of women with endometriosis. *Obstet Gynecol*. 2003;102:397–408.

CODES
ICD9-CM
- 617.0 Endometriosis of uterus
- 617.1 Endometriosis of ovary
- 617.2 Endometriosis of fallopian tube
- 617.3 Endometriosis of pelvic peritoneum
- 617.4 Endometriosis of rectovaginal septum and vagina
- 617.5 Endometriosis of intestine
- 617.6 Endometriosis in scar of skin
- 617.8 Endometriosis of other specified sites
- 617.9 Endometriosis, site unspecified

KEY WORDS

- Abdominal Pain
- Adnexal Pain
- Dysmenorrhea
- Pelvic Pain

EPILEPSY
Suzette M. LaRoche, MD

KEY CLINICAL POINTS

- Patients with a single seizure and risk factors for seizure recurrence should be considered for treatment.
- Newer antiepileptic drugs have similar efficacy as the older agents but are better tolerated due to fewer side effects and less drug interactions.
- Preconceptual counseling aids in optimizing the treatment to reduce maternal and fetal complications.

 BASICS

DESCRIPTION

- A seizure is defined as an abrupt alteration in behavior or perception and is often a symptom of underlying CNS or metabolic dysfunction.
- Epilepsy is a disease characterized by recurrent, unprovoked seizures (2 or more). Epilepsy is not a single disease, but a disorder with many possible underlying causes.

GENERAL PREVENTION

Avoid conditions that lower seizure threshold:
- Sleep deprivation
- Alcohol intoxication or withdrawal
- Illicit drugs: Cocaine, amphetamines
- Prescription drugs: Antipsychotics, tricyclic antidepressants, bupropion, selective serotonin reuptake inhibitors, demerol, penicillins

EPIDEMIOLOGY

The most common serious neurological disorder.

Incidence
- Seizures: 80/100,000
- Epilepsy
  - Average 45/100,000
  - Highest incidence <age 10 and >age 60 (>70 cases per 100,000)
  - Cumulative lifetime incidence 3.1% by age 80

Prevalence
- Seizures:
  - Lifetime prevalence: 9%
- Epilepsy:
  - Point prevalence: 0.5–1.0% (highest in underdeveloped countries)

RISK FACTORS

History of any of the following:
- Perinatal or gestational insults including prematurity
- Febrile seizures
- Family history of epilepsy
- Encephalitis or meningitis
- HIV+
- Stroke or subarachnoid hemorrhage
- Head trauma involving loss of consciousness
- CNS tumor

Genetics
- Contribution of genetics unknown in most epilepsy syndromes
- Some idiopathic epilepsy syndromes linked to defects in ion channels via mendelian or complex inheritance

PATHOPHYSIOLOGY

- Prolonged depolarization of neuronal cell membranes
- Many possible mechanisms
  - Dysfunction of excitatory (glutamate) or inhibitory (GABA) neurotransmitters
  - Alteration of Cl^- or Ca^{++} currents
  - Defective ion channels

ETIOLOGY

Idiopathic	65.5%
Vascular	10.9%
Congenital	8.0%
Trauma	5.5%
Neoplastic	4.1%
Degenerative	3.5%
CNS Infection	2.5%

- Underlying etiology varies by age
- Most common identified etiology (1):
  - <15 years: Congenital abnormalities
  - 15–24 years: Head trauma
  - 25–44 years: Brain tumor
  - >45 years: Stroke

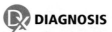 **DIAGNOSIS**

SIGNS AND SYMPTOMS
- Preceding the seizure (aura):
  - Déjà vu
  - Rising epigastric sensation
  - Olfactory hallucinations
- During the seizure (ictal):
  - Automatisms: Lip smacking, picking
  - Unresponsiveness or aphasia
  - Focal or generalized clonic movements
- After the seizure (post-ictal):
  - Confusion, agitation, psychosis
  - Amnesia for the event
  - Urinary incontinence
  - Oral laceration

History
- Assess for underlying risk factors
- Inquire about seizure frequency and duration
- Ask about catamenial pattern:
  - Increased seizures in periovulatory and perimenstrual period seen in up to 1/3 of women

Physical Exam
- Focal neurological findings may provide clues to underlying CNS etiology
- Post-ictal period: Todd's paralysis, positive Babinski, dilated pupils
- Nystagmus and ataxia often seen with toxicity from anticonvulsant medications

TESTS
Lab
Initial or acute onset seizures:
- Blood glucose

- Electrolytes: Sodium, calcium, magnesium, phosphate
- CBC
- Urine drug screen

Imaging
Initial or acute onset seizures:
- Head CT without contrast to exclude conditions requiring urgent intervention (hemorrhage, tumor)
- Brain MRI, seizure protocol may be done in follow-up as outpatient to exclude more subtle structural lesions

Diagnostic Procedures
- EEG:
  - Aids in classification of seizure type and localization of seizure onset
  - Initial EEG normal in up to 50%
  - Normal EEG does not exclude epilepsy
  - Higher yield if performed after sleep deprivation
- Lumbar puncture:
  - All HIV+ patients with new onset seizure(s)
  - Any patient with fever, elevated WBC or suspicion of infection

DIFFERENTIAL DIAGNOSIS
- Physiological:
  - Syncope
  - Transient ischemic attack (TIA)
  - Complicated migraine
  - Sleep disorder
  - Movement disorder: Tremor, tics
  - Transient metabolic disturbance
- Psychiatric:
  - Conversion disorder
  - Panic attacks
  - Attention deficit hyperactivity disorder (ADHD)

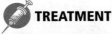 **TREATMENT**

GENERAL MEASURES
2/3 of patients can be controlled with medications

 MEDICATION (DRUGS)

- Traditional antiepileptic drugs
  - Phenobarbital, primidone, phenytoin, carbamazepine, valproate
  - Advantages
    - Once daily dosing available with most preparations (except carbamazepine)
    - Can be rapidly titrated or loaded intravenously (except carbamazepine)
    - Inexpensive/generic available (except valproate)
  - Disadvantages
    - Drug interactions
    - CNS side effects
    - Teratogenicity
    - Long-term effects
    - Serum monitoring required
- New antiepileptic drugs
  - Gabapentin, topiramate, lamotrigine, tiagabine, oxcarbazepine, levetiracetam, zonisamide, pregabalin
  - Advantages
    - Few drug interactions due to predominantly nonhepatic metabolism and low protein binding (2)

- Few side effects
- Broad spectrum coverage of both generalized and partial onset seizures (topiramate, lamotrigine, zonisamide, levetiracetam)
- Disadvantages
  - Slow titration rate (except levetiracetam, gabapentin, pregabalin)
  - No IV formulation available except levetiracetam
  - Cost
  - Degree of teratogenic risk unknown except for lamotrigine

ALERT
Antiepileptic drugs that decrease the efficacy of hormonal contraception: Phenobarbital, primidone, phenytoin, carbamazepine, oxcarbazepine, topiramate (>200 mg/day)

SURGERY
- Focal brain resection in patients with partial onset seizures refractory to trials of 2 or more medications (alone or in combination)
- Most successful in patients with focal lesions seen on MRI and/or temporal lobe seizures
- Up to 70% seizure freedom rate
- Other palliative surgical options are available for patients with multifocal onset seizures or generalized onset seizures

VAGUS NERVE STIMULATION
- For patients refractory to medications and not surgical candidates
- Stimulator implanted subcutaneously in the chest with electrode to the left vagus nerve
- Provides seizure reduction and shortened seizure duration but rarely complete seizure control

PREGNANCY CONSIDERATIONS
Maternal Risk
- Increased seizure frequency in up to 1/3 of patients during pregnancy
- Declining AED drug levels due to altered pharmacokinetics

Fetal Risk
- Major malformations in 4–8% (twice the general population)
  - Cleft lip/palate, congenital heart defects, neural tube defects, urogenital defects
  - Associated with use of all traditional agents but highest risk with valproate and polytherapy (up to 15%) (3)
  - Recent data shows lower risk with lamotrigine (2.9%) (3)
  - Data regarding use of other newer agents lacking
- Neonatal hemorrhage
- Low birth weight and prematurity
- Developmental delay

Recommendations
- Monotherapy at the lowest dose needed to control seizures
  - Fetal hypoxia from maternal seizures can have greater impact on fetal outcome than the teratogenic effects of antiepileptic drugs
- Avoid use of traditional antiepileptic drugs particularly valproate
- Folic acid supplementation 1–4 mg/day (start prior to conception)
- Monthly serum drug levels (total and free level) after conception
- Prenatal testing
  - Maternal serum alpha-fetoprotein at 15–20 weeks
  - Level II (structural) ultrasound at 16–20 weeks
- Vitamin K 10 mg/day during last month of gestation

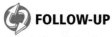

FOLLOW-UP

Admission Criteria
- Status epilepticus
  - Continuous seizure activity greater than 5–10 minutes or
  - 2 or more seizures without return to baseline in between
- Prolonged post-ictal state

Issues for Referral
Refer to neurologist or epileptologist if:
- Refractory to 1st or 2nd medication trial
- Suspicion of pseudoseizures
- Pregnant or considering pregnancy

PROGNOSIS
- Classification into appropriate epilepsy syndrome aids in prognosis
  - Some generalized epilepsy syndromes will remit in childhood (childhood absence, benign rolandic).
  - Juvenile myoclonic epilepsy and adult onset temporal lobe epilepsy are least likely to remit.

COMPLICATIONS
Infertility
- Number of births decreased by 33–66% (4)
- Anovulatory cycles increased
- Polycystic ovaries may be linked to valproate use.
- Occurs in women on no AEDs

Decreased Bone Mineral Density
- Reported with phenobarbital, mysoline, phenytoin, carbamazepine and valproate (5)
- Screen with DXA scan after 5 years of AED therapy in all patients and before initiating AED therapy in postmenopausal women
- Supplement calcium and vitamin D to ensure adequate daily intake

PATIENT MONITORING
- CBC and liver function tests
  - All patients taking phenobarbital, phenytoin, carbamazepine and valproate due to risk of agranulocytosis and hepatotoxicity
- Sodium
  - Risk of hyponatremia in patients taking carbamazepine and oxcarbazepine, especially elderly and patients on salt-wasting diuretics

- Serum drug levels
  - Available for all antiepileptic drugs
  - Aids in monitoring for toxicity, noncompliance

REFERENCES
1. Annegers JF. Epidemiology of epilepsy. In: Wyllie E, ed. *The Treatment of Epilepsy: Principles and Practice*. 3rd ed. Philadelphia: Lippincott, Williams & Wilkins; 2001;131–138.
2. LaRoche SM, Helmers SL. The new antiepileptic drugs: Scientific review. *JAMA*. 2004;291:605–614.
3. Pennell PB. Using current evidence in selecting antiepileptic drugs for use during pregnancy. *Epilepsy Curr*. 2005;5:45–51.
4. Morrell MJ, Montouris GD. Reproductive disturbances in patients with epilepsy. *Cleveland Clin J Med*. 2004;71:19–24.
5. Pack AM, Gidal B, Vazquez B. Bone disease associated with antiepileptic drugs. *Cleveland Clin J Med*. 2004;71:42–48.

ADDITIONAL READING
Morrell MJ. Epilepsy in women. *Am Fam Physician*. 2002;66:1489–1494.
Pennell PB. Pregnancy in the woman with epilepsy: Maternal and fetal outcomes. *Sem in Neurology*. 2002;22:299–307.

MISCELLANEOUS

WEBSITES
- Epilepsy Foundation: www.efa.org
- North American Pregnancy Registry: www.aedpregnancyregistry.org

CODES
ICD9-CM
- 345.3 Grand mal seizure
- 345.4 Partial seizure
- 780.39 Convulsion/seizure NOS

KEY WORDS
- Seizure
- Epilepsy
- Catamenial

E

EPSTEIN-BARR VIRUS INFECTION

Staci A. Fischer, MD, FACP

KEY CLINICAL POINTS

- Epstein-Barr Virus (EBV) is the most common cause of infectious mononucleosis in adolescents and adults.
- Chronic active EBV infection is rare and distinct from chronic fatigue syndrome.
- The oncogenic potential of EBV is being increasingly recognized in immunocompromised patient populations.

 BASICS

DESCRIPTION
EBV is a herpes family virus with worldwide distribution.

EPIDEMIOLOGY
EBV is spread via contact with infected saliva.

Like herpes simplex virus, EBV causes latent infection, with intermittent shedding of virus in the saliva of asymptomatic patients.

Prevalence
- Up to 95% of adults are infected with EBV.
- Up to 50% are infected before the age of 5.

RISK FACTORS
- EBV infection is acquired earlier in life in developing areas of the world and in lower socioeconomic settings.
- Immunocompromised patients are at higher risk for malignant complications.

PATHOPHYSIOLOGY
- EBV invades oral epithelial cells.
- An aggressive cytotoxic T cell response ensues, causing most of the symptoms.
- Splenomegaly occurs as a result of lymphocytic infiltration of the spleen.
- Latent infection in B cells occurs, providing a reservoir for viral shedding and immortalized cells at risk for malignant transformation with subsequent immune compromise.

ETIOLOGY
Human herpesvirus-4 (EBV)

ASSOCIATED CONDITIONS
Usually normal immune system

- HIV-infected patients may develop oral hairy leukoplakia.
- Overwhelming infection can occur in boys with X-linked lymphoproliferative disease (Duncan's disease), with fulminant hepatitis, hemophagocytosis, agammaglobulinema and eventual B-cell lymphoma.
- EBV-associated malignancy is seen in immunocompromised patients.
- Chronic infection with EBV is rare.

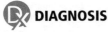 DIAGNOSIS

Infectious mononucleosis is a distinct clinical syndrome.

SIGNS AND SYMPTOMS
- Infection acquired in early childhood is often asymptomatic.
- Infectious mononucleosis is seen when primary infection is delayed into adolescence or adulthood.
- Mononucleosis presents with fever, sore throat, malaise, and adenopathy.

- Chronic active EBV infection is rare, with severe mononucleosis symptoms and signs present for over 6 months after documented primary infection.

History
- Infectious mononucleosis:
  - Prolonged fever (up to 14 days)
  - Malaise
  - Sore throat
  - Often no history of contact with infected person
- Abdominal pain or left scapular pain suggests splenic rupture and should be investigated immediately
- Oral hairy leukoplakia presents with asymptomatic hair-like projections on the lateral tongue, not removable by scraping

Physical Exam
- Fever
- Cervical adenopathy
  - Posterior adenopathy is characteristic
  - Mildly tender, mobile
- Symmetric tonsillar hypertrophy ("kissing tonsils" common)
- Palatal petechiae may be seen
- Splenomegaly (peaks during second week of symptoms)
- Hepatomegaly (10%)
- Jaundice (5%)
- Rash is uncommon except in those with recent ampicillin or amoxicillin exposure, in which 90% will develop a pruritic, maculopapular rash
  - If acute EBV infection is confirmed, these patients should not be labeled allergic to penicillins

TESTS
Lab
Routine Lab Findings:
- Lymphocytosis in 70% of patients
  - Up to 30% are atypical lymphocytes
- Thrombocytopenia in 50% (usually mild)
- Neutropenia can occur
- Up to 80% have elevated hepatic enzymes (AST, ALT, LDH, alkaline phosphatase)
- Microscopic hematuria, proteinuria can occur

Diagnostic Lab Testing:
- Viral culture for EBV is not widely available
- Heterophile antibody (Monospot) positive in ≥90% cases
  - May be absent in young children
  - Antibodies persist for 2 to 3 months
  - Up to 20% positive one year after infection
- EBV specific antibodies are indicated when clinical suspicion is high and Monospot is negative (see Figure 1 and Table 1)
  - Viral capsid antigen (VCA) antibodies detectable by two weeks
    - IgM is diagnostic of acute EBV infection and persists for 6–8 weeks
    - IgG persists for life
  - Early antigen (EA) antibodies develop in 70% of patients with acute EBV infection and disappear with recovery
    - Persistent anti-EA seen in some EBV-associated malignancies (nasopharyngeal carcinoma, Burkett's lymphoma)
  - Epstein-Barr nuclear antigen (EBNA) antibodies appear late in infection and persist for life

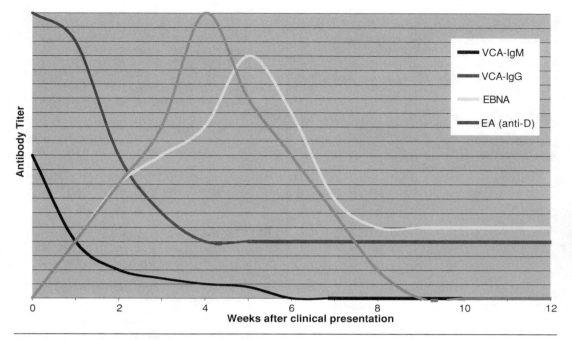

Figure 1 EBV-specific serologic testing in acute Epstein-Barr virus infection (infectious mononucleosis)

- PCR testing is available but of limited use in diagnosing acute EBV infection
- Patients with chronic active EBV infection have persistent, marked elevation of EA IgG and VCA IgM, often with markedly positive plasma PCR
  - Histopathologic examination of tissues (e.g., liver, bone marrow) with immunohistochemical staining for EBV can be diagnostic in these rare cases

Imaging
- Ultrasound or CT of the abdomen reveal splenomegaly in 50% of patients.

DIFFERENTIAL DIAGNOSIS
- Cytomegalovirus (CMV) infection
- Streptococcal pharyngitis (adenopathy is submandibular and anterior cervical)
- Acute HIV infection
- Viral hepatitis (AST, ALT markedly elevated)
- Rubella (rash is prominent)
- Acute toxoplasmosis

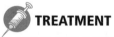

TREATMENT

GENERAL MEASURES
- Supportive care is indicated
- Patients rarely require hospitalization

Activity
- Bed rest
- No heavy lifting, strenuous exercise or contact sports for at least 4 weeks or until splenomegaly resolves
- Avoid repeated, aggressive palpation of the spleen for at least 4 weeks

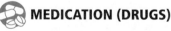

MEDICATION (DRUGS)

- Acetaminophen for fever
- Avoid aspirin (rare cases of Reye syndrome reported)
- Treat constipation when present

Table 1 Serologic Findings in Patients with EBV Infection

VCA-IgM	VCA-IgG	EA	EBNA	Interpretation
+	−	−	−	Early acute EBV infection
+	+	+	+	Acute EBV infection
+	+	−	+	Resolving acute EBV infection
−	+	−	+	Prior infection
+	++	+	+	Chronic active EBV infection (≥6 months fever, adenopathy)

VCA = viral capsid antigen, EA = early antigen; EBNA = Epstein-Barr nuclear antigen.

- Antivirals (acyclovir, ganciclovir, foscarnet) may be helpful in oral hairy leukoplakia.
- Antivirals are ineffective in the treatment of infectious mononucleosis and chronic active EBV infection.
- Acyclovir has no long-term effect on viral shedding.
- Corticosteroids may help with upper airway compromise and hemolytic anemia, but are otherwise not indicated.

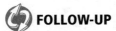 ## FOLLOW-UP

DISPOSITION
Admission Criteria
- Most patients do not require hospital admission for infectious mononucleosis.
- Impending upper airway compromise or suspicion of splenic rupture are indications for inpatient observation.

Issues for Referral
- Patients with suspected chronic active EBV infection should be referred to an infectious diseases subspecialist.
- Patients with suspected post-transplant lymphoproliferative disease (PTLD) or other EBV-associated malignancies should be referred to an oncologist.

PROGNOSIS
- Infectious mononucleosis resolves spontaneously within 3–4 weeks.
- Fatigue and hypersomnia can persist for 2–3 weeks after fever abates.
- Death from EBV is extremely rare, but can be the result of upper airway obstruction or splenic rupture.

COMPLICATIONS
- Cold agglutinins develop in 70–80% of patients
- Autoimmune hemolytic anemia (0.5–3%)
- Hemophagocytic syndrome reported
- Splenic rupture can occur, requiring splenectomy or splenorrhaphy
  – Up to 50% have a history of trauma
  – Rarely occurs spontaneously
- Fulminant hepatitis (rare)
- Hydrops of the gallbladder has been reported in children.
- Pericarditis and myocarditis reported
- Aseptic meningitis, acute encephalitis, Bell's palsy, transverse myelitis, Guillain-Barre' syndrome rarely reported.
  – Up to 85% recover completely
- EBV infection has been associated with endemic Burkett's lymphoma, nasopharyngeal carcinoma, some forms of Hodgkin's lymphoma, CNS lymphoma (in HIV-infected patients), and some gastric carcinomas.
- Post-transplant lymphoproliferative disease (PTLD) can occur in bone marrow or solid organ transplant recipients, most commonly following primary EBV infection in those receiving antithymocyte therapy or with graft-versus-host disease.
  – PTLD is treated by reduction in immunosuppression

- Surgical resection of localized tumors may be curative
- Antivirals are frequently given, although their role in the treatment of PTLD is unclear
- Rituximab has efficacy in the treatment of CD20+ B-cell tumors unresponsive to reduction in immunosuppression

Pregnancy Considerations
No teratogenicity has been reported as a result of acute EBV infection.

PATIENT MONITORING
- Patients with infectious mononucleosis should be evaluated 2–4 weeks after diagnosis for clearance to return to strenuous activity.
- Transplant recipients with documented primary EBV infection should be followed closely for the development of PTLD, with meticulous lymph node examinations.

REFERENCES
1. Baumforth KRN, Young LS, Flavell KJ, et al. The Epstein-Barr virus and its association with human cancers. *J Clin Pathol*. 1999;52:307–322.
2. Ebell MH. Epstein-Barr virus infectious mononucleosis. *Am Fam Physician*. 2004;70:1279–1287.
3. Johannsen EC, Schooley RT, Kaye KM. Epstein-Barr virus (Infectious Mononucleosis). In: Mandell GL, Bennett JE, Dolin R, ed. *Mandell, Douglas, and Bennett's Principles and Practice of Infectious Diseases*, 6th ed. Philadelphia: Elsevier; 2005:1801–1820.
4. Macsween KF, Crawford DH. Epstein-Barr virus—recent advances. *Lancet Infect Dis*. 2003;3:131–140.
5. Okano M, Kawa K, Kimura H, et al. Proposed guidelines for diagnosing chronic active Epstein-Barr virus infection. *Am J Hematol*. 2005;80:64–69.
6. Torre D, Tambini R. Acyclovir for treatment of infectious mononucleosis: A meta-analysis. *Scand J Infect Dis*. 1999;31:543–547.

CODES
ICD9-CM
- 075 Epstein-Barr infection (viral)
- 780.79 Chronic

KEY WORDS
- Fever
- Lymphadenopathy
- Mononucleosis
- Acute Hepatitis
- Lymphoma
- Post-transplant Lymphoproliferative Disease
- Oral Hairy Leukoplakia
- Chronic Epstein-Barr Virus Infection

FECAL INCONTINENCE

Rohini McKee, MD
Homayoon M. Akbari, MD, PhD, FRCS(C)

KEY CLINICAL POINTS

- May affect up to 7% of the general population
- Obstetrical trauma is the most common cause of fecal incontinence in women.
- Fecal incontinence is associated with significant social and mental health disability, stigmatization, and impaired quality of life.
- Many patients are home-bound due to fear of embarrassing public incontinence events.
- 2/3 of patients with incontinence do not seek medical attention.

 BASICS

DESCRIPTION
Inability to control passage of gas or stool.

EPIDEMIOLOGY
Prevalence
- Community prevalence: 2–15%
- Approximately 30% of incontinent patients are >age of 65.
- Prevalence of fecal incontinence or combined urinary/fecal incontinence in the elderly institutionalized population is about 50%.
- Approximately 60–70% of incontinent patients are women.

RISK FACTORS
- Obstetrical trauma to sphincter muscle or pudendal nerves
- Prior anorectal surgery with iatrogenic injury to sphincter muscle
- Diarrheal states particularly irritable bowel syndrome with diarrhea in women
- Diabetic neuropathy

PATHOPHYSIOLOGY
- Sphincter disruption secondary to obstetrical trauma, anal surgery, or trauma
- Pudendal nerve injury or neuropathy secondary to obstetrical trauma or neuropathy (i.e., diabetes)
- Congenital or acquired central nervous system deficits
- Diminished rectal compliance secondary to inflammatory bowel disease or radiation
- Diminished rectal sensation with altered rectoanal reflexes secondary to acquired or congenital central and peripheral nervous system dysfunction

ETIOLOGY
- Congenital anorectal anomalies
- Diarrhea
  - Inflammatory bowel disease
  - Irritable bowel syndrome
  - Short-gut syndrome
  - Radiation enteritis
  - Laxative abuse
- Overflow incontinence
  - Impaction
  - Encopresis
  - Neoplasms
- Neurologic conditions
  - Dementia, stroke
  - Congenital anomalies
  - Diabetes
  - Pelvic floor denervation
- Trauma
  - Accidental injury
  - Anorectal surgery
  - Obstetrical injury

ASSOCIATED CONDITIONS
- Urinary incontinence
- Rectovaginal fistula
- Pelvic organ prolapse

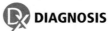 **DIAGNOSIS**

SIGNS AND SYMPTOMS
History
- Onset of incontinence and history of antecedent anorectal or gynecological surgery
- Detailed obstetrical history
- Degree of incontinence and progression of symptoms
- Presence or absence of passage of stool and of sensation of need to defecate
- Sensation of incomplete evacuation
- Quality of life questionnaire
- Bowel diary; incontinence score
- Detailed urologic history
- History of lower back pain, lower extremity sensory loss

Physical Exam
- Inspection: Patulous anus? Perineal body intact?
- Digital exam: Defects? Diminished resting/squeeze tone? Masses palpable?
- Stool impaction in rectal vault?
- Sensation intact? Test for "anal wink" reflex
- Examine for evidence of prior obstetrical trauma and anorectal surgery
- Examine for associated rectovaginal fistula with bimanual exam
- Examine for associated rectocele

TESTS
Lab
- Stool cultures if diarrhea present
- Metabolic
  - Thyroid function tests
  - Serum glucose

Imaging
- Transanal ultrasound
  - To assess sphincter atrophy
- MRI with endoanal coil (if available)
  - Assesses sphincter atrophy by measuring sphincter volume, which is more difficult with endoanal ultrasound
  - In addition, can be combined with dynamic pelvic MRI to assess the pelvic floor
- Defecogram
  - Allows for radiographic evaluation of the dynamics of defecation

- Can assess for concomitant pelvic organ prolapse
  - Barium paste is instilled into the rectum and the patient seated on a radiolucent commode
  - Fluoroscopic images are obtained during pelvic floor contraction and defecation
  - Amount of perineal descent, paradoxical contraction resulting in obstructed defecation, associated rectocele, and/or prolapse can be evaluated.

Diagnostic Procedures/Surgery
- Colonoscopy
- Pudendal nerve terminal motor latency
- Anorectal manometry
  - Quantifies pressures along sphincter
    - Resting tone correlates with internal sphincter function
    - Squeeze tone correlates with external sphincter function

DIFFERENTIAL DIAGNOSIS
- Causes of diarrhea, particularly irritable bowel syndrome
- Overflow incontinence
- Neurogenic incontinence

TREATMENT

GENERAL MEASURES
Diet
- Dietary modification
  - Limit foods that encourage loose/frequent bowel movements such as alcohol, caffeine, prunes, and fruit juices.
- Test for food intolerance to gluten and lactose.
- Fiber supplements: Firmer, bulkier stool

SPECIAL THERAPY
Physical Therapy
Biofeedback:
- Most beneficial in patients with intact rectal sensation and ability to contract external anal sphincter (EAS) voluntarily
- Response rates: 65–75%
- Success independent of patient age and initial severity of symptoms

MEDICATION (DRUGS)

First Line
Stool bulking agents:
Fiber supplements to increase dietary fiber intake to 30 g per day

Second Line
Antidiarrheals
- Adsorbents to decrease fluid content in the stool
  - Kaopectate commonly used
- Opium derivatives to decrease colonic motility
  - Loperamide (Imodium): Decreases frequency of incontinence; direct effect on basal sphincter tone

ALERT
- Patients whose symptoms do not adversely affect their quality of life and are controlled by dietary and medical measures can be followed on a regular basis by their primary care physician who can review food and bowel diaries and adjust treatment as needed.

- If lifestyle is impaired or there is progression of symptoms, referral should be made to colorectal surgery for surgical evaluation.

SURGERY
- Sphincter repair
  - Anterior sphincteroplasty:
    - Localized sphincter defect repaired with either direct apposition or overlapping sphincteroplasty
  - SECCA Procedure:
    - Radiofrequency energy used to create discreet submucosal thermal lesions circumferentially which results in remodeling of anal canal
    - Useful with multifocal injury not amenable to sphincteroplasty
- Artificial Bowel Sphincter:
  - Inflatable cuff with reservoir that can be deflated for passage of stool and gas
  - Useful when multifocal injury present or pudendal neuropathy present
- Sacral nerve stimulation:
  - Stimulation of sacral nerve afferent and efferent fibers by implantable device
  - Direct effect on sphincter tone and modulation of rectoanal reflex arc

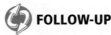

FOLLOW-UP

Issues for Referral
- Gastroenterology for colonoscopy/evaluation for colonic dysmotility and diarrhea
- Urogynecology for evaluation of concomitant urinary complaints such as incontinence
- Referral to colorectal surgery for surgical evaluation and possible sphincter repair if significant lifestyle impairment or progression of symptoms

PROGNOSIS
- Improved continence with overlapping sphincteroplasty: 70% to 90%
- Relapse incidence of incontinence 6–10 years following successful sphincteroplasty: 50–60%

COMPLICATIONS
Pregnancy Considerations
Cesarean section recommended for subsequent deliveries in women of child-bearing age after sphincter repair.

REFERENCES

1. Hinninghofen H, Enck P. Fecal incontinence: Evaluation and treatment. *Gastroenterol Clin.* 2003;32:685–706.
2. Congilosi Parker S, Thorsen A. Fecal incontinence. *Surg Clin North Am.* 2002;82:1273–1290.
3. Corman ML. Fecal Incontinence. In: Corman ML, ed. *Colon and Rectal Surgery.* 5th ed. Philadelphia: Lippincott, Williams and Wilkins; 2005.

ADDITIONAL READING

Rothholtz N, Wexner SD. Surgical treatment of constipation and fecal incontinence. *Gastroenterol Clin.* 2001;30:131–166.
Song AH, Advincula AP, Fenner DE. Common gastrointestinal problems in women and pregnancy. *Clin Fam Prac.* 2204; 6:(3).

Akbari HM, Bernstein MR. Diagnosis and management of postoperative fecal incontinence. In: Zbar A, Pescatori M, Wexner S, eds. *Complex Anorectal Disorders: Investigation and Management*. Springer-Verlag; 2005.

CODES
ICD9-CM
- 787.6 Incontinence of feces
- 664.2 Delivery complicated by laceration sphincter ani.

KEY WORDS
- Incontinence
- Anal Sphincter Injury
- Anal Sphincter Repair

F

FIBROCYSTIC BREAST DISEASE

Courtney A. Clark, MD
Susannah S. Wise, MD, FACS

KEY CLINICAL POINTS

- Fibrocystic breast "disease" is a misnomer as it is not a disease state, but a broad classification of benign breast tissue variations.
- Very commonly described
- Histology is benign on biopsy

 ## BASICS

DESCRIPTION

- Benign breast state that may include the signs and symptoms of swelling, pain, lumpiness, and nipple discharge.
- Fibrocystic breast change is the histologic term for the benign variations in breast tissue.
- Fibrocystic breast is the radiographic term for dense breast tissue found on imaging.
- Hughes classified the findings associated with this benign breast condition with ANDI (Aberrations of Normal Development and Involution).
- ANDI classifies breast states according to life stage up to age 55. After age 55, there is a greater risk of cancer associated with the signs and symptoms of fibrocystic breasts.

EPIDEMIOLOGY
Incidence
- Estimated >60% of all women
- Lower in women taking birth control pills

RISK FACTORS
Only considered to have increased cancer risk with fibrocystic changes if atypical cells are found on biopsy

PATHOPHYSIOLOGY
The female breast is made up of ducts, lobules, and stroma. Cyclical and age-related changes to these tissue types are manifested as benign fibrous changes and cysts.

ASSOCIATED CONDITIONS
- Cyclical mastalgia (pain occurring prior to onset of the menstrual cycle)
- Benign breast discharge

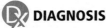 ## DIAGNOSIS

SIGNS AND SYMPTOMS
History
- The signs and symptoms of fibrocystic breast disease fluctuate with menstrual cycle and are typically worse just prior to menstruation.
- Patients may describe swollen, tender, and lumpy breasts.

Physical Exam
- The upper outer breast is the area most typically associated with fibrocystic changes.
- Providers should examine fibrocystic breasts in a similar manner as for cyclical mastalgia.
- If a lump is a concern, then repeating an exam after menstruation has completed may be of value, as the lump may have decreased or resolved.
- Any lump, mass, or nipple discharge deemed suspicious for malignancy should be evaluated as per standard of care.

TESTS
Imaging
For suspicious lumps or discharge:
- Mammography
- Ultrasound
- MRI is being used with increasing frequency

Diagnostic Procedures/Surgery
For suspicious lumps or discharge: Biopsy or aspiration

DIFFERENTIAL DIAGNOSIS
- Simple cysts (benign)
- Fibroadenoma (benign)
- Malignancy

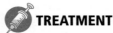 ## TREATMENT

GENERAL MEASURES
Diet
Reduction in caffeine intake has never been proven to decrease the incidence of fibrocystic changes.

Activity
A properly fitting bra may help reduce pain and swelling associated with fibrocystic breasts.

SPECIAL THERAPY
Complementary and Alternative Therapies
- Evening primrose: 1 to 3 g daily
- Medical management

First Line
Treatment for the pain associated with fibrocystic changes include:

Acetaminophen, aspirin and other nonsteroidal anti-inflammatory drugs.

Second Line
- Tamoxifen 10 mg daily for 3–6 months
- Danazole 200 mg daily (during luteal phase only)

SURGERY
Women rarely undergo breast reduction surgery for relief of symptoms.

 ## FOLLOW-UP

- Assurance
- Re-examination

DISPOSITION
Issues for Referral
Any suspicious breast mass should be referred to a breast surgeon.

REFERENCES

1. Donnegan WL, Spratt JS, eds. *Cancer of the Breast*. Philadelphia, PA: WB Saunders; 1995.
2. Love S. *Dr. Susan Love's Breast Book*. 3rd ed. Cambridge: Perseus Publishing; 2000.
3. Rastelli A. Breast pain, fibrocystic changes, and breast cysts. *Problems Gen Surg*. 2003;20:17–26.

4. Santen R, Mansel R. Current concepts: Benign breast disorders. *N Engl J Med*. 2005;353:275–285.
5. Smith M, Kent K. Breast concerns and lifestyles of women. *Clin Obstet Gynecol*. 2002;45:1129–1139.

CODES
ICD9-CM
610.1 Fibrocystic breast

KEY WORDS

- Ducts
- Lobules
- Cysts
- Mastalgia
- Dense Breasts

F

FIBROMYALGIA

Lori Lieberman-Maran, MD

KEY CLINICAL POINTS

- Chronic generalized pain in muscles and soft tissue
  - Middle-aged women
  - Fatigue and sleep disturbance
  - Lack of inflammation on exam
- Diagnosis made by history and physical
- Treatment includes education, low impact exercise, and medications to restore sleep

 BASICS

DESCRIPTION
- Chronic noninflammatory diffuse soft tissue pain syndrome
- Unremarkable physical examination except for tender points

EPIDEMIOLOGY
- 2nd most common rheumatic syndrome to OA
  - Women 10 times more affected than men
  - Mean age is 5th decade, but prevalence increases with age

Prevalence
- In general population: 1–4%
- In men, 0–4% and in women, 2.5–10.5%
  - Increases to 7–8% in women age 60–80

RISK FACTORS
See Associated Conditions

PATHOPHYSIOLOGY
Thought to be a more central cause than peripheral:
- "Central sensitization" theory
  - Exaggerated response of CNS to peripheral stimulus
  - Hyperexcitablily and hypersensitivity of neurons
  - Lowered CNS threshold to mechanical and thermal pain
- No evidence for abnormal pathology of muscle

ETIOLOGY
There is no clear etiology, but certain stressors may trigger fibromyalgia, such as:
- Trauma
- Emotional disturbances

ASSOCIATED CONDITIONS
Fibromyalgia can coexist with connective tissue diseases and has been associated with other syndromes including:
- Irritable bowel syndrome
- Migraine
- Interstitial cystitis
- Chronic fatigue syndrome
- Depression

 DIAGNOSIS

PRE-HOSPITAL
- Diagnosis is made by history and physical exam.
- Diagnostic criteria proposed from the American College of Rheumatology (1990) include:
  - Widespread musculoskeletal pain for at least 3 months
  - Excess tenderness in at least 11 of 18 predefined anatomic sites (tender points) by application of 4 kg/cm of pressure
    - Tender points (occur bilaterally): Occiput, low cervical, trapezius, supraspinatus, 2nd rib, lateral epicondyle, gluteal, greater trochanter, knee (see Figure 1)
  - If both criteria are present, there is 80% specificity and 88% sensitivity.

SIGNS AND SYMPTOMS
The most common symptom is diffuse, chronic, musculoskeletal pain in all 4 quadrants of the body. Other symptoms include:
- Fatigue (in 90% of cases)
- Sleep disturbance

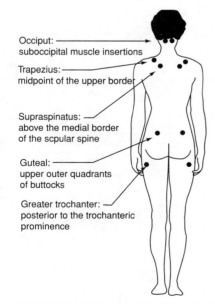

Occiput:
suboccipital muscle insertions

Trapezius:
midpoint of the upper border

Supraspinatus:
above the medial border
of the scpular spine

Guteal:
upper outer quadrants
of buttocks

Greater trochanter:
posterior to the trochanteric
prominence

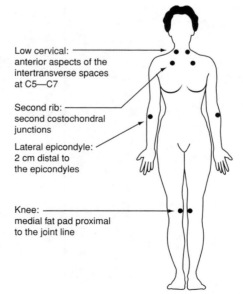

Low cervical:
anterior aspects of the
intertransverse spaces
at C5—C7

Second rib:
second costochondral
junctions

Lateral epicondyle:
2 cm distal to
the epicondyles

Knee:
medial fat pad proximal
to the joint line

Figure 1   Location of 18 tender points.

- Mood disturbance
- Cognitive dysfunction

History
Pain "all over":
- Subjective joint swelling
- Morning stiffness
- Sleep disturbances
- Parasthesias

Physical Exam
- Symmetric bilateral tender points
- Lack of joint swelling
- Normal muscle strength

TESTS
Lab
There is no laboratory test that is diagnostic for fibromyalgia, but often lab testing is performed to rule out other conditions. These include:
- CBC, ESR, TSH, complete metabolic profile, and CPK
  - These tests are normal in fibromyalgia.
- More extensive lab testing is not necessary and often leads to confusing results.

Imaging
Imaging is not helpful for the diagnosis and is not necessary.

DIFFERENTIAL DIAGNOSIS
There is a broad differential because many of these symptoms are present in other conditions:
- Endocrine disorders
  - Hypothyroidism
  - Hyperparathyroidism
- Inflammatory conditions
  - Polymyalgia rheumatica
  - Inflammatory arthritis
  - Myositis
- Malignancy
- Infection
  - Viral illness
  - Lyme disease

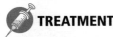 TREATMENT

INITIAL STABILIZATION
Treating patients with fibromyalgia requires a multidisciplinary approach including education and an exercise program; medications are considered second line.

GENERAL MEASURES
Diet
No restrictions

Activity
No restrictions; exercise is encouraged (see Physical Therapy).

SPECIAL THERAPY
Physical Therapy
Exercise has been proven to be beneficial in patients with fibromyalgia and should be encouraged.
- Low impact activities
  - Aquatic therapy
  - Walking
- Stretching exercises
  - Application of heat

Complementary and Alternative Therapies
Patient education has a proven therapeutic role and should be recommended.
- Group lectures
- Written educational materials
- Small sessions
Alternative therapies can be used, but have not been proven effective.
- Massage
- Acupuncture

 MEDICATION (DRUGS)

Medical management can be effective, but should be combined with patient education and an exercise plan.

First Line
- Amitryptyline 10–50 mg at bedtime–helps restore sleep and sense of well-being
- Cyclobenzaprine 10–30 mg at bedtime–similar response

Second Line
- Tramadol 200–300 mg/day in divided doses: Can administer with or without acetaminophen
- SSRIs
  - Fluoxetine is the only SSRI that has been evaluated. Dosage is 20–80 mg/day.
- NSAIDs
- There is no evidence regarding the efficacy of opioids, corticosteroids, or benzodiazepines.

 FOLLOW-UP

Can be followed regularly by their primary care physician

Issues for Referral
Referral to a rheumatologist is indicated if there is a question of an underlying inflammatory condition.

PROGNOSIS
- Variable between patients, but generally remains constant over time
- Improved outcome in younger patients
- Most patients have chronic, persistent symptoms; a complete remission is rare.

REFERENCES
1. Goldenberg D, Burckhardt C, Crofford L. Management of fibromyalgia. *JAMA*. 2004;292:2388–2395.
2. Hochberg M, et al. *Rheumatology*. 3rd ed. Edinburgh: Mosby, 2003.
3. Lieberman D. Fibromyalgia and myofascial pain. In: Lemke D, ed. *Current Care of Women: Diagnosis and Treatment*. New York, NY: Lange Medical Books/McGraw-Hill; 2004:429–439.
4. Wolfe F, Smythe H, Bennett R, et al. American College of Rheumatology 1990 criteria for the classification of fibromyalgia. *Arthritis and Rheumatism*. 1990;33:160–172.

CODES
ICD9-CM
729.1

KEY WORDS
- Fibromyalgia
- Chronic Pain
- Myalgias
- Muscle Aches

F

GALACTORRHEA

Geetha Gopalakrishnan, MD

KEY CLINICAL POINTS

- Hypersecretion of prolactin by the pituitary gland causes galactorrhea.
- There are numerous causes of galactorrhea including tumors, drugs, hypothyroidism, chronic renal failure, pregnancy, and chest wall injury.
- Prolactin levels between 20 and 200 ng/mL can be found in patients with any cause of hyperprolactinemia; however, values above 200 ng/mL usually indicate the presence of a prolactinoma.
- Dopamine agonists, including bromocriptine and cabergoline, are 1st line treatment for a symptomatic, large prolactinoma. Surgery is reserved for resistant prolactinoma and nonprolactin secreting pituitary macroadenomas.
- Patients on dopamine agonists should have serum prolactin levels checked after 1 month of treatment with an increase in the dose every month until serum prolactin level normalizes. An MRI to assess the size of the adenoma is recommended after 6 to 12 months of treatment.

BASICS

DESCRIPTION
Hypersecretion of prolactin by the pituitary gland causes galactorrhea.

EPIDEMIOLOGY
- More common in women
- Approximately 30–40% of pituitary adenomas are prolactinomas. Most are sporadic; however, some are associated with MEN Type 1.

ETIOLOGY
- Prolactin producing tumor: Prolactinoma (most common) and ectopic tumors (e.g., bronchogenic carcinoma)
- Conditions that decrease normal dopamine inhibition of prolactin secretion:
  - Hypothalamic and pituitary disease causing stalk injury or compression (e.g., tumors, infiltrative diseases, and trauma)
  - Drugs that block dopamine receptors or inhibit dopamine synthesis and storage (e.g., risperidone, phenothiazines, haloperidol, butyrophenones metoclopramide, sulpiride, domperidone, methyldopa and reserpine)
- Drugs that increase prolactin secretion: Estrogens, verapamil, cimetadine, and opiates
- Hypothyroidism can cause thyrotroph and lactrotroph hyperplasia. Prolactin levels are usually normal in most hypothyroid patients, but can be elevated in some. These levels normalize when hypothyroidism is corrected.
- Chronic renal failure: An increase in prolactin secretion and a decrease in prolactin clearance can occur. The levels normalize after renal transplantation.
- Pregnancy: Serum prolactin increases throughout pregnancy, peaks at delivery, and normalizes 6 weeks after delivery. High estrogen levels during pregnancy stimulate prolactin secretion. High prolactin is associated with galactorrhea during pregnancy and in the post partum period.
- Nipple stimulation: Nipple stimulation can result in galactorrhea by direct effect and by increasing serum prolactin concentrations. Nipple stimulation usually does not increase prolactin secretion in nonlactating women.

- Chest wall injury: Burns and trauma involving the chest wall can increase prolactin secretion via neural pathway and precipitate galactorrhea.
- Stress: Physical and psychological stress can cause an increase in the serum prolactin concentration and result in galactorrhea.

DIAGNOSIS

SIGNS AND SYMPTOMS
History
- Assess symptoms of pregnancy (e.g., nausea, amenorrhea), pituitary mass (e.g., vision loss, headache), hypothyroidism (e.g., fatigue, weight gain) and Hypogonadism (e.g., irregular cycles, infertility, decreased libido, hot flash, and vaginal dryness).
- Review medications, medical history (e.g., renal failure, chest wall injury) and psychological stress.

Physical Examination
Evaluate for breast discharge (clear, milky discharge is consistent with galactorrhea, but bloody discharge raises concern for breast cancer), visual field defects (e.g., bitemporal loss), chest wall injury, and signs of hypothyroidism (e.g., goiter, delayed reflexes).

TESTS
Lab
- Prolactin: Levels between 20 and 200 ng/mL can be found in patients with any cause of hyperprolactinemia and values above 200 ng/mL usually indicate the presence of a prolactinoma.
- Urine pregnancy test, thyroid function test, and creatinine to evaluate potential etiologies of prolactinemia.
- Evaluate pituitary hormone function if a pituitary hypothalamic lesion is noted on magnetic resonance imaging (MRI). Consider checking prolactin, TSH, Free thyroxine, LH, FSH, IGF-1, and 24-hour urine Cortisol.

Imaging
- MRI is recommended to evaluate for a hypothalamic pituitary lesion. Macroadenomas are >1 cm in size and microadenomas are <1 cm in size.
- Bone density to evaluate for osteoporosis since hypogonadism is a complication of elevated prolactin.

DIFFERENTIAL DIAGNOSIS
Breast cancer needs to be ruled out, especially in individuals with bloody breast discharge.

TREATMENT

The goal of treatment is to alleviate symptoms, lower prolactin levels, and decrease tumor size.

INITIAL STABILIZATION
- Galactorrhea due to stress, chest wall injury, and nipple stimulation usually does not need to be treated. Can consider a low dose dopamine agonist if severe galactorrhea and estrogen and progesterone therapy if menstrual irregularity
- Drug induced hyperprolactinemia resolves with discontinuation of the offending agent. If this is not an option, hypogonadism can be treated with estrogen and progesterone.
- Hypothyroidism induced hyperprolactinemia resolves when hypothyroidism is corrected with thyroid hormone replacement.

- Dopamine agonist is 1st line for a symptomatic, large prolactinoma. Surgery is reserved for resistant prolactinoma and nonprolactin secreting pituitary macroadenomas. Small asymptomatic pituitary tumors can be monitored without treatment. In these patients, estrogen and progesterone should be considered to prevent bone loss and for contraception.

 ## MEDICATION (DRUGS)

Dopamine agonists: Effective in improving symptoms, decreasing prolactin levels, and reducing the size of a prolactinoma. Visual symptoms start to improve within days of treatment and other symptoms such as menstrual irregularity resolve as prolactin levels fall to the normal range. Detectable decrease in tumor size can be noted within weeks to months of treatment.
- Bromocriptine: Bromocriptine should be taken b.i.d. with meals to lower prolactin levels. Starting dose of 1.25 mg is prescribed after dinner for 1 week. If no side effects, the dose is increased to 1.25 mg with breakfast and dinner. The dose is titrated every month until the prolactin level normalizes. Maximum dose is 5 mg b.i.d. Side effects include dizziness, nausea, and nasal stuffiness.
- Cabergoline: Cabergoline is taken once or twice a week to lower prolactin levels. Starting dose of 0.25 mg twice a week is prescribed and the dose is titrated every month to maintain normal prolactin levels. Maximum dose is 1.5 mg twice a week. Side effects such as nausea and dizziness are less common with Cabergoline.

Estrogen and progestin: Ovarian dysfunction is a common complication of elevated prolactin. Therefore, estrogen alone or in combination with progesterone should be considered to prevent bone loss in premenopausal women with hypogonadism.

SURGERY
Transsphenoidal surgical resection (TSS) is the initial treatment for a non-prolactin secreting pituitary marcoadenoma. TTS should be considered in prolactinomas if side effects develop or if symptoms, prolactin level or tumor size does not improve on dopamine agonists. Side effects include worsening of vision, hemorrhage, infection, and pituitary hormonal deficiencies.

RADIATION THERAPY
Radiation therapy (XRT) can shrink pituitary adenomas and lower serum prolactin levels. However, it takes several years to achieve maximum treatment effect. Therefore, XRT is reserved for the treatment of residual tumors that could not be removed after TSS in order to prevent tumor growth. Side effects include nausea, fatigue, loss of taste and smell, loss of hair, and pituitary hormone deficiencies.

Pregnancy Considerations
- Hypogonadotropic hypogonadism is a common complication of elevated prolactin. Normalizing prolactin levels with dopamine agonist can restore ovulation and improve fertility. If dopamine agonist does not improve prolactin levels, ovulation induction with clomiphene citrate or gonadotropin should be considered.
- Initial data reports Cabergoline to be safe in early pregnancy; however, bromocriptine is the recommended agent for women desiring pregnancy since more safety data is available on this agent. Once pregnant, all dopamine agonists must be discontinued and prolactin levels need to be monitored throughout pregnancy.

 ## FOLLOW-UP

Issues for Referral
Consider endocrine referral for pituitary or hypothalamic lesion and nephrology referral for chronic renal failure.

PATIENT MONITORING
- Monitor for side effects and assess serum prolactin levels after 1 month of dopamine agonist. Increase dose every month until serum prolactin level normalizes. Patients with visual symptoms need visual field assessment after 1 month of treatment to evaluate treatment effect. MRI to assess the size of the adenoma is recommended after 6 to 12 months. If the patient tolerates the dopamine agonist and the prolactin level normalizes, treatment dose can be continued for 1 year. The dose can be gradually decreased after 1 year as long as the prolactin levels stay normal and the tumor does not grow. After 2 years of normal prolactin levels and undetectable tumor on MRI, the dopamine agonist can be discontinued if the initial tumor was less than 1.5 cm in size. Large tumors (>1.5 cm) have greater recurrence if dopamine agonists are discontinued. Periodic prolactin levels and Pituitary MRI are recommended to evaluate for tumor recurrence in all patients with a prolactinoma.
- Another dopamine agonist should be tried if symptoms, prolactin levels and tumor size do not decrease or if side effects develop. TSS and XRT should be considered when both dopamine agonists have failed. Pituitary hormone function needs to be assessed after TTS or XRT.

REFERENCES

1. Schlechte J, Dolan K, Sherman B, et al. The natural history of untreated hyperprolactinemia: A prospective analysis. *J Clin Endocrinol Metab*. 1989;68:412–418.
2. Biller BM, Molitch ME, Vance ML, et al. Treatment of prolactin-secreting macroadenomas with the once-weekly dopamine agonist cabergoline. *J Clin Endocrinol Metab*. 1996;81:2338–2343.

CODES
ICD9-CM
- 253.1 Hyperprolactinemia
- 676.6 Galactorrhea

KEY WORDS
- Galactorrhea
- Prolactinoma
- Pituitary Gland

G

GALLBLADDER DISEASE

Chad Morse, MD
Fadlallah G. Habr, MD

KEY CLINICAL POINTS

- It is a common condition. Complications are rare.
- Initial conservative management works in the majority of cases.
- With complicated or recurrent disease, laparoscopic surgery or ERCP are safe in pregnant and nonpregnant patients.

 BASICS

DESCRIPTION
Wide spectrum of disease related to gallbladder dysfunction and cholelithiasis:
- Asymptomatic cholelithiasis
- Gallbladder sludge or microlithiasis
- Biliary pain: A result of a biliary distension
- Atypical pain with gallstones: Abdominal pain that is not clearly biliary-type pain is infrequently related to incidental gallstones.
- Acute cholecystitis: Inflammation of gallbladder
- Gallstone pancreatitis: Result of transient obstruction of the pancreatic duct by a stone
- Choledocholithiasis: Gallstone within the common bile duct, often causing obstruction with abnormal LFT's or ductal dilation
- Acute cholangitis: Ascending bactobilia resulting in bacteremia usually related to choledocholithiasis obstructing the bile duct

GENERAL PREVENTION
- Avoidance of risk factors
- Dietary factors that may prevent stones:
  - Ascorbic acid
  - Diet rich in polyunsaturated or monounsaturated fats
  - Vegetable protein
  - Coffee

EPIDEMIOLOGY
Incidence
The 5-year incidence for Danish women aged 30, 40, 50, and 60 years of age were 1.4%, 3.6%, 3.1%, and 3.7%, respectively. Likely higher in Hispanic, South American, and Native American populations and lower in African and Asian populations.

Cholelithiasis occurs in 4.5–12% of pregnancies of whom 30% progress to biliary pain usually in women with stones >10 mm. Progression to acute cholecystitis occurs in 0.04% and gallstone pancreatitis in 0.006% of pregnancies. It is the 2nd most common reason for nonobstetric surgery in pregnancy.

Prevalence
- High prevalence: 14.2 million adult women in United States have gallstones. The majority are asymptomatic.
- Women <30 years affected; 3:1 compared to men
- Gender gap equalizes by age 50

RISK FACTORS
- Strong (OR >2)
  - Multiparity, age >40, obesity, female gender when <40 years, rapid weight loss, cirrhosis
- Moderate (OR 1.5–2)
  - Diabetes mellitus, family history, ileal dysfunction (e.g., Crohn's disease, resection or bypass), estrogen therapy, first 5 years of oral contraceptive use
- Weak (OR 1–1.5)

- Drugs (ceftriaxone, clofibrate), sedentary lifestyle, total-parenteral nutrition

Genetics
- Patients with 1st-degree relative are 2–4× more likely to have gallstones than controls.
- The prevalence in the Pima Indian population is 73%.
- Inborn errors of metabolism

PATHOPHYSIOLOGY
- Bile is critical for digestion of fats.
- Most adult gallstones are made of cholesterol.
- Small proportions are pigment stones.
- Cholesterol gallstone formation
  - Cholesterol supersaturation
  - Alteration in ratio of bile acids favoring hydrophobic bile acids
  - Accelerated crystal nucleation
  - Diminished gallbladder motility with bile stasis
  - In acute cholecystitis, direct detergent action of bile salts on gallbladder mucosa stimulates inflammatory cascade and later superinfection

In pregnancy, altered physiology related to estrogen and progesterone exacerbates these factors leading to more lithogenic bile and hypomotility

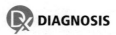 **DIAGNOSIS**

Diagnosis and management of gallbladder disease in pregnant and nonpregnant patients is nearly identical, except for their preference to use noninvasive techniques in pregnancy.

SIGNS AND SYMPTOMS
History
- Inquire about risk factors
- Location, quality, onset, timing, and severity of pain suggestive of biliary origin should prompt further evaluation.
  - Intermittent right upper quadrant pain +/− radiation to the shoulder
  - Rapid onset with plateau
  - Slow, gradual improvement over hours
  - Fatty food intolerance
  - Often associated with nausea
  - Exclude more serious complications or unrelated conditions

Physical Exam
- Benign exam with uncomplicated biliary pain
- Focus on excluding complications
  - Fever (abscess, cholecystitis, cholangitis)
  - Hypotension or tachycardia (cholangitis)
  - Murphy's sign
    - Inspiratory arrest with palpation of gallbladder fossa (cholecystitis)
  - Jaundice (obstruction)
  - Toxic appearance (cholangitis)

TESTS
Lab
- Liver function tests
  - Congruent elevations of alkaline phosphatase, bilirubin, and gamma glutaminase suggest biliary obstruction
- Complete blood count with differential
  - Leukocytosis may indicate cholecystitis or cholangitis.

- Amylase and lipase to exclude pancreatitis

Alkaline phosphatase is expected to be elevated in 3rd trimester often 2× the upper limit of normal.

Imaging
- Ultrasound
  - Prompt, noninvasive, safe, and cost-effective
  - Approximately 84% sensitivity for cholelithiasis
  - Evaluate for ductal dilation or cholelithiasis
  - Presence of pericholecystic fluid, thickened gallbladder wall or Murphy's sign indicates acute cholecystitis.
- Computed tomography
  - Given its increased accuracy, it may be helpful to evaluate for hepatic duct or intrahepatic duct dilation and exclude other pathologies.

Little role in pregnancy as majority of stones are radiolucent, unless heavily calcified

- Endoscopic ultrasound
  - High sensitivity but invasive
  - Consider in patients with recurrent classical biliary pain by history, but limited imaging secondary to anatomy or obesity

Safe in pregnancy, but rarely used

Cholecytokinin cholecystoscintigraphy (hepatobiliary iminodiacetic acid or HIDA scan):

- Non-visualization (no uptake of tracer) of gallbladder suggests acute cholecystitis

Unknown safety in pregnancy; reserve for postpartum evaluation

- Endoscopic retrograde cholangiography (ERCP)
  - Ability to diagnose and intervene on bile duct stones

Safest in 2nd and 3rd trimester. Shield pelvis, monitor fetus, and keep O2 saturation >96%. Monitor dosimetry. Average fetal dose is 164 millirads.

- Magnetic resonance cholangio-pancreatography (MRCP)
  - Highly accurate for choledocholithiasis

Gadolinium crosses the placenta, so safety in pregnancy is uncertain.

EXCLUDE CHOLANGITIS
Look for fever, evidence of sepsis, mental status changes, or evidence of biliary obstruction (i.e., jaundice or ductal dilation on imaging). Failure to treat with appropriate antibiotics may result in rapid deterioration of patient leading to sepsis and death.

DIFFERENTIAL DIAGNOSIS
- Acute hepatitis
- Hepatic abscess
- Biliary dyskinesia
- Sphincter of Oddi dysfunction
- Congenital choledochal cyst rupture/infection
- Irritable bowl syndrome
- Dyspepsia
- Peptic ulcer disease
- Empyema or pneumonia

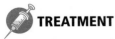# TREATMENT

INITIAL STABILIZATION
- For uncomplicated biliary pain, conservative management with pain meds, IVF, and NPO
- Evaluate for sepsis

GENERAL MEASURES
- Narcotic pain medication titrated to symptom control
- NSAIDs may be helpful in nonpregnant patients

Diet
Nothing by mouth until diagnosis is clear and pain resolved.

Activity
As tolerated

Nursing
- Monitor vital signs
- Supportive care

Appropriate fetal monitoring

IV Fluids
Electrolyte repletion, normal saline bolus followed by maintenance IVF if NPO

Complementary and Alternative Medicine
No evidence to support use

MEDICATION (DRUGS)

Ursodeoxycholic acid (UDCA) 5 mg/kg PO b.i.d.:
- Dissolution if <10 mm and adequate gallbladder motility
- Might be of benefit in recurrent pancreatitis secondary to bile microcrystals
- Indicated after bariatric surgery or in aggressive weight loss programs

UDCA has not been studied in pregnancy

- Ketorolac 30–60 mg IV or IM or ibuprofen 400 mg PO t.i.d. p.r.n. for acute attacks if no contraindications (age, renal failure, pregnancy)
- Broad spectrum antibiotics with enterococcal coverage are recommended if there is evidence of cholangitis or acute cholecystitis.

First Line
- Ampicillin and gentamicin
- Piperacillin-tazobactam
- Ciprofloxacin and metronidazole

Second Line
- Imipenem
- Levofloxacin

SURGERY
- Laparoscopic technique preferred
- Indications for nonurgent cholecystectomy
  - Recurrent biliary pain
  - Symptomatic biliary dyskinesia
  - Calcified gallbladder
- Indications for urgent cholecystectomy
  - Acute cholecystitis
  - Choledocholithiasis if ERCP failed to clear bile ducts

Recent surgical advances minimize risk to mother and fetus, but require multidisciplinary approach with perioperative fetal monitoring. Easiest to perform in the 2nd trimester

- ERCP
  - Indication
    - Nonimproving acute cholangitis, gallstone pancreatitis
  - Complications—rare: Pancreatitis, bleeding, perforation, cardiopulmonary. Risks are higher in therapeutic than diagnostic ERCP

Post-ERCP pancreatitis (5–7%) may cause abortion in pregnant woman

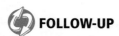 **FOLLOW-UP**

DISPOSITION
- After an acute attack, most patients may return home uneventfully.
- Education on recurrence risk and surgical management options

Admission Criteria
- Pain requiring intravenous narcotics
- Evidence of complications
  - Acute cholecystitis
  - Gallstone pancreatitis
  - Acute cholangitis

Discharge Criteria
- Pain controlled
- Tolerating diet
Stable fetus

Issues for Referral
Consult gastroenterology if biliary obstruction or pancreatitis

PROGNOSIS
For all patients with asymptomatic gallstones, 2% will become symptomatic every year for 5 years, with a cumulative rate of biliary colic of 18–28% and of complications of 3% at 10 years.

In pregnancy, after the 1st episode of biliary pain, 23% of women will progress to complications and 38% will have recurrent symptoms.

COMPLICATIONS
Rare complications of gallstone disease include:
- Gallstone ileus (erosion of stone into intestine causing obstruction)
- Fistula
- Gallbladder perforation with peritonitis

REFERENCES

1. Valdivieso V, Covarrubias C, Siegel F, et al. Pregnancy and cholelithiasis: Pathogenesis and natural course of gallstones diagnosed in early puerperium. *Hepatology*. 1993;17:1–4.
2. Glasgow RE, Visser BC, Harris HW, et al. Changing management of gallstone disease during pregnancy. *Surg Endosc*. 1998;12:241–246.
3. Tham TC, Vandervoort J, Wong RC, et al. Safety of ERCP during pregnancy. *Am J Gastroenterol*. 2003;98:308–311.
4. Lu EJ, Curet MJ, EL-Sayed YY, et al. Medical versus surgical management of biliary tract disease in pregnancy. *Am J Surg*. 2004;188:755–759.

CODES
ICD9-CM
- 574.2 Biliary pain
- 574.0 Nonobstructive cholelithiasis
- 574.1 Obstructive cholelithiasis
- 575.0 Acute cholecystitis
- 576.1 Acute cholangitis
- 574.3 Choledocholithiasis

KEY WORDS
- Abdominal Pain
- Gallstones
- Sepsis

HEADACHE

Elaine C. Jones, MD

KEY CLINICAL POINTS

- Migraine headaches are unilateral, throbbing, lasting 4–72 hours, and may be preceded by aura symptoms
- Red flags for headache may include:
  - Focal neurologic symptoms
  - "Worst headache ever"
  - Fever
  - Change in the headache type
  - Onset of headache with exertion, coughing, or sneezing
- Treatment consists of a combination of prophylactic and abortive therapies, addressing triggers, and reassurance.

 BASICS

DESCRIPTION
Headaches can be primary or secondary.
- Primary headaches include migraine with and without aura, tension-type headache, and cluster headache, for example.
- Secondary headaches are the result of other conditions such as tumors, infections, sinusitis, or TMJ, for example.

EPIDEMIOLOGY
- Migraine is often inherited with a female to male ratio of 2 to 3:1.
- Estrogen is a major trigger for migraine and so menstrual cycles, pregnancy, and menopause affect migraine frequency.
- Onset of migraine is most often in adolescence or early adulthood.

Incidence
Migraine incidence peaks in the 3rd decade of life.

Prevalence
- Migraine affects 18% of women and 6.5% of men.
- Less than 1/2 of those suffering with migraine are currently diagnosed.
- Approximately 90% of people will experience a headache at some point in their life.

Genetics
- There is a clear familial predisposition for migraine with >50% of migraneurs having at least 1 family member with migraine.
- Rare variants of migraine have identified and have autosomal dominant inheritance.
  - Familial Hemiplegic Migraine (chromosome 19p13 or 1q31)
  - Cerebral Autosomal Dominant Arteriopathy with Subcortical Infarcts and Leukoencephalopathy (CADASIL).

PATHOPHYSIOLOGY
- Trigeminovascular system: Activation of nerves around meningeal and cerebral blood vessels feeds back to the trigeminal ganglia and nuclei in the upper cervical cord.
- It is unclear what starts this cascade: Vasogenic vs. neurogenic theories exist.
  - Vasogenic: Intracranial vasoconstriction occurs followed by rebound vasodilation
  - Neurogenic: Chemical changes in the brain occur first and then cause vascular congestion.
- Migraine-specific abortive medications are known to work at the 5-HT1b/1d receptors (serotonin receptors fairly specific to brain vasculature).

Pregnancy Considerations
- Since migraines are often influenced by hormones, especially estrogen, they will be affected by pregnancy.
- Some women's migraines improve in pregnancy because estrogen levels are more constant; however, others may have worsening headaches.
- In the postpartum period, there is an increased risk for intracranial hemorrhage or cerebral venous thrombosis.
- New or different headaches may require evaluation with CT or MRV (venous phase MR angiography).

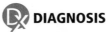 **DIAGNOSIS**

SIGNS AND SYMPTOMS
- Intermittent episodes of unilateral, pulsating head pain with gradual onset, building up to moderate to severe pain that lasts 4 to 72 hours
- Activity worsens the headaches
- Photophobia, phonophobia, and nausea/vomiting may be present.
- Prodromes may start days before the headache and include:
  - Mood changes
  - Food cravings
  - Fatigue
  - Yawning
  - Cognitive complaints
- Aura symptoms may precede the headache by 20 to 30 minutes and include:
  - Visual scotoma
  - Flashing lights
  - Loss of vision
  - Other focal neurologic symptoms
- Postdromes and other linger effects may last for days after the headache and include fatigue and cognitive complaints.

History
- Key features include a
  - Detailed description of a typical episode
  - Age of onset
  - Frequency of headaches
  - Duration
  - Associated symptomatology
- A change in headache type, frequency, or pattern may suggest concern for a new cause for headache and require investigation.
- Associated fever, constitutional symptoms, focal weakness, numbness, or tingling may require further investigation.
- A headache diary can be very helpful in monitoring headache patterns and triggers.

Physical Exam
- Neurologic and general physical exams should be normal.
- Look for papilledema, which suggests increased intracranial pressure and requires imaging.
- Any focal neurologic finding should be investigated further with imaging.

TESTS
If history consistent with migraine and exam is normal, then further testing may not be needed.

Lab
- Laboratory tests are generally not needed.
- Lumbar puncture indicated if:

- Meningeal findings suggestive of meningitis (stiff neck, fever, photophobia) or
- If headache is explosive and severe, suggesting intracranial hemorrhage

Imaging
- MRI is indicated when there are focal neurologic findings on exam.
  - Weakness
  - Hyper/hyporeflexia
  - Papilledema
  - Visual field defects
- CT scan is helpful for ruling out a bleed in the setting of sudden, acute, severe headache.

DIFFERENTIAL DIAGNOSIS
- Primary headaches
  - Tension: Bilateral, squeezing, little or no nausea/vomiting/photophobia, generally doesn't interfere with activities
  - Cluster: More frequent in men, sharp, unilateral, stabbing pain around the eye or temple, brief but comes in groups at once, often occurs at night
- Secondary headaches
  - Sinus: Unilateral or bilateral, throbbing, fever, nasal drainage; headache is not a major component of sinusitis.
  - Tumor: Recent onset of headaches, more diffuse pain, often worse in morning upon awakening.
  - Arteriovenous malformation (AVM)/aneurysm/subarachnoid hemorrhage
    - Sudden, explosive, severe head pain
    - Often diffuse, stiff neck,
    - May be brief loss of consciousness
  - Metabolic (thyroid, hepatic, renal, etc.)
    - Headache usually part of wide range of constitutional and systemic signs and symptoms

 ## TREATMENT

INITIAL STABILIZATION
Status migrainosis (migraine lasting a week or more) may require more urgent intervention
- Dihydroergotamine (DHE) IV
- Divalproex sodium (Depakote) IV
- Corticosteroids IV
- Prochlorperazine (Compazine) PR/IM

GENERAL MEASURES
- Establish realistic goals for treatment by
  - Reviewing benefits of therapy
  - How long it will take to see benefits
  - What side effects may arise
- Use a headache diary to monitor progress with treatments, to track patterns, and to identify triggers.
- Allow the patient to be actively involved in own management.
- All responses are not the same, so if one treatment fails try something else.
  - Medicines in the same class may work differently in different patients.
- Consider nonoral routes for patients with significant nausea or vomiting (nasal spray/IM).
- Avoid frequent use of abortive therapies.
  - All have been shown to cause rebound headaches.
  - Less frequent with the triptans but still can occur

Diet
- Certain foods can trigger migraine and should be avoided in susceptible individuals
  - Chocolate, aged cheeses, sausage, hot dogs, pate, pickled/dried foods, MSG, nuts, caffeine, alcohol (red wine, beer), artificial sweeteners

Physical Therapy
- Muscles of the neck and shoulders tighten when the trigeminal cervical systems are triggered.
- This can be secondary to the headache or may feedback and cause headache.
- Physical therapy to decrease cervical strain may benefit migraine patients.

Complementary and Alternative Medicine
- Herbal agents
  - Recent evidence suggests benefits from Feverfew, Butterbur, Magnesium, and B2 (riboflavin).
- Physical therapies
  - Acupuncture, cervical manipulation, massage, cervical mobilizations can be helpful but evidence-based recommendations are not yet possible.
- Relaxation training/biofeedback
  - Some evidence exists to suggest there is benefit from relaxation training and biofeedback therapies

 ## MEDICATION (DRUGS)

- Abortive: Start with medications most likely to work (triptans, DHE) and have rescue medications available for failures (butalbital, opioids, NSAIDs).
  - DHE nasal spray (Migranal)
    - 0.5 mg, max 24 hour = 2 mg
    - Good evidence for efficacy
    - Contraindicated in uncontrolled hypertension, coronary/peripheral or cerebrovascular disease, hepatic/renal dysfunction and pregnancy
  - Triptans: Common side effects are nausea, palpitations, chest pain; contraindicated in patients with coronary artery disease, uncontrolled HTN, hemiplegic migraine and basilar migraine
    - Almotriptan (Axert): 12.5 mg, max 24 hour = 25 mg
    - Eletriptan (Relpax): 40 mg, max 24 hour = 80 mg
    - Frovatriptan (Frova): 2.5 mg, max 24 hour = 7.5 mg
    - Naratriptan (Amerge): 2.5 mg, max 24 hour = 5 mg
    - Rizatriptan (Maxalt): 10 mg, max 24 hour = 30 mg; dose should be halved in patients on propranolol
    - Sumatriptan (Imitrex):
      ○ PO = 50 mg or 100 mg, max 24 hour = 200 mg;
      ○ NS = 20 mg in one nostril, max 24 hour = 40 mg;
      ○ IM = 6 mg, max 24 hour = 12 mg
    - Zolmitriptan (Zomig)
      ○ PO = 2.5 mg, max 24 hour = 10 mg;
      ○ NS = 5 mg, max 24 hour = 10 mg
- Prophylactic: Use when >2 to 3 headaches a month, goal is to prevent headaches.
  - Antihypertensives: Good in younger patients or if hypertension also a problem. Most common side effects are dizziness and lightheadedness.
    - Beta-blockers: Propranolol and timolol have the best evidence but atenolol, metoprolol, and nadolol also shown to have benefits
      ○ Propranolol: 60 mg/day starting dose
      ○ Timolol: 20 mg/day

- Calcium channel blockers: Verapamil and nimodipine have best evidence of benefit
  - Verapamil: 120 mg/day
- Antiepileptics
  - Divalproex sodium (Depakote): 500 mg/day
    - Has strongest evidence
    - Side effects include liver toxicity, weight gain and pregnancy risks
  - Gabapentin: 300 mg t.i.d., max 1,800–3,600 mg/day
  - Topiramate: 25 mg/day, max 100 mg/day
  - Carbamazepine: 200 mg t.i.d., max 1,200 mg/day
- Antidepressants: Common side effects include sleepiness, weight gain, urinary retention
  - Amitriptyline: 25 mg daily, max 150 mg/day
    - Has strongest evidence
  - Nortriptyline may be helpful
- Oral contraceptive pills (OCPs) may help some women with hormone affected migraines.
  - Occasionally, migraines may worsen with OCPs but lower dose estrogen pills have lessened this risk.
  - Currently it is unclear if there is an association between OCP use and increased risk of stroke in migraine sufferers.

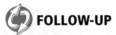

FOLLOW-UP

DISPOSITION
- Frequent monitoring is necessary for success.
- It may take 2 weeks or more to see benefit from prophylactic treatments.
- Doses should be maximized before moving on to another medication.

Admission Criteria
- Patients with status migrainosis and sometimes cluster headache may need admission for IV medications.
- Rarely patients with rebound headaches from analgesic overuse may require admission for detoxification.

Issues for Referral
Atypical headaches, focal neurologic abnormalities, and unresponsive headaches may require referral to a neurologist.

PROGNOSIS
- Migraines are extremely treatable, and there are a wide variety of options available.

- Combinations of treatments sometimes work better than monotherapy.
- Once headaches have improved or resolved, it is often possible to stop prophylactic treatments and maintain control with abortive therapies only.

COMPLICATIONS
Rebound headaches may occur with overuse of any and all analgesics, including triptans.
- Overuse is defined as taking them more than 2 days a week.
- Only treatment for rebound headaches is to abstain from any usage for 4–6 weeks.
- Other treatments may not work in the setting of rebound headaches.

REFERENCES

1. Goadsby PJ, Olesen J. Diagnosis and management of migraine. *Br Med J*. 1996;312(7041):1279–1283.
2. Lipton RB, Stewart WF. Migraine in the United States: A review of epidemiology and health care use. *Neurology*. 1993;43 (Suppl 3):S6–S10.
3. Silberstein SD. Practice parameter: Evidence-based guidelines for migraine headache (an evidence-based review). *Neurology*. 2000;55:754–762.
4. Silberstein SD, Young WB. Headache and facial pain. In: Goetz CG, ed. *Textbook of Clinical Neurology*. 2nd ed. Philadelphia, PA: Saunders; 2003:1187–1205.

CODES
ICD9-CM
- 784.0 Headache
- 346.00 Migraine w/o mention of intractable
- 307.81 Tension headache

KEY WORDS
- Headache
- Migraine
- Subarachnoid Hemorrhage
- Visual Loss

H

HEPATITIS B

Silvia D. Degli-Esposti, MD

KEY CLINICAL POINTS

- Acute hepatitis B resolves in 95% of adults with subsequent permanent immunity.
- In children <5 years old, it results in chronic infection in 85% of cases.
- Incidence has decreased dramatically since universal immunization of children.
- Passive and active immunization is recommended to stop transmission from infected individuals.
- Antiviral therapy in chronic infection decreases the risk of long-term complications (cirrhosis and hepatocellular carcinoma).

 BASICS

DESCRIPTION
Systemic viral infection by hepatotropic virus: Hepatitis B virus (HBV)
- Acute hepatitis: Occurs 6–12 weeks from contact with infectious individual
- Fulminant hepatitis: Rare; more common in the elderly or with hepatitis D virus (HDV) coinfection
- Chronic active hepatitis: >6 months persistence of replicating virus after an acute infection
  - Chronic inflammation present in the liver
  - Leads ultimately to cirrhosis and risk for hepatocellular carcinoma (HCC)
- Chronic inactive carrier state: >6 months persistence of virus after acute infection
  - Characteristic of infections acquired in childhood
  - Low level of replication
  - Minimal inflammation in the liver
  - Disease may reactivate during lifetime
  - Chronic infection may cause HCC even in absence of liver damage

GENERAL PREVENTION
Bloodborne pathogen spreads through bodily fluids or mucosal contact, enteric spread possible. Patients are infectious 2 weeks before the acute illness.
- General measures
  - Good sanitation and hygiene
  - Screening of blood products
  - Proper handling of medical instruments
- Vaccination is recommended
  - All infants and children <19 years old
  - All individuals with risks factors
  - Patients affected by liver disease
- Vaccination + Immunoprophylaxis (specific immunoglobulin or HBIG) is recommended.
  - Intimate contacts of infected individuals
  - Infants born from infected mothers
- Vaccines available
  - Single antigen (HBV only) : Recombivax, Energix-B
  - Multiple antigens other than HBV
    - Twinrix (adults only), Comvax, Pediatrix
- Vaccination schedules
  - Infants and children: 3 or more doses, 5 mcg intramuscularly (IM).
  - Adolescents and adults: 2 or more doses, 10 mcg IM.

- Immunocompromised patients: 3 or more doses, 20 mcg IM.
- Complications of vaccination
  - Anaphylaxis is rare: 1/1.1 million; alopecia
  - No conclusive evidence for causal association with Guillan-Barre syndrome, Multiple Sclerosis, Chronic Fatigue Syndrome
- Contraindications to vaccination
  - Yeast hypersensitivity
  - Previous reactions to vaccine components
  - Premature low birth infants (<2,000 grams)
- Vaccine efficacy
  - Vaccine produces greater than 95% seroprotection rate in immunocompetent subjects.
  - Vaccine-induced memory persists despite the decline of antibody titer. No further booster doses are recommended.

EPIDEMIOLOGY
Approximately 400 million individuals are infected with HBV worldwide.

Incidence
Overall incidence in United States has dramatically decreased since childhood immunization—currently 2.1 per 100,000 individuals

Prevalence
- In the North American population, 4.9% are infected with HBV or have been infected in the past.
- Foreign-born persons especially Asian and Pacific Islander populations are disproportionately affected by disease.

RISK FACTORS
- IV drug use
- Sexual partner of infected individuals
- Children born from HBV positive mothers
- Hemodialysis patients
- Individuals born in certain areas of the United States and in countries with high HBV prevalence (South Asia, Africa, Alaska)
- Household contacts of infected individuals
- Individuals with sexually transmitted diseases or multiple sex partners
- Blood products or organ recipients
- Workers exposed to bodily fluids

PATHOPHYSIOLOGY
HBV DNA virus replicates in hepatocytes and at low levels in bone marrow, lymphocytes and spleen
- Strong host cellular immune response against viral antigens causes the liver damage.
- Causes of chronicity of the infection are largely unknown.
- The chronic inflammatory response causes the production of mediators in the liver parenchyma leading to collagen deposition and end stage cirrhosis.
- HBV-DNA has been found integrated in the genome of HCC tissue and HBV seems to have direct carcinogenic potential.

ETIOLOGY
HBV is a DNA virus of the Hepadnavirus family structure:
- Outer shell (envelope protein or antigen s, HBsAg)
- Inner viral capside (180 subunit of core antigen protein, HBcAg)
- Partially double stranded DNA 3.2 kb length

ASSOCIATED CONDITIONS
- Polyarteritis nodosa
- Glomerulonephritis
- Cryglobulinemia
- Bone marrow aplasia
- Papular acrodermatitis

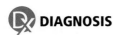 **DIAGNOSIS**

PRE-HOSPITAL
- Patients present with signs and symptoms of acute hepatitis.
  - Approximately 75% of all acute hepatitis B patients lack jaundice and are often missed.
- Chronically infected patients may be asymptomatic or present with signs and symptoms of chronic liver disease.

SIGNS AND SYMPTOMS
- Fever, anorexia, fatigue, nausea, arthralgia, vomiting, right upper quadrant pain, jaundice, dark urine, light stools
- Signs of chronic liver disease: Muscular wasting, confusion, ascites, bleeding

History
- For acute: Exposure to infected individuals or blood products over previous 12 weeks
- Risks factors: Country of birth, lifestyle hazards, occupational hazards

Physical Exam
- May be normal
- Jaundice, hepatosplenomegaly, rash
- Signs of advanced liver disease: Palmar erythema, spider nevi, gynecomastia, ascites, hyperreflexia

TESTS
Antibodies against HBV antigens (serological markers) are important diagnostic tools
- Acute Hepatitis: HBsAg+, HBsAb−, HBcAb IGM +, HBV DNA +
- Chronic Active Hepatitis: HBsAg+, HBsAb−, HBcAb IGG +, HBV DNA +
- Chronic Carrier State: HBsAg+, HBsAb−, HBcAb IGG+, HBV DNA − or low level +
- Recovered Individuals: HbsAg−, HBsAb+, HBcAb IGG+, HBV DNA −.
- Vaccinated Individuals: HBsAG−, HBsAb+, HBcIGG−, HBV DNA−.
  - The hepatitis B e antigen (HBeAg) and antibody (HBeAb) are useful in monitoring therapy; the presence of HBeAg correlates with infectivity.
  - Chronic carrier individuals are often HBeAg−.
  - Individuals infected with mutant strain of the virus (pre-core mutant) are HBeAg− and HBV DNA + with high infectivity.

Lab
- Acute Hepatitis:
  - ALT, AST >5× normal, alkaline phospatase (alk phos), and total bilirubin (TB) may be normal or mildly elevated.
  - HBcAb IGM +
- Fulminant hepatitis:
  - INR ≥6.5 correlates with poor prognosis
  - Test for Hepatitis D virus (HDV)
- Chronic Hepatitis:
  - AST, ALT 2 to 5 times normal
  - PT, gamma globulin may be increased.
  - Albumin, platelets may be low
  - Check alpha-fetoprotein every 6 months, if cirrhosis is present.

- Exclude other causes of liver disease:
  - Ceruloplasmin, ferritin, iron, Autoimmune markers, Hepatitis C (HCV), Herpes, Cytomegalovirus (CMV)

Imaging
- Abdominal ultrasound with Doppler to rule out other causes of liver disease
- CT scan with contrast if HCC is suspected

Diagnostic Procedures/Surgery
- Liver biopsy is necessary to differentiate chronic inactive carriers from patients with chronic active hepatitis.
- Liver biopsy is not indicated in acute hepatitis.

Pathologic Findings
- Chronic inactive carriers
  - Minimal to absent changes
  - Viral particles present in the hepatocytes (ground glass cells)
- Chronic active hepatitis
  - Inflammation extending in the liver lobule
  - Collagen deposition, bridging fibrosis, cirrhosis

DIFFERENTIAL DIAGNOSIS
Other causes of acute hepatitis
- Viral: Hepatitis C, Hepatitis A, Hepatitis E, Epstein Barr virus, Herpes viruses, CMV
- Toxic: Alcoholic, acetaminophen, poisonous mushrooms, Wilson's disease, autoimmune hepatitis
- 10% of acute hepatitis has an unknown cause.
- Other causes of chronic liver disease: HCV, alcohol, hemochromatosis, autoimmune hepatitis, NASH, drug-induced liver damage, primary biliary cirrhosis, primary sclerosing cholangitis, Alpha-1 antitripsin deficiency

 TREATMENT

INITIAL STABILIZATION
Hospitalize only severe cases of acute hepatitis B for observation, no specific treatment available:
- Monitor: INR, renal function, albumin, lactic acid
- Transfer to transplantation unit if neurological assessment worsens

GENERAL MEASURES
- Report all HBsAg+ patients to the State Health Department
- Offer post exposure prophylaxis to sexual and household contacts
- Vaccinate chronic hepatitis B patients for HAV
- Avoid hepatotoxic drugs

Diet
As tolerated. Avoid raw fish (risk of infections with Vibrio Vulnificus and HAV).

Activity
As tolerated

Complementary and Alternative Medicine
None effective. Avoid hepatotoxic herbal compounds (Kava Kava, Comfrey, Chaparall)

Pregnancy Considerations
- Mothers who are HBsAg + and HBeAg+ transmit to infants in 70–90% of cases without adequate immunoprophylaxis.
- All pregnant women are screened for HbsAg.
- Retest if risk factors persist during pregnancy.
- Women with high HBV DNA load may transmit HBV to infants despite adequate passive and active immunization.
- Test children born from HBsAg mothers after vaccination is completed.

H

- Acute HBV in 3rd trimester may cause premature labor.
- Pregnant women at risk of acquiring HBV should be vaccinated during pregnancy.

 ## MEDICATION (DRUGS)

Indicated for chronically infected patients with ongoing liver damage by histology, HBV DNA+, AST and ALT >2× normal
- End point of therapy: Suppression of viral load and clearance of HbeAg with or without development of anti-HBe antibodies
- Conversion from HBsAg+ to HBsAb+ is rare; occurs in about 10% of cases
- Duration of therapy not well established

First Line
Interferon alfa or pegylated interferon alfa × 24 weeks
- Contraindications: Pregnancy, low platelets, infants up to 3 years of age
- Complications: Depression, myelosuppression, cardiotoxicity, acute renal failure, seizures, autoimmune disorders, liver failure

Second Line
Alternatives to interferon therapy or as second line:
- Lamivudine, Adefovir
  - Development of resistant mutant strains of the virus limits the therapy.
  - Flares of the disease may occur upon discontinuation.
  - Lamivudine is probably safe in pregnancy.

SURGERY
Liver transplantation indicated for acute fulminant hepatitis, decompensated liver disease, HCC

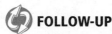 ## FOLLOW-UP

Issues for Referral
- Refer patients to hepatologist for staging, therapy, and management of chronic hepatitis B.
- Refer patients with end-stage liver disease for transplant evaluation.

PROGNOSIS
Recovery of acute infection depends on age; those who acquire infection at an earlier age much more likely to have chronic infection

- Fulminant hepatitis ~1%
- Chronic active hepatitis leads to end stage liver disease and HCC.
- Chronic inactive carriers have a significantly lower risk of disease progression, but are not free from disease progression and complications of hepatitis B.

PATIENT MONITORING
Monitor HBs Ag+ patients for HCC and progression of the disease every 3–6 months
- Liver ultrasound and alpha-fetoprotein
- ALT, AST, alk phos, TB, PT, albumin, platelet count , HBV serology and HBV DNA

REFERENCES

1. Mast E, et al. Comprehensive immunization strategy to eliminate transmission of hepatitis B virus infection in the United States. *MMWR Recomm Rep.* December 23 2005;54(RR-16):1–31.
2. Lok AS, McMahon BJ. Chronic hepatitis B. Practice Guideline on chronic hepatitis B. *Hepatology.* 2004;39:857–861.
3. Wright TL. Introduction to chronic hepatitis B infection. *Am J Gastroenterol.* 2006;101(Suppl 1):1–6.
4. McMahon BJ. Selecting appropriate management strategies for chronic hepatitis B: Who to treat. *Am J Gastroenterol.* 2006;101(Suppl 1):7–12.
5. Marcellin P, Chang TT, Lim SG, et al. Adefovir dipivoxil for the treatment of hepatitis B e antigen-positive chronic hepatitis B. *N Engl J Med.* 2003;348:808–816.

CODES
ICD9-CM
- 070.0 Acute viral hepatitis
- 070.2 Chronic viral hepatitis

KEY WORDS

- Hepatitis B
- Acute Hepatitis
- Chronic Hepatitis
- Fulminant Hepatitis

HEPATITIS C
Silvia D. Degli-Esposti, MD

KEY CLINICAL POINTS

- 5 million Americans are infected with hepatitis C virus (HCV).
- Hepatitis C is the leading cause of liver transplant in the United States.
- Disease generally manifests 20 to 30 years after the initial infection.
- Leads to cirrhosis in one quarter of cases
- The therapy is effective in 1/2 of the patients.
- Women respond better than men to the therapy.

 BASICS

DESCRIPTION
Systemic viral infection, involving mainly the liver:
- Of the infected individuals, 75% fail to clear the virus and become chronically infected.
- Only a fraction of those will develop complications: Liver cirrhosis and hepatocellular carcinoma (HCC).

GENERAL PREVENTION
HCV is a blood-borne pathogen. In absence of vaccine, prevention focuses on avoiding initial infection.
- Avoid contact with blood or bodily fluid.
- Universal precautions should be used.
- Avoid sharing syringes and drug paraphenalia, sharp objects, and razors.
- Screening of blood, blood product, and organs (available in the United States since 1992)
- Sexual transmission is rare and at present no specific recommendations are made for patients in a monogamous relationship with an HCV-infected partner.

EPIDEMIOLOGY
- Worldwide distribution: 3% of world population
- Prevalence: Male > Female: 1.5 to 1
- Racial distribution: Latinos and African-Americans have increased prevalence

Incidence
36,000 new cases of acute HCV infection per year

Prevalence
- Approximately 5 million infected in the United States
- 1.7% prevalence in the United States

RISK FACTORS
- Highest risk factors
  - IV drug use: 70% to 90% of all IV drug users are positive for HCV.
  - Recipients of blood, blood products, or solid organ before 1992
  - Hemodialyis patients
- Moderate risk factors
  - Sexual contact with infected HCV partner
  - Snorting cocaine without IV injection
  - Body piercing and tattooing
  - Children born from HCV positive mother
- Household contact does not constitute a risk factor.
- A significant number (9%) of infected individuals have unknown risk factors.

Genetics
Genetics may play a role in disease development and response to therapy, but it is still poorly understood.
African-Americans have milder disease, but respond poorly to therapy.

PATHOPHYSIOLOGY
HCV replication occurs mainly in the hepatocytes; acute hepatitis occurs 3 to 6 months after exposure
- Initial clearance of virus
  - HCV elicits a humoral and cell-mediated response.
  - Immunoresponse is inefficient and results in a low rate of viral clearance.
  - Rapidly mutating virus escapes immunosurveillance
  - Children and young women clear the virus better.
- Chronic infection
  - The causes of hepatocyte damage in chronic HCV infection are unknown.
  - Cirrhosis occurs in 10%–15% after 20 years of infection; overall probably only in 1/3 of all patients
  - Factors accelerating disease progression: Male gender, initial infection at >40 years of age, body mass index (BMI), confection with HIV and HBV, transfusion as modality of infection, excessive alcohol, and fatty liver
- HCC development
  - Occurs only when cirrhosis is present.
  - When cirrhosis is present, HCC arise at a rate of 1%–4% × year.

ETIOLOGY
- Hepatotropic single stranded RNA virus of the Flaviviridae family
- 6 known genotypes, 1A and 1B are most common in North America

ASSOCIATED CONDITIONS
- Fatty liver
- Autoimmune diseases (thyroiditis, rheumatoid arthritis, IDDM)
- Insulin resistance
- Porphyria cutanea tarda
- Urticaria
- Glomerulonephritis
- Cryoglobulinemia
- Depression and cognitive disorders
- Polyneuritis
- Vasculitis
- Autoimmune hepatitis type 2

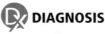 **DIAGNOSIS**

PRE-HOSPITAL
Outpatient management recommended:
- Initial acute hepatitis is almost always asymptomatic.
- HCV infection is often discovered during routine testing.
- May present as advanced liver disease

SIGNS AND SYMPTOMS
Mostly asymptomatic:
- Acute infection
  - Fatigue, anorexia, jaundice, dark urine, light stools
- Chronic infection

- Signs and symptoms of chronic liver disease: Difficulty in concentration, irritability, arthralgia, neuropathy, rashes, muscle wasting, gastrointestinal bleeding, weight changes

History
- IV drug use and other substance abuse even if remote
- Family history of liver disease
- Blood or blood products prior to 1992
- Sexual contacts
- Alcohol consumption

Physical Exam
Normal or
Jaundice, hepatosplenomegaly, palmar erythema, muscle wasting, gynecomastia.

TESTS
Maintain high index of suspicion and screen all patients with risk factors
- HCV ELISA 3rd generation as screening test: High specificity and sensitivity
- RIBA confirmatory test: To confirm + ELISA in a low risk population
- HCV qualitative PCR: Follows a + ELISA in a high risk population checking for presence of the virus
- HCV ELISA+ and HCV PCR: Patients (aviremic) may have virus hidden in tissue reservoirs or they may have cleared the infection with residual circulating antibodies.
- Check HCV PCR during acute infection: Antibodies directed against HCV appear up to 6 months after initial infection and are negative during acute hepatitis phase.

Lab
- CBC with platelets, ALT and AST, total bilirubin, alkaline phosphatase, INR, albumin, alfa-fetoprotein
  - Rule out associated conditions.
    - Fasting glucose, TSH, cryoglobulin, creatinine, BUN, Urinalysis, 24 hour urine for uro- and coproporphyrin
    - Nonorgan specific auto-antibodies often present: Antinuclear antibody (ANA), antimitochondrial antibody (AMA), smooth muscle antibody (SMA), liver kidney microsomal type I antibody (LKM1)
  - Rule out other causes of liver disease.
    - Iron, ferritin, ceruloplasmin, alpha 1 antitripsin

Imaging
- Liver ultrasound with doppler to rule out other causes of liver disease
- CT scan with contrast when HCC is suspected

Pathologic Findings
Histology is the best predictor of disease severity and progression, not pathognomonic

Biopsies are graded to score liver damage; Metavir system: 1 to 3 for inflammatory activity and 1 to 4 for fibrosis

DIFFERENTIAL DIAGNOSIS
Other causes of acute and/or chronic liver disease
- Viral infections: Hepatitis B, A, E, Epstein-Barr virus, cytomegalovirus
- Toxic and metabolic: Alcohol, drug-induced liver disease, poisonous mushrooms, hemochromatosis, Wilson's disease
  - Autoimmune hepatitis, primary biliary cirrhosis (PBC)

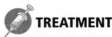

TREATMENT

PRE-HOSPITAL
Outpatient evaluation and treatment is recommended.

GENERAL MEASURES
- HBV and hepatitis A (HAV) vaccination for HCV infected patient
- Avoid alcohol, smoking and any hepatotoxic drugs

Diet
- BMI influences progression of the disease and response to therapy. Weight reduction for the obese patient
- Avoid raw fish for risk of HAV and Vibrio Vulnificus infections

Activity
Active lifestyle to restore insulin sensitivity

Nursing
- Education regarding prevention of spreading of infection
- Education and support regarding compliance with therapy

MEDICATION (DRUGS)

Goal of therapy: Sustained virologic response (SVR): Negative qualitative PCR after discontinuation of therapy sustained over time
- Acute hepatitis C
  - No liver biopsy required for these patients
  - Pegylated Interferon monotherapy given as soon as 8 weeks from initial contact for 24 weeks will induce SVR in >80% of cases
- Chronic HCV
  - Criteria for treatment for genotype 1 and 4:
    - Abnormal ALT and/or AST at least once, Metavir score >2 for fibrosis
    - Treat for 48 weeks
- Criteria for treatment for genotype 2 and 3
  - Need for liver biopsy or abnormal AST and ALT controversial given the high response rate (84%)
  - Treat for 24 weeks
- Contraindications or relative contraindications to treatment
  - Unstable mental illness
  - Pancytopenia, thrombocytopenia
  - Severe cardiopulmonary disease
  - Decompensated liver disease
  - Pregnancy (self or partner)
  - Ribavin use is contraindicated in renal insufficiency

First Line
Pegylated Interferon alpha subcutaneously once a week and daily oral Ribavirin.
- Weight-based Ribavirin more effective
- Frequent monitor of patient physical signs, symptoms and laboratory values is mandatory during therapy
- Side effects:
  - Anemia, leukopenia, fatigue, depression, nausea, diarrhea, fever, body ache, weight loss, hair loss, sleep disturbance, short-term memory impairment
  - Treatment for side effects
    - Growth factors for hematological alterations and fatigue
    - Selective serotonin reuptake inhibitors for depression
    - Proton pump inhibitors for dyspepsia
- Response to therapy (50% to 60% overall)
  - Patients classified as:
    - Responders: SVR obtained for >3 years from discontinuation of treatment
    - Nonresponders: Fail to achieve >2 log decrease in viral load at 12 weeks of treatment; in this case, discontinuation of therapy is recommended

- Relapsers: Achieve response at 12 weeks but fail to maintain response after discontinuation of therapy
- Factors which predict a poor response to therapy
  - Cirrhosis, older age, males, genotype 1, high pretreatment viral load, increased BMI

Second Line
New drugs are under investigation (proteases, polymerase, helicase inhibitors)

SURGERY
Decompensated cirrhosis and HCC may require a liver transplant.

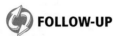 FOLLOW-UP

Admission Criteria
Patients with decompensated liver disease may require hospitalization.

Issues for Referral
Refer patient to hepatologist for:
- Staging of disease and HCV treatment
- Complications of advanced liver disease (gastrointestinal bleeding, refractory ascites, encephalopathy)
- Evaluation for liver transplant

PROGNOSIS
- Patients that do not respond to therapy may progress to end stage liver disease and require liver transplant.
- Indefinite treatment with Interferon may halt this process.

COMPLICATIONS
- HCC
- Decompensated liver disease
- Renal disease
- Diabetes mellitus
- Autoimmune diseases

PATIENT MONITOR
- Monitor HCV+ patients every 6 months for disease progression.
- Monitor cirrhotic patients for the development of HCC – obtain an alpha fetoprotein and abdominal ultrasound every 6 months

Pregnancy Considerations
- Screen all pregnant patients with risk factors for HCV.
- 3% of infants born from HCV+ mother are vertically infected.
- Risk factors for vertical transmission: High viral load of mother, HIV coinfection, rupture of membrane > than 6 hours, and invasive monitoring during delivery.
- Screen all infants born from HCV+ mother with PCR × 2 in the 1st 12 months and HCV ELISA after 18 months.
- Maternal antibodies persist in the infant's circulation up to 18 months.
- Breast feeding is safe in the absence of open sores.

REFERENCES

1. Strader DB, Wright T, Thomas DL, et al. AASLD Practice Guidelines: Diagnosis, management and treatment of hepatitis C. *Hepatology.* 2004;39:1147–1171.
2. Marcellin P, Asselah T, Boyer N. Fibrosis and disease progression in hepatitis C. *Hepatology.* 2002;36:47–56.
3. National Institute of Health Consensus development conference panel statement: Management of hepatitis C: 2002. *Hepatology.* 2002;36:3–20.
4. Lonardo A, Adinolfi LE, Loria P, et al. Steatosis and hepatitis C virus: Mechanisms and significance for hepatic and extrahepatic disease. *Gastroenterology.* 2004;126:586–597.
5. Mast EE, Hwang LY, Seto DS, et al. Risk factors for perinatal transmission of hepatitis C virus (HCV) and the natural history of HCV infection acquired in infancy. *J Infect Dis.* 2005;192:1880–1889.

CODES
ICD9-CM
- 070.0 Acute liver disease
- 070.9 Chronic viral liver disease
- 571.0 Cirrhosis

KEY WORDS

- Hepatitis C
- Viral Hepatitis

H

HIRSUTISM

Geetha Gopalakrishnan, MD

KEY CLINICAL POINTS

- Hirsutism may represent 1 end of a spectrum of normal hair development, but it can also be a marker of an underlying disorder of androgen excess.
- Most cases of hirsutism are secondary to idiopathic hirsutism or PCOS. In order to make this diagnosis, other rare causes of hirsutism need to be ruled out including hyperprolactinemia, congenital adrenal hyperplasia, and androgen secreting tumors.
- Later age of onset and a rapid rate of progression of hirsutism should raise concern for an adrenal or ovarian tumor especially if DHEA-S >700 mcg/dL or total testosterone >150 ng/dL respectively. Surgical resection of the androgen secreting tumor will alleviate symptoms.
- Hair removal, weight reduction, OCPs, and spironolactone will improve hirsutism in PCOS and idiopathic hirsutism.

 BASICS

DESCRIPTION

Hirsutism refers to excessive terminal (long, coarse and pigmented) hair growth in androgen responsive areas such as upper lip, chin, chest, back, and abdomen. Often hirsutism represents one end of a spectrum of normal hair development, but it can also be a marker of an underlying disorder of androgen excess. In combination with other signs of masculinization such as clitoromegaly, deepening of voice and temporal balding, hirsutism can be a sign of ovarian or adrenal tumor. Excessive growth of total body androgen independent vellus (fine, soft, and not pigmented) hair is hypertrichosis. It does not represent true hirsutism.

EPIDEMIOLOGY

- Women of reproductive age: 5% to 10%
- More common in individuals of Mediterranean and Middle Eastern origin

PATHOPHYSIOLOGY

Hirsutism is a result of:
- Excess production of androgens by the ovary or the adrenals
- Increased conversion of androgens from steroid precursors
- Increased rate of utilization by androgen-responsive tissue

ETIOLOGY

- Idiopathic hirsutism: Diagnosed in women with normal serum androgen, regular menstrual cycle, and no other cause for hirsutism.
- Polycystic ovary syndrome (PCOS): Elevated levels of serum androgens or symptom of hyperandrogenism (i.e., hirsutism and acne) in a woman with menstrual irregularity characterizes PCOS. This condition starts at puberty and progresses with age and is associated with obesity and insulin resistance.
- Hyperthecosis: Nonmalignant ovarian disorder characterized by an increased production of testosterone. This condition may be an exaggerated variation of PCOS.
- Severe insulin resistance syndromes: Hyperinsulinemia is associated with genetic or antibody mediated defects in the insulin receptor and syndromes of lipoatrophy and lipodystrophy. These syndromes include leprechaunism, Rabson-Mendenhall syndrome, lipoatrophy, type A syndrome and type B syndrome. Hyperinsulinemia can cause ovarian hyperandrogenism.

- Congenital Adrenal Hyperplasia (CAH): Usually diagnosed at birth or in early infancy because of sexual ambiguity, but nonclassical late-onset CAH can present at time of puberty or later. In late onset CAH, women present with menstrual irregularity and hirsutism without cortisol deficiency. 21-hydroxylase deficiency is the most common cause of late onset CAH.
- Ovarian and Adrenal Tumors: Hirsutism caused by an androgen-secreting tumor is most likely to occur later in life and progress rapidly. Should be considered in hirsute women with symptoms of virilization such as deepening of the voice, breast atrophy, temporal balding, increased muscle bulk, clitoromegaly, and increased libido.
- Adrenal tumors: Adenomas (rare) secrete excess testosterone and carcinomas secrete excess DHEA/DHEA-S and Cortisol.
- Ovarian tumors: Most ovarian tumors will have serum testosterone concentrations greater than 150 ng/dL. These tumors are usually derived from sex cords or stromal cells and can secrete other hormones including estrogens, hCG, serotonin, and thyroxine.
- Hyperprolactinemia: May stimulate adrenal DHEA-S concentrations and cause mild hirsutism.
- Cushing syndrome: Amenorrhea and hirsutism can be associated with Cushing syndrome resulting from an ectopic tumor, pituitary tumor, adrenal adenoma, or adrenal carcinoma.
- Menopause: Physiologic change in ratio of estrogen to androgen can cause facial hirsutism.
- Drugs: Testosterone, DHEA, danazol, and oral contraceptives with androgenic progestins (norgestrel and levonorgestrel) can cause hirsutism.
- Hypertrichosis: Excessive growth of total body androgen independent vellus (fine, soft and not pigmented) hair is hypertrichosis. It does not represent true hirsutism. It is usually familial, but can be associated with certain medical conditions such as hypothyroidism, anorexia nervosa, and dermatomyositis and medications including phenytoin, penicillamine, diazoxide, minoxidil, and cyclosporine.

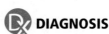 **DIAGNOSIS**

Most cases of hirsutism are secondary to idiopathic hirsutism or PCOS. In order to make this diagnosis, other rare causes of hirsutism need to be ruled out including hyperprolactinemia, CAH, and ovarian and adrenal tumors.

SIGNS AND SYMPTOMS

- Hirsutism: Long, coarse and pigmented hair growth in androgen responsive areas such as upper lip, chin, chest, back, and abdomen.
- Virilization: Hirsutism, clitoromegaly, deepening of voice, increased muscle mass, frontal balding, breast atrophy, and loss of female body contour are characteristic of virilization. It can be a sign of ovarian or adrenal tumor.
- Hyperandrogenism: Hirsutism, seborrhea, acne, menstrual irregularity and virilization can be seen with hyperandrogenism.
- Hypertrichosis: Excessive growth of fine, soft and not pigmented total body androgen independent vellus. It does not represent true hirsutism.

History
- Assess family history, medical history including diabetes and hypertension, medications, weight, menstrual regularity, breast

discharge, hot flashes, pregnancy, infertility, estrogen use, acne, change in voice, hair loss and symptoms of ovulation including ovulatory pain, premenstrual symptoms and breast tenderness.

- Age of onset, rate of progression, and associated symptoms of virilization or hyperandrogenism can help guide the diagnosis.
- In PCOS, hirsutism starts at puberty and steadily progresses with age.
- Later age of onset and a rapid rate of progression of hirsutism associated with symptoms of virilization should raise concern for adrenal or ovarian tumors.

Physical Exam

Evaluate location, pigmentation and intensity of hair growth.
Assess patterns of hair loss (e.g., frontal balding), acne, seborrhea, muscle mass, breast atrophy, weight, fat distribution (e.g., truncal, buffalo hump, supraclavicular fat), acanthosis nigricans (insulin resissitance), striae (Cushing syndrome), and galactorrhea (hyperprolactinemia).
Pelvic examination is recommended to evaluate clitoral size and ovarian mass.

TESTS
Lab

- Check total testosterone, free testosterone, DHEA-S, 17-hydroxyprogesterone, Prolactin, LH, FSH, TSH, Free T4 and 24-hour urine Cortisol.
- Consider ovarian tumor in women with total testosterone >150 ng/dL or free testosterone >2 ng/dL and adrenal tumor in DHEA-S >700 mcg/dL.
- If elevated 17-hydroxyprogesterone, consider CAH; elevated prolactin, consider hyperprolactinemia; elevated FSH, consider menopause; elevated TSH, consider hypothyroidism; and elevated 24-hour urine cortisol, consider Cushing syndrome as possible etiology of hirsutism.

Assess fasting blood glucose and lipids to evaluate complications of PCOS and insulin resistance. PCOS is a clinical diagnosis, made after other conditions are excluded.

Imaging

- Transvaginal ultrasound of the ovary to evaluate ovarian tumor if elevated testosterone levels
- CT scan of the adrenals to evaluate adrenal tumors if elevated DHEA-S and if ovarian ultrasound normal in women with elevated testosterone

DIFFERENTIAL DIAGNOSIS

Hirsutism represents 1 end of a spectrum of normal hair development. Approximately 25% of women develop terminal hair in the upper lip, abdomen, and back. Certain races (Caucasians) and genetic backgrounds (Mediterranean origin) are more prone to hirsutism. Therefore, the normal variation in hair growth needs to be considered during a hirsutism evaluation.

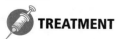 **TREATMENT**

Goal of treatment is to remove hair, decrease hair growth, and address associated heath conditions, such as menstrual irregularities and infertility.

GENERAL MEASURES

- Hair removal and lightening: Shaving, waxing, chemical depilation, bleaching, electrolysis, and laser hair removal.
- Weight reduction: In PCOS, androgen levels decrease with weight loss resulting in regular cycles and improved symptoms of hirsutism.

 MEDICATION (DRUGS)

- Eflornithine hydrochloride facial cream: Slows facial hair growth
- Oral contraceptives (OCP): Improves hirsutism and regulates cycle. Preparations with low estrogen dose and nonandrogenic progestin are ideal. Women with PCOS may be at an increased risk of endometrial hyperplasia and carcinoma. Estrogen in combination with progesterone or progesterone alone is recommended to induce menses in these women. Side effects include high blood pressure, deep venous thrombosis and high cholesterol levels.
- Antiandrogens: In the United States, spironolactone is the only antiandrogen approved by the Food and Drug Administration (FDA) for hirsutism. Other antiandrogens (e.g., flutamide and finasteride) have been approved for other conditions, but not hirsutism. In combination with OCP, antiandrogens may be more effective in improving hirsutism than given alone.
- Spironolactone: Inhibits the binding of testosterone to its receptors. It also decreases the ovarian production and the clearance of testosterone. It is effective in 60% to 70% of women with hirsutism. Starting dose is 50 mg once daily and the dose can be increased after several months. Maximum dose is 200 mg per day. Side effects include hyperkalemia, abdominal discomfort, and irregular menstrual bleeding.
- Flutamide: Inhibits the binding of testosterone to its receptors. Flutamide 250 mg b.i.d. may be more potent than spironolactone for the treatment of hirsutism. However, it can be hepatotoxic and has been associated with deaths.
- Finasteride: Inhibits the conversion of testosterone to dihydrotestosterone. Finasteride 5 mg/day is as effective as spironolactone in women with hirsutism.
- Gonadotropin-releasing hormone (GnRH) agonist: Inhibits gonadotropin and therefore ovarian androgen and estrogen secretion. Hirsutism improves with GnRH agonist, but the adverse effect of estrogen deficiency needs to be countered with low-dose estrogen and progesterone in premenopausal women. It can be considered for women with moderate to severe ovarian hyperandrogenism in whom oral contraceptive and antiandrogen therapy have not been effective. Low-dose estrogen and progesterone should also be prescribed to women treated with a GnRH agonist to avoid the adverse effects of estrogen deficiency.
- Metformin: Regulates cycles and improves fertility in women with PCOS. It is not as effective for the treatment of hirsutism. Side effects include lactic acidosis and abdominal discomfort.
- Glucocorticoid: Lowers adrenal androgen production in women with CAH. Side effects include weight gain, osteoporosis and impaired glucose tolerance.
- Dopamine agonist: Cabergoline and bromocriptine can improve hyperprolactinemia. Refer to chapter on galactorrhea.

SURGERY

Surgical resection of androgen secreting adrenal and ovarian tumors is recommended. In hyperthecosis resistant to medical therapy, oophorectomy can be considered especially in women with high testosterone levels.

Pregnancy Considerations

Because of unknown teratogenic risks associated with all medications currently used to treat hirsutism, oral contraceptives are recommended for all sexually active women. Discontinuation of these medications is recommended before becoming pregnant.

H

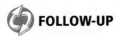

FOLLOW-UP

DISPOSITION
Idiopatic hirsutism and PCOS are chronic conditions and require life long therapy. Continuation of treatment is a personal decision and is determined by the women's comfort level.

Issues for Referral
Referral to a weight management program is critical in PCOS. Endocrine and cardiology referrals to address complications of PCOS such as diabetes and heart disease can be considered.

PROGNOSIS
Most of these medications must be taken for at least 6 months before improvement is detectable and not all medications are equally effective in all women.

COMPLICATIONS
Women with PCOS are at increased risk for diabetes, hypertension, hyperlipidemia, and cardiovascular disease. Risk reduction is achieved with weight loss.

REFERENCES

1. Hatch R, Rosenfield RS, Kim MH, et al. Hirsutism: Implications, etiology, and management. *Am J Obstet Gynecol*. 1981;140:815–830.
2. Derksen J, Nagesser SK, Meinders AE, et al. Identification of virilizing adrenal tumors in hirsute women. *N Engl J Med*. 1994;331:968–973.
3. McKenna TJ. Screening for sinister causes of hirsutism. *N Engl J Med*. 1994;331:1015–1016.
4. Rittmaster RS. Medical treatment of androgen-dependent hirsutism. *J Clin Endocrinol Metab*. 1995;80:2559–2563.

CODES
ICD9-CM
704.1 Hirsutism

KEY WORDS

- Hirsutism
- Hyperandrogenism
- Virilization
- Hypertrichosis

HIV

Jennifer R. Hur, MD

KEY CLINICAL POINTS

- Women represent 1 of the fastest growing populations being diagnosed with HIV infection.
- Treatment of HIV includes HAART therapy, but equally important must include addressing risk factors, prevention of transmission, and screening for AIDS-related illnesses.

 BASICS

DESCRIPTION

- Acquired Immune Deficiency Syndrome (AIDS) was first recognized in the United States in 1981. It was then discovered to be due to infection by Human Immunodeficiency Virus (HIV).
- The CDC maintains elaborate case definitions for definitive and presumptive diagnoses of AIDS based upon the clinical presence of AIDS defining illnesses with or without laboratory evidence of HIV infection.

GENERAL PREVENTION

In the absence of a cure for HIV, prevention is the most effective strategy for reducing the number of new cases.

Avoidance/Modification of High Risk Behaviors

- Abstinence from sexual intercourse (oral, vaginal, anal) with multiple partners who are themselves at risk of being infected with HIV
- Use of barrier contraception
- Testing of new partners prior to intercourse
- Avoiding intravenous drug use
- Use of needle exchange programs
- Universal Body Fluid Precautions for those at risk of occupational exposure

ALERT

20–35% women with undetectable plasma viral loads are positive for HIV in cervicovaginal secretions and therefore are able to transmit infection. Therefore, any selected method of contraception should include barrier protection to prevent transmission.

EPIDEMIOLOGY

Sexual transmission

- Per episode of receptive intercourse: 0.1–3%; in insertive intercourse: 0.06–0.1%
- Case reports exist for transmission occurring with oral intercourse, female-to-female sexual activity, and digital intercourse.

Bloodborne transmission

- Transfusion: 95% risk from transfusion of a single unit of HIV infected whole blood. In the United States, risk of HIV infected blood products is 1:100,000.
- Needlestick: 0.3–0.4% risk per exposure
- IVDU needle sharing: 0.67% risk per exposure

Perinatal transmission

Overall, 25–30%, but varies based on maternal stage of disease, use of HAART, duration of ruptured membranes, and practice of breast-feeding.

Incidence

- Estimated 40,000 new cases per year remains steady despite overall decrease in number of AIDS related deaths per year.
- Women constitute over 11,000 new cases of HIV annually.

- Women account for 21% of people living with AIDS in the United States and are one of the fastest growing populations infected with HIV.
- The rate of HIV among minority women, especially African American and Latino, and young women between the ages of 13 to 39, is rising more rapidly than in other populations.

Prevalence

- Prevalence of HIV infection: 136.7 per 100,000 at the end of 2004.
- As of 2003, women represented 1/2 of all people living with HIV globally. In the United States, women represent roughly 20% of people living with HIV.

RISK FACTORS

- Lack of recognition of partner's risk: Approximately 80% HIV infected women report acquisition via heterosexual contact.
- Sexual inequality in relationships with men
- Biologic vulnerability and high-risk STIs (gonorrhea, syphilis, genital ulcer disease, esp. HSV-2, trichomoniasis)
- Substance abuse (crack cocaine and IVDU)
- Poverty
- History of unwanted pregnancy
- Incarcerated sex partner
- Vaginal infections

PATHOPHYSIOLOGY

HIV infects all cells expressing the T4 (CD4) antigen. Once HIV enters a cell, it replicates and causes cell death or integrates into the cell's genome to become latent. Disordered CD4 lymphocyte function then causes B cell dysfunction and infected macrophages carry the virus throughout the body. The end results of HIV proliferation are immunodeficiency, rendering the host susceptible to potentially life-threatening infection, autoimmunity, giving rise to increased malignancies, as well as neurologic damage.

ETIOLOGY

HIV is a retrovirus that depends on a reverse transcriptase enzyme (RNA-directed DNA polymerase) to replicate in cells. HIV-1 is the classic AIDS virus. HIV-2 is a different strain that exists mostly in West Africa.

ASSOCIATED CONDITIONS

- AIDS defining illnesses
  - Invasive cervical cancer (more common with lower CD4 count but not protected by HAART): 40% incidence of cervical dysplasia in HIV-infected women
  - Recurrent Pneumonia
  - Candidiasis of bronchi, trachea, lungs, esophageal candidiasis
  - Coccidiomycosis, disseminated or extrapulmonary
  - Cryptococcosis, extrapulmonary
  - Cryptosporidiosis, chronic intestinal
  - Cytomegalovirus (other than liver, spleen, nodes), cytomegalovirus retinitis
  - Encephalopathy, HIV-related
  - HSV bronchitis, pneumonitis, esophagitis, or chronic ulcers
  - Histoplasmosis
  - Isosporiasis, chronic intestinal
  - Kaposi's sarcoma
  - Lymphoma: Burkitt, immunoblastic, primary brain
  - Mycobacterium avium complex or *M. kansasii*
  - Mycobacterium tuberculosis, pulmonary or extrapulmonary
  - Mycobacterium, other species
  - Pneumocystis carinii pneumonia

- Progressive multifocal leukoencephalopathy
- Salmonella septicemia, recurrent
- Toxoplasmosis of brain
- Wasting syndrome due to HIV
- Aside from invasive cervical cancer, general gynecologic issues, such as amenorrhea, menorrhagia, and fertility problems, are more common in HIV+ women.

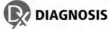 **DIAGNOSIS**

SIGNS AND SYMPTOMS
- Primary/Acute HIV Infection
  - Fever
  - Rash
  - Lymphadenopathy
- HIV-associated symptoms
  - Fatigue
  - Lymphadenopathy
  - Weight loss
  - Skin problems
  - Bacterial pneumonia
  - Thrush (oral or vaginal)
- More advanced HIV/AIDS
  - Fevers
  - Night sweats
  - Persistent diarrhea
  - Severe headache
  - Progressive dyspnea on exertion and cough
  - Mental status changes
  - Dysphagia or odynophagia
  - Visual changes (especially floaters or visual field defects)

History
- Symptoms
- Medication history
- Social history
- **If HIV diagnosis known:**
  - Time of diagnosis?
  - Mode of acquisition and/or risk behaviors?
  - CD4 count at time of diagnosis?
  - Prior therapy? Reasons for changing therapy?
  - Resistance testing?
  - History of opportunistic infection and/or prophylaxis?
  - History of STDs, TB, viral hepatitis
  - Complete gynecologic history, including PID, PAP smears.
- **If HIV diagnosis suspected:**
  - History of symptoms suggestive of acute seroconversion in last 6–9 months: Fever, aches, pharyngitis, lymphadenopathy, frequently a rash

Physical Exam
- Vital signs and weight
- Wasting and fat redistribution (truncal obesity)
- Skin and conjunctival exams for purplish spots of Kaposi sarcoma (KS)
- Fundoscopy may show "cotton wool" spots of retinal microinfarcts vs. "eggs and ketchup" infiltrates of CMV retinitis, which is usually accompanied by visual field defects.
- Oropharyngeal exam for thrush, oral hairy leukoplakia, bacillary angiomatosis, or KS
- Lymph node exam
- Lung exam for rales of Pneumocystis carinii pneumonia
- Hepatosplenomegaly may be seen with disseminated MAI, TB, Histoplasmosis, or lymphoma.

- Pelvic exam for STDs, malignancy (vulvar intraepithelial neoplasia), candidal infection, PAP smear to rule out cervical dysplasia
- Neurologic exam for neuropathy from HIV or HAART, evaluation for AIDS dementia, and depression

TESTS
Labs
The CDC recommends routine testing for all patients:
- In clinical settings where HIV prevalence >1%
- With risks for HIV in low HIV-prevalence clinical settings
- All cases of acute or nonacute occupational exposure to HIV
- All persons who request testing

Pregnancy Considerations
All pregnant women, regardless of risk, should be tested for HIV as a part of their routine prenatal screening to ensure any necessary perinatal prophylaxis is given to prevent perinatal transmission.

Serologic Tests
- Usually become positive 3–12 weeks after infection.
- >99% sensitivity and specificity of serologic testing
- All tests require informed consent and pre and post test counseling.
- Initial Enzyme-Linked Immunoabsorbent Assay (ELISA)
- Confirmatory Western blot assay: Require a band pattern indicating antibodies to 2 of the following proteins: p24, gp41, and gp120/160.

Nucleic Acid Amplification (PCR) Tests
Should be used for diagnosis in any ELISA/Western blot indeterminate cases, to evaluate for risk of progression to AIDS, and to track response to therapy.
- Quantitative RNA PCR assay: 90–95% sensitivity, 98–100% when CD4 counts <200/mm^3. False positive rates 2–3%.
- Qualitative DNA assay: Usually used to detect neonatal infection and with indeterminate serology. Sensitivity >99%, specificity approximately 98%.

Rapid Tests
- OraQuick Rapid HIV-1 Antibody Test – FDA approved. The CDC has recommended a negative test result be given the same day, and any positive tests go on for a confirmatory test. Sensitivity approaches 100%, specificity >99%.
- Home Access Express Test. Filter paper with blood sent to lab and tested with ELISA/Western blot. Sensitivity and specificity approach 100%.
- OraSure saliva test uses ELISA/Western blot to detect HIV antibodies in saliva. Sensitivity and specificity similar to standard serology.

DIFFERENTIAL DIAGNOSIS
Primary HIV infection may be mistaken for infectious mononucleosis with fever, malaise, lymphadenopathy, and sometimes rash.

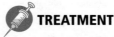 **TREATMENT**

BASELINE LAB EVALUATION
- CBC, basic chemistries, liver panel, renal function, lipid profile
- CD 4 Lymphocyte Count: Indicates level of immunosuppression. Usually see an initial, transient drop and rebound followed by gradual decline.
- Viral load: Predicts how fast disease will progress and how infectious someone is. Women have approximately 50% lower mean viral loads as compared with men at comparable CD4 counts.

- Drug resistance testing: Should be considered before initiating therapy with established infection, with acute HIV infection, and should definitely be done to guide therapy in cases of treatment failure and for pregnant women
- PPD: >5 mm is positive for HIV+ individuals
- PAP smear every 6 months and if normal × 1 year, annually If positive, refer to colposcopy
- STD screening
- G6PD level testing in select individuals may predispose to hemolytic anemia with some medications
- Serologies
  - Syphilis: RPR, if positive, FTA
  - Toxoplasmosis: IgG. 30% prevalence for latent toxo infection in the United States
  - CMV antibody
  - Varicella-zoster
  - Viral hepatitis: A, B, C. Will guide vaccination

INITIAL STABILIZATION
Treatment of any active AIDS defining illnesses

GENERAL MEASURES
Initiate HAART if:

- Symptomatic AIDS
- Asymptomatic, CD4 <200 mm^3, and strongly consider if <350/mm^3
- CD4 >350/mm^3 and Viral load >50 to 100,000 (risk to progression to AIDS >30%) – some advocate starting women at an even lower viral load threshold.
- Monitor if CD4 >350/mm^3 and viral load <50,000 (risk to progression to AIDS <15%)

Complementary and Alternative Therapies
A daily multivitamin may be helpful and should be recommended.

 MEDICATION (DRUGS)

Highly Active Anti-Retroviral Therapy (HAART)
General principles

- Mutations that may confer resistance to antiretroviral therapy arise rapidly.
- Treatment should be initiated before symptoms develop and should be maintained to prevent resistance.
- The goal of therapy is achieving the lowest viral load possible.
- Combination therapy has been shown to be superior to monotherapy at controlling viral replication and limiting resistance to medications.
- Choice of therapy is based on: Efficacy, durability of antiretroviral activity, tolerability, and adverse side effects, convenience, drug-drug interactions, and potential salvageability of initial regimen.
- There is no single recommended initial therapeutic regimen but common combinations include:
  - NNRTI + 2 NRTIs
  - 3 NRTIs
  - PI + 2 NRTIs +/− low-dose ritonavir
  - PI + NNRTI + 1–2 NRTIs +/− low-dose ritonavir – only in advanced disease with high near-term mortality. Otherwise not ideal initial therapy as development of resistance to all 3 classes limits future options.

Nucleoside Analogue Reverse Transcriptase Inhibitors (NRTIs)
Nucleoside analogues that incorporate into DNA thereby blocking HIV reverse transcriptase enzyme:

- Zidovudine (AZT), didanosine (ddI), stavudine (d4T), lamivudine (3TC), abacavir (ABC), emtricitabine (FTC), zalcitabine (ddC), tenofovir.
- Combination drugs: Combivir (lamivudine/zidovudine), Trizivir (abacavir/lamivudine/zidovudine), Truvada (emtricitabine/tenofovir).
  - Common side effects: Peripheral neuropathy, GI intolerance, pancreatitis, lactic acidosis with hepatic steatosis

Non-Nucleoside Reverse Transcriptase Inhibitors (NNRTIs)
Bind to HIV reverse transcriptase enzyme:

- Nevirapine, delavirdine, efavirenz
  - Common side effects: Rash, hepatitis, headache

Protease Inhibitors (PIs)
Bind to protease to inhibit viral protein cleavage thereby preventing release of virus from cell:

- Saquinavir, ritonavir, indinavir, nelfinavir, amprenavir, atazanavir, fosamprenavir
- Combination drug: Lopinavir/ritonavir
- Metabolized by cytochrome P450 system and therefore multiple drug interactions
  - Common side effects: Diarrhea, nausea, abdominal discomfort, dyslipidemia, lipodystrophy, glucose intolerance
- Other common complications of HAART therapy
  - Lactic acidosis/Hepatic steatosis
  - Dyslipidemia
  - Lipodystrophy (fat maldistribution)
  - Hepatotoxicity
  - Hyperglycemia
  - Avascular necrosis of hips and decreased bone density

Opportunistic Infection Prophylaxis
- CD4 <100 MAI prophylaxis
Consider CMV prophylaxis
- CD4 <200 PCP prophylaxis

Vaccination
All HIV-infected patients should receive:

- Pneumococcal vaccine every 5 years if CD4 count <200, otherwise first at diagnosis and a booster at 65 years of age
- Influenza vaccine annually
- Hepatitis vaccines as guided by serologies
- Haemophilus influenzae b vaccination

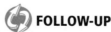 **FOLLOW-UP**

DISPOSITION
- Routine evaluation
  - Initially at 4, 8, 12, and 16 weeks and once 2 sequential measurements of viral load are below the limits of detection, monitor every 8–12 weeks.
    - CBC with differential
    - CD4 count
    - Viral load
- Frequency of follow-up
  - Asymptomatic patient not on HAART, CD4 >500/mm^3, follow-up every 6 months.
  - Symptomatic and/or on HAART, follow every 3 months.

Issues for Referral
- CDC HIV guidelines emphasize that patients should be referred to services that can respond best to their most important needs, appropriate to their gender, culture, language, sexual orientation, age, and developmental level.

H

- Patients should be referred to a specialist if they are:
  - Failing treatment
  - Intolerant of standard antiretroviral drugs
  - In need of systemic chemotherapy
  - Diagnosed with complicated opportunistic infections, especially if invasive procedures or experimental therapies are needed
- A resource guide should be maintained in the office to assist staff in making appropriate referrals.
- A partial list of resources include:
  - CDC hotlines
  - AIDS hotline in English: 800-342-2437
  - AIDS hotline in Spanish: 800-344-7432
  - AIDS hotline TTY (teletypewriter): 800-243-7889
  - STD Hotline: 800-227-8922
  - National Clinicians' Post-Exposure Prophylaxis Hotline: www.ucsf.edu/hivcntr/, Telephone: 888-448-4911

Prognosis
- Without treatment, 50% of seropositive persons will develop AIDS within 10 years.
- CD4 count typically increases by >50 cells/mL at 4–8 weeks after starting HAART, followed by an increase of 50–100 cells/mL per year thereafter. Virologically effective therapy generally reduces viral load by >90% (10-fold reduction) within 8 weeks of treatment.

REFERENCES

1. Cejtin H. Gynecologic issues in the HIV-infected woman. *Obstet Gynecol Clin North Am*. 2003;30:711–729.
2. Gallant J. HIV counseling, testing, and referral. *Am Fam Physician*. 2004;70:295–302.
3. Gilad J, Walfisch A, Borer A, et al. Gender differences and sex-specific manifestations associated with human immunodeficiency virus infection in women. *Eur J Obstet Gynecol Repro Bio*. 2003;109:199–205.
4. Yeni P, Hammer SM, Carpenter CC, et al. Antiretroviral treatment for adult HIV infection in 2002: Updated recommendations of the International AIDS Society – USA Panel. *JAMA*. 2002;288:222–235.
5. Centers for Disease Control and Prevention. 1993 revised classification for HIV infection and expanded surveillance case definition for AIDS among adolescents and adults. *MMWR Morb Mortal Wkly Rep*. 1992;41:1–19.

ADDITIONAL READING

Centers for Disease Control and National Prevention Information Network website: www.cdcnpin.org/scripts/population/women.asp

U.S. Department of Health and Human Services, Health Resources and Services Administration (HRSA), HIV/AIDS Bureau. www.hab.hrsa.gov/publications/womencare05/index.htm

HIV Medicine Association (physicians who treat patients with AIDS/HIV; affiliated with Infectious Diseases Society of America): www.hivma.org

CDC's National Center for HIV, STD, and Tuberculosis Prevention: www.cdc.gov.revproxy.brown.edu/nchstp/od/nchstp.html

CDC HIV counseling, testing, and referral guidelines: www.cdc.gov.revproxy.brown.edu/hiv

CODES
ICD9-CM
- 042 Human immunodeficiency virus (HIV) Infection, symptomatic HIV infection, AIDS
- v08 Asymptomatic HIV infection, HIV positive, NOS
- v1.79 Exposure to HIV
- 795.71 Nonspecific serologic evidence of HIV, inconclusive HIV test
- v65.44 HIV counseling
- 079.53 Human immunodeficiency virus, type 2 (HIV-2)

KEY WORDS

- HIV
- HAART
- AIDS
- AIDS Defining Illness

HYPERCHOLESTEROLEMIA

Purva Agarwal, MD
Joseph A. Diaz, MD

KEY CLINICAL POINTS

- Dyslipidemia is one of the most important modifiable risk factors for CAD.
- LDL cholesterol is the major atherogenic lipoprotein and is the primary target of therapy.
- Aggressive lowering of LDL and early use of statins with therapeutic lifestyle changes can significantly reduce risk of CAD.

 ## BASICS

DESCRIPTION
Hyperlipidemia is defined as abnormally high levels of plasma fats (such as cholesterol and triglycerides) in the blood, as per the National Cholesterol Education Program (NCEP).

- Total cholesterol: A total cholesterol of <200 mg/dL is considered desirable; 200–239 mg/dL borderline high, and ≥240 mg/dL high.
- LDL cholesterol: LDL <100 mg/dL is considered optimal; 100–129 mg/dL near optimal/above optimal; 130–159 mg/dL borderline high; 160–189 mg/dL high, and ≥190 mg/dL very high.
- HDL cholesterol: HDL cholesterol of <40 mg/dL is considered low and ≥60 mg/dL high.
- Low HDL itself is an independent cardiac risk factor. For every 1% decrease in HDL cholesterol, the risk for CHD increases by 2–3%.
- Triglycerides: A triglyceride level of <200 mg/dL is considered normal, 200–400 mg/dL borderline high, and >400 mg/dL high.
- VLDL Cholesterol: Normal VLDL cholesterol level is <30 mg/dL.

EPIDEMIOLOGY
- Overall prevalence of hyperlipidemia in women is about 29% and increases with age from 20% in 20–44 age group to 47.5% in >65 age group.
- Cardiovascular disease is the primary cause of death in American women, accounting for more than 500,000 deaths per year.
- Women become at increased risk for death from coronary heart disease approximately 10 years later than men.
- Approximately 38% of women die within a year after a heart attack as compared to 25% of men.
- For the first 6 years after a heart attack, the rate of having a 2nd attack is 35% for women and 18% for men.

PATHOPHYSIOLOGY
Cholesterol filled macrophages composed mainly of LDL cholesterol form fatty streak in the arteries. These later develop into atherosclerotic plaques. Unstable plaques can rupture, causing acute coronary syndromes, whereas fibrous and calcified plaques contribute to the development of chronic stable angina.

ETIOLOGY
- Primary
  - Genetic/Familial (rare)
  - Types I–V hyperlipoproteinemias
- Secondary
  - Diet
  - Smoking
  - Obesity
  - Physical inactivity
  - Alcohol abuse
  - Drugs: Anabolic steroids, oral contraceptives, β-Blockers, thiazides, isotretenoin
- Associated conditions: Hypothyroidism, nephrotic syndrome, chronic renal failure

SIGNS AND SYMPTOMS
- Majority with no symptoms or signs
- Some may present with:
  - Atherosclerosis: Coronary artery disease, cerebrovascular disease, peripheral artery disease
- PE findings:
  - Tendon xanthomas
  - Xanthelesma: Fat deposits beneath the surface of the skin, most common on the eyelids, seen commonly in familial hyperlipidemias
  - Arcus Corneae: A white or grey opaque ring in the corneal margin resulting from cholesterol deposits, mostly seen in familial hyperlipidemia

 ## DIAGNOSIS

- NCEP recommends fasting lipoprotein profile obtained at least once every five years in women ≥20 years.
- The United States Preventive Services Task Force recommends screening starting at the age 35 for men and age 45 for women, if no risk factors for CAD are present. Younger men and women (>20 years) may be screened earlier, if risk factors are present.
- Assessment of other risk factors for CAD
  - Cigarette smoking
  - Hypertension (BP ≥140/90 mmHg or on antihypertensive medication)
  - Low HDL cholesterol (<40 mg/dL)
  - Family history of premature CAD (CAD in male first-degree relative <55 years; CAD in female first-degree relative <65)
  - Age (women ≥55 years)
- For persons with multiple (2+) risk factors, a 10-year risk assessment is carried out with Framingham scoring to assess the risk, goals, and intensity of therapy.
- Diabetes, peripheral vascular disease, and cerebrovascular disease are considered CAD equivalents when determining treatment goals.

EMERGING TESTS
The following tests are currently under evaluation for use in further risk stratification of patients for intensity of lipid lowering therapy:
- Serum C-reactive protein
- Serum homocysteine

 ## TREATMENT

- LDL (mg/dL) goals and treatment options
- CAD and CAD equivalents (10-year risk >20%)
  - Goal: 100 mg/dLl
  - In high risk (acute coronary syndrome, diabetes + CVD, CVD if baseline LDL <100), goal: 70 mg/dL
  - Lifestyle changes at 100–130 mg/dL
  - Consider drug therapy at >130 mg/dL
- Multiple 2+ risk factors (10-year risk 10–20%)
  - Goal: <130 mg/dL

- Lifestyle changes at 130–160 mg/dL
- Consider drug therapy at >130 mg/dL
- Multiple 2+ risk factor (10-year risk <10%)
  - Goal: <130 mg/dL
  - Lifestyle changes at 130–160 mg/dL
  - Consider drug therapy at >160 mg/dL
- 0–1 risk factor
  - Goal: <160 mg/dL
  - Lifestyle changes at 160–190 mg/dL
  - Consider drug therapy at >190 mg/dL
- Non-HDL cholesterol (LDL + VLDL cholesterol): Secondary target of therapy in persons with high triglycerides.
  - Goal for non-HDL cholesterol in persons with high serum triglycerides can be set at 30 mg/dL higher than that for LDL cholesterol
- Triglycerides
  - High triglyceride levels are more dangerous for women than men and appear to increase CAD risk in women, but not in men.
  - Borderline high triglycerides levels are treated by weight reduction, exercise, and diet.
  - High triglyceride levels need to be treated by drug therapy in addition to lifestyle changes.
- Nonpharmacologic therapy
  - Lifestyle changes encompass diet, physical activity, and weight loss.

Diet
- Diet and exercise can reduce serum cholesterol by 10–20%.
- Diet should include <7% calories from saturated fat, up to 10% from polyunsaturated fat, up to 20% from monounsaturated fat. Total fat should contribute to 25–35% of total calories.
- Enhance LDL lowering with plant stanols/sterols (2 g/day) and increased viscous (soluble) fiber (10–25 g/day).

Activity
Aerobic exercise: 20–30 minutes of mild-to-moderate intensity (including walking) 3 times per week is recommended to raise HDL cholesterol and lower TG levels.

Additional Therapy
Smoking cessation (can increase HDL by 30%)
For every increase of 1 mg per dL in the HDL cholesterol level, a 2–3% decrease in CAD risk may occur, independent of changes in the LDL cholesterol level.

Pharmacologic Therapy
- HMG CoA Reductase inhibitors
  - Lower LDL by 18–55%; lower TG by 7–30%; raise HDL by 5–15%
  - Rosuvastatin 5–40 mg
  - Simvastatin 20–80 mg
  - Lovastatin 20–80 mg (>20 mg give b.i.d.)
  - Fluvastatin 20–80 mg (>40 mg, give b.i.d.)
  - Pravastatin 20–80 mg
  - Atorvastatin 10–80 mg
  - Side effects: Myopathy, increased liver enzyme, rhabdomyolysis
  - Contraindications: Active/chronic liver disease
  - Pregnancy category X, contraindicated in pregnant and lactating women
  - Monitor liver function tests at baseline, 12 weeks after starting therapy, then annually
- Bile acid sequestrants
  - Lower LDL by 15–30%; raise HDL by 3–5%; No change/raise TG
  - Cholestyramine: 4–16 g/day; within 30 minutes of meals (per day or b.i.d. dosing)

- Colestipol: 5–30 g/day; within 30 minutes of meals (per day or b.i.d. dosing)
- Colesevelam: 2.6–3.8 g/day, with meals (per day or b.i.d. dosing)
- Side effects: GI distress, constipation, decreased absorption of other drugs
- Contraindication: Dysbetalipoproteinemia, TG >400 mg/dL, TG >200 mg/dL (relative)
- Pregnancy Category-C
- Nicotinic acid
  - Lower LDL by 5–25%; raise HDL by 15–35%; lower TG by 20–50%
  - Immediate-release (crystalline): 1.5–3 g (with meals, start with 100 mg b.i.d. and titrate up to t.i.d. dosing)
  - Extended-release (Niaspan): 1–2 g/day
  - Side effects: Flushing, hyperglycemia, hyperuricemia (gout), upper GI distress
  - Contraindications: Known hypersensitivity to Niacin, chronic liver disease, severe gout, active peptic ulcer disease, arterial bleeding
  - Relative contraindications: Diabetes, hyperuricemia, peptic ulcer disease
  - Use with caution in patients with alcohol abuse.
  - To avoid flushing, use of Tylenol 30 minutes prior to administration is indicated.
  - Pregnancy Category C
- Fibric acid:
  - Lower LDL 5–20%; raise HDL 10–20%; lower TG 20–50%
  - Gemfibrozil: 600 mg b.i.d.
  - Fenofibrate: 200 mg/day
  - Side effects: Dyspepsia, gallstones, myopathy, unexplained non-CAD deaths
  - Contraindications: Severe renal and hepatic disease, hypersensitivity reactions, preexisting gall bladder disease, primary biliary cirrhosis
  - Pregnancy Category C
- Selective Cholesterol Absorption Inhibitor:
  - Lower LDL 18%; raise HDL 1%; lower TG 8%
  - Ezetimibe: 10 mg
  - Side effects: Abdominal pain, tiredness
  - Contraindications: Hypersensitivity to any component of the medication
  - Pregnancy Category C

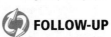 **FOLLOW-UP**

After initiating LDL-lowering therapy, lipid profile should be monitored at 6-week intervals. If the LDL goal based on established risk is not achieved, therapy should be intensified with an increase in drug dosage or the addition of another LDL-lowering drug. Once the LDL goal is attained, other lipid risk factors should be addressed on an ongoing basis. Once LDL levels are at the target, a patient's lipoprotein profile should be monitored every 6–12 months.

PROGNOSIS
The prognosis for cardiovascular disease is worse in women than in men in part because less aggressive lipid-modifying strategies are used when treating women compared to men with similar risk profiles. Coronary artery disease (CAD) and heart attacks are erroneously believed to occur primarily in men, which leads to underdiagnosis and inattention to risk factors in women. In addition, women are more likely to encounter delays in establishing the diagnosis of cardiovascular disease than men because of the atypical nature of their symptoms.

REFERENCES

1. Adult Treatment Panel III. Executive summary of the third report of the National Cholesterol Education Program (NCEP) expert panel on detection, evaluation, and treatment of high blood cholesterol in adults (adult treatment panel III). *JAMA*. 2001;285:2486–2497.
2. Grundy SM, Cleeman JI, Bairey Merz N, et al. Implications of recent clinical trials for the National Cholesterol Education Program Adult Treatment Panel III Guidelines. *Circ*. 2004;110: 227–239.
3. Trends in cholesterol screening and awareness of high blood cholesterol–United States, 1991–2003. *MMWR Morbidity Mortality Weekly Rep*. 2005;54:865–870.

CODES
ICD9-CM
- 272.0 Hypercholesterolemia
- 272.1 Hypertriglyceridemia
- 272.2 Hyperlipidemia, mixed

KEY WORDS

- Hyperlipidemia
- Dyslipidemia

H

HYPERTENSION

Anne W. Moulton, MD

KEY CLINICAL POINTS

- Over the lifespan, hypertension (HTN) is more common in women than men.
- HTN is the most common cardiovascular risk factor in women.
- In general anti-HTN medications are equally effective in males and females.

 ## BASICS

DEFINITION (JNC VII)
- Normal blood pressure (BP): Systolic <120 and diastolic <80.
- Prehypertension: Systolic 120–139 or diastolic 80–89.
- HTN:
    - Stage I: Systolic 140–159 or diastolic 90–99.
    - Stage II: Systolic ≥160 or diastolic ≥100.

DEFINITIONS-OTHER
- Primary (essential) HTN:
    - Defined as persistently increased blood pressure for which no specific cause can be identified
    - Accounts for over 95% of all cases of HTN
- Secondary HTN: Etiology of HTN is secondary to another disease (see list).
- White Coat HTN (WC HTN):
    - Mild HTN detected in provider's office, but not when taken outside office
    - Accounts for 20% to 25% patients with mild HTN in office
    - More common in women

EPIDEMIOLOGY
Incidence
- Women <50 years have lower systolic BP than men.
- After age 50 the rates of HTN increase more rapidly in women.
- After age 60 the rates of HTN are higher in women than men.

Prevalence
- HTN occurs earlier and more frequently in African-American women than in white or Hispanic women.
- Occurs in 75% African-American women above age of 75

RISK FACTORS: ESSENTIAL HYPERTENSION
- Family history
- Sodium intake
- Alcohol intake
- Obesity
- Black race

Genetics
- Evidence of genetic influence seen in twin studies and population studies for females and males
- Several unique genetic abnormalities account for a very small percentage of HTN.
- Potential interaction between gender and gene polymorphisms

PATHOPHYSIOLOGY
Multiple mechanisms implicated:
- Increased sympathetic tone
- High dietary salt intake
- Inadequate dietary intake of potassium and calcium
- Increased or inappropriate renin secretion
- Deficiencies of vasodilators
- Alterations in expression of the Kallikrein-Kinin system
- Abnormalities of resistance vessels

Gender Differences in HTN
- Possible role of sex hormones
- Lower plasma renin levels in women
- Autonomic dysfunction in women

ASSOCIATED CONDITIONS: SECONDARY HYPERTENSION
- Primary renal disease
- Drug induced (e.g., oral contraceptives, NSAIDs)
- Renovascular disease: Strong female risk 8:1
- Obstructive sleep apnea
- Pheochromocytoma
- Primary hyperaldosteronism
- Cushing disease
- Other endocrine diseases (thyroid disease, hyperparathyroidism)

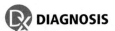 ## DIAGNOSIS

SIGNS AND SYMPTOMS
Women presenting with new onset HTN are more likely to experience symptoms: headache, dizziness, palpitations, dyspnea on exertion.

History: Goals
- Determine etiology of HTN and potential aggravating factors.
- Assess duration of HTN and presence of end-organ damage.
- Identify other cardiac risk factors.

Physical Exam
- 3 to 6 separate high BP readings in a provider's office spaced over weeks to months
- Fundoscopy: Assess retinopathy
- Neck: Palpation and auscultation carotids, thyroid
- Heart: Size, rhythm, sounds
- Lungs: Assess for evidence of CHF
- Abdomen: Renal masses, bruits, femoral pulses
- Extremities: Peripheral pulses, edema
- Neurologic evaluation

TESTS
Lab
- Hematocrit
- Urine analysis
- BUN
- Creatinine
- Electrolytes
- Fasting lipid panel
- Calcium
- Creatinine clearance
- Urine microalbumin
- Consider additional testing for secondary causes of HTN if suspected (i.e., BP: sudden onset or not easily controlled).

Other
- 12-lead electrocardiogram
- 24-hour ambulatory BP monitor provides multiple readings during patient's usual activities
- Indicators:
    - Suspected WC HTN
    - Hypotensive symptoms
    - Episodic hypertension
    - Autonomic dysfunction

- More accurate picture of BP control required
- Echocardiogram:
  - Helpful for more accurate assessment of LVH
  - The presence of LVH carries an increased risk of cardiac events in women similar to the risk in men.

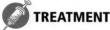

TREATMENT

GENERAL MEASURES

Diet
- Low sodium: Less than 100 meq (2.3 gm sodium or 6 gm salt/day) more effective in women than men
- Weight loss (see below)
- Reduce or eliminate alcohol: Less than 4–7 drinks/week (lower than recommendations for men).

Exercise
- Regular aerobic exercise can lower BP 5–15 mm Hg in 4 weeks.
- Recommend 30 minutes of regular physical exercise most days of the week.
- Benefits noted with strength training as well as aerobic exercise

Weight Loss
- Weight loss accompanied by diet and exercise or medication reduces BP.
- Body fat reduction (even without significant weight loss) can decrease BP.
- Average reduction of 0.5–1.0 mm Hg for every kilogram of weight loss.

MANAGEMENT
- Initiate diet and exercise for all patients with HTN (see above).
- Indications for addition of medication:
  - Persistent elevation in systolic >140 and diastolic >90.
  - Patients with diabetes or chronic renal insufficiency (goal = 130/80).
  - Patients with pre-existing cardiovascular disease (goal = 130/80).

MEDICATION (DRUGS)

- Most anti-HTN drugs provide same degree of cardiovascular protection in women as in men.
- Majority of patients with HTN will require 2 or more drugs.
- Women are more likely to experience medication side effects.
- Sexual side effects in women: Limited data
- Thiazide diuretic:
  - Best 1st line drug in women and African Americans
  - Smaller doses – Fewer side effects
- Angiotension converting enzyme (ACE):
  - Useful in patients with diabetes or renal disease
  - Approximately 20% of women will develop dry cough.
- Angiotension II receptor blocker (ARB):
  - Useful in patients with diabetes or renal disease
- Beta blockers:
  - Preferred if migraine headaches or recurring tachycardia
  - Contraindicated with Raynaud's Syndrome
  - Higher rates of side effects; fatigue and depression in women
- Calcium channel blockers (CCB):
  - Not 1st line of treatment
  - Use only long-acting CCB
  - Side effects more common in women (especially dizziness, peripheral edema)

FOLLOW-UP

ALERT
The guidelines for evaluation and treatment of hypertension in pregnancy are substantially different. See chapter.

Indications for Referral to Nephrology
- Patient poorly controlled on 3 or more meds.
- Concern for secondary HTN.
- Evidence of renal disease and HTN.

PROGNOSIS – WITH TREATMENT
No gender difference overall in cardiovascular complications or mortality for appropriately treated patients

COMPLICATIONS
- Stroke: More common in women
- Congestive heart failure: More common in women
- Coronary heart disease: Less common in women
- Renal insufficiency/end stage renal disease
- Dementia: Increasing evidence between heart and brain health

PATIENT MONITORING
- BP well-controlled: Office visits every 3–6 months
- BP poorly controlled: More frequent office visits until stabilized on medication

REFERENCES

1. Chobanian AV, Bakris GL, Black HR, et al. Seventh report of the Joint National Committee on Prevention, Detection, Evaluation, and Treatment of High Blood Pressure JNC 7 – Complete Version. *Hypertension.* 2003;42:1206–1252.
2. Quan A, Kerlikowske K, Gueyffier F, Boissel JP. INDANA investigators. Pharmacotherapy for hypertension in women of different races. *The Cochrane Database of Systematic Reviews 2000.* Issue 2. Art. No.: CD002146.DOI: 10.1002/14651858.CD002146.
3. Huang Z, Reddy A. Weight change, ideal weight and hypertension [Review]. *Curr Opin Nephrol Hypertens.* 1999;8:343–346.
4. Hayes SN, Taler SJ. Hypertension in women: Current understanding of gender differences [Review]. *Mayo Clin Proc.* 1998;73:157–165.
5. Os I, Oparil S, Gerdts E, et al. Essential hypertension in women. *Blood Pressure.* 2004;13:272–278.

WEBSITES FOR PATIENTS

- www.americanheart.org
- www.nhlbi.nih.gov/guidelines/hypertension
- www.womenshealth.gov/OWH

CODES
ICD9-CM
- 401.9 Essential hypertension
- 405 Secondary hypertension

KEY WORDS

- Essential Hypertension
- Secondary Hypertension
- Hypertension
- Renal Insufficiency

H

HYPERTHYROIDISM

Geetha Gopalakrishnan, MD

KEY CLINICAL POINTS

- There are numerous causes of hyperthyroidism including Graves' disease and toxic multinodular goiter.
- Thyroid stimulating hormone (TSH), free thyroxine (FT4) and free tri-iodothyronine (FT3) should be checked to confirm diagnosis and help determine etiology.
- The goal of treatment is to alleviate symptoms and to return blood levels of FT4 and FT3 to the normal range.
- Treatment may include beta blockers (for symptoms), antithyroid medications, radioactive iodine, or surgery.

DESCRIPTION

Excess thyroid hormone results in thyrotoxicosis. An increase in thyroid hormone production by the thyroid results in hyperthyroidism.

EPIDEMIOLOGY

- More common in women than men (5:1 ratio)
- More common in Whites
- Graves' more common in women 20–40 years old
  Toxic multinodular goiter more common in women >55 years old

PATHOPHYSIOLOGY

- Hyperthyroid thyrotoxicosis: Increase in thyroid hormone production by thyroid follicular cells
  - Primary: An increase in thyroid hormone production as a result of thyroid gland dysfunction.
  - Secondary: An increase in thyroid hormone production as a result of an increase in thyroid-stimulating hormone (TSH), thyrotrophin-releasing hormone (TRH) or human chorionic gonadotropin (HCG).
- Non-hyperthyroid thyrotoxicosis: Thyroid hormone excess that does not result from an increase in thyroid hormone production

ETIOLOGY

- Hyperthyroid thyrotoxicosis
  - Primary hyperthyroidism
    - Graves: Autoimmune disorder resulting in antibody mediated thyroid hormone synthesis and release. Precipitated by stress and iodine.
    - Toxic multinodular goiter (TMG) or solitary toxic nodule: Diffuse or focal autonomously functioning follicular cells. Precipitated by iodine. Activating receptor mutation has been associated with both TMG and toxic adenoma.
    - Iodine load (i.e., amiodarone, contrast agents and angiography): Can lead to excess thyroid hormone synthesis. Risk factors include goiter and iodine deficiency.
    - Struma Ovarii: Ovarian neoplasm with functioning thyroid tissue.
    - Functional metastases: Follicular thyroid cancer metastases that secrete thyroid hormone
    - Activating mutation of TSH receptor: Autosomal dominant disorder that results in thyroid hormone production
  - Secondary hyperthyroidism
    - TSH or TRH secreting tumor involving the pituitary or hypothalamus.
    - Chorionic gonadatropic tumor (i.e., hydatidiform mole, choriocarcinoma, and testicular germ cell tumors): Human chorionic gonadotropin (HCG) mediated TSH receptor stimulation.
    - Gestational thyrotoxicosis (hyperemesis gravidum): Human chorionic gonadotropin (HCG) mediated TSH receptor stimulation.
    - Mutation in the triiodothyronine (T3) receptor: Resistance to the feedback effect of T3 on pituitary TSH production
- Non-hyperthyroid thyrotoxicosis
  - Thyroiditis (i.e., viral illness, postpartum, amiodarone, palpation or radiation): Inflammation of the thyroid resulting in the release of preformed thyroid hormone.
  - Exogenous intake of thyroid hormone

ASSOCIATED CONDITIONS

- Evaluation of other autoimmune conditions should be considered in Graves (e.g., adrenal insufficiency)
- Evaluation of other pituitary hormone dysfunction should be considered in central hyperthyroidism.

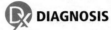 DIAGNOSIS

SIGNS AND SYMPTOMS

Thyrotoxicosis is related to increased metabolic activity.

History

Fatigue, weight loss, heat intolerance, sweating, increase appetite, eye symptoms (i.e., tearing, redness, double vision, etc), frequent bowel movement, decreased libido, menstrual cycle irregularities, infertility, proximal muscle weakness, tremors, palpitations, angina, shortness of breath, insomnia, anxious, irritable and in severe cases mental status change. Neck pain is usually associated with thyroiditis.

Physical Exam

Weight loss, lid lag, fine hair, moist skin, onycholysis, wide pulse pressure, tachycardia, irregular rhythm (i.e., atrial fibrillation), CHF, hyper-reflexia, fine tremor, muscle wasting, myopathy (i.e., hypokalemic periodic paralysis in Asian men), gynecomastia, goiter, and thyroid bruit. Ophthalmopathy (i.e., exophthalmos and lid retraction) and pretibial myxedema are seen only in Graves' disease.

Pregnancy Considerations

Women with hyperthyroidism may have difficulty becoming pregnant. Once pregnant they are at increased risk for spontaneous abortion, premature labor, preeclampsia, and heart failure.

TESTS

Lab

Check thyroid stimulating hormone (TSH), free thyroxine (FT4) and Free triiodothyronine (FT3) to start.

- Thyrotoxicosis: Elevated free thyroxine (FT4) and Free triiodothyronine (FT3)
  - Hyperthyroid thyrotoxicosis
    Primary hyperthyroid: Elevated FT3 and/or FT4 associated with a suppressed TSH. Thyroid stimulating immunoglobulin (TSI) elevated in Graves.
    Secondary hyperthyroid: High TSH or human chorionic gonadotropin (HCG) associated with an elevated FT3 and/or FT4.
- Non-hyperthyroid thyrotoxicosis
  - Elevated FT3 and/or FT4 associated with a suppressed TSH. Thyroglobulin (TG) elevated in thyroiditis and suppressed with exogenous intake.

Subclinical thyrotoxicosis: TSH suppressed, but T3 and T4 are normal.

Imaging
Radioactive Iodine (RAI) Uptake Scan: In general, conditions and regions associated with increased thyroid hormone production increase RAI uptake. Iodine load (e.g., contrast agents) limits RAI uptake. Low uptake is also seen in conditions associated with low endogenous thyroid hormone production.

- Hyperthyroidism: Increased uptake
  - Primary
    - Graves: Diffuse uptake in the neck
    - TMG: Patchy uptake in the neck
    - Toxic nodule: Focal uptake in the neck
    - Iodine load: Low uptake
    - Struma Ovarii: Uptake in the pelvis
    - Functional metastases: Uptake in region of thyroid metastases
    - Activating mutation: Uptake in the neck
  - Secondary: Diffuse uptake in the neck
- Nonhyperthyroid thyrotoxicosis: Low uptake
- Consider MRI in secondary hyperthyroidism to evaluate pituitary and hypothalamic lesions. Ultrasound to evaluate struma ovarii and chorionic gonadotropic tumors. Consider DXA to assess bone loss in thyrotoxic individuals.

DIFFERENTIAL DIAGNOSIS
Pheochromocytoma, carcinoid syndrome, menopause and anxiety disorder can mimic symptoms of thyrotoxicosis. Thyroid function test during severe illness, dopamine use and corticosteroid therapy can be associated with a suppressed TSH.

TREATMENT

Treatment is considered in individuals with overt thyrotoxicosis. The goal of treatment is to alleviate symptoms and to return blood levels of FT4 and FT3 to the normal range. In subclinical disease, consider treatment if TSH <0.1 mU/l or if symptoms of cardiac compromise and bone loss are noted.

- Hyperthyroid thyrotoxicosis
  - Primary hyperthyroidism
    - Graves: Antithyroid or radioactive iodine (RAI) ablation
    - TMG: RAI ablation
    - Solitary toxic nodule: RAI ablation
    - Iodine induced hyperthyroidism: Self-limited if iodine is discontinued. Prophylactic antithyroid drug may be considered in nodular goiter prior to an iodine load such as cardiac catheterization.
    - Struma Ovarii: Surgical removal of the tumor
    - Functional metastases: RAI ablation
    - Activating mutation of TSH receptor: Thyroid surgery or RAI ablation
  - Secondary hyperthyroidism
    - TSH or TRH secreting tumor: Treat the tumor and consider antithyroid drugs, RAI ablation and thyroid surgery to control persistent hyperthyroid symptoms.
    - Chorionic gonadotropic tumor: Treat the tumor and consider antithyroid drugs as adjuvant therapy.
    - Gestational thyrotoxicosis: Self-limited. Beta blockers if symptomatic.
    - Mutation in the triiodothyronine (T3) receptor: Thyroid surgery or RAI ablation
- Non-hyperthyroid thyrotoxicosis
  - Thyroiditis: Self-limited. Beta blockers if symptomatic.
  - Exogenous intake of thyroid hormone: Resolves when thyroid hormone is discontinued.

MEDICATION (DRUGS)

- Beta-blockers (e.g., Atenolol and Propanolol) control symptoms such as rapid heart rate, tremors, anxiety, and heat intolerance. Starting dose of Atenolol 25 mg daily and propranolol 20 mg q6h. Dose titrated to alleviate symptoms. Side effects include bronchospasm and heart failure.
- Antithyroid drugs: Methimazole (MMI) and propylthiouracil (PTU) decrease thyroid hormone production. PTU also prevents peripheral conversion of T4 to T3. Can be used in the initial treatment of hyperthyroidism; however, long-term use is only recommended for Graves'. After 1 year of antithyroid drugs, remission occurs in 20–30% of individuals with Graves'. Despite initial remission, need to monitor thyroid function test regularly to evaluate for recurrence. Starting dose of PTU 50–100 mg TID and MMI 10–20 mg daily. Dose is titrated to maintain TFT in the normal range. Side effects include agranulocytosis, and liver toxicity. If side effects develop, discontinuation of antithyroid drug is recommended.

Radiotherapy
- Radioactive iodine (RAI) ablation: Destroys the thyroid in 6–18 weeks. Consider antithyroid drugs prior to ablation in high-risk symptomatic individuals such as the elderly and those with heart disease.
- Most become hypothyroid after ablation and require lifelong thyroid hormone replacement. About 10% will require a second dose of RAI ablation. Therefore, regular monitoring thyroid function test is critical post ablation. Side effects include progression of Graves' Ophthalmopathy and parotiditis.

SURGERY
Surgery to remove the thyroid should be considered only if antithyroid drugs are not tolerated and radioactive iodine ablation is not an option. Complications include hypothyroidism, laryngeal nerve damage and hypoparathyroidism.

ALERT
More aggressive management is required in thyroid storm, a life-threatening condition in which patients may present with mental status changes, hyperthermia and hemodynamic instability.
- Treat hyperthermia with cooling blankets and acetaminophen.
- Beta blockers to control heart rate and symptoms.
- Consider D5 NS if hypotensive and intubation followed by mechanical ventilation if respiratory compromise.
- Antithyroid drugs (PTU or MMI) decrease thyroid hormone synthesis. PTU is 1st line because of its additional effect on peripheral conversion. PTU loading dose 300–600 mg followed by 150–300 mg q8h may be required.
- Iodide (e.g., iopodate, SSKI, Lugol's) prevents thyroid hormone release. Important to give antithyroid drugs approximately 1 hour before iodide in order to prevent utilization of iodide in thyroid hormone synthesis.
- Consider stress dose corticosteroids until adrenal insufficiency can be ruled out. Corticosteroids also prevent thyroid hormone release and impair peripheral conversion of T4 to T3.
- Evaluate for precipitating events.

Pregnancy Considerations
In pregnancy, RAI ablation and MMI are contraindicated. PTU is the treatment of choice. Surgery should be considered for those who cannot tolerate PTU. β-blocker can be used to control symptoms. Breast feeding is safe with MMI and PTU; however, PTU is preferred because it is less concentrated in breast milk.

H

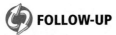 **FOLLOW-UP**

Admission Criteria

- Thyroid storm should prompt an ICU admission and an endocrine consultation.
- Atrial Fibrillation precipitated by thyrotoxicosis requires admission to telemetry floor for rate control and anticoagulation.

Issues for Referral

Consider endocrine consultation for evaluation and management of thyrotoxicosis.

PROGNOSIS

In general, prognosis is excellent with early diagnosis and treatment. However, mortality rate associated with storm is 20–50%.

Pregnancy Considerations

Consequences to the fetus/infant of hyperthyroid mothers include higher perinatal mortality and low birth weight. Fetal thyrotoxicosis is noted in 1–5% of women with Graves' due to transplacental transfer of TSH-receptor stimulating antibody. High fetal heart rate, fetal goiter, poor growth, craniosynostosis, cardiac failure, and hydrops have been reported with fetal thyrotoxicosis. Fetal goiter and hypothyroidism are complications of antithyroid drugs during pregnancy.

PATIENT MONITORING

Monitor thyroid function tests (TFT) at initial visit and every 6–8 weeks until normal. Once normal, individuals on antithyroid drugs should be monitored every 3 months until anti thyroid drugs are discontinued. In remission, TFT should be monitored every 6–12 months. Post surgery and RAI ablation, TFT should be monitored regularly to evaluate for hypothyroidism and recurrence of thyrotoxicosis.

REFERENCES

1. ACOG Practice Bulletin. Clinical management guidelines for obstetrician-gynecologists. Number 37, August 2002. Thyroid disease in pregnancy. *Obstet Gynecol*. 2002;100:387.
2. Auer J, Scheibner P, Mische T, et al. Subclinical hyperthyroidism as a risk factor for atrial fibrillation. *Am Heart J*. 2001; 142:838.
3. Singer PA, Cooper DS, Levy EG, et al. Treatment guidelines for patients with hyperthyroidism and hypothyroidism. *J Am Med Assoc*. 1995;273:808.

CODES

ICD9-CM

- 242.9 Thyrotoxicosis
- 242.9 Hyperthyroidism
- 245.9 Thyroiditis
- 242.8 Thyrotoxicosis factitia
- 242.9 Thyroid storm

KEY WORDS

- Hyperthyroidism
- Graves' Disease
- Goiter

HYPOTHYROIDISM

Geetha Gopalakrishnan, MD

KEY CLINICAL POINTS

- The prevalence of hypothyroidism increases with age. Women are more commonly affected than men.
- Primary hypothyroidism accounts for 95% of the cases of hypothyroidism.
- Thyroid stimulating hormone (TSH) and free thyroxine (FT4) should be checked to confirm diagnosis.
- Most cases of hypothyroidism will require thyroid hormone replacement for treatment.
- The goal of treatment is to alleviate symptoms and to return TSH and/or free T4 to the normal range.
- TSH and/or free T4 should be monitored 6–8 weeks after meds are adjusted until the values normalize.

 BASICS

DESCRIPTION
Hypothyroidism is caused by an inadequate production of thyroid hormone.

EPIDEMIOLOGY
- More common in women than men (4:1 ratio)
- Increases with age
- More common in whites

PATHOPHYSIOLOGY
- Primary hypothyroidism: A decrease in thyroid hormone production as a result of thyroid gland dysfunction; accounts for 95% of cases
- Secondary or central hypothyroidism: A decrease in thyroid hormone production as a result of pituitary or hypothalamic dysfunction causing a deficiency in thyroid-stimulating hormone (TSH) or thyrotrophin-releasing hormone (TRH)
- Tissue resistance to thyroid hormone: Autosomal dominant disorder resulting in decreased ligand binding and receptor function

ETIOLOGY
- Primary hypothyroidism
  - Iodine deficiency
  - Autoimmune (i.e., hashimoto thyroiditis)
  - Iatrogenic: Thyroidectomy, radioactive iodine and external radiation to the neck
  - Medications including iodine excess, lithium, sulfonamides, amiodarone, thiourea, interleukin-2, and interferon alpha.
  - Infiltrate disease including sarcoidosis, amyloidosis, hemochromatosis, and fibrous thyroiditis
  - Congenital including agenesis, defect in hormone production, or TSH-receptor mutation
- Secondary or central hypothyroidism
  - Pituitary or hypothalamic disease including tumors, cysts, infarctions, bleeding, trauma, surgery, radiation, and infiltrative diseases such as sarcoidosis and hemochromatosis
  - Bexarotene, a retinoid X receptor ligand that selectively inhibits TSH secretion
  - Genetic mutation including an inactivating mutation in the TRH-receptor gene and mutations in the gene coding for the TSH-beta subunit
- Tissue resistance to thyroid hormone

ASSOCIATED CONDITIONS
- Evaluation of other autoimmune conditions including pernicious anemia, vitiligo, Type 1 diabetes, and adrenal insufficiency should be considered in Hashimoto's thyroiditis.
- Evaluation of other pituitary hormone dysfunction including hypogonadism and adrenal insufficiency should be considered in central hypothyroidism.

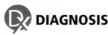 **DIAGNOSIS**

SIGNS AND SYMPTOMS
Hypothyroidism causes slowing of the metabolic processes.

History
Fatigue, cold intolerance, hoarse voice, dry skin, hair loss, brittle nails, decreased hearing, dyspnea on exertion, constipation, weight gain, menstrual cycle irregularities, decreased libido, glactorrhea, infertility, myalgia, paresthesias, arthralgia, depression, poor memory, decreased concentration and psychosis

Physical Exam
- Dry skin, coarse or thin hair, brittle nails, loss of outer eyebrows, periorbital edema, hoarse voice, slow speech, macroglossia, bradycardia, hypertension, pericardial effusion, pleural effusion, ascites, glactorrhea, carpal tunnel, non-pitting edema involving hands and feet, delayed relaxation of deep tendon reflexes, slow movement, cerebellar ataxia, slow thought process, psychosis, and dementia. Thyroid may or may not be palpable depending on the etiology of the hypothyroidism.
- Congenital hypothyroidism is associated with mental retardation. Juvenile hypothyroidism is associated with short stature and pubertal delay. Central hypothyroidism can be associated with headache, vision loss, and other pituitary hormone dysfunction.

TESTS
Lab
Check thyroid stimulating hormone (TSH) and free thyroxine (FT4) to confirm the diagnosis.
- Primary hypothyroidism
  - Increased TSH and decreased FT4
  - Increased antimicrosomal or thyroid peroxidase antibody associated with autoimmune thyroiditis
- Central hypothyroidism
  - Decreased/normal TSH and decreased FT4
- Resistance to thyroid hormone
  - Increased FT4 and normal/increased TSH
- Subclinical hypothyroidism: TSH elevated, but T3 (triiodothyronine) and FT4 are normal. Anti-thyroid peroxidase (TPO) antibody may be positive in autoimmune thyroid disease.
- Hypothyroidism can result in hyperlipidemia, hyperprolactinemia and hyponatremia.

ALERT
Consider ruling out adrenal insufficiency in critically ill patients.

Imaging
- Consider MRI to evaluate the pituitary and hypothalamus in central hypothyroidism.

- Consider an ultrasound of the thyroid to confirm diagnoses such as infiltrative disease of the thyroid and congenital agenesis.

DIFFERENTIAL DIAGNOSIS
Thyroid function test during severe illness, dopamine treatment, or corticosteroid use can mimic hypothyroidism.

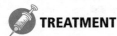

TREATMENT

The goal of treatment is to alleviate symptoms and to return blood levels of TSH (in primary hypothyroidism) and FT4 (in secondary hypothyroidism) to the normal range.

INITIAL STABILIZATION
Oral thyroid hormone replacement should be considered in all patients with hypothyroidism except:
- Medication induced hypothyroidism
  - Usually resolve when the drug is discontinued. If discontinuation is not an option, thyroid hormone replacement may be considered.
- Subclinical hypothyroidism
  - Consider thyroid hormone replacement if anti-thyroid Peroxidase (TPO) antibody, TSH >10 mU/l, or signs and symptoms of hypothyroidism such as goiter can be documented. Otherwise, no treatment is required.
- Myxedema coma
  - Cover patients to avoid heat loss.
  - Consider IV thyroid hormone replacement.
  - Consider stress dose steroid until adrenal insufficiency can be ruled out.
  - Consider intubation followed by mechanical ventilation if respiratory compromise.
  - Normal saline and pressers may be required if hypotensive

MEDICATION (DRUGS)

Thyroxine (T4), triiodothyronine (T3) or a combination of T3 and T4 can be used.

First Line
Thyroxine (T4) therapy is the treatment of choice in most circumstances. Starting dose of T4 is between 25–75 mcg/day based on age, weight, and comorbid conditions. In an elderly patient with coronary artery disease consider a starting dose of 25 mcg/day.

Second Line
In certain circumstances, Triiodothyronine (T3) can sometimes be used alone or in combinations with T4. Advantage of combination T3-T4 over T4 alone has been reported; however, several other studies have not shown this advantage (2).

Pregnancy Considerations
Replacement doses of thyroid hormone increase by as much as 50% during pregnancy. The goal of therapy is to maintain TSH concentration within the normal range. After delivery, the dose can be reduced to prepregnancy levels.

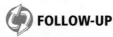

FOLLOW-UP

DISPOSITION
Most patients with hypothyroidism will require lifelong treatment with thyroid hormone replacement; exceptions include medication induced hypothyroidism and subacute thyroiditis.

Admission Criteria
Myxedema coma should prompt an ICU admission and an endocrine consultation. Central hypothyroidism may require a hospital admission for treatment of the underlying condition or its complications, such as adrenal crisis.

Issues for Referral
Consider endocrine consultation for myxedema, hypothyroidism in pregnancy, central hypothyroidism, and in a patient with difficulty reaching therapeutic goals.

PROGNOSIS
In general, prognosis is excellent with early diagnosis and treatment. However, mortality rate associated with myxedema is 20–50%.

COMPLICATIONS
Stress induced by sepsis and trauma, for example, can trigger a life-threatening condition called myxedema coma in hypothyroid patients. Patients present with mental status change and hypothermia. The condition can result in respiratory failure, hemodynamic instability and death.

Pregnancy Considerations
Consequences to the fetus/infant of hypothyroid mothers include higher perinatal mortality, low birth weight and impaired cognitive/psychomotor development.

PATIENT MONITORING
- Primary hypothyroidism: Monitor TSH at initial visit and every 6–8 weeks until TSH normalizes. Monitor every 6–12 months once TSH has normalized.
- Central hypothyroidism: Monitor FT4 every 6–8 weeks until FT4 normalizes. Monitor every 6–12 months once FT4 has normalized.

Pregnancy Considerations
TSH should be measured 4–6 weeks after conception and at least once each trimester.

REFERENCES

1. ACOG Practice Bulletin. Clinical management guidelines for obstetrician-gynecologists. Thyroid disease in pregnancy. *Obstet Gynecol*. 2002;100:387–396.
2. Bunevicius R, Kazanavicius G, Zalinkevicius R, et al. Effects of thyroxine as compared with thyroxine and triiodothyronine in patients with hypothyroidism. *N Engl J Med*. 1999;340: 424–429.
3. Oppenheimer JH, Braverman LE, Toft AD, et al. Thyroid hormone treatment: When and what? *J Clin Endocrinol Metab*. 1995;80:2873–2883.

CODES
ICD9-CM
- 245.2 Hashimotos
- 244 Acquired hypothyroidism
- 243 Congenital hypothyroidism
- 244.1 Surgical hypothyroidism
- 244.3 Iatrogenic hypothyroidism
- 244.8 Pituitary hypothyroidism
- 246.1 Sporadic hypothyroidism

KEY WORDS

- Hypothyroidism
- Hashimotos
- Myxedema

INFERTILITY

Christine Duffy, MD, MPH

KEY CLINICAL POINTS

- Evaluation includes assessment of the couple.
- The pace and extent of the evaluation should consider the woman's wishes, age, duration of infertility, medical history, and physical exam.
- Early referral for women who are ≥35, have history of oligo/amenorrhea, known or suspected tubal disease
- Infertility can result in substantial emotional, financial, and relationship stress; consider referral for counseling and support groups when appropriate.

BASICS

DESCRIPTION
- Defined as the inability to conceive after 1 year of intercourse without contraception
- Normally 85% of fertile couples will conceive within this period

GENERAL PREVENTION
Major preventable causes of infertility or subfertility include pelvic inflammatory disease (PID) and lifestyle habits such as obesity and smoking.
- Prevent sexually transmitted infections (STIs)
- Optimize weight
- Avoid excessive alcohol
- Smoking cessation

EPIDEMIOLOGY
Incidence
- ~20% of all couples are infertile
- ~14% of women are infertile
- Estimated 25% of women will experience fertility problems during childbearing years
- ~1% of women experience premature ovarian failure (ovarian failure occurring age <40)

Prevalence
Approximately 6 million couples are affected in the United States

RISK FACTORS
- History of anovulation, polycystic ovarian syndrome (PCOS), endometriosis, PID, previous infertility
- Toxic exposures such as chemotherapy and radiation to pelvic organs

Genetics
Most cases have no genetic cause

ETIOLOGY
- Ovulation disorders: 20–35%
- Tubal disease: 20–25%
- Endometriosis: 5–15%
- Cervical factors: 3%
- Unexplained infertility: 20–30%
- Ovulation disorders
  - PCOS
  - Hyperprolactinemia
  - Thyroid dysfunction
  - POF
  - Hypothalamic dysfunction
- Tubal disorders
  - Occlusion
  - Adhesions

- Endometriosis
- Cervical disorders
  - Abnormalities of cervical mucous production
  - Sperm/mucous interaction
- Unexplained Infertility

ASSOCIATED CONDITIONS
- STIs
- PCOS
- Endometriosis

DIAGNOSIS

Diagnosis is straightforward, identifying cause can be complicated

SIGNS AND SYMPTOMS
- Frequently no signs and symptoms
- Oligomenorrhea
- Amenorrhea

History
Focus on identifying common or reversible causes of infertility
- Reproductive health:
  - Previous pregnancy
  - Menstrual cycle irregularity (anovulatory cycles)
  - Dysmenorrhea (endometriosis)
  - STIs (PID)
  - Frequency and timing of sexual activity
- Medical history:
  - Hyperthyroid or hypothyroid symptoms
  - Abnormal hair growth, weight gain
  - Current medical problems
- Social history
  - Use of alcohol, tobacco and other drugs
  - Exposure to chemotherapy or radiation
  - Exercise and eating habits
- Surgical history
  - Fallopian tube surgery
  - Ectopic pregnancy, appendectomy or other pelvic surgery

Physical Exam
- Weight and BMI
- Thyroid exam
- Breast secretions
- Signs of androgen excess (hirsutism, acne, acanthosis nigricans)
- Pelvic or abdominal tenderness, enlargement or mass
- Vaginal or cervical abnormality, secretions, or discharge
- Uterine size, shape, position and mobility

TESTS
Testing should be guided by the results of the history and physical.

Lab
In women with irregular menses or oligomenorrhea:
- TSH, FSH, prolactin
- Serum progesterone (luteal phase values over 3 ng/mL suggest ovulation)
- If ≥35 years old, prior ovarian surgery, chemotherapy or radiation, FSH day 3 testing. Elevated FSH (>12–20 IU/L) associated with poor ovarian response

Imaging

- Hysterosalpingogram (HSP) or sonohyhysterogram for unexplained infertility and evidence or suspicion of endometriosis, intra-pelvic adhesions or fallopian tube disease
- Laparoscopy is indicated in unexplained infertility and suspicion of endometriosis/tubal disease that is amenable to repair.

Pathologic Findings

- HSP can identify tubal blockages and other structural malformations that can impair conception.
- Laparoscopy can identify endometriosis, adhesions, and tubal blockages that impair conception.

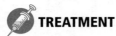 ## TREATMENT

- Dependent on cause of infertility, age, partner infertility, resources, and patient preferences
- All women should be counseled regarding appropriate weight, tobacco cessation, limiting caffeine (2 cups/day) and eliminating or limiting alcohol (no more than 4 drinks per week).
- Ovulatory disorders (majority have PCOS)
  - Weight modulation
  - Clomiphene citrate
  - Gonadotropins
  - Metformin
  - In vitro Fertilization (IVF)
  - Bromcriptine/dopamine agonists in women with hyperprolactinemia
  - In POF, no treatment is effective for women desiring conception with own oocytes
- Tubal factors
  - Tubal flushing
  - Tubal reconstruction (distal obstruction)
  - Adhesiolysis
  - Salpingectomy (in women with hydrosalpinges)
  - IVF
- Endometriosis
  - Laparoscopic surgery if mild disease
  - Clomiphene citrate and intrauterine insemination
  - IVF
- Uterine factors
  - Surgical removal if submucosal or obstructing leiomyomas
  - Cervical factor infertility
  - Intrauterine insemination or IVF
- Unexplained
  - Trial of clomiphene citrate and intrauterine insemination
  - Gonadotropins and intrauterine insemination
  - IVF

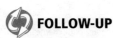 ## FOLLOW-UP

Issues for Referral

Refer early to reproductive health specialist:
- Age 35 or older
- History of oligo/amenorrhea
- Known or suspected uterine/tubal disease or endometriosis
- Partner known to be subfertile

PROGNOSIS

Live birth depends on:
- Underlying cause of infertility

- Ovulation disorders: 42%
- Tubal disease: 22%
- Endometriosis: 30%
- Unexplained: 32%
- Age of the woman
  - Deliveries per retrieval range from 37% in women <35 to 11% in women over 40
- Treatment method employed
  - Clomiphene citrate pregnancy per cycle is 9.5%.
  - IVF live birth per cycle is ~25%.
  - Tubal surgery for distal/partial occlusion successful in 15% to 35% of the cases.
  - Surgical ablation for mild endometriosis ~30% pregnancy at 9 months

COMPLICATIONS

- Nulliparity is associated with increased risk of breast and ovarian cancers
- Risks associated with infertility treatments:
  - Clomiphene
    - Hyperstimulation syndrome: 1.3%
    - Multiple gestations: ~10%
    - Hot flashes: 10% to 20%
  - IVF
    - Hyperstimulation syndrome: 5%
    - Multiple gestations: 37%
    - Preterm delivery: 20%
    - Spontaneous abortion: 17%
- Surgical procedures: All treatments carry the risks associated with anesthesia and laparoscopic/general surgery
  - Tubal reconstruction surgery
    - Increased risk of ectopic pregnancy (20%)
  - Salpingectomy
    - Theoretical risk of diminishing blood supply to ovaries
  - Endometriosis ablation
    - Adhesions
  - Myomectomy
    - Increased risk of uterine rupture

REFERENCES

1. Frey KA, Patel KS. Initial evaluation and management of infertility by the primary care physician. *Mayo Clin Proc.* 2004;79:1439–1443.
2. Practice Committee of the American Society for Reproductive Medicine. Optimal evaluation of the infertile female. *Fertil Steril.* 2004;82 (Suppl 1):169–172.
3. Smith S, Pfeifer SM, Collins JA. Diagnosis and management of female infertility. *JAMA.* 2003;290:1767–1770.

 ## MISCELLANEOUS

For patient information website sponsored by the National Fertility Association: http://www.Resolve.com

CODES
ICD9-CM
- 628 Infertility
- 628.0 Infertility associated with anovulation
- 628.1 Infertility of pituitary-hypothalamic origin
- 628.2 Infertility of tubal origin
- 628.3 Infertility of uterine origin
- 628.4 Infertility of cervical or vaginal origin
- 628.8 Infertility of other specified origin
- 628.9 Infertility of unspecified origin

KEY WORDS

- Infertility
- Subfertility
- IVF

INFLAMMATORY BOWEL DISEASE

Rossana Moura, MD

KEY CLINICAL POINTS

- Inflammatory bowel disease (IBD) is characterized by a tendency for chronic or relapsing immune activation and inflammation within the gastrointestinal tract.
- Crohn disease (CD) and ulcerative colitis (UC) are the two major forms of idiopathic IBD.
- No single symptom, sign, or diagnostic test establishes the diagnosis. Etiology remains unknown.

 BASICS

DESCRIPTION

- CD potentially involves any location of the alimentary tract from mouth to anus, but with propensity for the distal small bowel and proximal large bowel. Inflammation is often discontinuous, but may involve all layers from mucosa to serosa.
- UC affects the rectum and extends proximally to affect a variable extent of the colon. The inflammatory response in UC is largely confined to the mucosa and submucosa.
- In indeterminate colitis, the clinical picture falls between the two diseases.

EPIDEMIOLOGY

- More common in whites than in blacks and Asians
- Jewish population has an incidence 3–6 times greater than that of non-Jewish
- CD: Small excess risk among women, female-to-male ratio between unity and 1.2:1
- UC: Nearly equal to slight male predominance
- Higher rates in northern climates and in well developed areas
- Peak age of onset is between 15–25 years, with a second lesser peak between ages 55–65

Incidence
- UC: Incidence has remained relatively constant, ranging from 3–15 cases per 100,000 population
- CD: Incidence has risen progressively; 6–7:100,000, but the incidence can be equivalent to UC in certain areas of North America and Europe

Prevalence
- UC: 50–80 cases per 100,000 population
- CD: 20–40 per 100,000 population

RISK FACTORS

- Environment
- Higher socioeconomic level
- Oral contraceptives (conflicting data)
- NSAIDs/COX-2 selective inhibitors
- Refined sugars, paucity of fresh fruits and vegetables
- Smoking
  - UC is largely a disease of ex-smokers and nonsmokers
  - CD is associated with smoking
- Stress
- Infectious: A correlation (Mycobacteruim paratuberculosis, measles virus) remains unproven
- Appendectomy may be protective against UC

Genetics

- Approximately 10–25% of patients with IBD have first-degree relatives who also have IBD.
- Concordance for the same disease category within families, especially with CD, which shows concordance for disease location, type and severity
- Monozygotic twins have a higher concordance for IBD than dizygotic twins.
- Mutations within the NOD2 gene (IBD1) on chromosome 16 is linked to CD. NOD 2 mediates the innate immune response to microbial pathogens, leading to activation of nuclear factor kappa B.
- HLA-DR2 is associated with UC, particularly in the Japanese.
- Extraintestinal manifestations of CD are more commonly seen in HLA-A2, HLA-DR1, and DQw5.

PATHOPHYSIOLOGY

- Immunologic mechanism within lamina propria implicated in pathogenesis of inflammation and involves both humoral and cellular responses
- An immunologic sequence postulated to account for inflammatory response starts with an exogenous sensitization to luminal antigens, presumably bacterial, possibly facilitated by undefined genetic influences

ASSOCIATED CONDITIONS

- Rheumatologic: Arthralgia, arthritis, ankylosing spondylitis, sacroiliitis
- Gastrointestinal: Sclerosing cholangitis, bile duct carcinoma, fatty liver
- Dermatological: Erythema nodosum, pyoderma gangrenosum, aphthous stomatitis
- Ophthalmological: Iritis, uveitis, episcleritis

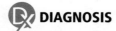 **DIAGNOSIS**

SIGNS AND SYMPTOMS

History
- Diarrhea, usually bloody in UC
- Abdominal pain
- Tenesmus with rectal involvement
- Fever
- Weight loss
- Fatigue and malaise

Physical Exam
- Abdominal tenderness or distention
- Fever
- Tachycardia
- Hypotension
- Perforation
- In CD
  - Perianal disease (fissures, abscesses, fistulae)
  - Intestinal obstruction from inflammation or fibrotic stenosis

TESTS

Lab
- Anemia
- Leukocytosis with a left shift

- Hypoalbuminemia
- Elevated erythrocyte sedimentation rate or C-reactive protein
- Electrolyte abnormalities
- Abnormal liver function tests
- Stool examination (positive leukocytes)
- Antineutrophil cytoplasmic antibodies with perinuclear staining (p-ANCA) in 50–70% of patients with UC, 15% in CD
- Antibodies to *S. cerevisiae* (ASCA) in 60–70% of patients with CD, 5% in UC

Imaging
- Plain abdominal films
  - To rule out toxic megacolon, perforation, obstruction, sacroiliitis
- Air-contrast barium enema/upper GI/small bowel series/CT
  - Loss of smooth mucosa, thickened bowel wall, undermined ulcers, dilated bowel, abscess, stricture, fistula and perirectal disease in CD

Diagnostic Procedures/Surgery
- Flexible sigmoidoscopy/colonoscopy
  - UC
    - Loss of mucosal vascularity, diffuse erythema, friability, granularity, mucosal edema, small punctate ulcers, and exudates consisting of mucus, blood and pus.
    - Uniform involvement extending proximally from the rectum in a continuous fashion but for a variable distance
    - Extent of disease:
      - Approximately 50% have disease confined to the rectosigmoid region, 30% extend to the splenic flexure, and <20% extend more proximally.
      - Backwash ileitis: Minimal involvement of a few centimeters of the terminal ileum when entire colon is involved with UC
  - CD
    - Focal intestinal inflammation, transmural, discontinuous (skip areas), ulcerations, which may be tiny, aphthous erosions or deep, serpiginous ulcers.
    - Cobblestone appearance
    - 1/3 of the cases involve only the small bowel, most commonly the terminal ileum.
      - Approximately 50% have ileocolitis
      - Approximately 20% have disease limited to the colon

Pathologic Findings
- Architectural distortion, cryptitis and crypt abscesses, infiltration with inflammatory cells
- Granulomas, sinus tracts, fistula and fibrosis, fat wrapping (encroachment of mesenteric fat onto the serosal surface of the bowel) in CD

DIFFERENTIAL DIAGNOSIS
- Hemorrhoids
- Colonic neoplasms
- Colonic diverticula
- Arteriovenous malformations
- Radiation proctitis
- Behcet syndrome
- Infectious colitis
- Ischemic colitis (rectum usually spared)
- Irritable bowel syndrome
- Lymphoma, NSAIDs, eosinophilic gastroenteritis (small bowel disease)

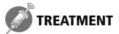

TREATMENT

GENERAL MEASURES
- Maintain weight and nutrition
- Control inflammation, prevent complications

Diet
Specific nutritional replacement therapy is determined by patient's nutritional status and if clinical course expected to be protracted
- NPO in severely ill patients +/- parenteral nutrition
- Diet may be advanced from clear liquids to low residue and then regular as tolerated
- Lactose free diet if lactose intolerant

MEDICATION (DRUGS)

First Line
- 5-aminosalicylates (5-ASA):
  - Sulfasalazine (azulfidine): 500–1000 mg q.i.d.
  - Mesalamine (asacol: 800 mg t.i.d.; pentasa: 1000 mg q.i.d.)
  - Balsalazide (colazal): 2–25 g t.i.d.
  - Olsalazine (dipentum): 500 mg b.i.d.
  - Mesalamine enemas (rowasa) or suppositories (canasa) or hydrocortisone enemas for topical therapy for distal UC
- Glucocorticoids
  - Moderate to severe disease
  - No benefit to continuing steroids after remission
  - Steroid therapy can be tapered and discontinued over a 2–3-month period.
    - Oral prednisone (40–60 mg/day)
    - Budesonide (9 mg/day) for CD involving the terminal ileum and/or ascending colon
    - Intravenous prednisolone 45–60 mg/d or IV hydrocortisone (300 mg/day) or methylprednisolone (36–48 mg/day) in severely ill patients

Second Line
- Immunosuppressive therapy when glucocorticoids fail or as steroid-sparing therapy
  - Azathioprine, 6-mercaptopurine or methotrexate
    - Positive response may take 3–4 months
  - Cyclosporine IV in severely ill patients with UC
- Antibiotics usually used in CD include: Metronidazole, ciprofloxacin, and rifaximin, which is under investigation.
- Anti-tumor necrosis factor antibody
  - Infliximab 5 mg/Kg at weeks 0, 2, and 6 with maintenance infusions every 8 weeks, approved for both UC and CD

SURGERY
- Reserved for specific complications, intractable disease, dysplasia or carcinoma
  - UC
    - Colectomy is curative.
      - Approximately 20–25% of patients with UC require colectomy during the course of their disease.
    - Total proctocolectomy with permanent ileostomy
    - Total colectomy with ileorectal anastomosis (patients will require surveillance of the rectal mucosa) or ileoanal anastomosis
    - Emergency surgery for massive hemorrhage, perforation, or toxic megacolon that does not respond to treatment in 48–72 hours

- CD
  - Should be reserved for complications
  - Approximately 70% of the patients require at least one operation during course of their disease.
  - Surgery may be required for bowel narrowing or obstruction, fistula formation, anal or intraabdominal abscesses, toxic dilation of colon, or perforation.
  - High rate of recurrence after small bowel resection, with risk for short bowel syndrome

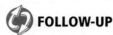 ## FOLLOW-UP

Issues for Referral
- To gastroenterology to establish diagnosis
- All patients with IBD should be under the care of a gastroenterologist
- To surgery for complications, such as perforation, obstruction, fistula, or hemorrhage

PROGNOSIS
- UC
  - Approximately 80% have intermittent attacks, but length of remission varies from few weeks to many years
  - Patients with extensive colitis
    - More likely to have severe attacks
    - Colectomy rate is higher
  - Patients with proctitis have a favorable course
  - More extensive disease can develop with time:
    - More extensive disease develops in 11% of the patients in 5 years, 19% of the patients in 10 years, and 29% of the patients after 19 years.
    - Most patients (70%) remain with only rectal involvement.
  - Mortality rate for a severe attack of UC <2% with the use of more potent medications.
- CD
  - Over a 4-year period
    - Patients that remain in remission: 22%
    - Patients that have chronically active symptoms: 25%
    - Patients that have a course that fluctuates between active and inactive disease: 53%
  - Modest increase in mortality
    - Highest in first 4 or 5 years after diagnosis
    - Most deaths from peritonitis and sepsis
  - Patients with proximal small bowel disease may have a higher risk of mortality.
  - Risk of colorectal cancer is similar in Crohn's colitis and UC of similar extent. Annual surveillance colonoscopy is recommended after 8–10 years of pancolitis.

COMPLICATIONS
- Nutritional and metabolic (weight loss, decreased protein and electrolytes)
- Anemia (iron, folate, or B12 deficiency)

- Fistulae, abscess formation, strictures, perforation, hemorrhage
- Toxic megacolon
- Bile salt diarrhea with ileal disease
- Venous thrombosis
- Uric acid and oxalate renal stones
- Osteoporosis
- Carcinoma
- Extraintestinal manifestations (see associated conditions)

Pregnancy Considerations
- Fertility does not seem to be impaired
- Course of IBD during pregnancy is determined in part by the disease activity at conception. Recommend delaying pregnancy until the disease is inactive.
- Endoscopy with conscious sedation (meperidine and midazolam) can be performed during pregnancy, if needed.
- 5-ASA drugs, corticosteroids, and even azathioprine appear to be safe.
- Methotrexate is contraindicated.
- Mode of delivery in CD is controversial. Avoid episiotomy in active perianal disease due to concerns of fistula formation.

REFERENCES

1. ASGE Guideline: Guidelines for endoscopy in pregnant and lactating women. *Gastrointest Endosc*. 2005;61:357–362.
2. Garcia Rodriguez LA, Gonzalez-Perez A, Johansson S, et al. Risk factors for inflammatory bowel disease in the general population. *Aliment Pharmacol Ther*. 2005;22:309–315.
3. Katz JA. Pregnancy and inflammatory bowel disease. *Curr Opin Gastroenterol*. 2004;20:328–332.
4. Navarro F, Hanauer SB. Treatment of inflammatory bowel disease: Safety and tolerability issues. *Am J Gastroenterol*. 2003;98:S18–23.
5. Sleisenger MH, Fordtran JS. *Gastrointestinal and Liver Disease*. 7th ed. Philadelphia: Elsevier Science; 2002.

CODES
ICD9-CM
- 555.0 Regional enteritis of small intestine
- 555.1 Regional enteritis of large intestine
- 555.9 Regional enteritis of unspecified site
- 556.9 Ulcerative colitis, unspecified

KEY WORDS

- Diarrhea
- Abdominal Pain
- Rectal Bleeding
- Colitis/Proctitis
- Crohn's Disease
- Ulcerative Colitis

INSOMNIA

Christine Duffy, MD, MPH

KEY CLINICAL POINTS

- Among the most common complaints in primary care
- Health care utilization is higher for patients with insomnia.
- Thorough history and physical essential to rule out potential secondary causes
- Primary insomnia: No underlying medical/psychiatric disorder
- Secondary: Insomnia caused by comorbid condition
- Cognitive Behavioral Therapy (CBT) effective
- Pharmacologic therapy effective for short-term use
- Little data on long-term treatment outcomes

 BASICS

DESCRIPTION

- Disorder, not a disease
- Characterized by inadequate quantity or quality of sleep, difficulty initiating or maintaining sleep, early awakenings, and/or interrupted or nonrestorative sleep
- Acute insomnia: No more than 2 weeks duration, usually caused by emotional or physical distress
- Chronic insomnia: Lasting 1 month or more, affecting more than 2–3 nights per week
- Primary insomnia (not due to an underlying medical or psychiatric diagnosis)
  - Idiopathic: Insomnia arising in infancy or childhood, persistent and unremitting
  - Psychophysiologic insomnia: Due to a maladaptive conditioned response
  - Paradoxical insomnia: Sleep-state misperception
- Secondary Insomnia or "comorbid" insomnia (sleep disorder caused by some psychiatric or medical condition)
  - Adjustment insomnia (psychosocial stressors)
  - Psychiatric disorders
  - Medical conditions
  - Drugs/substance abuse

GENERAL PREVENTION

- Avoid stimulants
- Avoid alcohol
- Exercise regularly

Employ good sleep hygiene: See Non-pharmacologic treatment of insomnia)

EPIDEMIOLOGY

- Most common sleep disorder in the United States
- More common in women
- More common in those with medical or psychiatric disorders

Incidence

- Approximately 1/3 of the adult population suffers from insomnia in a given year.
- Persistent in ~10% of the population
- There are approximately 50–70 million Americans affected by insomnia.

RISK FACTORS

- Medical disorders
  - COPD, musculoskeletal disorders, chronic pain, heart disease, renal disease
- Psychiatric disorders
  - Depression, anxiety

- Inactivity
- Medications or stimulants
  - Consumption or discontinuation of medication (i.e., benzodiazepines)
  - Drugs of abuse, caffeine, and alcohol

PATHOPHYSIOLOGY

- Primary insomnia
  - Evidence suggests probably related to a state of hyperarousal
- Secondary insomnia
  - Precipitating disease or condition interrupts or disturbs normal sleep architecture

ETIOLOGY

- Primary insomnia:
  - Unknown
- Secondary insomnia:
  - Depends on underlying cause
    - Behavioral practices
    - Medications or drugs
    - Symptoms/sequelae of disease
  - All of which can result in difficulty initiating sleep, maintaining sleep, or affect sleep quality

ASSOCIATED CONDITIONS

- Chronic debilitating medical conditions
  - COPD
  - CHF
  - Renal failure
- Obstructive sleep apnea (OSA)
- Vasomotor instability (menopause)
- Depression/anxiety
- Chronic pain
- Substance abuse
- Periodic limb movement disorder (PLMD)/restless leg syndrome (RLS)

 DIAGNOSIS

- Diagnosis of insomnia is generally based on a careful history and physical.
- Polysomnography (sleep study) may be required for certain types of sleep disorders.

SIGNS AND SYMPTOMS

- Daytime sleepiness, fatigue
- Nonrestorative sleep
- Accidents or irritability
- Cognitive deficits

History

- Determine the onset, frequency, duration and severity of sleep complaints
  - Chronology
  - Transient, intermittent or persistent
  - Problems with initiation and/or maintenance of sleep
  - Functional status during the day
- Precipitating events, ameliorating or exacerbating factors
  - Psychological stressors
  - Inadequate sleep hygiene
  - Psychiatric disorders such as anxiety or depression
  - Shift work

INSOMNIA

- Assess for:
  - Chronic pain, nocturnal cough, dyspnea, hot flashes
  - OSA (snoring, reports of apnea, driving accidents)
  - Chronic lung, heart, renal disease, thyroid disease
  - RLS, PLMD
  - Prescription drugs (bronchodilators, steroids, diuretics, stimulants, activating antidepressants, hypnotic rebound), drugs of abuse (cocaine, methamphetamines), alcohol and caffeine

Physical Exam
The physical exam is directed at the identification of medical disorders that may result in secondary insomnia, such as heart, lung, kidney and thyroid disease, as well as evidence of illicit drug use and chronic alcohol use.

TESTS
Testing should be guided by a thorough history and physical, which may suggest an underlying medical or psychiatric cause of the insomnia.

Lab
- No specific lab test for insomnia
- Lab testing geared to identify underlying medical problems that may cause or contribute to insomnia

Imaging
Imaging should be pursued when the history and physical suggest imaging for other medical conditions or problems (i.e., evaluation of chronic lung disease).

Diagnostic Procedures/Surgery
Polysomnography is generally not indicated except under the following circumstances:
- Sleep-related breathing disorder such as OSA
- Narcolepsy is suspected
- Violent sleep behaviors
- Atypical or unusual parasomnias (abnormal behavioral or physiologic events which occur during sleep or sleep-wake transitions)
- Seizure-related sleep disorders
- Periodic limb movement disorder is suspected (NOT needed for RLS unless uncertainty exists as to the diagnosis)

DIFFERENTIAL DIAGNOSIS
- Differential diagnosis should be focused on determining whether there are underlying medical conditions that are causing insomnia.
- Patients may complain of insomnia for a secondary gain (e.g., to obtain medications such as benzodiazepines).

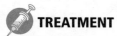 TREATMENT

GENERAL MEASURES
- Primary insomnia/idiopathic:
  - For primary insomnia, nonpharmacologic and pharmacological treatments have been shown to be effective
  - Comparative benefits or combination of these treatments is largely unknown.
- Secondary insomnia/comorbid insomnia:
  - Proper diagnosis and management of underlying disorders (i.e., optimal management of CHF, OSA, ESRD, etc)
  - Little research has explored the effectiveness of therapy for secondary causes of insomnia.

Non-pharmacologic Treatment of Idiopathic Insomnia
- Sleep hygiene
  - Sleep only until rested
  - Keep regular sleep schedule
  - Avoid forcing sleep
  - Exercise regularly (but not within 3 to 4 hours of bedtime)
  - Avoid caffeinated beverages after noon
  - Avoid alcohol
  - Avoid smoking in evening
  - Do not go to bed hungry
  - Comfortable room environment
- Relaxation therapy
- Stimulus control therapy
  - Go to bed only when sleepy
  - Only sleep and have sex in bed
  - Get up if unable to sleep and return only when sleepy
  - Set an alarm clock to same time every day (including weekends)
  - Do not nap
- Sleep restriction
  - Determine average sleep time (not time in bed)
  - Patient is allowed only that amount of time in bed which will decrease the amount of time for sleep and increase pressure to sleep
- CBT: Uses a combination of techniques described above

 MEDICATION (DRUGS)

- Medication is generally recommended only for short-term treatment of insomnia.
- Careful monitoring in elderly
- Contraindicated in patients with undiagnosed sleep apnea, those who need to maintain maximum alertness during their sleep period, and pregnant or breast-feeding women.
- Treatment with sleep-inducing aids should include careful monitoring of side effects and efficacy, especially in the elderly.
- All agents can cause dizziness or drowsiness.
- Nonbenzodiazepine hypnotics:
  - Zolpidem, zaleplon
  - Eszopiclone (approved for up to 6 months)
    - Advantages: Improves sleep latency, minimal next-day sedation, rebound insomnia and rebound insomnia
    - Disadvantages: Sensory/perceptual distortions, abuse, dependence possible
- Benzodiazepines
  - Temazepam, flurazepam, triazolam, estazolam, quazepam
    - Advantages: Improve TST, anxiolytic effect
    - Disadvantages: Next day sedation, impaired memory, falls, tolerance, abuse and dependence
- Antidepressants
  - Amitryptylline
  - Trazedone
  - Doxepin
    - Advantages: Improves TST, low risk of abuse, may be helpful with coexisting depression
    - Disadvantages: Potential serious side effects depending on agent used (e.g., cardiac arrythmias, priapism)

- Melatonin-receptor agonist
  - Ramelteon
- Advantages: Improves sleep latency
- Disadvantages: Increases prolactin levels, caution in those with coexisting depression, few published studies evaluating efficacy or long-term safety
- Nonprescription products
  - Diphenhydramine
  - Doxylamine
    - Advantages: Improves sleep latency, duration, low risk of abuse, inexpensive
    - Disadvantages: Cognitive side effects, tolerance develops quickly (days)

Complementary and Alternative Medicine
Common CAMs used for sleep.
- Valerian root: No well-controlled studies have been conducted to ascertain its usefulness
- Melatonin: Results conflicting, may have efficacy in jet-lag

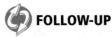 FOLLOW-UP

Issues for Referral
Referral to a sleep specialist may be indicated in the following circumstances:
- OSA is suspected
- Narcolepsy is suspected
- Individuals do not respond to therapy

PROGNOSIS
- Patients typically experience waxing and waning symptoms.
- Approximately 10% of the patients will have persistent insomnia.

COMPLICATIONS
- No long-term adverse medical complications of insomnia (not related to comorbid conditions) have been consistently described, but research is lacking.
- QOL may be adversely affected, although studies measuring the impact of insomnia on QOL are lacking.
- Insomnia may result in short-term impairment of cognitive function and mood, increased accidents, and reduced QOL.
- Insomnia may increase appetite and decrease immune function.

REFERENCES

1. Kushida CA, Littner ME, Morgenthaler T, et al. Practice parameters for the indications for polysomnography and related procedures: An update for 2005. *Sleep*. 2005;28:499–521.
2. Sateia MJ, Nowell PD. Insomnia. *Lancet*. 2004;364: 1959–1973.
3. Silber MH. Chronic insomnia. *N Engl J Med*. 2005;353: 803–810.
4. Morin CM, Hauri PJ, Espie C, et al. Nonpharmacologic treatment of chronic insomnia. *Sleep*. 1999;22:1134–1156.
5. Winkelman J, Pies R. Current patterns and future directions in the treatment of insomnia. *Ann Clin Psychol*. 2005;17:31–40.
6. Report of the June 2005 Conference on insomnia, sponsored by the National Institutes of Health http://consensus.nih.gov/ta/026/InsomniaDraftStatement061505.pdf

ADDITIONAL READING

http://www.nhlbi.nih.gov/about/ncsdr/index.htm
Report of the June 2005 Conference on insomnia, sponsored by the National Institutes of Health http://consensus.nih.gov/ta/026/InsomniaDraftStatement061505.pdf

 MISCELLANEOUS

QOL-quality of life

CODES
ICD9-CM
- 780.52 Sleep disturbance, unspecified
- 291.82 Sleep disorder, alcohol-induced
- 292.85 Sleep disorder, drug-induced
- 307.40 Non
- Organic sleep disorder, unspecified
- 307.41 Nonorganic sleep disorder, transient
- 307.42 Nonorganic sleep disorder, persistent
- 327.00 Sleep disorder, organic
- 327.01 Organic insomnia, due to medical condition elsewhere classified
- 327.02 Organic Insomnia, due to mental disorder
- 327.20 Organic sleep apnea, unspecified
- 327.23 Obstructive sleep apnea

KEY WORDS

- Insomnia, Primary
- Insomnia, Secondary
- Sleep Disorders

IRRITABLE BOWEL SYNDROME

Rossana Moura, MD

KEY CLINICAL POINTS

- Cluster of chronic symptoms consisting most commonly of abdominal pain, bloating, constipation or diarrhea
- Functional bowel disorder and more common in women
- Associated with significant emotional distress, impaired health-related quality of life and high health care costs

 BASICS

DESCRIPTION
- Group of functional bowel disorders in which abdominal discomfort or pain is associated with defecation or a change in bowel habit, and with features of disordered defecation
- The diagnosis of a functional bowel disorder always presumes the absence of a structural or biochemical explanation for the symptoms.

EPIDEMIOLOGY
Prevalence
- Up to 20% of the United States population
- Prevalence: Female > Male (2:1)
- Seems to be similar in whites and blacks, but may be lower in Hispanics
- Symptoms typically begin early in life (teens to early 20s).
- Patients generally first complain about symptoms to a health care professional between the ages of 30–50 years.

RISK FACTORS
See Pathophysiology section

PATHOPHYSIOLOGY
IBS is not caused by a single factor, rather it is a complex disorder in which a number of physiologic processes are involved:
- Altered gut motility and secretion in response to luminal or provocative stimuli
- Enhanced visceral sensitivity
- Postinfectious
- Dysregulation of the brain-gut axis
  - Serotonin appears to be the common link in GI motility, intestinal secretion, and pain perception
- Hormonal factors
- Food intolerance
- Psychosocial factors
  - Although not etiologic to IBS, relevant to understanding patient's adjustment to IBS, the clinical outcome and the plan of treatment

ASSOCIATED CONDITIONS
Psychological disorders
- Depression and anxiety are the most common
- Phobias, obsessional behavior, sleep disturbance, panic attacks
- Multiple somatic symptoms
- History of abuse

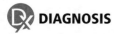 **DIAGNOSIS**

SIGNS AND SYMPTOMS
ROME criteria

- Pain or discomfort for 12 weeks, which need not be consecutive, in the preceding 12 months, associated with 2 of the following 3 features:
  - Relief with defecation
  - Change in stool frequency
  - Change in stool appearance or form
- Symptoms that cumulatively lend support to the diagnosis:
  - Abnormal stool passage (straining, urgency or feeling of incomplete evacuation)
  - Passage of mucus
  - Bloating or feeling of abdominal distention

History
Patients are usually categorized according to their primary bowel habits as:
- IBS-C (<3 bowel movements per week, presence of hard stools, straining, and lumpy stools)
- IBS-D (>3 bowel movements per day, loose watery stools, and urgency)
- IBS-A (alternating constipation and diarrhea)

Physical Exam
- Usually reveals no abnormalities
- Helpful in detecting or ruling out other conditions
- Useful to meet the patient's expectations of a thorough evaluation
- Rectal examination should be performed, particularly in patients reporting incontinence or rectal bleeding

TESTS
Lab
- Routine blood tests are usually normal
- May help rule out other medical conditions
- Check CBC, ESR, TSH, celiac sprue serology and stool studies depending on the presenting symptoms

Imaging
- Usually normal and not necessary to establish a diagnosis of IBS
- Plain radiography in patients with infrequent bowel movements may be performed to evaluate for obstructive signs
- Sitzmark study to evaluate for colonic inertia or pelvic dyssynergia in patients with severe constipation and/or defecation difficulties
- Defecography to evaluate for enterocele or rectocele

Diagnostic Procedures/Surgery
- IBS previously considered diagnosis of exclusion, but now diagnosis can be made clinically based on ROME criteria in patients without red flags
- Colonoscopy or flexible sigmoidoscopy:
  - Findings are usually normal
  - Colonoscopy reserved for patients with "red flags": Anemia, rectal bleeding, severe or nocturnal diarrhea, unintentional weight loss, family history of colon cancer or onset of symptoms in a older patient
  - Random biopsies done in patients with diarrhea to rule out microscopic colitis
- Anorectal motility testing with balloon expulsion

DIFFERENTIAL DIAGNOSIS
- Lactose intolerance
- Celiac sprue

- Inflammatory bowel disease
- Microscopic colitis
- Bacterial overgrowth
- Colorectal cancer

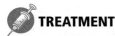

TREATMENT

GENERAL MEASURES
- Establish an effective physician-patient relationship
- Educate and reassure patient

Diet
- Dietary fiber, increased slowly to avoid excessive intestinal gas
- Avoidance of foods known to aggravate symptoms
- Excessive intake of legumes and cruciferous vegetables, sorbitol, and carbonated drinks should be avoided in patients who complain of gas/bloating.
- Temporary elimination of dairy products to exclude possible lactose intolerance

Activity
Daily exercise can be extremely helpful.

Complementary and Alternative Therapies
- Considered in IBS patients with moderate to severe symptoms, when patients have failed medical treatment, or when there is evidence of stress or psychological factors contributing to GI symptom exacerbations
  - Counseling
  - Hypnosis
  - Biofeedback
  - Massage
  - Acupuncture
- Herbs and natural therapies (most of unproven benefit)
  - Peppermint oil
  - Acidophilus
  - Chamomile tea
  - Primrose oil

MEDICATION (DRUGS)

- Medications do not cure IBS
- Different treatments can be prescribed according to type and severity of symptoms

First Line
- Diarrhea-predominant
  - Alosetron (lotronex), 5-HT$_3$ receptor antagonist
  - Anticholinergic drugs (antispasmodic effect)
    - Dicyclomine (bentyl)
    - Hyoscyamine (levsin)
  - Antidiarrheal drugs
    - Loperamide (Imodium)
    - Diphenoxylate with atropine (lomotil)
  - Cholestyramine, a bile acid binding agent
    - In patients with diarrhea and prior cholecystectomy
- Constipation-predominant
  - Tegaserod (Zelnorm), partial 5-HT$_4$ agonist
  - Lubiprostone (Amitiza), chloride channel activator
  - Magnesium hydroxide, lactulose, polyethylene glycol solutions (Miralax)

Second Line
Antidepressants, due to a pain relieving effect that is independent of a depression relieving effect

SURGERY
- Surgery is not indicated for treatment of IBS.
- Female patients with IBS are more likely to undergo cholecystectomy, appendectomy, hysterectomy, and back surgery.
- Such operations may complicate the condition with scar pain, adhesions, and further alteration in bowel habit.

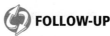

FOLLOW-UP

DISPOSITION
Issues for Referral
To gastroenterology to help establish diagnosis

PROGNOSIS
- Although IBS can produce substantial physical and emotional distress, most people do not develop serious long-term health conditions.
- The majority of patients learn to control their symptoms.
- Once diagnosed, nearly 75% of patients will carry the IBS diagnosis 5 years later.
- IBS does not decrease life expectancy.

Pregnancy Considerations
IBS symptoms may be exacerbated during pregnancy.

REFERENCES

1. Chang SY, Jones M. Consulters and nonconsulters in irritable bowel syndrome: What makes an IBS patient a patient? *Pract Gastroenterol.* 2003;12:15–26.
2. Drossman DA, Camilleri M, Mayer EA, et al. AGA technical review: Irritable bowel syndrome. *Gastroenterol.* 2002;123:2108.
3. Hwang C, Chang L, IBS. Gender differences. *Pract Gastroenterol.* 2004;12:13–28.
4. Lacy BE. Irritable bowel syndrome: An overview. *Gastroenterol Endosc.* 2004;2:27–33.
5. Rome II. In: Drossman DA, Corazziari E, Talley NJ, et al., eds. *The Functional Gastrointestinal Disorders.* 2nd ed. McLean, VA: Degnon Associates; 2000:355.
6. Sleisenger MH, Fordtran JS. *Gastrointestinal and Liver Disease.* 7th ed. Philadelphia: WB Saunders; 2002.

ICD9-CM
564.1 Irritable bowel syndrome

KEY WORDS

- Abdominal Pain
- Constipation
- Diarrhea
- Bloating
- Urgency
- Spastic Colon

LESBIAN HEALTH

Kelly A. McGarry, MD
Megan Hebert, MA

KEY CLINICAL POINTS

- Health care providers must avoid assuming heterosexuality.
- Health care providers need to be aware that some of their patients will identify as lesbians. Some patients may be engaging in same-sex relationships but will not want to identify as a lesbian.
- Create a safe health care environment for all patients by using gender-neutral language.
- Employ the same screening guidelines and lifestyle advice for lesbians as for heterosexual women (i.e., appropriate PAP smear, mammogram, and colonoscopy screening, exercise, diet, and alcohol moderation).
- Because same-sex partners are not legally recognized in most states, health care providers should discuss durable power of attorney for health care and finances with their lesbian patients.

 BASICS

DESCRIPTION

- There are an estimated 2.3 million women living in the United States who identify themselves as lesbian.
- The 2000 United States Census reported a total of 293,000 households headed by female same-sex partners.
  –Likely an underestimate
- Being lesbian is not a homogeneous experience.
  –Racial, ethnic, and socioeconomic diversity of the United States is mirrored in the lesbian community.
- In its 1996 report from the Council on Scientific Affairs, the American Medical Association stated "the physician's nonjudgmental recognition of sexual orientation and behavior enhances his or her ability to render optimal patient care in health as well as illness. . . the physician's failure to recognize homosexuality or the patient's reluctance to report his or her sexual orientation and behavior can lead to failure to screen, diagnose, or treat important medical problems." Physicians must be educated to "recognize the physical and psychological needs of their homosexual patients."
- Not all women who have had or are engaging currently in same-sex intimate contact label themselves as a lesbian and many women, regardless of sexual orientation, identity, and behavior, are uncomfortable discussing sexual histories with providers. Conveying respect for lesbians' lives and their partners will help to facilitate an open, honest medical encounter.

INTERACTING WITH THE HEALTH CARE SYSTEM

- Lesbians are significantly more likely than heterosexual women to experience discrimination during health care visits.
- In a 1999 study, 50% of lesbians rarely or never sought care despite being highly educated professionals with adequate access to health care due to negative experiences.
- Many lesbians do not disclose their sexual orientation to their health care providers for fear of receiving inadequate health care.
- Avoidance of routine medical care may be the most significant health risk for many lesbians.
- Many providers do not take a sexual history or inquire about sexual orientation
  - One study of general practitioners found that the most common reason cited for not asking about sexuality was that it was unimportant or that it was the patient's responsibility to mention.

- Another study found that physicians reported not being knowledgeable about sexual practices of lesbians and thus felt a barrier existed during discussions about sexual health.

CREATING A SAFE ENVIRONMENT

- Heterosexism is the ideology that denies the existence of and stigmatizes any nonheterosexual form of behavior and identity, analogous to sexism and racism.
- Health care providers may inadvertently assume heterosexuality and communicate heterosexist attitudes towards patients, making it more difficult for patients to disclose their sexual orientation.
- Examples of heterosexism in the provider's office include:
  - Medical intake forms that acknowledge only single, married, widowed and divorced patients
  - Omitting cervical cancer screening when a woman acknowledges she is a lesbian
  - Asking all women what form of birth control they need
- Health care providers can create a safe environment for lesbian patients through:
  - Ensuring that all office personnel use gender-neutral language
  - Making questions on intake forms inclusive (i.e., married, single, partnered, etc.)
  - Taking histories and communicating in a gender-neutral manner (i.e., "do you have a significant other?")
  - Refer to Table 1: "Developing A Patient Friendly Environment"

SPECIFIC HEALTH CONCERNS

- Although not true of all lesbians, many lesbians may have a higher prevalence of certain risk factors for diseases compared to their heterosexual peers, including:
  - Nulliparity/fewer pregnancies
  - Higher dietary fat intake
  - Higher prevalence of being overweight
  - Higher rates of alcohol consumption
  - Higher rates of cigarette smoking
- This may confer higher risk for certain diseases, including:
  - Coronary artery disease
  - Liver disease
  - Cancers, including breast, colon, lung, endometrial and ovarian cancer
- Counseling about lifestyle issues and screening for the above diseases should occur in lesbians just as in heterosexual women.

SPECIFIC DISEASES

- Sexually transmitted infections
  - Lesbians have been felt to be at low risk.
  - However, more than 10% of women with exclusively female partners have a history of STIs.
    - Viral STIs, including herpes and human papillomavirus, Treponema pallidum, and Trichomonas have been transmitted between women.
    - Bacterial vaginosis is often found in monogamous lesbian couples, suggesting it may be sexually transmitted.
    - Less reports on the transmission of gonorrhea, Chlamydia, and HIV, but there is a need to test in the appropriate clinical scenario.
  - Screening and counseling around safe sex depends on a thorough behavioral/sexual history and requires knowledge of lesbian sexual practices.

Table 1 Developing a Patient-Friendly Environment

Office environment
- Have a nondiscrimination policy visible to patients.
- Provide reading materials (magazines, health education pamphlets) that address the specific needs of lesbian patients.
- Ensure that the staff is comfortable with lesbian patients and their families.
- Ensure confidentiality.
- Make sure intake forms include options for nonmarried partners.

Interviewing

- Use gender neutral language:
  - "Do you have a significant other?"
- Use language free of heterosexist assumptions. Avoid questions like:
  - "Are you married?"
  - "What form of birth control do you use?"
- Ask about prior heterosexual intercourse and assess safe sex behavior.
  - "Have you ever been sexually active with men, women, or both?"
  - "Are you presently in a sexual relationship with a woman or a man or both?"
- Ask with whom the patient lives, who is important to them, and who would care for them if they were sick.
- Ask the patient how they would like to be referred to and/or how to refer to their partner.
- Encourage lesbians to have legal documents regarding who can make medical and/or legal decisions for them (Durable Power of Attorney for Healthcare and Finances).

- Lesbian sexual practices include:
  - High risk: Oral-vaginal contact, tribadism (genital-to-genital contact), digital stimulation, oral-anal contact, and sharing of sex toys
  - Lower risk: Kissing, rubbing genitals to partner's body
- Safer sex includes use of dental dams, surgical gloves, or plastic wrap with a water-based lubricant
  - Serve as a barrier to vaginal secretions or rectal exposure
- Cervical cancer
  - Rate of PAP testing may be lower in lesbians
  - Both lesbians and their health care providers may see them at low risk for the disease and not recommend screening.
  - Risk of cervical cancer is highest in lesbians who:
    - Have been treated for abnormal PAP in the past or have a history of HPV
    - Have had sex with men (between 50 and 80% of lesbians report heterosexual intercourse at some point in their lives)
    - Have a history of incest or early age at 1st coitus with men
    - Smoke cigarettes
  - Screen for cervical cancer using the same guidelines as for heterosexual women.

- Ovarian cancer
  - Lesbians may be at higher risk because of a lower likelihood of getting pregnant or using oral contraceptive pills (OCPs) for a prolonged period of time.
  - Lesbians with a family history of ovarian cancer may want to consider the potential benefits of using OCPs to reduce their risk.

PSYCHOSOCIAL CONSIDERATIONS
- Coming out/self-acceptance
  - Given that the larger culture is unaccepting of homosexuality, lesbians consistently receive the message that same-sex attraction is wrong and should be "fixed."
  - The process of self-acceptance, "coming out," requires that an individual recognize their same-sex attraction, act on their feelings, and be willing to negotiate preexisting relationships (with those who previously thought the individual was heterosexual).
  - The risk in "coming out" is the potential rejection from family, friends, colleagues, and self ("internalized homophobia").
  - Evidence suggests that "out" lesbians are more satisfied in their personal lives.
- Depression
  - Lesbians in the Women's Health Initiative (WHI) were more likely to have depression and to be taking antidepressants than their heterosexual counterparts.
  - Reasons cited by lesbians for their depression include:
    - Stress from isolation
    - Inferior social status
    - Lack of support from family and friends
  - Physicians should counsel lesbians around social supports as well as social stressors and inquire about symptoms of depression.
- Alcohol and tobacco use
  - Tobacco use is more prevalent in the lesbian population, however, the data regarding alcohol use is conflicting.
  - Recent studies suggests lesbians may drink more often than heterosexual women but the rates of heavy, abusive drinking may be no different.
  - Data from the WHI, however, found a higher incidence of heavy drinking among lesbians.
- Family/child rearing
  - Lesbians encounter obstacles when desiring to become parents including:
    - Potential rejection by family
    - Stigmatization from society as unfit parents
    - Limited availability of insurance coverage—many states offer no coverage for semen, office insemination, and infertility services to unmarried women, whether heterosexual or homosexual.
    - Difficulty accessing sperm banks
  - Children raised in lesbian households develop normally in the domains of sexual orientation, self-esteem, moral judgment, and intelligence.
  - Lesbians may also become parents through adoption or foster care.
  - Health care providers should discuss parenting issues with their lesbian patients, including encouraging both parents to adopt the child to ensure a permanent legal relationship to the child, durable power of attorney for health care and finances, and custody issues in the event of death or separation.
    - Consultation with a knowledgeable attorney should be advised.

L

- Domestic violence
  - Lesbians are not immune from domestic violence and should be screened for abusive relationships.

LEGAL ISSUES

- Lesbians in committed relationships are not granted the same legal and financial protection the U.S. laws confer to heterosexual couples:
  - Civil marriage contracts exist only in Massachusetts.
  - Civil unions exist in only 3 states.
  - 38 states have passed laws to prohibit recognition of same sex marriages.
  - 3 states have prevented recognition of any other state's domestic partnerships or civil unions.
  - Without legal recognition, same-sex partners are not entitled to many state and over 1,100 federal laws that protect married couples.
  - Despite legally sanctioned inequality:
    - Approximately 75% of Americans support laws to protect lesbians from prejudice and discrimination in employment and housing and to provide them with employment benefits, inheritance rights, employer-provided health insurance, and social security benefits.
    - The Kaiser Foundation survey found that 66% of Americans believe that homosexual behavior is a normal part of an individual's sexuality.

REFERENCES

1. Institute of Medicine. Lesbian health: Current assessment and directions for the future. Washington, DC: National Academy Press; 1999.
2. American Medical Association. Health care needs of gay men and lesbians in the United States. *JAMA*. 1996;275: 1354–1359.
3. Westerstahl A, Segesten K, Bjorkelung C. GPs and lesbian women in the consultation: Issues of awareness and knowledge. *Scand J Prim Health Care*. 2002;20:203–207.
4. Hinchliff S, Gott M, Galena E. 'I daresay I might find it embarrassing': General practitioners' perspectives on discussing sexual health issues with lesbian and gay patients. *Health Soc Care Community*. 2005;13:345–353.
5. Eliason MJ, Schope R. Does "Don't ask don't tell" apply to health care? Lesbian, gay and bisexual people's disclosure to health care providers. *Journal of the Gay and Lesbian Medical Association*. 2001;5:125–134.
6. Valanis BG, Bowen DJ, Bassford T, et al. Sexual Orientation and Health. *Arch Fam Med*. 2000;9:843–853.
7. Bailey JV, Farquhar C, Owen C, Whittaker D. Sexual behavior of lesbians and bisexual women. *Sex Transm Infect*. 2003;79:147–150.
8. Marrazzo JM, Stine K, Koutsky LA. Genital human papillomavirus infection in women who have sex with women. *Am J Obstet Gynecol*. 2000;183:770–774.
9. Oetjen H, Rothblum ED. When lesbians aren't gay: Factors affecting depression among lesbians. *J Homosex*. 2000;39:49–73.
10. Anderssen N, Amlie C, Ytteroy EA. Outcomes for children with lesbian or gay parents. A review of studies from 1978 to 2000. *Scand J Psychol*. 2002;43:335–351.

 MISCELLANEOUS

www.glma.org—Gay and Lesbian Medical Association: Organization for health care professionals providing information about lesbian and gay health research, public policy, advocacy, and patient information.

KEY WORDS

- Lesbian
- Same-sex Relationships
- Heterosexism

MASTITIS

Julie S. Taylor, MD, MSc

KEY CLINICAL POINTS

- The clinical diagnosis of mastitis is made when a lactating woman has a tender, hot, swollen, wedge-shaped area of breast associated with fever and chills.
- Women with mastitis should continue to breast-feed.
  - Stasis is often the initiating fact
  - Most important management is frequent and effective milk removal.
- Often a 10–14 day course of cephalexin, dicloxicillin, flucloxicillin, or clindamycin is needed to treat penicillin-resistant *Staphylococcus aureus*.

 BASICS

DESCRIPTION
- Inflammation of the breast, whether or not there is a bacterial infection present.
- Tender, hot, swollen, wedge-shaped area of breast associated with fever of 38.5 C or greater, chills, flu-like aching, and systemic illness

GENERAL PREVENTION
- Effective management of breast fullness and engorgement:
  - Improve latch
  - Do not restrict feeds.
  - Teach mothers to hand-express milk:
    - Before the feed, if the breasts are too full for the baby to attach
    - After the feed, if the baby does not relieve breast fullness
- Prompt attention to any signs of milk stasis:
  - Teach mothers to check their breasts for lumps, pain, or redness.
  - Any signs of milk stasis, mother needs to:
    - Increase the frequency of breastfeeding.
    - Apply heat to breast.
    - Massage any lumpy areas towards the nipple.
- Attention to other difficulties with breastfeeding by skilled professionals in a timely fashion.
- Rest as much as possible.

EPIDEMIOLOGY
- Common condition in lactating women
- Majority of cases occur in the 1st 6 weeks postpartum
- Prevalence of 20% in the 1st 6 months postpartum
- Mastitis can occur any time during lactation.

RISK FACTORS
- Poor latch
- Infrequent feeds
- Missed feeds
- Scheduled frequency or duration of feeds
- Milk oversupply
- Rapid weaning
- Pressure on the breast (e.g., tight bra)
- Damaged nipple
- Blocked nipple duct
- Maternal or infant illness
- Maternal stress and fatigue

ETIOLOGY
- Milk stasis is often the initiating factor, for whatever reason.

- There have been few research trials in this area.
- Evidence for associations other than milk stasis is inconclusive.

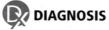 **DIAGNOSIS**

SIGNS AND SYMPTOMS
- Red, painful breast
- Usually unilateral
- Subjective fever/chills
- Most often within 6 weeks postpartum

Physical Exam
- Fever
- Ill-appearing
- Exquisitely tender, firm, red breast
- +/− Nipple abnormality

TESTS
- Primarily a clinical diagnosis.
- Laboratory investigations and other diagnostic procedures are NOT routinely needed.

Lab
- Breast milk culture and sensitivity testing should be undertaken only if:
  - There is no response to antibiotics within 48 hours
  - Mastitis recurs
  - Mastitis is hospital-acquired
  - Case is severe or unusual
- To obtain a culture:
  - Cleanse the nipple
  - Collect a mid-stream, clean-catch sample of hand-expressed breast milk into a sterile cup.
  - Take care not to touch the inside of the container.

DIFFERENTIAL DIAGNOSIS
- Breast abscess
- Breast mass
- Inflammatory or ductal carcinoma

 TREATMENT

INITIAL STABILIZATION
Focuses primarily on frequent and effective milk removal.

GENERAL MEASURES
- Effective milk removal
  - Breastfeed more frequently, starting on the affected side
  - If pain interferes, start breast-feeding on the unaffected side and promptly switch to the affected side as soon as milk let down occurs.
  - Position the infant so that the chin or the nose points to the blockage.
  - During the feed, massage the breast from blocked area toward the nipple.
  - After the feed, consider expressing by hand or pumping.
- Supportive measures
  - Rest
  - Adequate fluids and nutrition
  - Practical help at home
  - Direct application of heat prior to feeding may help milk flow.
  - Direct application of cold packs after feeding may reduce pain and swelling.

MEDICATIONS (DRUGS)

- Analgesia:
  - Antiinflammatory agents, such as ibuprofen, may help with the milk ejection reflex and be more effective than simple analgesics, such as acetaminophen.
    - Ibuprofen is safe during breast-feeding.
    - Doses up to 1.6 g/d are not detected in breast milk.
- Antibiotics:
  - A 10- to 14-day course is indicated if:
    - Symptoms are not improving after 12–24 hours of conservative measures or if a woman is acutely ill
  - The most common pathogen is
    - Penicillin-resistant *Staphylococcus aureus*
    - Less common are *streptococcus* or *Escherichia coli*
  - Possible treatment regimens include:
    - Cephalexin 500 mg PO b.i.d. OR
    - Dicloxacillin 500 mg PO q.i.d. OR
    - Flucloxicillin 500 mg PO q.i.d. OR
    - Clindamycin 300 mg PO q.i.d. (for women with severe penicillin hypersensitivity)

FOLLOW-UP

- Initial clinical response to antibiotics is usually rapid, within 1–2 days.
- Consider hospital admission for intravenous antibiotic therapy if a woman is extremely ill or has inadequate support at home.
  - If hospitalized, rooming of the baby with the mother is mandatory so that breast-feeding can continue.

Issues for Referral
- Consider a lactation consultation for anyone with mastitis.
- Consider surgical or infectious disease evaluation for the mother if she does not improve in 48 hours or has had more than 1 episode.

COMPLICATIONS
- Early cessation of breast-feeding (which may actually exacerbate mastitis)
- Breast abscess (diagnosed on physical exam and confirmed with breast ultrasound)
- Fungal infection (in which case treatment is needed for both mother and baby)

ALERT
Mastitis more than twice in the same location warrants evaluation for an underlying mass.

REFERENCES

1. Academy of Breastfeeding Medicine Clinical Protocol #4: Mastitis, February 2, 2002. Accessed April, 2005 at http://www.bfmed.org/protocol/mastitis.pdf.
2. World Health Organization 2000. Mastitis: Causes and management. Department of Child and Adolescent Health and Development. WHO/FCH/CAH/00.13, Geneva.
3. Hale T. *Medications and Mother's Milk: A Manual of Lactational Pharmacology.* 11th ed. Texas: Pharmasoft Medical Publishing; 2004.

CODES
ICD9-CM
- 675.14 Mastitis (purulent)
- 675.24 Mastitis (nonpurulent)
- 611.71 Breast pain

KEY WORDS

- Mastitis
- Postpartum
- Breast-feeding
- Lactation
- Nipple Pain
- Abscess, Breast

MENOPAUSE

Michele G. Cyr, MD, FACP

KEY CLINICAL POINTS

- Menopause is the permanent cessation of menstruation resulting from loss of ovarian function.
- Symptoms include changes in menstrual cycle, vasomotor symptoms, and urogenital atrophy.
- Medical and surgical treatment options are available for the symptoms associated with menopause.
- Hormone therapy for vasomotor symptoms should be at the lowest dose needed for the shortest duration of time.

BASICS

DESCRIPTION
- Menopause is the permanent cessation of menstruation that results from loss of ovarian function.
  Spontaneous menopause refers to the expected loss of ovarian function associated with aging.
  Induced menopause refers to the cessation of ovarian function from bilateral oophorectomy (surgical menopause) or from chemotherapy or pelvic irradiation.
  Premature menopause is menopause occurring before the age of 40.
  Perimenopause is the 2–8 years preceding menopause and one year after the final menstrual period.
- System(s) affected: Endocrine, urogenital, reproductive, and vasomotor.

EPIDEMIOLOGY
- Mean age of menopause: 51.4 years
- Typical range: 48–55 years
- Female only

Prevalence
- Incidence/Prevalence in United States: In the year 2000, 45.6 million women were menopausal. Of these 39.9 million were >51 years old, 3.12 million were spontaneously menopausal between 40- and 50-years-old, 2 million were surgically menopausal, and 0.5 million had experienced premature menopause <40 years of age.
- It is estimated that in the year 2000, 1.8 million women >51 years of age became menopausal and 263,000 experienced surgical menopause.
- By the year 2020, it is expected that over 50 million women in the United States will be menopausal.

RISK FACTORS
- Current smoking is a risk factor for earlier menopause (~1.5 years) and increased risk of hot flashes.
- Age of maternal menopause predicts age of menopausal transition.
- Less physical activity is a risk factor for hot flashes.

PATHOPHYSIOLOGY
- Symptoms associated with menopause are directly or indirectly related to declining estrogen levels.
- The precise cause of hot flashes is not known.

ETIOLOGY
Loss of ovarian function
- Spontaneous
- Induced
  - Surgical-bilateral oophorectomy
  - Chemotherapy
  - Pelvic irradiation

ASSOCIATED CONDITIONS
- Osteoporosis
- Incontinence, possibly
- Coronary artery disease, possibly
- Depression, possibly

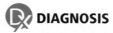 DIAGNOSIS

SIGNS AND SYMPTOMS
- Menstrual changes
  - ~90% women experience 4–8 years of menstrual changes before spontaneous menopause
  - Change in menstrual flow, duration of bleeding, cycle length, and skipped periods
  - Presumed caused by anovulatory cycles
- Vasomotor symptoms: Hot flashes and night sweats
  - ~66–75% of menopausal women experience hot flashes
  - Women experience hot flashes severe enough to seek treatment: ~25%
  - Increase during menopausal transition with greatest frequency 2 years after menopause
  - ~50–75% of women experience hot flashes for <5 years after menopause.
- Urogenital atrophy
  - ~25% of menopausal women, 5 years after menopause, have symptoms related to urogenital atrophy.
  - Of the women with urogenital symptoms, only 25% seek treatment
  - Symptoms may include: Vaginal dryness or irritation, discomfort during sexual activity, dyspareunia, urinary symptoms of frequency, dysuria and incontinence, and vaginal discharge.

History
- Absence of menstrual periods for >12 months in nonpregnant women >45 years of age is diagnostic of menopause.
- Hot flashes, night sweats, insomnia, and menstrual changes are symptoms of perimenopause. These are helpful in diagnosis when menstrual changes cannot be assessed after hysterectomy.

Physical Exam
- Vital signs
- Thyroid examination
- Breast examination
- Pelvic examination

TESTS
Bone densitometry: Postmenopausal women <65 years old with additional risk factors for osteoporosis and all women ≥65 years old

Lab
- May not be required if history consistent with diagnosis
- FSH >40 iu/mL
- Estradiol <20 pg/mL
- TSH: To rule out thyroid disease

Imaging
- Vaginal ultrasound to evaluate abnormal vaginal bleeding (endometrial biopsy if endometrial stripe ≥4 mm)

- Mammography
  - For women 40–50 years of age: Every 1–2 years
  - For women ≥50 years of age: Annually
  - Annually for all women on HT

Diagnostic Procedures
Endometrial biopsy for abnormal vaginal bleeding

DIFFERENTIAL DIAGNOSIS
- Menstrual changes
  - Pregnancy
  - Endometrial cancer
  - Pituitary failure
  - Thyroid disease
- Hot flashes
  - Hyperthyroid
  - Carcinoid syndrome
  - Panic attacks
- Urogenital symptoms
  - Vaginitis
  - Urinary tract infection

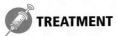 TREATMENT

GENERAL MEASURES
Vasomotor symptoms
- Layered clothing
- Avoid identified triggers
- Paced respirations
- Relaxation response

Urogenital atrophy
- Continued sexual stimulation/activity helps to prevent/treat urogenital atrophy

Diet
Vasomotor symptoms:
- Avoid foods that trigger hot flashes; e.g., spicy foods, caffeine, alcohol, and hot foods.
- Diets high in soy may decrease hot flashes, but evidence is conflicting.
- Vitamin E supplements (<400 IU daily, generally safe) have been shown to have only a marginal effect on hot flashes.

Activity
- Vasomotor symptoms
  - Increased physical activity may decrease hot flashes
- Urogenital atrophy
  - Kegel exercises help stress incontinence

 MEDICATION (DRUGS)

- Menstrual Changes
  - Low dose oral contraceptives can be continued in nonsmokers without other contraindications.
    - Check FSH after 6 days off oral contraceptives to diagnose menopause transition.
- Vasomotor symptoms
  - Choice depends on severity of hot flashes, response to other measures, patient preference, and relative contraindications.
  - If hormone therapy is used, it should be at the lowest effective dose for the shortest duration of time.

- Systemic estrogen alone for women without a uterus (pills, patches, or vaginal ring that gives systemic levels of hormone) or estrogen plus progestin (cyclic or continuous) for women with a uterus.
  - SSRIs and SNRIs – venlafaxine* (37.5–75 mg/daily), paroxetine CR* (12.5 or 25 mg/daily), and fluoxetine* (20 mg/daily)
  - Gabapentin* (300–900 mg/daily)
  - Megestrol (20–80 mg/daily)
  - Clonidine* (.2–.3 mg) patches or (0.1–0.2 mg PO daily or b.i.d.)
- Contraindications
  - To estrogen and/or progestin – any estrogen sensitive tumor, h/o DVT or PE, active liver disease, undiagnosed abnormal vaginal bleeding, and coronary artery disease
- Urogenital atrophy
  - Over-the-counter vaginal preparations
    - Water soluble lubricants
    - Bioadhesive moisturizers
  - Prescription
    - Estrogen: Vaginal (creams, tablets, rings), if treating only vaginal symptoms. Use systemic estrogen, if also treating vasomotor symptoms. Use lowest effective dose for shortest duration needed.

Complementary and Alternative Medicine
Vasomotor symptoms

Black cohosh (20–40 mg of extract, b.i.d., for up to 6 months)

SURGERY
Menstrual changes: Generally not required
- Endometrial ablation
- Hysterectomy

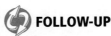 FOLLOW-UP

PROGNOSIS
- Menstrual cycle irregularity and changes in menstrual flow should cease at menopause.
- Vasomotor symptoms should improve with time; therefore, tapering treatment, at least annually, is advisable to determine whether it can be stopped or the dose decreased.
- Urogenital symptoms are likely to continue and potentially worsen after menopause unless measures are employed to prevent and/or treat.

COMPLICATIONS
Depending on treatment choice

HT: Abnormal mammograms, endometrial hyperplasia or carcinoma, breast cancer, coronary events, DVT/PE

PATIENT MONITORING
For patients on hormone therapy:
- Vaginal bleeding diary
- Mammograms annually
- Lipid profile
- Monitor for DVT, PE
- Monitor for coronary artery disease events with history, EKGs, and further testing as warranted by symptoms

*Off label indication

REFERENCES

1. Guthrie JR, Dennerstein L, Taffe JR, et al. The menopausal transition: A 9-Year prospective population-based study. The Melbourne Women's Midlife Health Project. *Climacteric*. 2004;375–389.
2. Kronenberg F, Fugh-Berman A. Complementary and alternative medicine for menopausal symptoms: A review of randomized, controlled trials. *Ann Int Med*. 2002; 137:805–813.
3. NAMS – The North American Menopause Society, with assistance from Santoro NF, Clarkson TB, Feedman RR, et al. Treatment of menopause-associated vasomotor symptoms: Position statement of the North American Menopause Society. *Menopause*. 2004;11:11–33.
4. Nelson HD. Commonly used types of postmenopausal estrogen for treatment of hot flashes. *JAMA*. 2004; 291:1610–1620.
5. Nelson HD. Postmenopausal estrogen for treatment of hot flashes: Clinical applications. *JAMA*. 2004;291:1621–1625.
6. NIH State-of-the-Science Panel. National Institutes of Health state-of-the-science conference statement: Management of menopause-related symptoms. *Ann Int Med*. 2005;142: 1003–1013.
7. The NIH state-of-the-Science conference on management of menopause-related symptoms. *Am J Med*. 2005;118: 1401–1412.
8. NAMS – The North American Menopause Society. Menopause practice: A clinician's guide. Cleveland, OH; The North American Menopause Society; 2004.
9. Websites: www.4women.org
10. www.menopause.org
11. www.nhlbi.nih.gov/health/women/pht_facts.htm

ADDITIONAL READING

The Women's Health Initiative Steering Committee. Effects of conjugated equine estrogen in postmenopausal women with hysterectomy. The Women's Health Initiative Randomized Controlled Trial. *JAMA*. 2004;291:1701–1712.

Writing Group for the Women's Health Initiative Investigators. Risks and benefits of estrogen plus progestin in healthy postmenopausal women: Principal results from the Women's Health Initiative Randomized Controlled Trial. *JAMA*. 2002;288:321–333.

 MISCELLANEOUS

CODES
ICD9-CM
- 256.31 Premature menopause
- 627.2 Symptomatic menopause or female climacteric states
- 627.8 Other specified menopausal and postmenopausal disorders

KEY WORDS

- Menopause
- Hot Flashes
- Vasomotor Symptoms
- Hormone Therapy
- Menstrual Changes
- Urogenital Atrophy
- Vaginal Atrophy

M

MITTELSCHMERZ

Michelle A. Stozek Anvar, MD

KEY CLINICAL POINTS

- History of midcycle pelvic pain is key to diagnosis
- Need to rule out other causes of pelvic pain

 BASICS

DESCRIPTION
Midcycle left or right lower quadrant pain associated with ovulation that lasts 24–48 hours

EPIDEMIOLOGY
Prevalence
Approximately 20% of menstruating women experience mittelschmerz either each month or intermittently

RISK FACTORS
Menstruating females

PATHOPHYSIOLOGY
- The mechanism is not clearly understood.
- Theories include:
  - An ovarian follicle releasing blood, follicular fluid, and prostaglandins causing local irritation
  - Increased fallopian tube peristalsis during ovulation, and
  - Rapid expansion of the dominant follicle causing pain

ASSOCIATED CONDITIONS
None

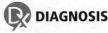 **DIAGNOSIS**

SIGNS AND SYMPTOMS
History
- Sudden onset of RLQ or LLQ pain that occurs on days 12–16 of the menstrual cycle.
- Occasionally there is midcycle vaginal bleeding
- Pain can be described as intense, dull, or aching pelvic pain.
- Symptoms typically last 24–48 hours.

Physical Exam
- Tenderness to palpation in the right or left lower quadrants.
- Normal gynecologic exam except for occasional midcycle bleeding

TESTS
Lab
- Serum β-human chorionic gonadotropin (β-hCG)
  +/– transvaginal ultrasound to rule out ectopic pregnancy
- Rule out infection (cervicitis, pelvic inflammatory disease)
  - Chlamydia
  - Gonorrhea
  - Trichomonas

Imaging
- May need pelvic ultrasound to rule out other ovarian or uterine pathology
- CT to rule out appendicitis, if RLQ tenderness, or other GI pathology

DIFFERENTIAL DIAGNOSIS
- Ectopic pregnancy
- Pelvic inflammatory disease

- Adnexal cysts or masses with bleeding, torsion, or rupture
- Uterine infection
- Infarction or torsion of leiomyomas
- Appendicitis if pain is in RLQ
- Endometriosis

 TREATMENT

GENERAL MEASURES
Patient education regarding diagnosis

Activity
As tolerated

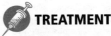 **MEDICATION (DRUGS)**

First Line
Analgesics, generally NSAIDs or acetaminophen, are sufficient.

Second Line
For recurrent symptoms, oral contraceptives, which suppress ovulation, are helpful.

 FOLLOW-UP

DISPOSITION
Once diagnosed, patients can be treated as an outpatient.

Issues for Referral
Referral is necessary only if diagnosis is uncertain.

PROGNOSIS
- Symptoms may recur.
- Patients should be educated regarding symptoms and treatment.

COMPLICATIONS
None

REFERENCES

1. Gerber-Zimmerman P. Triaging lower abdominal pain. *RN*. 2002;65:52–58.
2. *Mittelschmerz in Stenchever: Comprehensive Gynecology*, 4th ed. Mosby Inc. St. Kouis, MO. 2001.
3. Myers DL, Aguilar VC. et al. Gynecologic manifestations of interstitial cystitis. *Clin Obst Gyn*. 2002;45:233–241.

CODES
ICD9-CM
625.2 Mittelschmerz

KEY WORDS

- Pelvic Pain
- Ovulation
- Midcycle Pelvic Pain

MULTIPLE SCLEROSIS

Elaine C. Jones, MD

KEY CLINICAL POINTS

- Multiple sclerosis (MS) can present with a wide variety of symptoms and complaints.
- History and magnetic resonance imaging (MRI) will usually confirm the diagnosis.
- Various treatments are available that decrease disease activity and may decrease long-term disability.

BASICS

DESCRIPTION

- An autoimmune disease that attacks the myelin on neurons in the central nervous system (brain and spinal cord)
- Types include:
  - Relapsing remitting (RRMS)
    - Intermittent symptoms which resolve completely between episodes
  - Primary progressive (PPMS)
    - Slow decline in functioning from the onset of symptoms
  - Secondary progressive (SPMS)
    - Symptoms initially consistent with RRMS, but then followed by slow decline in functioning

EPIDEMIOLOGY

- Women affected 3 times more than men
- World-wide: Caucasians more affected than Asian or Black populations
- Appears to be hemispheric contribution, such that frequency of disease increases as distance from equator increases (at least to a point)

Incidence

Age at onset follows unimodal distribution with a peak onset between 20 and 30 years of age.

Prevalence

- Approximately 250,000–350,000 cases of MS in the United States currently.
- In tropical regions, prevalence is 5 per 100,000.
- In areas further from the equator, prevalence can be 30–100 per 100,000.
- Migration from high to low prevalence areas before age 15 lowers risk of developing MS, but migration after age 15 has no effect on risk.

RISK FACTORS

- There is much debate about environmental causes for MS.
- Viral infection in a susceptible individual is the most commonly proposed mechanism but a common viral cause has not been identified.
- Head injury and trauma have been suggested but linkage has not been proven.

Genetics

- Genetic studies suggest an inherited susceptibility to MS.
- Siblings of MS patients have a 2.6% and children of MS patients have a 1.5% increased risk over the general population.
- Monozygotic twins have a 26% concordance rate for MS.
- Specific genes for MS have not been identified but there is a high correlation with HLA haplotypes DR15, DQ6.

PATHOPHYSIOLOGY

- Cellular immunity is focused on as the problem in MS because infiltration of T cells is seen in plaques.
- Specifically changes in CD8+ T cells seem to play an important role in MS.
- Perivascular lymphocyte and macrophage infiltration is also common in CNS plaques.
- Type and amount of inflammation that occurs may be directly related to the amount of damage and therefore the severity of symptoms.
- Result of the cellular infiltration is breakdown of the myelin sheaths surrounding the axons.
- Although MS is categorized as a demyelinating process we now know that the axons are often involved as well.

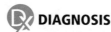 DIAGNOSIS

SIGNS AND SYMPTOMS

- Motor
  - Weakness
  - Spasticity
  - Hyperreflexia
- Sensory
  - Decreased pain/temp
  - Positive Romberg test
  - Decreased vibration/position sense
- Cerebellar
  - Ataxia
  - Tremor
  - Dysarthria
- Cranial Nerves
  - III/Optic Neuritis: Monocular vision loss, color blindness (red affected most)
  - V, VII: Facial numbness, weakness
  - VIII: Hearing changes
- Autonomic
  - Bladder dysfunction
  - Bowel dysfunction
  - Hypo/hypertension
  - Sweating
- Cognitive
  - Memory, concentration, judgment

History

- History is the key to diagnosis
  - History of more than one event is necessary
  - Review events in the past that may have been ignored or attributed to other causes.
- History will help with diagnosing type of MS
  - Episodes that come and resolve completely suggest Relapsing Remitting MS.
  - If from the onset of symptoms there is a slow decline in functioning this might suggest Primary Progressive MS.
  - A patient who begins with RRMS and then has a slow decline in function may have Secondary Progressive MS.

Physical Exam

- Physical findings will be consistent with areas of white matter that are affected – motor, sensory, cerebellar, etc.

- Questions about autonomic symptoms are important.
- MMSE and cognitive testing can demonstrate impairment in memory and language.

TESTS

- MRI: 2nd only to history in importance.
- Lumbar puncture: May be normal.
  - Mild elevations of lymphocytes (5–20 cells/mm^2) seen in 40% of MS patients
  - IgG index increased in 90% of patients
  - Oligoclonal bands seen in 90%
  - Myelin basic protein elevated in 80%
- Visual Evoked Potentials
  - Sensitive for detecting optic nerve lesions
- Somatosensory Evoked Potentials
  - May be useful in diagnosing spinal lesions that can be missed by MRI

Lab

Rule out other etiologies: Lyme, B12 deficiency, HIV, sarcoid, inflammatory disorders

Imaging

MRI:

- Positive in approximately 90% of cases
- Proton density and T2 weighted images show lesions best
- Gadolinium enhancement occurs in new lesions and lasts 4–6 weeks
- T1 hypointensities suggest more severe damage and may reflect axonal loss
- Various locations of the lesions make MS more likely: Flame-shaped lesions in or around the corpus callosum, brainstem lesions, and juxtacortical lesions.

DIFFERENTIAL DIAGNOSIS

- Stroke
- Hemiplegic migraine
- Lyme disease
- HIV
- Acute disseminated encephalomyelitis (ADEM)
- Neurosyphilis
- SLE
- Sarcoidosis
- B12 deficiency
- Guillain-Barre syndrome

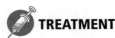 TREATMENT

GENERAL MEASURES

- In the setting of an acute exacerbation IV steroids are the mainstay of treatment.
- Currently there are a number of disease-modifying treatments. These work best for relapsing remitting forms of MS, but recent advances in secondary progressive treatments have come out.
- More attention needs to be paid to physical and cognitive symptoms associated with MS, and treatment should be offered for these as well.

Diet

- No clear association between diet and MS
- Well-balanced, healthy diet will maintain general good health.

Activity

- Maintaining an active lifestyle is important to prevent worsening weakness, help with mood issues, and decrease disability.
- Activity may need to be modified to take into account periods of increased fatigue.

Physical Therapy

- Can be very important in patients with MS
- Pool therapy has been especially helpful
  - Significant benefit for spasticity
  - Can help decrease pain
  - Improves ADLs

 MEDICATION (DRUGS)

- Acute Treatments
  - Methylprednisolone 1 gm IV per day for 3–7 days
  - Plasmapheresis every other day, 7 treatments
    - Shown to be helpful in acute attacks when steroids have failed,
- Chronic Treatments
  - RRMS
    - Interferon Beta-1b (Betaseron)
      - 0.25 mg every other day
      - Common side effects include flu-like symptoms, myalgias, fever, and injection site reactions.
      - Liver enzyme elevation is possible and should be monitored. Monitor liver function tests.
    - Interferon Beta-1a (Avonex, Rebif)
      - Avonex: 30 μg IM a week
      - Common side effects: Flu-like symptoms, myalgias, fever, and injection site reactions.
      - Monitor liver function tests
      - Rebif: 44 μg sq tiw
      - Common side effects: Flu-like symptoms, myalgias, fever, injection site reactions
      - Monitor liver function tests
    - Glatiramer Acetate (Copaxone): 20 mg sq per day
      - Most common side effect is injection site reactions
  - Progressive MS
    - Cyclophosphamide: May be helpful in progressive MS.
    - Mitoxantrone (Novantrone): 12 mg/m^2 once every 3 months, max cumulative dose 140 mg/m^2.
      - Also used for worsening RR MS that is not responding to other therapies
      - Pretreatment patients must undergo echocardiogram for cardiac output monitoring, CBC, and when appropriate pregnancy testing
- Treatment of associated symptoms
  - Spasticity: ~ 70% of MS patients
    - Baclofen: 5 mg b.i.d./t.i.d., max 80 mg daily recommended (higher doses can be used if tolerated). Can be given intrathecally which minimizes side effects.
    - Tizanidine: 2–4 mg t.i.d., max 36 mg daily.
    - Botulinum toxin (Botox, Myobloc): Injected IM to relieve spasticity/pain.
  - Depression: Extremely common in MS but usually responds very well to treatment.
    - SSRIs: Better tolerated and effective for depression in MS.
      - Celexa: 20 mg PO every day
      - Lexapro: 10–20 mg PO every day
      - Prozac: 20–60 mg PO every day
      - Zoloft: 50–200 mg PO every day
    - TCAs: Often worsen fatigue and can affect bladder/bowel function
  - Fatigue: One of most common and problematic symptoms
    - Lifestyle: Good sleep and routine exercise important, limit activities, rest when fatigue worse, plan activities when better

- Amantidine: 100 mg daily or b.i.d.
- Modafinil: 100–400 mg daily in divided doses
- Cognitive dysfunction: ~65% of MS patients
  - Short-term memory loss, visuospatial and/or verbal difficulties, and problems with attention, concentration, information processing
  - No proven therapies yet. In some preliminary studies donepizil (Aricept) showed possible benefit and is currently being studied more formally.
- Bladder dysfunction: ~75% of MS patients
  - Oxybutynin (Ditropan): 5 mg b.i.d./t.i.d. or extended release daily
  - Tolterodine (Detrol): 2 mg b.i.d.
  - Doxazosin (Cardura): 1 mg every day
  - Prazosin (Minipress): 1 mg b.i.d.
  - Tamsulosin (Flomax): 0.4 mg every day
  - Terazosin (Hytrin): 1 mg q.h.s.

Pregnancy Considerations
- Pregnancy does not alter risk of developing MS but does influence disease activity
- Relapse rates drop by 1/3 during the last 2 trimesters but increases in postpartum.
- Most studies conclude that there are no long-term effects of pregnancy on MS.
- Patients with MS who become pregnant should not be considered "high risk" pregnancies based solely on their MS.
- No contraindication to vaginal delivery in a healthy MS patient, however fatigue during labor can occur.
- Most medications used in MS have not been studied in pregnancy and therefore should NOT be used during pregnancy or breast-feeding.

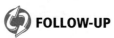 # FOLLOW-UP

Issues for Referral
To neurologist to aid in diagnosis and treatment

PROGNOSIS
- Amount of disease seen on MRI at time of presentation correlates with amount of disability over time.
  - Higher disease burden at presentation is associated with worse disability.
  - MRI disease burden at other times of the disease are less predictive of outcome.
- Positive indicators include minimal disability at 5 years after onset, complete and rapid remission of initial symptoms, age ≤35 years at onset, only 1 exacerbation in the 1st year, sensory symptoms, and optic neuritis.
- Negative indicators include polysymptomatic at onset (suggesting multiple systems involved), cerebellar signs, and spinal involvement.

- Life expectancy has not been shown to be shortened by a diagnosis of MS.

PATIENT MONITORING
- Periodic neurologic examination is important to assess for worsening symptoms.
- Little evidence supports routine MRI monitoring in MS patients.
  - It may be useful if new symptoms arise that cannot be explained by MS or if decisions are being made regarding response to treatment.
- Some patients have been shown to develop neutralizing antibodies to the interferon therapies.
  - Unclear importance of these antibodies
  - Routine monitoring or screening for antibodies is not currently recommended.

REFERENCES

1. Frohman EM, Goodin DS, Calabresi PA, et al. The utility of MRI in suspected MS: Report of the therapeutics and technology assessment subcommittee of the American Academy of Neurology. *Neurology.* 2003;61:602–611.
2. Lublin, FD. Treatments for multiple sclerosis. *Continuum: Lifelong learning in Neurology.* 2004;10:120–141.
3. McDonald WI, Compston A, Edan G, et al. Recommended diagnostic criteria for multiple sclerosis: Guideline from the international panel on the diagnosis of multiple sclerosis. *Ann Neurology.* 2001;50:121–127.
4. Tullman M. Symptomatic therapy in multiple sclerosis. *Continuum: Lifelong learning in Neurology.* 2004;10:142–172.

ADDITIONAL READING

Cook SD, ed. *Handbook of Multiple Sclerosis.* 3rd ed. New York, NY: Marcel Dekker, Inc Publishers; 2001.

CODES
ICD9-CM
340 Multiple sclerosis

KEY WORDS

- Cerebral Demyelinating Diseases
- Hemiplegia
- Optic Neuritis
- Spasticity

M

NABOTHIAN CYSTS

Agnieszka K. Bialikiewicz, MD
Melissa Nothnagle, MD

KEY CLINICAL POINTS

- Nabothian cysts are common benign cysts of the uterine cervix that do not spontaneously regress.
- They are rarely symptomatic unless very large
- Symptomatic cysts may be treated in the office setting with electrocautery or cryotherapy.
- Deep cysts may be difficult to differentiate from minimal-deviation adenocarcinoma of the cervix.

BASICS

DESCRIPTION
- First described by German anatomist Martin Naboth in 1707
- Also called inclusion cysts or retention cysts
- Visible on speculum exam as round or oval cervical lesions, translucent or opaque with ivory-yellow tinge
- Range in size from microscopic to 2–4 cm in diameter
- May be single or multiple in number
- Almost always superficial but can be deep, extending to serosa or surrounding paracervical connective tissue
- Numerous or very large cysts can produce enlargement of the cervix resulting in dyspareunia
- Cysts farthest from cervical os indicate the extent of the "transformation zone" (the area of squamous metaplasia between the endocervical columnar epithelium and ectocervical squamous epithelium).

RISK FACTORS
- Nabothian cysts are associated with increased age and higher parity
- Chronic cervicitis may predispose to development of Nabothian cysts

PATHOPHYSIOLOGY
- The uterine cervix consists of the endocervix, with mucous secreting columnar epithelium, and the ectocervix, with squamous epithelium.
- Inflammation at the squamo-columnar junction induces a continuous repair process.
- This healing process results in the growth of squamous epithelium over the columnar cells of the ectocervix, which continue to secrete mucus, resulting in cystic dilatation.
- Chronic inflammation (i.e., cervicitis) also leads to stenosis of endocervical glands, resulting in retention of mucous and cystic enlargement.

ETIOLOGY
Benign lesions resulting from normal squamous metaplasia at the squamo-columnar junction or chronic inflammation of the cervix

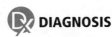 DIAGNOSIS

- Nabothian cysts can be diagnosed clinically, based on their appearance on vaginal speculum exam.
- Colposcopic examination and biopsy may be useful to diagnose lesions with atypical features.

SIGNS AND SYMPTOMS
- Nabothian cysts are most often asymptomatic.
- Increased size or number can cause clinical symptoms such as:
  - Sensation of fullness in vagina
  - Dyspareunia
  - Low back pain
  - Spotting if associated with chronic cervicitis

Physical Exam
- Smooth, tense, round or oval cysts
- Slightly raised from the surface of the cervix
- Few millimeters to 2–4 cm in size
- Translucent or opaque with ivory or bluish tinge; may be hemorrhagic
- Single or grouped
- Branching network of vessels visible over the surface in a regular pattern
- With numerous large or deep cysts, cervical enlargement palpable on bimanual exam

TESTS
Lab
Cytology:
For evaluation of lesions with atypical features

Imaging
- Transvaginal ultrasound
  - For diagnosis of deep cysts or those that are not visible on speculum exam
- Computed Tomography (CT)
  - To differentiate Nabothian cysts from endometriosis, Gartner duct cysts or mucoceles
  - Not useful for cysts >2 cm, as CT may confuse them with cystic adnexal mass
- Magnetic resonance imaging (MRI)
  - Cysts appear smooth-walled and do not enhance with intravenous gadolinium
  - For evaluation of deep Nabothian cysts (to differentiate from cystic adnexal mass)
  - For evaluation of large diameter (>2 cm) cysts

Diagnostic Procedures/Surgery
- Speculum and bimanual exam usually sufficient
- If atypical appearance:
  - Colposcopy with or without biopsy
  - Drainage with cytological analysis
  - Excision for histopathological assessment

Pathologic Findings
- Gross examination:
  - Round or oval mucin-filled cysts extending from mucosa to endocervical stroma
- Microscopic features:
  - Round cysts, lined by single layer of columnar epithelial cells containing variable amounts of cytoplasm
  - Basally situated nuclei with fine chromatin and small nucleoli without cytologic atypia

DIFFERENTIAL DIAGNOSIS
- Cervical pregnancy
- Gartner duct cyst: Remnant of Wollfian duct, seen on lateral wall of vagina
- Cervical stenosis
- Mesonephric cyst: Remnant of Wollfian duct found deep within cervical stroma forming cysts up to 2.5 cm in size

- Endometriosis: May form cystic structures on cervix that appear red-black and are non-blanching
- Minimal-deviation adenocarcinoma (MDA): Adnexal adenocarcinoma which mimics cystic mass of cervix with benign appearing glands

 ## TREATMENT

GENERAL MEASURES

Treatment is rarely needed as Nabothian cysts are generally asymptomatic.

 ## MEDICATION (DRUGS)

SURGERY

- For symptomatic large Nabothian cysts:
  - Electrocautery
  - Cryotherapy
  - Aspiration
- For abnormal appearing lesions requiring histopathological assessment:
  - Conization
  - Excisional biopsy

FOLLOW-UP

No follow up necessary unless surgical intervention needed.

PROGNOSIS

- No malignant potential
- No spontaneous resolution

COMPLICATIONS

Enlargement of the cervix

REFERENCES

1. Burghardt E. *Colposcopy-Cervical Pathology Textbook and Atlas*. 2nd ed. New York, NY: Thieme Medical Publishers, Inc.; 1991.
2. Fogel SR, Slasky BS. Sonography of nabothian cysts. *AJR* 1982;138:927–930.
3. Clement PB, Young RH. Deep Nabothian Cysts of the uterine cervix. A possible source of confusion with minimal-deviation adenocarcinoma. *Int J Gynecol Pathol*. 1989;8:340–348.
4. Merrill JA. Benign lesions of the cervix uteri. In: Danforth DN, Scott JR, eds. *Obstetrics and Gynecology*. 5th ed. Philadelphia, PA: JB Lippincott,1986:1037–1041.
5. Oguri H, Maeda N, Izumiya C, et al. MRI of endocervical glandular disorders: Three cases of a deep nabothian cyst and three cases of a minimal-deviation adenocarcinoma. *Magn Reson Imaging*. 2004;22:1333–1337.

CODES
ICD9-CM

- 622.8 Other specified noninflammatory disorders of cervix (includes cyst)
- 616.0 Cervicitis and endocervicitis including Nabothian (gland) cyst or follicle

KEY WORDS

- Uterine Cervix
- Dyspareunia
- Cervicitis
- Minimal Deviation Adenocarcinoma
- Nabothian Cyst

N

NONALCOHOLIC FATTY LIVER DISEASE

Silvia D. Degli-Esposti, MD

KEY CLINICAL POINTS

- Spectrum of diseases with common histological features and presumed etiology: Simple nonalcoholic fatty liver (steatosis), nonalcoholic steatohepatitis (NASH), nonalcoholic fatty liver with cryptogenic cirrhosis
- NASH carries significant potential to progress to cirrhosis
- Most common cause of abnormal liver function test (LFTs) in United States
- NAFLD represents the hepatic component of metabolic syndrome. Suspect in patients with obesity and insulin resistance
- Current therapeutic measures focus on risk factors: Obesity, diabetes and hyperlipidemia

 BASICS

DESCRIPTION
Spectrum of diseases with different clinical significance: It is a histological diagnosis: Accumulation of large fat droplets in the hepatocytes (macrovescicular steatosis) in absence of excessive alcohol consumption

- Patients are asymptomatic
- Only patients with abnormal LFTs during routine testing come to medical attention
- Viral etiology, alcohol abuse and other causes of liver disease must be ruled out
- NAFLD
  - Includes simple fatty liver, NASH and cryptogenic cirrhosis with fatty liver
  - Fat in the liver >5–10% by weight
  - Compatible imaging studies and biopsy
- NASH
  - Subset of NAFLD that may progress to cirrhosis
  - Histology: Fat, necroinflammatory changes and hepatocellular injury (steatohepatitis)
- Cryptogenic cirrhosis: Fatty liver disease most common cause of cryptogenic cirrhosis
- Natural history
  - Natural history of the disease is still controversial
  - The progression from steatosis without inflammation to steatohepatitis is debated
  - NASH may progress to cirrhosis, although timing and percent of those who progress has not been established.

GENERAL PREVENTION
Hyperinsulinemia and diabetes are important predisposing factors: Prevention includes weight control, diet and exercise.

EPIDEMIOLOGY
Prevalence parallels obesity epidemic. Good epidemiologic data are lacking.

- Females represent 60–80% of patients in clinical studies
- Common in 3rd–4th decade
- Occurs in 2.6% of all children and 22–52% of children that are obese
- Mexican Americans and African Americans may have increased prevalence.

Incidence
Unknown

Prevalence
Prevalence of NAFLD in the United States is 20–30% as estimated by ultrasound.
- By autopsy review
  - NAFLD in 35% of lean patients, and in 70% of obese patients
  - NASH in 6.3% of patients with NAFLD

RISK FACTORS
- Obesity
  - In patients with BMI >51: 90% have steatosis and 34% NASH
- NIDDM
- Hyperlipidemia
- Can occur in nonobese patients

Genetics
- Family clusters have been described
- Presence of hemochromatosis gene mutations may accelerate the disease process

PATHOPHYSIOLOGY
Proposed mechanism
- Fatty liver: Insulin resistance (IR) causes an increase of free fatty acid (FFA) in the blood stream that overwhelms the liver's ability to metabolize them causing fatty accumulation in the liver
- NASH: A second hit is required (Oxidative stress? Endotoxin? Metabolic syndrome?) which causes inflammatory cytokines to promote liver damage and fibrosis deposition

ETIOLOGY
- Remains controversial. Metabolic syndrome plays a major role.
- Metabolic syndrome is an inflammatory condition modulating proinflammatory cytokines.
- Fat tissue, especially truncal, is metabolically active, secreting some of the key cytokines and neuroendocrine mediators involved in the pathogenesis of NAFLD: Tumor necrosis factor-alpha, adiponectin, leptin
- The role of each cytokine in the process is the subject of intense investigation.

ASSOCIATED CONDITIONS
- Obesity
- Metabolic syndrome
- Diabetes mellitus
- Hyperlipidemia
- Hypertension
- Lipodystrophy

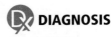 **DIAGNOSIS**

PRE-HOSPITAL
Diagnostic goals:
- Establish diagnosis of NAFLD
- Differentiate simple fatty liver from NASH with or without cirrhosis
- The majority of patients are asymptomatic

SIGNS AND SYMPTOMS
Vague right upper quadrant pain, fatigue, malaise

History
- Inquire about alcohol consumption (>40 mg/alcohol per day)
  - Inquire about alcohol consumption with family members and other providers
- Toxin exposure
- Medications and recreational drugs
- Concomitant illness: NIDDM, IR
- Gastric bypass

Physical Exam
- Obesity, hepatomegaly
- With Cirrhosis
  - Splenomegaly, spider angiomata, palmar erythema, ascites, jaundice

TESTS
Lab
- NAFLD
  - ALT and AST 2–4 times normal, alkaline phosphatase and GGT 2 to 3 times normal, ferritin elevated
  - Fasting glucose and insulin level to calculate insulin resistance
- NAFLD with cirrhosis
  - Albumin, platelets decreased
  - INR, total bilirubin increased
- Exclude other causes of liver disease
  - Genetic test for hemochromatosis, autoimmune markers: Antinuclear (ANA), antimitocondrial Ab (AMA), antismoothmuscle Ab (SMA), antiliver/kidney/microsomial Ab (LKM), ceruloplasmin,alpha1antitripsin, viral serologies for Hepatitis B, C

Imaging
Liver ultrasound and CT scan may be helpful in diagnosis of NAFLD
- Ultrasound sensitive and specific for diagnosis of fatty deposition in the liver
- Imaging technique cannot discriminate between steatosis and NASH

Diagnostic Procedures/Surgery
Liver biopsy is the gold standard and has the best prognostic value
- It differentiates steatosis from NASH and NASH with cirrhosis
- The need for liver biopsy is controversial
  - It has associated morbidity and mortality
  - There are limited specific therapeutic options regardless of the biopsy results
  - Excluding other potential causes and careful monitoring for disease progression is advocated by many
- Aggressive therapy with novel agents should be done only for selected group of patients with established histological diagnosis of NASH

Pathologic Findings
- NAFLD
  - Macrovescicular steatosis
  - Diffuse or centrolobular
- NASH
  - Parenchymal inflammation, pleomorphic, lipogranulomas
  - Ballooning hepatocytes degeneration
  - Hepatocyte necrosis
  - Mallory bodies
  - Perivenular, perisinusoidal or periportal fibrosis
  - Stainable iron

- NAFLD with cirrhosis
  - Fibrous septa, bridging fibrosis
  - Decreased steatosis

DIFFERENTIAL DIAGNOSIS
- Secondary fatty liver disease
  - Alcoholic liver disease
  - Wilson disease
  - Hepatitis C
  - Starvation
  - Surgical procedures
    - Gastroduodenal bypass, biliopancreatic diversion, extensive small bowel surgical resection
  - Parenteral nutrition
  - Drugs
    - Amiodarone, metotrexate, corticosteroid, estrogen in high dose
  - Genetic diseases
    - Sphingolipidosis, abetalipoproteinemia, tyrosinemia
- If biopsy is not obtained, exclude all other causes of abnormal LFTs

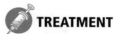

TREATMENT

PRE-HOSPITAL
- Correction of known underlying risk factors: Obesity, hyperlipidemia, glucose intolerance
- Avoidance of hepatotoxic drugs and substances (alcohol)

GENERAL MEASURES
- Weight loss and exercise form the cornerstone of initial therapy
- The aim is to increase insulin sensitivity, decrease truncal body fat tissue, and improve lipid profile

Diet
Weight loss as a treatment for NASH has been examined in a few small trials.
- The value of caloric or specific food group restriction has not been evaluated
- Current common practice is to advise a low fat, low simple carbohydrate diet
- Achieving significant weight loss with dietary modification alone is difficult

Activity
Benefits of exercise include: Weight loss, increase in insulin sensitivity, modulation of inflammatory cytokines
Small studies have confirmed a beneficial role of exercise in the therapy of NAFLD

Complementary and Alternative Medicine
Among antioxidants, vitamin E and SAMe and its precursor Betaine have been used.
- Vitamin E was evaluated in various liver diseases
- Preliminary results are promising
- Caution: Vitamin E may increase overall mortality at high dose (>400 IU day)

 ## MEDICATION (DRUGS)

Optimize medical regimen and lifestyle changes for underlying morbidity (diabetes, hyperlipidemia, and hypertension)
- IR is associated with NAFLD independent of body mass
- Insulin sensitizing drugs have been used even in non-diabetic patient with NASH, however, they are still investigational

N

First Line
- Metformin has been studied in humans and animals: Improves biochemical profile but no clear improvement in histology
- Thiazolidinedione drugs are promising agents
  - Improve IR
  - Decrease plasma lipids
  - Have anti-inflammatory and immunomodulatory properties
  - Improve histology in pilot human studies

SURGERY
- Bariatric surgery can be considered for morbid obesity (BMI ≥40 or ≥35 with comorbidities)
- Contraindications: High portal pressure, intra-abdominal or esophageal varices, ascites, decompensated liver disease
- Liver transplant for end stage, decompensated liver disease

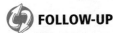 FOLLOW-UP

DISPOSITION
- No end point of therapy has been established
- Lifestyle modifications should be life long

Admission Criteria
Decompensated liver disease may require hospitalization

Discharge Criteria
When stabilization is achieved

Issues for Referral
Refer to hepatologist for diagnosis and treatment of NAFLD
- Refer to transplant center for evaluation of patient with decompensated liver disease
- Refer to endocrinologist for treatment of metabolic syndrome, diabetes mellitus
- Refer obese patients to weight loss center

PROGNOSIS
- The risk of progression of NAFLD is variable. Predictors of fibrosis in NAFLD:
  - Older age (>50 years), obesity, diabetes mellitus, insulin resistance, hypertension
  - AST/ALT >1, triglyceride >1.7 mmol/L, ALT >2 times upper limit of normal
  - Necroinflammation and iron deposition in liver biopsy

COMPLICATIONS
Cirrhosis and hepatocellular carcinoma

PATIENT MONITORING
Monitor patients at intervals for:
- Disease progression
- Evaluate fat content with ultrasound and if indicated with liver biopsy
- Alphafetoprotein and liver ultrasound to monitor for HCC in cirrhotic patients
- Imaging and noninvasive measures to monitor therapy results

REFERENCES

1. Matteoni CA, Younossi ZM, Gamlich T, et al. Nonalcoholic fatty liver disease: A spectrum of clinical pathological severity. *Gastroenterology*. 1999;116:1413–1419.
2. Marchesini G, Bugianesi E, Forlani G, et al. Nonalcoholic fatty liver, steatohepatitis and the metabolic syndrome. *Hepatology*. 2003;37:917–923.
3. Xu A, Wang Y, Keshaw H, et al. The fat derived hormone adiponectin alleviates alcoholic and non alcoholic fatty liver disease in mice. *J Clin Invest*. 2003;112:91–100.
4. Angulo P, Keach JC, Batts KP, et al. Independent predictors of liver fibrosis in patients with nonalcoholic steatohepatitis. *Hepatology*. 1999;30:1356–1362.
5. Promrat K, Lutchman G, Uwaifo GI, et al. A pilot study of pioglitazone treatment for nonalcoholic steatohepatitis. *Hepatology*. 2004;39:188–196.

CODES
ICD9-CM
- 571.8 Chronic liver disease non alcoholic
- 571.8 Cirrhosis of the liver without mention alcohol
- 789.1 Hepatomegaly NOS

KEY WORDS

- Fatty Liver
- NAFLD
- Obesity
- NASH
- Metabolic Syndrome
- Cryptogenic Cirrhosis

OBESITY

Jennifer R. Hur, MD

KEY CLINICAL POINTS

- Obesity is an extremely prevalent problem with serious medical consequences.
- Effective treatment for obesity depends on simultaneous interventions in diet, physical activity, behavioral modification, and for some patients, medication and/or surgery.
- Even modest weight loss can be associated with tremendous health benefits.

 BASICS

DESCRIPTION

- Defined as a Body Mass Index (BMI) of greater than 30. Extreme obesity ("morbid") is defined as BMI ≥40.
- BMI is calculated as weight (kg)/height (m)^2

EPIDEMIOLOGY

Approximately $100 billion healthcare dollars were spent in 1995, more than 1/2 of which represented medical expenses related to obesity related illness.

Prevalence

- 20.9% of the adults in the United States are considered obese.
- Obesity is more prevalent among women than men. Approximately 33.4% of women are obese compared with 27.5% of men in the 1999–2000 NHANES survey. 1 in every 30 women fall into the category of extreme obesity.
- Each year, an estimated 300,000 United States adults die of causes related to obesity.

RISK FACTORS

- Overweight or obese during childhood
- Increased intake of refined carbohydrates
- Decreased fresh fruit and vegetable intake
- Decreased physical activity
- Increased time spent watching television
- Lower socioeconomic status
- Risk factors for secondary causes

Genetics

Studies of twins, adoptees, and families indicate that as much as 80% of the variance in BMI may be related to genetic factors. However, obesity is rarely ever due to isolated genetic causes but rather, due to interactions between genetic and environmental factors.

PATHOPHYSIOLOGY

- Increased adipose tissue leads to increased insulin resistance, increased tissue insulin levels, increased basal and stimulated insulin, leading to chronic hyperinsulinemia with resultant secondary hypertension and hyperlipidemia.
- Leptin, insulin, adiponectin, ghrelin, α-melanocyte-stimulating hormone, as well as many other neurohormonal factors, interact to influence food intake and energy expenditure.
- Estrogen has been found to interact with leptin and its role in the regulation of eating behavior and fat distribution is being studied.

ETIOLOGY

- Multifactorial interactions between genetic and environmental factors.

- Women are disproportionately affected by obesity due to the effects of female sex hormones, the menstrual cycle, the use of contraceptive hormones, and weight gains associated with pregnancy and menopause.

COMPLICATIONS

- Cardiovascular disease, obstructive sleep apnea; obesity-hypoventilation syndrome (Pickwickian Syndrome), Type 2 diabetes mellitus, dyslipidemia; hypertension; cerebrovascular disease; nonalcoholic fatty liver disease (NAFLD) formerly NASH; cholelithiasis/choledocholithiasis, accelerated osteoarthritis; increased rates of breast, prostate, colon, and endometrial cancer; stress incontinence; GERD; psychological disorders (depression, eating disorders, body image disorders, low self-esteem); and the
- Metabolic Syndrome, defined by 3 or more of following 5 risk factors:
  - Abdominal obesity (waist >35 inches)
  - Elevated triglycerides (>150 mg/dL)
  - Decreased HDL (<50 mg/dL in women)
  - Hypertension (>130/85)
  - Hyperglycemia (>110 mg/dL)

Pregnancy Considerations

- Obesity is associated with increased risk of pregnancy complications such as: Gestational diabetes, hypertension, spontaneous abortion, pre-eclampsia, cesarean section and DVT
- Infants of obese women are more likely to suffer: Fetal growth abnormalities, macrosomia, and intrauterine growth retardation
- Obese women are also more likely to have problems with reproduction such as: Menstrual irregularities, infertility, and anovulation.

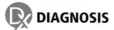 **DIAGNOSIS**

SIGNS AND SYMPTOMS

Obesity is often overlooked as a distinct medical problem. If a patient's BMI meets criteria, obesity should be listed as a discreet issue on their problem list.

History

- Sudden weight gain should prompt a work-up for secondary causes of weight gain (see differential diagnosis).
- A food diary and review of any particular stressors that provoke eating.
- Motivation and readiness to commit to losing weight.
- Careful screening for comorbidities associated with obesity.
- Review for any medications that might contribute to weight gain.
- Review of systems to check for any undiagnosed conditions that might contribute to obesity.

Physical Exam

- Height and weight to calculate BMI
- If BMI <35, measure waist circumference
  - Central obesity, defined as waist circumference >35 inches in women, is strongly associated with associated medical conditions. If BMI >35, risk already high and this measurement adds no additional information.
- Blood pressure
- Distribution of adipose tissue and other physical exam findings may be clues to undiagnosed endocrinopathies.

TESTS

Lab

- If any underlying endocrine disorders are suspected, those specific lab tests may be ordered.
- Otherwise, lab tests ordered are geared at diagnosing common complications.
  - Fasting cholesterol panel
  - Fasting glucose (>112 insulin resistance, >126 diabetes)
  - Liver function tests

Imaging

RUQ Ultrasound may show a fatty liver

DIFFERENTIAL DIAGNOSIS

It is important to rule out secondary causes of weight gain that may be amenable to treatment.

- Endocrine
  - Hypothyroidism
  - Polycystic ovarian syndrome (PCOS)
  - Congenital adrenal hyperplasia
  - Cushing syndrome
  - Growth hormone deficiency
- Perimenopause
- Hypothalamic lesions
- Syndrome X
- Medications: Antihyperglycemics, antidepressants, mood stabilizers, antipsychotics, antiepileptics, hormones

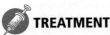

TREATMENT

GENERAL MEASURES

- As with any intervention that requires profound lifestyle modification, a discussion about weight loss must begin with an assessment of readiness to change.
- In general, the most successful weight loss treatment plans are multidisciplinary and combine diet modification with exercise regimens and occasionally medications.
- Aim for a 1–2 pound weight loss per week for 6 months. After 6 months, the focus is on maintenance of new weight and lifestyle changes.
- Set reasonable goals. A loss of 5–10% of initial body weight can provide significant health benefits.

Diet

Should be advised to anyone whose BMI >25, and as a general preventive measure for everyone.

- Diet as the primary intervention has been reported to result in a weight loss of approximately 7 kg at 6 months and maintained for 12 months.
- Diets emphasizing carbohydrate restriction produce better weight loss, lipid, and glucose control than do conventional diets, although the bottom line for any effective diet is overall caloric restriction.
- One of the most challenging aspects of weight control interventions is the difficulty adhering to a meal plan.
  - Portion controlled foods (i.e., meal replacements) have been shown to have positive results with regard to weight loss.

EXERCISE PROGRAMS

- Despite the additional health benefits of exercise, little evidence supports its use as the solitary means of losing weight.
- Combined with dietary and behavioral changes, significant benefits are seen.
- Somewhere between 20 and 60 minutes per day of moderate physical activity is required to maintain a healthy body weight.

- Higher levels of exercise appear to be needed to maintain long term weight loss and maintenance; 40 minutes a day.
- Care must be taken to tailor exercise programs as high impact activities may be inadvisable in very obese persons. Aquatic exercise or walking may be preferable low-impact alternatives.

MEDICATION (DRUGS)

Should be considered when BMI >30, BMI >27 with comorbidities, and if dietary/exercise programs have failed.

- Sibutramine (Meridia or Reductil), given 10 mg/day and may be increased to 15 mg/day after a month if tolerated.
  - Serotonin, norepinephrine, and dopamine reuptake inhibitor. Promotes satiety and increases energy expenditure.
  - Efficacy related to dose and simultaneous diet and behavioral intervention.
  - Approximately 75% treated with sibutramine at maximal doses will lose >5% weight loss and most impressively, 80% of those patients maintain their new weight for at least 2 years.
  - Approximately 5% will not tolerate the drug. Side effects include tachycardia, hypertension, seizures, and allergic reactions. Approximately 20% will not respond.
- Orlistat (Xenical), given 120 mg t.i.d. before meals.
  - Blocks action of pancreatic lipase resulting in blocked fat digestion and absorption.
  - Efficacy related to dose and combination with a diet that includes about 30% fat; a very low fat diet will not result in any weight loss benefit.
  - Approximately 70% patients achieve >5% weight loss and 70% of them maintain their new weight at 2 years.
  - LDL reduction is often impressive.
  - With advance patient education, orlistat is fairly well tolerated. Side effects may include abdominal pain, steatorrhea (especially after high fat meals), fecal incontinence, fat-soluble vitamin deficiencies (supplemental vitamins A, D, E, K need to be taken at least 2 hours before or after orlistat).
- Phentermine (Adipex-P), still widely used but only approved for short term (several weeks) use.
  - Schedule IV drug. Potential for abuse appears low.
  - Not much data on its use so routine use not recommended.
  - Side effects include insomnia, dry mouth, asthenia, constipation, and hypertension.
- Off-label use has been reported using bupropion, venlafaxine, and topiramate.

SURGERY

Patients that should be considered for bariatric surgical referral have failed a nonsurgical program integrating diet, exercise, behavior modification, and psychological support, are well-informed, motivated, able to tolerate the procedure and have:

- BMI >40
- BMI >35 + serious coexisting medical problem
  - Severe sleep apnea
  - Pickwickian syndrome
  - Obesity related cardiomyopathy
  - Severe Type 2 diabetes
  - Joint disease
- 2 types dominate practice in the United States.
  - Gastric bypass: Results in more weight loss and more likely to reverse the medical problems associated with obesity. Currently, the more common procedure to be done laparoscopically.
  - Gastric-banding

- Common complications with both include vomiting, dumping syndrome, nutritional deficiencies.
- Major complications include pulmonary embolism, respiratory failure, gastrointestinal leaks, stromal obstruction or stenosis, and bleeding.
- Postoperative mortality rates range from 0.1% to as high as 1–2%. Postoperative surgical complication rates can be as high as 15%.

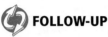 FOLLOW-UP

Behavioral Tools
- Contact time with brief visits and phone help keep the patient engaged and feeling motivated.
- Social support can be critical for success, both short- and long-term, via Weight Watchers and friends/family.
- Self-monitoring with diaries, psychotherapy
- Behavioral contract with setting of precise, reasonable goals.

Stimulus Control Procedures
- Eating at the same time and place at each meal.
- Slowing eating by putting utensils down between bites.
- Resisting the urge to have seconds.
- Limiting portion size.
- Using smaller dishes.
- Not eating in front of the television.

Follow-Up After Bariatric Surgery
- Monitor for strictures that may require endoscopic dilation.
- Gallstones can occur in up to 30% patients and so need to be suspected with the appropriate presenting symptoms.
- Nutrition needs to be closely monitored to avoid dehydration and protein malnutrition.
- Risk for micronutrient deficiencies is high and independent of protein and caloric deficiencies. Supplement and monitor for deficiencies of: Vitamin B12, iron, folic acid, and calcium
- Pregnancy after bariatric surgery: Pregnancy may be associated with fewer complications after bariatric surgery than while obese. Close monitoring is required and pregnancy is generally not recommended until 12–18 months after surgery once weight loss has stabilized.

PROGNOSIS
- Even modest weight reduction can produce substantial health benefits.
- Loss of less than 7% of baseline weight has been shown to produce 58% reduction in risk for diabetes in people with impaired glucose tolerance.
- The biggest challenge is maintenance of weight loss; as many as 90–95% of persons who lose weight subsequently regain it.

REFERENCES
1. Moore T. Adolescent and adult obesity in women: A tidal wave just beginning. *Clin Obstet Gynecol*. 2004;47:884–889.
2. Ryan D, Stewart T. Medical management of obesity in women: office-based approaches to weight management. *Clin Obstet Gynecol*. 2004;47:914–927.
3. Nagle A, Prystowsky J. Surgical management of obesity. *Clin Obstet Gynecol*. 2004;47:928–941.
4. Clegg D, Woods S. The physiology of obesity. *Clin Obstet Gynecol*. 2004;47:967–979.
5. Hedley A, Ogden C, Johnson C. Prevalence of overweight and obesity among U.S. children, adolescents, and adults, 1999–2002. *JAMA*. 2004;291:2847–2850.
6. Ford E, Giles W, Pietz W. Prevalence of the metabolic syndrome among U.S. adults—findings from the Third National Health and Nutrition Survey. *JAMA*. 2002;287:356–359.
7. Rosenbaum M, Leibel R, Hirsch J. Obesity. *N Engl J Med*. 1997;337:396–407.

CODES
ICD9-CM
- 278.00 Obesity, unspecified
  - 278.01 Morbid obesity
  - 278.0 Overweight
- 783.1 Abnormal weight gain

KEY WORDS
- Obesity
- Morbid Obesity
- Overweight
- Bariatric Surgery

O

OBSTRUCTIVE SLEEP APNEA

Alice E. Bonitati, MD

KEY CLINICAL POINTS

- Common sleep disorder, more prevalent in men but common in women as well
- Associated with nocturnal and daytime symptoms, including daytime hypersomnolence, neurocognitive deficits, and mood changes
- High index of suspicion
  - In patients who are overweight or obese
  - In postmenopausal women
  - In patients with craniofacial abnormalities
- Consider in anyone with suggestive symptoms and reported snoring

 BASICS

DESCRIPTION

- Obstructive sleep apnea falls under the broad heading of sleep-disordered breathing, which represents a spectrum of abnormal breathing patterns during sleep including obstructive sleep apnea-hypopnea syndrome (OSAHS), central sleep apnea syndrome, Cheyne-Stokes respiration, and sleep hypoventilation syndrome.
- The obstructive sleep apnea-hypopnea syndrome (OSAHS) or obstructive sleep apnea syndrome (OSAS) consists of repetitive collapse of the upper airway during sleep, in conjunction with symptoms, including nonrefreshing sleep, daytime sleepiness and sleep fragmentation.
- Definitions
  - Obstructive apneas: Respiratory events associated with complete or near complete cessation of airflow and lasting at least 10 seconds
  - Obstructive hypopneas: Respiratory events characterized by partial reductions in airflow and associated with oxygen desaturation >3% and/or EEG arousals from sleep.
  - Arousal: A shift in EEG frequency lasting at least 3 seconds. A measure of sleep fragmentation.
  - Apneic hypopneic index (AHI): Number of episodes of apnea and hypopnea per hour of sleep
    - Standard parameter used to report overall severity of OSA
    - Rough but not consistent correlation with presence of symptoms
    - Does not encompass other aspects of sleep apnea such as arousals and oxygen desaturation
- Classification of severity based on AHI:
  - Normal or 1° snoring AHI <5 events/hour
  - Mild OSA AHI: 5 to 15 events/hour
  - Moderate OSA AHI: 15 to 30 events/hour
  - Severe OSA AHI: >30 events/hour

EPIDEMIOLOGY

There has been a marked increase in the number of cases diagnosed each year due to increased recognition of the disorder and actual increase in prevalence due to increased obesity in population.

Incidence

- 108,000 cases diagnosed/year in 1990 in the United States.
- 1.3 million cases diagnosed/year in 1998

Prevalence

Dependent on diagnostic criteria used:

- Approximately 9% of women and 24% of men age 30–60 using AHI cutoff of ≥5 events/hour
- Approximately 2% of women and 4% of men age 30–60 using AHI of ≥5 events/hour and daytime hypersomnolence (Wisconsin Sleep Cohort)
- More recent data suggests prevalence may be higher
- Significantly increased in postmenopausal women and appears to be reduced with hormonal replacement therapy

RISK FACTORS

- Male gender
- Overweight/obesity
- Wide neck circumference
- Increasing age
- Postmenopausal status
- Positive family history of OSA
- Craniofacial abnormalities

Genetics

Family and genetic studies suggest there is a genetic predisposition to OSA, but magnitude of genetic influence not well determined.

- Familial aggregation is common
- Factors influencing genetic predisposition likely include:
  - Obesity/fat distribution
  - Presence of upper airway abnormalities
  - Patterns of ventilatory control

PATHOPHYSIOLOGY

- Narrowed upper airway susceptible to collapse during sleep when upper airway dilator muscle tone is reduced, despite compensatory increase in activity of these muscles.
- Occlusion of upper airway associated with several ventilatory, hemodynamic, and metabolic effects
- Obstructive apneas and hypopneas are associated with acute hypoxemia and hypercarbia, arousals from sleep, and reductions in intrathoracic pressure.
  - Increased sympathetic nervous system activation and catecholamine release
  - Increased heart rate and blood pressure
  - Decreased stroke volume
  - Insulin resistance and increased release of proinflammatory mediators

ETIOLOGY

- Overweight and obesity, especially central obesity
- Wide neck circumference major predictor
- Postmenopausal state
- Increasing age

ASSOCIATED CONDITIONS

Increased incidence in:

- Hypothyroidism
- Cushing syndrome
- Down syndrome
- Marfan syndrome
- Pierre Robin syndrome
- Polycystic ovarian syndrome
- Emerging as a manifestation of metabolic syndrome
- Any syndrome associated with macroglossia

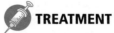 DIAGNOSIS

SIGNS AND SYMPTOMS
- Snoring
- Witnessed apnea
- Gasping or choking arousals
- Morning tiredness/nonrefreshing sleep
- Excessive daytime sleepiness
- Morning headaches
- Neurocognitive defects of attention, concentration, and/or memory
- Mood changes, irritability
- Sleep fragmentation
- Nocturia
- Enuresis
- Impotence/sexual dysfunction

History
Classic presentation is that of a patient with reported snoring and witnessed apnea accompanied by morning tiredness and excessive daytime sleepiness.
- Caution is needed when evaluating hypersomnolence, as some patients become habituated to chronic sleepiness and do not perceive themselves as being hypersomnolent, but have improved alertness and wellbeing following therapy of OSA.
- Some patients with severe OSA may truly not be hypersomnolent.
- Some patients may present with prominence of nocturnal symptoms such as sleep fragmentation and/or choking arousals.
- Depression or problems with memory and/or concentration may be part of the clinical presentation.
- Refractory hypertension, nocturnal angina pectoris, and new onset atrial fibrillation are possible reasons for presentation.
- OSA may exacerbate migraine headaches, seizure disorders, and chronic pain syndromes.

Physical Exam
- Presence or absence of hypertension
- BMI: Overweight >25 kg/m^2; obese >30kg/m^2
- Wide neck circumference
  - ≥ 16 inches in women
  - ≥ 17 inches in men
- Upper airway abnormalities
  - Nasal obstruction: Septal deviation or nasal mucosal and turbinate edema
  - Posterior pharyngeal narrowing
    - Tonsillar hypertrophy/lateral narrowing from prominent tonsillar pillars
    - Deep set palate/elongated, thick uvula
- Retrognathia/micrognathia
- Macroglossia
- Presence or absence of peripheral edema

TESTS
Lab
Check TSH to screen for hypothyroidism.

Diagnostic Procedures/Surgery
All night polysomnography in sleep disorders laboratory is gold standard for diagnosis. Sensitivity and specificity of home studies is significantly lower.
- Simultaneous monitoring of several physiologic signals including snoring, respiration, oxygen saturation, airflow via nasal and oral sensors, sleep stage distribution via EEG, and cardiac rate and rhythm.

DIFFERENTIAL DIAGNOSIS
Differential diagnosis of excessive daytime sleepiness:
- Insufficient sleep
- Sleep fragmenting process other than OSAS, such as Periodic Limb Movement Disorder
- Disorder of sleep drive such as narcolepsy
- Circadian rhythm disorder such as Shift Work Sleep Disorder
- Sedating medication or drug effect
- Depression may present with excessive daytime sleepiness

TREATMENT

GENERAL MEASURES
- Weight loss
- Positional management: Patient conditions self to sleeping in lateral decubitus position
- Treatment of nasal congestion
- Consider repair of deviated nasal septum
- Avoidance of evening alcohol consumption
- Avoidance of sedating medications, especially benzodiazepines
- Screening for hypothyroidism
- For patients with OSAS who are hospitalized:
  - Continue CPAP or BIPAP therapy during their hospitalization
  - Minimize sedative hypnotics and narcotics

SPECIAL THERAPY
Positive airway pressure (PAP) is most effective treatment modality available and is considered first line therapy for moderate to severe OSAS. Oral appliances and upper airway surgery are other potential therapies.
- PAP therapy: Positive pressure is applied to the upper airway via a nasal or oronasal interface, thereby maintaining airway patency.
  - Nasal CPAP: Continuous positive airway pressure is the standard treatment.
  - Compliance with PAP therapy has been shown to be higher in moderate to severe disease; however, patients with mild disease whose symptoms warrant can benefit from PAP therapy.
  - Compliance may be improved with new features to enhance comfort, such as Cflex, which reduces expiratory pressure.
  - In patients in whom the sleep-disordered breathing cannot be controlled with CPAP, bilevel positive airway pressure (BIPAP) may be effective.
  - Treatment with CPAP has been shown to have a multitude of beneficial effects including improvement in daytime sleepiness and wellbeing, neurocognitive deficits and mood, hypertension, and cardiovascular risk reduction.
- Therapy with oral appliance
  - Consider in patients with:
    - Mild to moderate OSA
    - Patients intolerant of CPAP
    - Patients with retrognathia
    - Patients without markedly narrowed posterior pharynx
    - Need to have fair to good dentition
    - For treatment of OSA, as opposed to primary snoring only, an adjustable oral appliance is needed, fitted by a qualified orthodontist. A "one-size-fits-all" snoreguard can be effective for snoring alone.
- Surgical therapy
  - Uvulopalatopharyngoplasty: Success rate 40% to 50%
  - Laser assisted uvuloplasty (LAUP) only effective for snoring, not OSAS
  - Radiofrequency ablation at palate level or retrolingual (RFA, somnoplasty): Final recommendations not yet available

O

- More advanced maxillomandibular surgery
  - Genioglossal advancement, genioglossal advancement with hyoid myotomy, or maxillomandibular osteotomy and advancement
- Surgery often performed in staged fashion with UPPP first, followed by reevaluation of OSA, and then additional jaw advancement procedure if warranted
- Tracheostomy: Considered therapy of last resort for patients with severe OSAS who cannot tolerate CPAP or BIPAP or in whom such therapy is ineffective
- Bariatric surgery: Likely will make major impact in reducing OSAS in patients with severe obesity, but long term efficacy data not yet available.

 MEDICATION (DRUGS)

Modafinil: Can be used as adjunctive therapy in patients with residual symptoms after primary treatment of the OSA.
- Minimal risk of cardiovascular side effects
- Not found to be habit forming
- Common side effect is headache, more likely to occur in patients with preexisting headaches.
- Potential for reduced steroidal contraceptive action, including depot and implantable agents; avoid use of this drug in patients on steroidal contraceptives.
- Use with caution in patients with Bipolar Affective Disorder or other psychiatric illness.
- Pregnancy category C

COMPLICATIONS
- Cardiovascular
  - Hypertension: Significant independent risk even when controlling for obesity, smoking, diabetes mellitus.
  - CAD: Increased prevalence of OSA in patients with myocardial infarction and angina pectoris
  - CHF: In Sleep Heart Health Study, odds ratio was 4.37 for patients in highest quartile of OSAS severity
  - Arrhythmias
    - Bradycardias and episodes of asystole
    - Ventricular arrhythmias
    - Increased prevalence of atrial fibrillation
  - Stroke: High prevalence of OSA; causative role not definitively proven
  - Pulmonary hypertension
    - More likely in patients with daytime hypoxemia
    - OSAS alone does not generally cause severe pulmonary hypertension

- Patients with coexistent obstructive lung disease, the Overlap Syndrome, can develop pulmonary hypertension with less severe degrees of OSA
  - Hypercapnia: The vast majority of patients with OSAS do not have daytime hypercapnia. Its presence suggests associated obesity hypoventilation or hypoventilation of other cause.
- Sleepiness while driving and increased risk of motor vehicle accidents
  - Risk of MVA increased as much as 7-fold
  - Higher risk in patients with near misses
  - Physician responsibility to counsel patients on risks of driving while sleepy

REFERENCES

1. Caples SM, Gami AS, Somers VK. Obstructive sleep apnea. *Ann Int Med.* 2005;142:187–197.
2. Young T, Finn L, Austin D, et al. Menopausal status and sleep-disordered breathing in the Wisconsin Sleep Cohort Study. *Am J Respir Crit Care Med.* 2003;167:1181–1185.
3. Bixler E, Vgontzas AN, Lin HM, et al. Prevalence of sleep-disordered breathing in women – effects of gender. *Am J Respir Crit Care Med.* 2001;163:608–613.
4. Leung RST, Bradley TD. Sleep apnea and cardiovascular disease. *Am J Respir Crit Care Med.* 2001;164:2147–2165.
5. Peppard PE, Young T, Palla M, et al. Prospective study of the association between sleep-disordered breathing and hypertension. *NEJM.* 2000;342:1378–1384.
6. Black JE, Hirshkowitz M. Modafinil for treatment of residual excessive sleepiness in nasal continuous positive airway pressure-treated obstructive sleep apnea/hypopnea syndrome. *Sleep.* 2005;28:464–471.

CODES
ICD9-CM
780.53 Obstructive sleep apnea

KEY WORDS

- Obstructive Sleep Apnea
- Sleep-Disordered Breathing
- Excessive Daytime Sleepiness
- Snoring

OSTEOPOROSIS
Kelly A. McGarry, MD

KEY CLINICAL POINTS

- Osteoporosis is asymptomatic until a fracture occurs
  - Goal is to make diagnosis prior to fractures occurring
- Dual energy x-ray absorptiometry (DXA) is screening test of choice
- Bisphosphonates are the most efficacious treatment and are first-line if no contraindications and tolerated by the patient

 BASICS

DESCRIPTION
- Osteoporosis is a "silent disease" characterized by:
  - Low bone mass
  - Microarchitectural deterioration of bone tissue
  - Increased skeletal fragility
- Symptomatic once a fragility fracture occurs

GENERAL PREVENTION
- Adequate calcium (1,200–1,500 mg/day) and vitamin D intake (400–600 IU/day) through diet or supplementation
- Weight-bearing exercise at least 3 times per week (more is better)
- Smoking cessation
- Fall prevention counseling (especially in elderly women)
  - Includes modifying:
    - Environment (loose rugs, dim lights);
    - Physiologic factors (poor vision, postural instability);
    - Adjusting medications (psychoactive medications, polypharmacy)

EPIDEMIOLOGY
- More than 1.5 million Americans experience osteoporotic fractures each year.
- Disproportionately affects postmenopausal women: 80% of those affected are women
- 1 out of 2 white women aged 50 can expect to sustain a hip, forearm, or spine fracture in their lifetime.
- Only 50% of women who suffer a hip fracture regain their premorbid level of independence.
- Asian and African American women have a lower fracture risk than white women at every level of BMD; race-specific normative databases may be appropriate for defining osteoporosis.

Incidence
Osteoporotic fractures/year:
- 500,000 vertebral fractures
- 300,000 hip fractures
- 200,000 wrist fractures
- 300,000 other bones
  - 80% are from minor falls

Prevalence
- Prevalence rate 1 in 9
- Affected Americans: 28 million
  - With osteoporosis: 10 million
    - Women: 8 million
    - Men: 2 million
  - With low bone mass: 18 million
- Approximately 55% of people >age 50 have low bone mass.

- National Osteoporosis Risk Assessment Observational Study of >200,000 asymptomatic postmenopausal women:
  - Of these, 47% had low BMD and 7% met the criteria for osteoporosis.
    - At 1-year follow-up, women with osteoporosis had a 4-fold risk of fracture compared to women with normal BMD.

RISK FACTORS
- Major risk factors:
  - Personal history of fracture as an adult
  - History of fragility fracture in a 1st degree relative
  - Low body weight (<127 lbs)
  - Current smoking
  - Use of corticosteroid therapy for more than 3 months
- Additional risk factors:
  - Impaired vision
  - Early estrogen deficiency (<45 years)
  - Dementia
  - Poor health/frailty
  - Recent falls
  - Low calcium intake (lifelong)
  - Low physical activity
  - Alcohol ≥2 drinks per day

Genetics
The genetic study of osteoporosis has been based on research into candidate genes relevant to bone metabolism:
- No clear clinical utility at this point
- Most intensively studied
  - VDR gene
  - Collagen type I (COLIA1) gene
  - Estrogen receptor-alpha gene

PATHOPHYSIOLOGY
- Bones are made of trabecular networks surrounded by a cortical shell.
- Osteoporotic bone is characterized by loss of trabecular bone and thinning of the cortical shell.

ETIOLOGY
- Age-related: About 80% of cases
- Secondary causes: About 20% of cases
  - GI diseases
    - Malabsorption syndromes (Crohn's disease, celiac sprue)
    - Severe liver disease, especially PBC
    - Gastrectomy
    - Hemochromatosis
    - Parenteral nutrition
  - Rheumatologic diseases
    - Osteogenesis imperfecta
    - Rheumatoid arthritis
    - Ankylosing spondylitis
    - Sarcoidosis
  - Hematologic diseases
    - Lymphoma and leukemia
    - Mastocytosis
    - Multiple myeloma
    - Pernicious anemia
    - Hemophilia
    - Thalassemia
  - Endocrine diseases
    - Hyperthyroidism
    - Cushing's disease
    - Addison's disease

- Acromegaly
- Insulin-dependent DM
- Gonadal insufficiency
– Drugs
  - Anticonvulsants
  - Excessive thyroid replacement therapy
  - Glucocorticoids
  - Heparin
  - Lithium
  - Premenopausal tamoxifen use

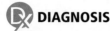 **DIAGNOSIS**

SIGNS AND SYMPTOMS
- Asymptomatic until a fracture occurs
- Nonvertebral fractures most often clinically apparent
- Vertebral fractures often found incidentally
  - Symptoms include:
    - New or worsened midline back pain
    - Band-like discomfort in dermatomal pattern

History
Inquire about relevant risk factors and family history of osteoporosis/fracture.

Physical Exam
- No specific physical exam sign can rule in or rule out osteoporosis.
- Low body weight (<51 kg) favors earlier screening
- Rib-pelvis distance less than 2 finger breadths and wall-occiput distance (done with patient standing with back against the wall) greater than 0 cm suggest the presence of occult fracture and, therefore, screening and probable treatment.
- Assess ADLs, stability, and strength in elderly patients – strength may reduce falls

TESTS
Lab
- Generally none required except in the work-up of secondary causes
  - Secondary causes may be evident historically
  - Basic work-up of secondary causes:
    - TSH, CBC, LFTs, PTH level, vitamin D, urine calcium levels, SPEP/UPEP
- Urinary N-telopeptide
  - Measures rate of bone turnover
  - Generally not necessary in the routine clinical encounter, but may be useful in patients not responding to treatment

Imaging
- Dual energy x-ray absorptiometry (DXA)
  - Most often used screening and diagnostic test
  - Very precise measurements at clinically meaningful sites (hip and spine)
  - Most useful to follow treatment response
  - 1/10 the radiation of a chest x-ray
  - Costs approximately $200
  - Covered by most insurances
- US (forearm or calcaneal)
  - Predicts risk of vertebral and hip fractures
  - Cannot be used to follow treatment response
  - Can be used in provider's office for screening with follow-up DXA if treatment is warranted
- T-score used to determine need for treatment with DXA and US methods
  - T-score > −1 is normal
  - T-score −1 to −2.5 indicates osteopenia

- Treatment should be considered in light of patient's other risk factors (consider earlier treatment if many risk factors)
  - T-score ≤ −2.5 indicates osteoporosis and warrants treatment

DIFFERENTIAL DIAGNOSIS
Vertebral compression fractures may be most difficult to diagnose
- Musculoskeletal strain
- Metastatic cancer to bone
- Osteomyelitis/epidural abscess
- Herpes zoster

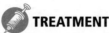 **TREATMENT**

GENERAL MEASURES
Activity
- Vertebral fractures
  - Encourage patients to continue ADLs
- Nonvertebral fractures
  - Activity recommendations depends on location of fracture

Physical Therapy
- Nonvertebral fractures generally require PT for regaining function and strength
- PT may increase strength and stabilization in any patient with osteoporosis
  - Can reduce falls and, hence, fractures

 MEDICATION (DRUGS)

- All currently available meds work by decreasing bone resorption
  - Only one, Teriparatide, increases bone formation
- Fracture reduction
  - Vertebral fractures
    - All meds decrease the incidence of vertebral fractures between 40% and 65%.
  - Hip fractures
    - Bisphosphonates and teriparatide reduce the risk of hip fractures about 50%.
    - Raloxifene and calcitonin have not yet been proven to reduce the risk of hip fractures.
- Some meds come in different doses depending on indication: Prevention vs. treatment (established osteoporosis)
- Pain medications (NSAIDs, opiates) may be required, especially for the management of acute fracture pain.

First Line
Bisphoshonates
- Alendronate
  - Prevention: 5 mg/day or 35 mg/week
  - Treatment: 10 mg/day or 70 mg/week
- Risedronate
  - Prevention/Treatment: 5 mg/day or 35 mg/week
- Ibandronate
  - Prevention/Treatment: 150 mg/month
- Side-effects mainly GI disturbances: Abdominal pain, nausea, dyspepsia, and rarely esophageal ulcer

Second Line
- Selective Estrogen Receptor Modulators
  - Raloxifene
    - Prevention/Treatment: 60 mg/day
    - Side effects: Deep venous thrombosis/PE, hot flashes, leg cramps

- Calcitonin
  - Treatment: 200 IU/day intranasally
    - Side effects: Nasal irritation, rhinitis
    - Alternate nostrils to decrease side effects
    - Less effective than other agents
    - Used when other agents not tolerated or in combination treatments
- Teriparatide (Parathyroid hormone)
  - Treatment: 20 micrograms/day SC
  - Side-effects: Arthralgias, leg cramps, dizziness, GI disturbances (constipation, diarrhea, dyspepsia, nausea), sweating, hypertension, syncope, rash, cough, pharyngitis
  - Reserved for those who cannot tolerate other meds, those who have an inadequate treatment response to other treatments, and those with severe disease
- Estrogen
  - Dose depends on formulation of estrogen
  - Only indicated for prevention, not treatment
  - Risks of other illnesses (breast cancer, coronary artery disease, thromboembolic disease) outweighs benefits of fracture reduction for most patients, thus, has fallen out of favor as osteoporosis treatment
  - Side effects: Vaginal bleeding, breast tenderness, gall bladder disease, risk of above illnesses

SURGERY
Percutaneous vertebroplasty
- Minimally invasive technique to help stabilize osteoporotic fractured vertebrae, decreasing pain and improving the function
- Cement mixture is injected through a needle into the fractured bone
- Outcome of procedure may not depend on duration of fracture
- Outcome may be better in individuals with a vertebral body height loss of less than 70%
- No clear agreement concerning inclusion and exclusion criteria
- Requires orthopedic referral

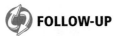 **FOLLOW-UP**

Issues for Referral
Consider referral to an endocrinologist for:
- Work-up of secondary causes, particularly if osteoporosis is detected in a premenopausal woman or Z-score < -2 in any woman (≥ 2 standard deviations away from her age-matched cohort)
- Further treatment if bone loss occurs while on therapy

PROGNOSIS
- Treatment of osteoporosis with medications may reduce vertebral fractures by 30–65% and reduce nonvertebral fractures by 25–50% (both raloxifene and calcitonin not yet proven to reduce nonvertebral fractures).
- Those who experience fractures are at highest risk of subsequent fractures.
- Thus, health care providers should be aggressive in treating this population.

PATIENT MONITORING
- DXA scan 12–24 months after treatment initiated
- The frequency of BMD testing depends on the treatment response, but no more frequently than every 1–2 years.
- Given expected rate of bone loss, if BMD is normal on 1st assessment, may choose to rescreen about 5 years later
- Assess for side effects from medications at each visit.

REFERENCES

1. Alvarez L. Predictors of outcomes of percutaneous vertebroplasty for osteoporotic vertebral fractures. *Spine*. 2004;30:87–89.
2. Cauley J. Bone mineral density and the risk of incident nonspinal fractures in black and white women. *JAMA*. 2005;293:2102–2108.
3. Eastell R. Treatment of postmenopausal osteoporosis. *N Engl J Med*. 1998;338:736–746.
4. Green A. Does this woman have osteoporosis? *JAMA*. 2004;292:2890–2900.
5. Neer RM. Effect of parathyroid hormone on fractures and bone mineral density in postmenopausal women with osteoporosis. *N Engl J Med*. 2001;344:1434–1441.
6. Yao-Zhong L. Molecular studies of identification of genes for osteoporosis: The 2002 update. *J Endocrinology*. 2003;177:147–196.

CODES
ICD9-CM
733.0 Osteoporosis

KEY WORDS

- Osteoporosis
- Fractures
- DXA Scan
- Vertebroplasty

O

OVARIAN CANCER

Etsuko Aoki, MD, PhD

KEY CLINICAL POINTS

- Ovarian cancer is primarily a disease of postmenopausal women; the majority of cases occur between 50- and 75-years-old.
- Increased risk in women with low parity or infertility and defects in BRCA1, BRACA2, or hereditary nonpolyposis colorectal cancer (HNPCC) genes
- Majority of cases are advanced at time of diagnosis because the symptoms are vague and nonspecific in early stage
- Prognosis in women with advanced disease depends on the amount of residual tumor burden after the initial operation

 BASICS

DESCRIPTION
- Ovarian cancer is the 2nd most common gynecologic malignancy.
- Derives from ovarian epithelial cells (>90%), germ-cell or sex cord-stroma
  - Pathology of epithelial cell cancer: Papillary serous (75%), mucinous (10%), endometrioid (10%), clear cell tumors, Brenner tumors, undifferentiated, mixed

GENERAL PREVENTION
Oral contraceptives appear to have a protective effect: In women who have used oral contraceptives for 7 years or more, approximately 50% risk reduction.

EPIDEMIOLOGY
- The incidence is highest in 75- to 79-year-old age group at the rate of 62/100,000 women.
- The average population risk of developing ovarian cancer is 1.5%.
- The incidence varies by race and geography; there is a higher incidence in whites and developed countries.
  - High incidence in Eastern European Jewish ancestry, probably related to high incidence of BRCA1 and BRCA2 gene mutations

Incidence
Whites: 18/100,000; African-Americans: 12/100,000

RISK FACTORS
- High animal fat diet
- Exposure to talc used on diaphragms and sanitary napkins
- Low parity
- Infertility
- Prolonged use of ovulation-inducing drugs (possibly)
- Hereditary cancer syndrome (breast-ovarian cancer syndrome, site-specific ovarian cancer syndrome and Lynch II syndrome)

Genetics
Familial susceptibility with mutation of BRCA1 gene

Risk of developing ovarian cancer is 40% in women who have mutated BRCA1 and a strong family history and 15–20% in women who have mutated BRCA1 without a strong family history.

ETIOLOGY
Ovarian cancer results from the accumulation of multiple discrete genetic defects and environmental factors.

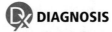 **DIAGNOSIS**

SIGNS AND SYMPTOMS
In early stage, symptoms are vague and nonspecific:
- Lower abdominal discomfort, pressure or pain
- Bloating or gas
- Constipation
- Nausea/vomiting
- Constitutional symptoms: Low grade fever, fatigue, and weight loss

In advanced stage;
- Abdominal bloating or swelling (ascites)
- Bladder or rectal symptoms caused by large pelvic mass
- Respiratory distress
- Abnormal vaginal bleeding (infrequent)

History
- History of breast cancer
- Family history of ovarian cancer

Physical Exam
- Palpable adnexal mass
  - Solid, irregular and fixed mass
- Upper abdominal mass (advanced)
- Ascites (advanced)

TESTS
Lab
- Serum CA-125:
  - >65 U/mL in 80% of women with epithelial ovarian cancer
  - More useful in postmenopausal women
- Consider AFP, LDH, and hCG when a germ cell tumor is suspected.
- Potential new biomarkers/method; osteopontin, YKL-40, CA15-3, gene expression profile (still investigational, limited reports of clinical use)

Imaging
- Ultrasound has not proven to be useful for screening, but is useful in the evaluation of pelvic mass
  - Sonographic criteria suggestive of malignancy
    - Solid component that is not hyperechoic and is often nodular or papillary
    - Thick septations (>2–3 mm)
    - Color or power Doppler flow in the solid component
    - Ascites
    - Peritoneal masses, lymphadenopathy
- Chest X-ray or chest CT to assess for metastatic disease
- Abdominal CT and MRI; may be useful to assess extent of disease preoperatively
- To exclude extraovarian primary (metastases)
  - Barium enema if occult blood in the stool
  - Upper GI series if indicated
  - Bilateral mammography if breast mass is present
  - Endocervical curettage and/or biopsy if abnormal vaginal bleeding is present

Diagnostic Procedures/Surgery
- Exploratory laparotomy is definitive
- Stage of the disease can only be determined by surgery (see Surgery in Treatment)

DIFFERENTIAL DIAGNOSIS
- Endometriomas
- Nonepithelial primary ovarian tumors (sex cord-stromal tumors, germ-cell tumors, mixed cell type tumors)
- Pedunculated uterine fibroid
- Functional ovarian cyst
- Tuboovarian abscess
- Benign ovarian tumor
- Primary peritoneal cancer
- Ovarian metastases
- Ectopic pregnancy

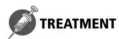

TREATMENT

SURGERY
- Early stage
  - Surgical staging (exploratory laparotomy) including
    - Multiple cytologic washing
    - Intact tumor removal
    - Complete abdominal exploration
    - Hysterectomy with bilateral salpingo-oophorectomy
    - Omentectomy
    - Lymph node sampling
    - Random peritoneal biopsies, including the diaphragm
- Advanced disease
  - Surgical staging plus optimal cytoreduction followed by chemotherapy/irradiation
    - Goal of residual tumor diameter <1 cm

Radiotherapy
Consider in early stage women with high risk (higher histologic grade and/or stage) disease and advanced stage women, especially when the disease is chemotherapy-refractory

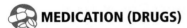

MEDICATION (DRUGS)

- Except in some early stage disease, chemotherapy after optimal surgical cytoreduction is considered as a standard therapy.
- Chemotherapy regimens continue to change as research continues.
  - Early stage
    - Platinum- and taxane-based chemotherapy should be considered the standard treatment in patients with high risk features (moderately to poorly differentiated tumors, stage IC or II and clear cell histology)
  - Advanced stage
    - Combination chemotherapy with platinum and taxane provides survival benefit

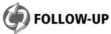

FOLLOW-UP

DISPOSITION
For the gynecologist, need gynecologic oncology backup when there is a suspicion of malignancy.

PROGNOSIS
Epithelial cell cancers
- Disease stage is strongly associated with the prognosis.
  - Overall 5-year survival
    - Stage I and II: 80–100%
    - Stage III: 15–20%
    - Stage IV: 5%
- In advanced stage, the amount of residual tumor at the conclusion of the initial surgery is of most importance (<1 cm is goal).
- Histologic cell types have weaker effect on prognosis, but clear cell and mucinous tumors may have the worst prognosis.

PATIENT MONITORING
- 7-fold to logarithmic drop of CA-125 suggest good response to therapy. If it is not achieved by 3 courses of chemotherapy, change the therapy.
- Physical and pelvic examination every 3 months for 2 years, every 4 months for the 3rd year, and then every 6 months
- CA-125 at every visit. If it increases, suspect recurrence.

REFERENCES

1. Modan B, Hartge P, Hirsh-Yechezkel G, et al. Parity, oral contraceptives and the risk of ovarian cancer among carriers and noncarriers of a BRCA1 or BRCA2 mutation. *N Engl J Med.* 2001;345:235–240.
2. Goff BA, Mandel L, Muntz HG, et al. Ovarian carcinoma diagnosis. *Cancer.* 2000;89:2068–2075.
3. Goff BA, Mandel LS, Melancon CH, et al. Frequency of symptoms of ovarian cancer in women presenting to primary care clinics. *JAMA.* 2004;291:2705–2712.
4. National Institutes of Health Consensus Development Conference Statement. Ovarian cancer: Screening, treatment, and follow-up. *Gynecol Oncol.* 1994;55:S4.
5. International Collaborative on Ovarian Neoplasm (ICON) Group. Paclitaxel plus carboplatin versus standard chemotherapy with either single agent carboplatin or cyclophosphamide, doxorubicin, and cisplatin in women with ovarian cancer: The ICON 3 randomized trial. *Lancet.* 2002;360:505–515.

CODES
ICD9-CM
183.0 Ovarian cancer

KEY WORDS

- Adnexal Mass
- Lower Abdominal Pain
- Ovarian Cancer

O

OVARIAN CYSTS

Etsuko Aoki, MD, PhD

KEY CLINICAL POINTS

- Most common adnexal mass in reproductive age and adolescence
- Ovarian cysts are rare in prepubescent and postmenopausal women, should consider neoplastic tumors when adnexal mass is found in these age groups
- Etiology of cystic lesion of ovary varies by age group
- Diagnosis can be made based on history, physical examination, and characteristic ultrasound findings

 BASICS

DESCRIPTION
Ovarian cysts are benign cystic tumors of the ovary.
- Physiologic (functional) cysts: Follicular, corpus luteum and theca lutein cysts
- Others: Endometriotic cysts

EPIDEMIOLOGY
- Follicular cysts
  - Rare in childhood, frequent in reproductive age, never occur in postmenopausal women
- Corpus luteum cysts
  - Occasionally occur in reproductive age
- Theca lutein cysts
  - Occur in adolescence and reproductive age, association with gonadotropin or clomiphene therapy, and also with hydatidiform mole/choriocarcinoma
- Endometriotic cysts
  - Most common in women at age 20–40, never seen in preadolescent and postmenopausal women

Prevalence
Found in 7% of pre- and postmenopausal women in screening studies

RISK FACTORS
Theca lutein cysts:

Occur with gonadotropin or clomiphene therapy, also can occur with hydatidiform mole/choriocarcinoma

PATHOPHYSIOLOGY
Physiologic cysts occur related to normal ovulation process

ETIOLOGY
- Infants
  - Usually follicular cysts, resulting from ovarian stimulation by maternal hormones
- Prepubescent
  - Physiologic cysts are uncommon
  - Suspect malignancy when adnexal mass is found in this age group
  - Recurrent, large, multiple ovarian cysts with signs of early sexual development may result from precocious puberty
- Adolescents
  - Majority are physiologic cysts related to normal ovarian activity
- Reproductive age
  - The majority of physiologic cysts are related to normal ovarian activity

- Consider polycystic ovary syndrome when patient has multicystic ovaries; other characteristics include obesity, hirsutism, prolonged amenorrhea and infertility.
- Postmenopausal women
  - High gonadotropin levels may cause ovarian cysts.
  - Always consider the possibility of malignancy.

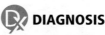 **DIAGNOSIS**

SIGNS AND SYMPTOMS
- Usually asymptomatic
- Midcycle pain in premenopausal women (physiologic cysts)
- Occasional anovulation (follicular cysts)
- Chronic pain during intercourse (endometriotic cyst)
- Pain immediately after intercourse (ruptured cyst)
- Severe lower abdominal pain associated with nausea and vomiting, when cyst is torsed

Physical Exam
Adnexal mass on pelvic examination

TESTS
Lab
- Serum CA-125 for excluding epithelial ovarian carcinoma
- AFP, LDH and hCG for excluding germ cell tumors of ovary
- Pregnancy test if ectopic pregnancy is suspected

Imaging
Ultrasound:
- Physiologic cysts are generally solitary, thin walled, unilocular and less than 10 cm diameter
  - Follicular cysts: <6 cm, often bilateral
  - Corpus luteum cysts: 4–6 cm, unilateral
  - Theca lutein cysts: 4–5 cm, multiple, bilateral
- Endometriotic cysts: 10–12 cm, may have thicker walls, may be multilocular, and may be occasionally bilateral
- In 1 study, only 0.3% of unilocular cysts were malignant, whereas the rate of malignancy was 8% in multilocular cysts.

DIFFERENTIAL DIAGNOSIS
- Malignant ovarian/fallopian tube/colon tumors
- Ectopic pregnancy
- Diverticular abscess
- Appendiceal abscess/appendicitis
- Tuboovarian abscess
- Paraovarian cyst
- Retroperitoneal cyst
- Polycystic ovary syndrome

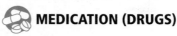 **MEDICATION (DRUGS)**

Oral contraceptives
- Follicular cysts often disappear after a 2-month regimen of oral contraceptives.
- Endometriosis cysts also may be managed with oral contraceptives.

SURGERY

Indications for surgery;

- Postmenopausal women
  - Symptomatic cyst
  - Cyst size greater than 3–5 cm diameter
  - Elevated CA-125 level
  - Multilocular cyst
  - Family history of breast or ovarian cancer in the first degree relatives
- Premenopausal women
  - Cyst size greater than 10 cm diameter
  - No resolution or an increase in size of cyst during the period of observation
- Ruptured or torsed cyst

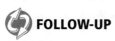 **FOLLOW-UP**

PROGNOSIS
Spontaneous resolution: May occur in physiologic cysts

COMPLICATIONS
- Ovarian torsion
- Rupture of cyst with intraperitoneal hemorrhage
- Bleeding into cyst

PATIENT MONITORING
- Infants and prepubescent
  - When physiologic cyst is suspected, follow up with serial ultrasound every 4–8 weeks. If it does not resolve within 3–6 months, consider laparoscopic surgery or ultrasound guided cyst aspiration.
- Adolescents
  - An asymptomatic simple cyst less than 10 cm diameter can be followed with ultrasound examination for 3 months.
  - If the size increases or does not change during the period of observation, or the cyst is >10 cm or symptomatic, perform laparoscopic cystectomy.

- Reproductive age
  - Cyst size <10 cm diameter can be observed, often with 2-month regimen of oral contraceptives. If it does not resolve after this period of time, surgical exploration is indicated.
- Postmenopausal women
  - Patients who have asymptomatic, simple unilateral cyst with normal Pap smear and CA-125 level can be observed with serial ultrasound examination and CA-125 measurement. Most of these cysts resolve spontaneously within 12–24 months. Otherwise, surgical exploration should be performed.

REFERENCES

1. Borgfeldt C, Andolf E. Transvaginal sonographic ovarian findings in a random sample of women 25–40 years old. *Ultrasound in Obstet Gynecol*. 1999;13:345–350.
2. Granberg S, Wildand M, Jansson I. Macroscopic characterization of ovarian tumors and the relation to histological diagnosis: Criteria to be used for ultrasound evaluation. *Gynecologic Oncol*. 1989;35:139–144.
3. Ekerhovd E, Wienerroith H, Staudach A, et al. Preoperative assessment of unilocular adnexal cysts by transvaginal ultrasonography: A comparison between ultrasonographic morphologic imaging and histopathologic diagnosis. *Am J Obstet Gynecol*. 2001;184:48–54.
4. Levine D, Gosink BB, Wolf SI, et al. Simple adnexal cysts: The natural history in postmenopausal women. *Radiology*. 1992;184:653–659.
5. Roman LD, Muderspach LI, Stein SM, et al. Pelvic examination, tumor marker level and gray-scale and Doppler sonography in the prediction of pelvic cancer. *Obstet Gynecol*. 1997;89:493–500.

CODES
ICD9-CM

620.2 Ovarian cyst

KEY WORDS

- Adnexal Mass
- Benign Ovarian Tumor

O

OVARIAN TORSION

Etsuko Aoki, MD, PhD

KEY CLINICAL POINTS

- Ovarian torsion can occur in all age groups: It is most common during a woman's reproductive years.
- Should be suspected in any women with sudden onset of lower abdominal pain, which is often associated with nausea and vomiting, an adnexal mass, and decreased or absent blood flow in the ovarian vessels.
- Pregnant women and women placed on ovarian hyperstimulation for infertility treatment are at increased risk.
- 3-dimensional ultrasonography or 2-dimensional ultrasonography with Doppler are the most useful diagnostic tests.

 ## BASICS

DESCRIPTION
Ovarian torsion is the twisting of the ovary on its ligamentous supports, often resulting in the obstruction of its blood supply. It is more common in the right ovary.

EPIDEMIOLOGY
In 1 hospital's 10-year review, ovarian torsion accounted for 2.7% of surgical emergencies.

RISK FACTORS
- Pregnancy
- Ovarian hyperstimulation for infertility treatment
- Tubal ligation (intermittent partial torsion)

PATHOPHYSIOLOGY
- Venous, arterial, and lymphatic flows are impeded due to the obstruction of blood vessels in the ligament of the torsed ovary.
- First, because of the impedance of venous flow, the affected ovary enlarges significantly, and subsequently ovarian ischemia can occur.

ETIOLOGY
- Ovarian cyst (48%)
- Tumor (46%)
  - Approximately 90% are benign; however, in children < age 15, 80% are malignant.
- Vigorous exercise or sudden increase in abdominal pressure may cause torsion.

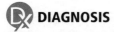 ## DIAGNOSIS

SIGNS AND SYMPTOMS
Symptoms are usually nonspecific. Most common presentations are:
- Stabbing or sharp lower abdominal pain (83%)
- Adnexal mass (72%)
- Nausea and vomiting
- Pain radiating to back, groin, or flank
- Peritoneal signs

History
- Vigorous exercise
- Chronic, intermittent lower abdominal pain after tubal ligation

Physical Exam
- Abdominal tenderness
- Palpable adnexal mass
- Fever

TESTS
Lab
- Complete blood cell count with differential
  - Anemia: Resulting from hemorrhage
  - Leukocytosis: Resulting from necrosis

Imaging
- Ultrasound:
  - Pelvic ultrasound can detect adnexal mass, ovarian enlargement, but it is difficult to determine if torsion of these structures is present.
    - Cystic or solid adnexal mass: >70%
    - Free fluid: 50%
  - Doppler ultrasound may be able to detect diminished or absent blood flow in the ligament of affected ovary.
- MRI and CT
  - Can detect ovarian lesions, limited ability to diagnose torsion

Diagnostic Procedures/Surgery
Definitive diagnosis is made with surgical exploration

DIFFERENTIAL DIAGNOSIS
- Ectopic pregnancy
- Appendicitis
- Hemorrhagic cyst
- Pelvic inflammatory disease
- Endometriosis

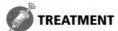 ## TREATMENT

SURGERY
Historically, removal of the torsed ovary has been a standard therapy. More recently, it has been shifted to ovary evaluation and preservation (Detorsion).
- Intraoperative evaluation
  - Evaluate the potential viability using a fluorescent injection or ovarian bivalving.
  - If malignancy is suspected or ovary appears to be nonviable, salpingo-oophorectomy should be done.
- Detorsion can be performed laparoscopically.

Pregnancy Considerations
The treatment of ovarian torsion in pregnancy is similar to that in nonpregnant women.

COMPLICATIONS
- Peritonitis and systemic infection can occur if the detorsed ovary is necrotic. Observe 24 hours after detorsion.
- Recurrence
  - Prevention
    - Relatively high dose oral contraceptives (≥50 mcg estrogen); OCPs are not effective in decreasing the risk of recurrence in younger women.
    - Oophoropexy (a procedure to fix [immobilize] ovary) in selected cases

REFERENCES

1. Varras M, Tsikini A, Polyzos D, et al. Uterine adnexal torsion: Pathologic and gray-scale ultrasonographic findings. *Clin Exp Obstet Gynecol*. 2004;31:343–348.
2. Houry D, Abbott JT. Ovarian torsion: A fifteen-year review. *Ann Emerg Med*. 2001;38:156–159.
3. Bayer AI, Wiskind AK. Adnexal torsion: Can the adnexal be saved? *Am J Obstet Gynecol*. 1994;171:1506–1510.
4. Ben-Ami M, Perlitz y, Haddad S. The effectiveness of spectral and color Doppler in predicting ovarian torsion. A prospective study. *Eur J Obstet Gynecol Reprod Bio*. 2002;104:64–66.
5. Oelsner G, Soriano D, Cohen SB, et al. Minimal surgery for the twisted ischaemic adnexal can preserve ovarian function. *Human Reprod*. 2003;18:2599–2602.

CODES
ICD9-CM
620.5 Ovarian torsion

KEY WORDS

- Lower Abdominal Pain
- Adnexal Mass
- Ovarian Cyst
- Ovarian Tumor
- Ovarian Torsion

PAGET'S DISEASE
Geetha Gopalakrishnan, MD

KEY CLINICAL POINTS

- Paget's disease causes bones to become enlarged and deformed.
- The disease is often asymptomatic. It is often diagnosed after alkaline phosphatase is found to be elevated on routine chemistries or by finding evidence of Paget's disease on an x-ray.
- Complications of abnormal bone growth includes nerve compression (may lead to hearing loss, facial droop, and vision loss), high output heart failure, osteosarcoma, and arthritis.
- Suppression of the pagetic process with an antiresorptive agent should be considered in all symptomatic individuals and some asymptomatic individuals who are at risk for complications such as nerve compression or fracture.

 ## BASICS

DESCRIPTION
Paget's disease of bone (osteitis deformans) is a skeletal disorder characterized by a focal increase in bone turnover (i.e., breakdown and formation). In this condition, bone structure and modeling are not normal. Affected bones become enlarged and deformed.

EPIDEMIOLOGY
- Approximately 3–4% of the individuals are over 40 years of age.
- Increases with age
- Men and women equally affected
- More common in Anglo-Saxons

ETIOLOGY
The exact cause is unknown; however, there seems to be a genetic component and a viral association. 1st degree relatives of Paget's patients are 7–10 times more likely to develop the disease. Viruses such as the canine distemper virus, measles virus and Paramyxoviridae family of viruses have been linked to the disease. Current thinking hypothesizes that individuals genetically predisposed to Paget's disease may develop the disease when they come in contact with a particular virus.

 ## DIAGNOSIS

Paget's disease is usually asymptomatic. An elevated alkaline phosphatase level on a routine chemistry panel or evidence of Paget's on x-ray conducted for some other reason usually leads to the diagnosis of this condition.

SIGNS AND SYMPTOMS
- Signs and symptoms of Paget's disease are related to the disease itself and its complications (i.e., abnormal bone growth and increased blood flow to the affected areas).
- Any bone can be affected by Paget's disease; however, pelvis, spine, skull, and long bones of the arms and legs are the most common sites of involvement. These sites are prone for bone deformity (i.e., bow legs, skull enlargement), bone pain (worsens with weight bearing) and fractures.
- Abnormal bone growth can cause nerve compression. Hearing loss, facial droop, and vision loss are common complications.
- A pagetic site has increased blood flow and therefore, the affected area is warm to touch. Increased blood flow can also cause high output heart failure and other cardiac complications in severe disease.
- Individuals with Paget's disease are also at an increased risk of bone tumors (osteosarcoma) and arthritis.

TESTS
Lab
- Alkaline phosphatase: An elevated level in an individual without liver problems raises concern for Paget's disease.
- N-telopeptide (NTX): Increased bone turnover noted with Paget's disease is associated with elevated levels of NTX.
- Calcium and phosphate: Normal in most patients, but can increase in the presence of a second disorder such as immobilization.

Imaging
- Radionuclide bone scan: Focal areas of increased uptake ("hot") spots are seen in Paget's disease.
- Plain radiographs: X-ray of suspected regions noted on bone scan can confirm the diagnosis and evaluate the extent of the disease. Bone thickening, enlargement, lytic areas, deformity and fractures can be seen on plain films.

DIFFERENTIAL DIAGNOSIS
Metastatic bone disease needs to be ruled out in individuals with new lab or x-ray findings. Bone biopsy can confirm the diagnosis.

 ## TREATMENT

Asymptomatic individuals generally do not need treatment for Paget's disease. Pain due to osteoarthritis may benefit from NSAIDs or acetaminophen. Suppression of the pagetic process with an antiresorptive agent should be considered in all symptomatic individuals and some asymptomatic individuals who are at risk for complications such as nerve compression or fracture.

 ## MEDICATION (DRUGS)

- Non-narcotic analgesics such as acetaminophen and NSAIDs will relieve pain symptoms in most patients.
- In symptomatic individuals, antiresorptive agents such as calcitonin and bisphosphonate therapy should be considered to suppress bone breakdown.
- Calcitonin: Subcutaneous injection of calcitonin at bedtime has been approved by the FDA for the treatment of Paget's disease. Salmon calcitonin 100 units or 0.5 mg of human calcitonin is the usual starting dose. Symptoms can start to improve after 2 weeks, but remission can be achieved after 22 months of therapy. Severe disease may require indefinite treatment or the addition of another agent.
  - Side effects: Nausea, facial flushing, metallic taste, diarrhea, abdominal pain, and allergic reactions. These symptoms diminish as treatment progresses. Serum anticalcitonin antibodies develop in 20% of individuals treated with salmon calcitonin. These individuals can become resistant to therapy.
- Bisphosphonates: Oral and IV preparation can inhibit bone resorption. Intravenous pamidronate (single 60 mg IV infusion over 4 hours for mild disease and 20–60 mg IV every 3 months in more severe disease), alendronate (40 mg/day for 6 months), risedronate (30 mg/day for 2 months) and Etidronate (400 mg/day for 6 months) have all been approved by the FDA for treatment of Paget's disease.
  - Side effects: Pill-induced esophagitis has been reported with oral bisphosphonates. Therefore proper intake (fasting, with 8 oz of water, in the upright position for at least 1/2 hour without other oral intake) is recommended.

IV bisphosphonates are associated with low-grade fever and flu-like symptoms for 1–2 days after the infusion. Hypocalcemia can occur with high-dose bisphosphonate therapy. Calcium supplementation (1,000 mg) will alleviate this problem. Ocular side effects such as conjunctivitis, uveitis, and scleritis and osteonecrosis of the jaw have been described with bisphosphonate therapy.

SURGERY
Surgery to stabilize fractures, nerve decompression, and joint replacement should be considered if complications such as vision loss and arthritis develop. In patients undergoing elective surgery, recommend prophylaxis with a drug that suppresses pagetic activity for 2–3 months. This should reduce hypervascularity and therefore blood loss during the procedure.

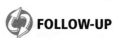 **FOLLOW-UP**

DISPOSITION
Remission is achieved when symptoms improve and a 50% reduction in markers of bone resorption such as NTX and alkaline phosphatase is noted. If relapse, retreatment is as effective.

Issues for Referral
Endocrine referral should be considered for symptomatic individual with Paget's disease. ENT, ophthalmology and orthopedic evaluation should be considered on an individual basis according to symptoms (i.e., hearing loss, vision loss, and fractures).

COMPLICATIONS
Patients need to be monitored for osteosarcoma, fractures, nerve compression, and cardiac abnormalities such as high output failure.

PATIENT MONITORING
Monitor symptoms and serum alkaline phosphatase levels periodically. Consider repeat bone scans and x-rays only if new symptoms develop. Treatment should be considered in symptomatic individuals with elevated alkaline phosphatase. Levels and symptoms should improve with treatment.

REFERENCES

1. Polednak AP. Rates of Paget's disease of bone among hospital discharges, by age and sex. *J Am Geriatr Soc*. 1987;35: 550–553.
2. Siris ES. Epidemiological aspects of Paget's disease: Family history and relationship to other medical conditions. *Semin Arthritis Rheum*. 1994;23:222–225.
3. Delmas PD, Meunier PJ. The management of Paget's disease of bone. *N Engl J Med*. 1997;336:558–566.

CODES
ICD9-CM
- 731.0 Paget's disease (osteitis deformans)

KEY WORDS
- Paget's Disease
- Osteoarthritis
- Hearing Loss
- Vision Loss
- Bony Deformity

PARVOVIRUS B19 INFECTION

Laura M. Ofstead, MD

KEY CLINICAL POINTS

- In adults, suspect if fever, mild URI, and polyathritis, and anemia
- Suspect if patient has close contact with children (who may have had Fifth's disease)
- Fetal morbidity/mortality is significant in pregnancy.

 BASICS

DESCRIPTION

- Human Parvovirus B19, also known as Erythrovirus B19, is a DNA virus.
- Causes an acute viral illness typically in adults exposed to school-age children who have erythema infectiosum ("slapped cheek" rash with mild cold-like symptoms)
- Presenting illness typically include:
  - Acute mild upper respiratory symptoms
  - Fever
  - Acute inflammatory polyathritis
- Polyathritis can last 2–3 months after the upper respiratory symptoms have resolved.
- Bone marrow suppression with moderate transient anemia is common.
- Special populations:
  - Sickle-cell patients can have aplastic crises.
  - Immunocompromised patients can have more severe illness with encephalitis, chronic anemia, and possible pancytopenias.
  - In pregnancy, fetal morbidity/mortality is significant leading to 5–10% fetal mortality from anemia and heart failure.

GENERAL PREVENTION

- Virus transmission is typically through respiratory droplets.
  - Hand-washing may help.
- Transmission is also possible through blood product transfusion.
  - Most blood banks currently screen blood products for the virus, although this is not mandatory.

EPIDEMIOLOGY

- Parvovirus B19 infection is seen globally.
- Many children (age 5–15) are exposed and experience mild clinical syndromes.
- As many as 60% of adolescents have positive antibody status by 19 years or age.
- Typical outbreaks occur in the late winter to early spring months.

Incidence

- Incidence and prevalence are difficult to estimate, because it is a very common infectious agent among children.
- In adults, it is common to see presentation of illness in the late winter/early spring.
- Typically in adults that work in schools, daycare centers, or with young children at home
- Estimates of seropositivity:
  - Children ages 1–5 years: 2–15%
  - Children ages 5–19 years: 15–60%
  - Adults: 40–60%
- During pregnancy, 1–2% seroconversion is typical

RISK FACTORS

- Exposure to school-age children:
  - School teachers
  - Daycare workers
  - Health care workers in pediatrics
  - Parents of school-age children
- Blood transfusion risks should be extremely limited as most blood products are currently screened (however screening is not mandatory for all blood banks at the current time).

Genetics

No specific genetic predisposition for infection is known.

PATHOPHYSIOLOGY

- The cellular receptor for the virus is based on a "P antigen" that is present on erythroid precursor cells, endothelial cells, megakaryocytes, and fetal myocardial cells.
- Given the distribution of affected cells above, typical clinical findings include:
  - Anemia
  - Arthralgia
  - Rash (less common in adults)
  - Pancytopenia
  - Myocarditis (rarely)
- Patient with high red-cell turnover states such as sickle cell anemia and hereditary spherocytosis may present with profound anemia such as aplastic crisis.

ETIOLOGY

- Human Parvovirus B19

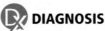 **DIAGNOSIS**

SIGNS AND SYMPTOMS

History

- Typically exposure to children
- Mild upper respiratory symptoms
- Polyathritis
- Fever common
- Fatigue (probably related to the anemia)
- Rash
  - Less common in adults
  - Vasculitic appearance
  - Classically petechal/purpuric glove and sock syndrome

Physical Exam

- Fever
- Mild URI findings on exam
- Erythematous, mildly swollen, warm joints
  - Typically hands, wrists, knees, ankles

TESTS

Often a clinical diagnosis, but laboratory testing available

Lab

- Parvovirus B19 antibody testing (IgM, IgG levels)
- Parvovirus B19 PCR testing
- Several associated laboratory testing abnormalities seen:
  - Isolated anemia, with low reticulocyte counts
  - Mild pancytopenia can be seen, particularly if immunosuppressed

– Aplastic anemia, with crisis, is seen in patients with sickle cell disease because of dependency of high bone marrow productivity.

– Mild transaminitis can be seen.

Imaging
- X-rays of affected joints shouldn't reveal destructive changes.
- EKG and echocardiogram can reveal myocarditis/pericarditis changes.

Diagnostic Procedures/Surgery
Bone marrow biopsy will confirm red cell aplasia.

DIFFERENTIAL DIAGNOSIS
- Consider other viral causes of upper respiratory illnesses that are associated with arthralgias such as
  - CMV
  - Adenovirus
  - HIV
- Consider initial presentation of rheumatologic conditions such as
  - Rheumatoid arthritis
  - Systemic lupus erythematosis

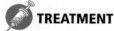

TREATMENT

GENERAL MEASURES
- Generally, a self-limited condition
- Supportive therapies with NSAIDs for arthralgia and fever
- Potentially routine laboratory monitoring of CBC

Diet
No specific dietary issues related to the disease process are known.

Activity
No specific required limitations, although mild anemia and arthralgia may limit activities until resolved.

SPECIAL THERAPY
- Blood transfusions may be necessary for:
  - Patients with high red-cell turnover states such as sickle cell disease, hereditary spherocytosis
  - Patients whose cardio-pulmonary status may not tolerate the transient anemia
- Immunoglobulin therapy may be indicated with patients with immunocompromised states such as
  - HIV disease
  - Immunoglobulin deficiency
  - Chemotherapy causing immunosuppression

Physical Therapy
Consider if patients have prolonged arthralgia, although no conclusive data to support

Complementary and Alternative Medicine
- None known
- Consider general immune-boosting herbal remedies that have been used for other viral illnesses.

MEDICATION (DRUGS)

- For symptomatic arthralgias, consider acetaminophen or NSAIDs.
- Immunosuppressed patients may benefit from IVIG if prolonged or symptomatic anemia or pancytopenia.

FOLLOW-UP

DISPOSITION
- Typically a self-limited disease in a previously healthy adult
- May require short-term use of NSAIDs for arthralgia

Admission Criteria
- It is typically an outpatient disease except in those patients at risk for complications.
- Consider if profound anemia, including symptomatic anemia in patients at risk for cardiopulmonary complications such as coronary artery disease, COPD, etc.
- Sickle-cell patients with aplastic crisis will need monitoring and likely transfusions.

Discharge Criteria
Stable blood counts, as noted above.

Issues for Referral
Consider referral to Hematology in patients at higher risk:
- Pregnancy (see Pregnancy Considerations)
- Sickle-cell disease or high red-cell turnover states
- Immunosuppressed states including HIV disease

PROGNOSIS
- Generally self-limited disease without long-term sequelae
- In immunosuppressed states, the potential for long-term bone marrow suppression with chronic anemia is possible.

PATIENT MONITORING
- In sickle-cell disease, may require more regular laboratory testing (CBC periodically) to evaluate need for transfusion
- Consider serial monitoring of CBC in all patients with anemia at presentation.
- Consider monitoring LFT, although transient transaminitis is unusual.

Pregnancy Considerations
- Anticipate about 1–2% seroconversion rate during pregnancy (not all women will be symptomatic).
- In pregnancy, 5–10% fetal mortality is estimated.
- Fetal risks appear to be higher if the infection occurs earlier in the pregnancy.
- Fetal ultrasound can show hydrops fetalis.
- Fetal ultrasound can indicate high cardiac output with congestive heart failure.
- In utero transfusion has been attempted to help correct fetal anemia.

REFERENCES

1. Young N, Brown K. Mechanisms of disease: Parvovirus B19. *N Eng J Med*. 2004;350:586–597.
2. Koch W. Fifth (human parvovirus) and sixth (herpesvirus 6) diseases. *Curr Opin Infect Dis*. 2001;14:343–356.
3. Burrow, Ferris. Medical Complications during Pregnacy. 4th ed. 1999:392–394.

MISCELLANEOUS

For patient education, see www.cdc.gov, directed to Diseases and Conditions, keyword Parvovirus.

CODES

ICD9-CM

- 057.0 Erythema infectiosum (fifth disease)
- 079.99 Unspecified viral infection
- 719.4 Arthralgia
- 284.8 Other specified aplastic anemias

KEY WORDS

- Parvovirus B19
- Erythema Infectiosum
- Fifth Disease
- Nonimmune Fetalis Hydrops
- Aplastic Anemia

PELVIC INFLAMMATORY DISEASE

Amy Boardman, MD

KEY CLINICAL POINTS

- Pelvic inflammatory disease (PID) is a serious health risk to young, sexually active, reproductive-age women and may be complicated by tubo-ovarian abscess, Fitz-Hugh-Curtis Syndrome, infertility, ectopic pregnancy, and chronic pelvic pain.
- Most cases are due to the sexually transmitted agents *Chlamydia trachomatis* and *Neisseria gonorrhoeae*, although non-sexually transmitted infection (STI)-related PID is an established and recognized entity.
- Although the clinical diagnosis of PID is imprecise, the morbidity associated with PID can be decreased by maintaining a high index of suspicion, considering the likelihood of an anaerobic infection, and providing prompt treatment of patients and partners with appropriate antibiotics.
- Early follow-up is essential.

BASICS

DESCRIPTION
- Pelvic inflammatory disease consists of a spectrum of inflammation and infection of the upper female genital tract, including any combination of endometritis, salpingitis, tubo-ovarian abscess, and pelvic peritonitis.
- Uncomplicated cervicitis or lower genital tract infection with *C. trachomatis* and *N. gonorrhoeae* can lead to PID if left untreated.

GENERAL PREVENTION
Prevention represents a significant opportunity to improve women's health given the major morbidity and long term sequelae associated with PID.
- Primary prevention includes:
  - Education of young women and at-risk teenagers via brochures, videos, and patient education programs
- Secondary prevention includes:
  - Screening asymptomatic women for lower genital tract infection
  - Screening for chlamydial infection by DNA amplification studies through cervical or urine specimens, which is cost-effective in at-risk populations
- Current U.S. recommendations are that all sexually active women younger than 25 years of age be screened yearly.
- Population-specific data may help to determine the ages of at-risk women in specific populations.
- Sexual partners should be examined and treated if they had sexual contact with the patient within 60 days before onset of symptoms.
  - Screening and treatment of partners should be empiric, because men are often asymptomatic for *N. gonorrhoeae* and *C. trachomatis*.
  - Treatment should cover these two likely pathogens.
- Untreated partners pose a high risk of reinfection.
  - Additional STI testing should include HIV, hepatitis B and C, and syphilis, because of possible coinfection or cotransmission.

EPIDEMIOLOGY
- PID is the most common infectious disease that affects young women aged 15–25 years.

- PID accounts for 94% of the morbidity that is associated with sexually transmitted infections in developed nations.
- Costs approximately $1 billion per year in the United States due to the disease and sequelae, such as infertility and chronic pelvic pain.
- PID is responsible for 250,000 hospital admissions per year.

Incidence/Prevalence
Exact estimates of incidence and prevalence in the United States are uncertain because PID is not a reportable disease and because the disease cannot be diagnosed reliably from clinical symptoms and signs.
- The most recent estimate of incidence from the Centers for Disease Control and Prevention (CDC) is that approximately 1 million cases of acute PID occur annually.
- In the United States, an estimated 600,000 new *N. gonorrhoeae* infections occur each year.
- The overall prevalence of chlamydial infection in the United States is 4.19%.
  - Prevalence among white women: 2.52%
  - Prevalence among African-American women: 14%

RISK FACTORS
Several demographic, behavioral, and contraceptive factors are risk factors for PID.
- Adolescents tend to have cervical ectopy (large zones of columnar epithelium for attachment of *C. trachomatis* and *N. gonorrhoeae)* and demonstrate high-risk sexual behavior.
- Multiple sexual partners
- ≥2 sexual partners in the past 4 weeks
- New partner in the past 4 weeks
- Prior history of PID
- Sexually transmitted infections (gonorrhea, chlamydia)
- Nonbarrier contraceptive use
- Inconsistent condom use
- Smoking
- Instrumentation of the cervix:
  - Sonohysterogram
  - Hysteroscopy
  - Hysterosalpingogram
  - IUD insertion within the past 20 days
- Possible douching

PATHOPHYSIOLOGY
- Acute PID results from ascending infection of the bacterial flora vaginal and cervical mucosa of the vagina and cervix
- Bacteria colonize and infect the endometrium and fallopian tubes
- PID is rare in women without menstrual periods, i.e., pregnant, premenarchal or postmenopausal women.
- The process sometimes extends to the surface of the ovaries and adjacent peritoneum. Less commonly nearby soft tissues of broad ligament and pelvic blood vessels are involved.
- Other rare forms of transmission include transperitoneal spread of infectious material from a perforated appendix or intraabdominal abscess, hematogenous or lymphatic spread to the tubes or ovaries.
- Acute PID is a *polymicrobial* infection that is a mixture of aerobic and anaerobic bacteria.
- Most long-term sequelae of PID result from destruction of the tubal architecture by the infection.

MICROBIAL ETIOLOGY

PID is caused by a polymicrobial infection that arises from ascent of vaginal and cervical microorganisms to the upper genital tract and peritoneal cavity. Such etiologic agents include:

- Sexually transmitted organisms
  - *C. trachomatis*
  - *N. gonorrhoeae*
- Vaginal flora microorganisms
  - *Bacteroides* sp
  - *Gardnerella vaginalis*
  - *Peptostreptococcus* sp
  - *Ureaplasma* sp
  - *Haemophilus influenzae*
  - Enteric Gram-negative rods
  - *Streptococcus agalactiae*
  - *Mycoplasma genitalium*

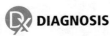 **DIAGNOSIS**

SIGNS AND SYMPTOMS OF MUCOPURULENT CERVICITIS (MPC)

MPC is characterized by purulent or mucopurulent discharge present in the endocervical canal or in an endocervical swab specimen. Although most patients are asymptomatic, other signs and symptoms include:

- Cervical contact friability
- Abnormal vaginal discharge
- Postcoital bleeding
- Intermenstrual bleeding

MPC can be caused by *C. trachomatis* and *N. gonorrhoeae*; however, in most cases, neither organism is isolated. Alternatively, *C. trachomatis* and *N. gonorrhoeae* infection may occur in the absence of mucopurulent discharge.

SIGNS AND SYMPTOMS OF PID

- Diagnosis of PID may be difficult because the signs and symptoms vary, often overlap with other disease entities, and may vary according to the type of pathogen.
- The CDC guidelines base treatment on a specific set of findings; occasionally, in the course of clinical evaluation, other studies will be needed to clarify the diagnosis.
- The CDC criteria for diagnosis are divided to increase sensitivity and specificity. The minimum criteria improve the sensitivity of the diagnosis; but requiring all three minimum criteria in patients who are at high risk (in whom the prevalence, or pretest probability, will be greater) may decrease sensitivity.
- The additional criteria may improve diagnostic specificity, which is useful in patients who are low risk (in whom the prevalence will be lower).

2006 Centers for Disease Control Criteria for Diagnosis of Pelvic Inflammatory Disease

- *Minimum Criteria (only one of the following findings is required for diagnosis)*
  - Uterine tenderness
  - Adnexal tenderness
  - Cervical motion tenderness
  - No other cause of above signs noted
- *Additional criteria that support diagnosis*
  - Oral temperature of greater than 101°F (>38.3°C)
  - Abnormal cervical or vaginal mucopurulent discharge
  - Presence of copious white blood cells on saline microscopy of vaginal secretions
  - Elevated erythrocyte sedimentation rate
  - Elevated C-reactive protein

  - Laboratory documentation of cervical infection with *N. gonorrhoeae* or *C. trachomatis*
- *Specific criteria that support diagnosis*
  - Endometrial biopsy with histopathologic evidence of endometritis
  - Transvaginal sonography or magnetic resonance imaging techniques showing thickened, fluid-filled tubes with or without free pelvic fluid or tubo-ovarian complex, or doppler studies suggesting pelvic infection
  - Laparoscopic findings consistent with PID

History

In addition to the CDC criteria, patients may describe or complain of the following:

- Dull abdominal pain
  - Variable character and intensity of pain
  - Usually bilateral
  - Duration >3 weeks
- Fevers
- Pelvic pain and pressure
- Vaginal discharge
- Onset of symptoms after menstruation
- Dyspareunia
- Abnormal vaginal bleeding
- Nausea and vomiting in >50%
- Dysuria or suprapubic pain during micturition only

Physical Exam

In addition to the CDC criteria, the physical examination may include the following:

- Fever
- Abdominal tenderness
- Peritoneal signs
- Perihepatic irritation with right upper quadrant irritation
- Pelvic examination
  - Vaginal discharge
  - Cervical motion tenderness
  - Uterine tenderness
  - Adnexal tenderness
  - Palpable adnexal mass

TESTS

Lab

- Pregnancy test
- Complete blood count with differential
- Erythrocyte sedimentation rate or C-reactive protein
- Urinalysis
- Saline microscopy
- Gonorrhea and chlamydial nucleic acid amplification testing
- Additional STD evaluation with HIV, syphilis screening (RPR or VDRL), Hepatitis B surface antigen, and Hepatitis C antibody

Imaging

- Transvaginal ultrasound
  - Sensitivity of 80% for diagnosis of PID
  - Useful to rule out other diagnoses, such as TOA, ovarian cyst and ovarian torsion
- MRI
  - Sensitivity of 93% for diagnosis of PID
  - Expensive
  - Less widely available
- Enhanced CT

Pathological Findings

The appearance of the pelvic organs may vary from red, indurated, edematous oviducts, to pockets of purulent material, to a large pyosalpinx or tubo-ovarian abscess.

DIFFERENTIAL DIAGNOSIS

- Appendicitis
- Ectopic pregnancy, ruptured or non-ruptured
- Endometriosis
- Hepatitis
- Gallbladder disease
- Gastrointestinal conditions
  - Gastroenteritis
  - Diverticulitis
  - Inflammatory bowel disease
  - Mesenteric adenitis
- Menstrual disorders
  - Abnormal uterine bleeding
  - Myomata
  - Mittelschmerz
- Ovarian conditions
  - Cyst
  - Cyst rupture
  - Torsion
- Renal conditions
  - Colic
  - Cystitis/UTI
  - Nephrolithiasis
  - Pyelonephritis

 TREATMENT

 MEDICATION (DRUGS)

Uncomplicated Lower Genital Tract Infection (Cervicitis and Mucopurulent Cervicitis—MPC)

- Treatment prevents transmission to sex partners and in pregnant women usually prevents transmission of *C. trachomatis* and *N. gonorrhoeae* to infants during birth. Treatment of sex partners also prevents reinfection of the index patient and infection of other sex partners.
- The recommended treatment regimens from the 2006 CDC Guidelines cure infection and typically relieve patient symptoms.

Chlamydial Infections in Adolescents and Adults

- Recommended Regimens
  Azithromycin 1 gram PO in a single dose; *or*
  Doxycycline 100 mg PO b.i.d. for 7 days
- Alternative Regimens
  Erythromycin base 500 mg PO q.i.d. for 7 days; *or*
  Erythromycin ethylsuccinate 800 mg PO q.i.d. for 7 days; *or*
  Ofloxacin 300 mg PO b.i.d. for 7 days; *or*
  Levofloxacin 500 mg PO q.d. for 7 days

ALERT

Results of clinical trials indicate that azithromycin and doxycycline are equally efficacious. Individuals should abstain from intercourse for 7 days after single dose therapy or until the end of a 7-day regimen *and* all their partners have been treated.

Chlamydial Infections in Pregnancy

- Recommended Regimens
  Azithromycin 1 gram PO in a single dose; *or*
  Amoxicillin 500 mg PO t.i.d. for 7 days
- Alternative Regimens
  Erythromycin base 500 mg PO q.i.d. for 7 days; *or*
  Erythromycin base 250 mg PO q.i.d. for 14 days; *or*
  Erythromycin ethylsuccinate 800 mg PO q.i.d. for 7 days; *or*
  Erythromycin ethylsuccinate 400 mg PO q.i.d. for 14 days

Pregnancy Considerations

- Doxycycline, ofloxacin, and erythromycin estolate are contraindicated during pregnancy. However, clinical experience and research date indicate that azithromycin is safe and effective in pregnancy.

Gonococcal Cervical Infections in Adolescents and Adults

- Recommended Regimens
  Ceftriaxone 125 mg IM in a single dose, *or*
  Cefixime 400 mg PO in a single dose; *or*
  Ciprofloxacin 500 mg PO in a single dose, *or*
  Ofloxacin 400 mg PO in a single dose, *or*
  Levofloxacin 250 mg PO in a single dose

PLUS, IF CHLAMYDIAL INFECTION IS NOT RULED OUT

Azithromycin 1 gram PO in a single dose, *or*
Doxycycline 100 mg PO b.i.d. for 7 days

- Alternative Regimens
  Spectinomycin 2 g IM in a single dose; *or*
  Ceftizoxime 500 mg IM in a single dose; *or*
  Single-dose cephalosporin regimens; or single-dose quinolone regimens *or*
  Cefotaxime 500 mg IM in a single dose

ALERT

Women infected with *N. gonorrhoeae* often are coinfected with *C. trachomatis*. This association led to the recommendation that patients with gonococcal infection be treated routinely for uncomplicated chlamydial infection as well. The prevalence of chlamydial coinfection with gonorrhea is approximately 10–30%. Routine dual therapy is cost effective in a high prevalence population because cost of therapy for chlamydia is less than cost of testing.

ALERT

Women who cannot tolerate cephalosporins or quinolones should be treated with spectinomycin.

Pregnancy Considerations

Quinolones and tetracyclines are contraindicated in pregnancy. Pregnant women should be treated with a recommended or alternative cephalosporin or spectinomycin.

ALERT

Fluoroquinolones have not been recommended in adolescents aged <18 years because of possible risk for articular cartilage damage seen in animal studies. However, no joint damage has been observed in children treated with long-term ciprofloxacin regimens. Therefore, children >45 kg can be treated with any regimen recommended for adults.

Pelvic Inflammatory Disease

Pharmacologic therapy should provide broad-spectrum coverage for *N. gonorrheae*, *C. trachomatis*, gram-negative facultative bacteria, streptococci, as well as anaerobes, depending on the clinical circumstances. Current CDC regimens are listed below.

- *Parenteral Regimen A*
  Cefotetan, 2 g IV q12h; OR cefoxitin, 2 g IV q6h AND doxycycline, 100 mg PO or IV q12h
- *Parenteral Regimen B*
  Clindamycin, 900 mg IV q8h AND gentamicin, loading dose IV or IM (2 mg/kg of body weight) followed by maintenance dose (1.5 mg/kg) q8h (single daily dosing may be substituted)
- *Alternative Parenteral Regimens*
  Levofloxacin 500 mg IV q.d. WITH OR WITHOUT Metronidazole 500 mg IV q8h, OR Ofloxacin 400 mg IV q12h WITH OR

WITHOUT Metronidazole 500 mg IV q8h, OR Ampicillin/Sulbactam 3 g IV q6h PLUS Doxycycline 100 mg PO or IV q12h

- *Oral Regimen A*
  Levofloxacin, 500 mg PO q.d. for 14 days; OR Ofloxacin, 400 mg PO b.i.d. for 14 days with or without metronidazole, 500 mg PO b.i.d. for 14 days
- *Oral Regimen B*
  Ceftriaxone, 250 mg IM in a single dose; OR cefoxitin, 2 g IM in a single dose AND probenecid, 1 g PO in a single dose; OR other third-generation cephalosporin PLUS doxycycline, 100 mg PO b.i.d. for 14 days with or without metronidazole, 500 mg PO b.i.d. for 14 days

ALERT

Because of pain associated with infusion, doxycycline should be administered PO when possible, even when patient is hospitalized. Both oral and IV administration of doxycycline provide similar bioavailability.

IV Fluids

- Administer appropriate parenteral fluids for hydration.
- Some patients may not tolerate oral intake and require parenteral hydration, antibiotics, and antiemetics.

First Line

- Outpatient therapy with oral antibiotics may be attempted initially.
- Patients should be re-examined within 48–72 hours and should demonstrate significant clinical improvement (e.g., defervescence; reduction in direct or rebound abdominal tenderness; and reduction in uterine, adnexal, and cervical motion tenderness) within 3 days of initiation of therapy.
- Patients who do not respond within this period usually require hospitalization, additional diagnostic tests, and surgical intervention.
- Single daily dosing of aminoglycoside antibiotics is acceptable for treatment.
- Anaerobic coverage with metronidazole or clindamycin is necessary for organisms associated with bacterial vaginosis or with tubo-ovarian abscess.

SURGERY

Laparoscopy is considered the gold standard for diagnosis. Generally reserved for severe cases, in patients who have tubo-ovarian abscess, or when the diagnosis is uncertain.

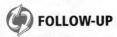 **FOLLOW-UP**

DISPOSITION

Chlamydial Cervicitis:

- Patients do not need a test of cure (TOC) after treatment with azithromycin or doxycycline unless symptoms persist or reinfection is suspected.
- A TOC may be considered after 3 weeks with treatment with erythromycin.
- *Nonculture* tests performed at <3 weeks after completion of therapy for patients treated successfully could lead to false-positive results due to excretion of dead organisms.
- Rescreening women is encouraged 3–4 months after treatment because of the likelihood of high prevalence of C. trachomatis, leading to reexposure and reinfection.
- Adolescents should also be rescreened at 3–4 months after treatment.
- All pregnant women should undergo TOC 3 weeks after completion of therapy.

Gonococcal Cervicitis:

- Patients do not need a TOC with culture after treatment with any of the recommended regimens unless symptoms persist or reinfection is suspected.
- If needed, culture with antimicrobial susceptibilities should be performed.
- All pregnant women should undergo TOC 3 weeks after completion of therapy.

PID:

There is no good evidence on optimal duration of duration of treatment of PID.

- Many RCTs have demonstrated efficacy of both parenteral and oral regimens.
- Transition to oral therapy is usually after 24–48 hours following significant clinical improvement on parenteral antibiotics.
- Oral antibiotics should then be continued for a total of 14 days.

Admission Criteria

The following criteria for hospitalization are based on observational data and theoretical concerns:

- Surgical emergencies (i.e., appendicitis) cannot be excluded.
- Pregnancy
- Poor clinical response to oral antimicrobial therapy
- Inability to follow or tolerate outpatient oral regimen
- Severe illness, nausea and vomiting or high fever
- Tubo-ovarian abscess
- Unreliable follow-up

Discharge Criteria

- Parenteral therapy may be discontinued 24 hours after a patient improves clinically, and oral therapy continued with doxycycline (100 mg b.i.d.) to complete 14 days of therapy.
- If a TOA is present, then clindamycin (450 mg PO q.i.d.) or metronidazole (500 mg b.i.d.) should be added to doxycycline for continued therapy rather than doxycycline alone.

PROGNOSIS

PID has a high morbidity:

- About 20% of affected women become infertile.
- About 20% develop chronic pelvic pain.
- Approximately 10% of those who subsequently conceive have an ectopic pregnancy.
- Uncontrolled observations suggest that clinical symptoms and signs resolve in a significant proportion of untreated women.
- Repeated episodes of PID are associated with a 4–6 times increase in the risk of permanent tubal damage.
- One case control study found that delaying treatment by even a few days is associated with impaired fertility (OR 2.6).

ACUTE COMPLICATIONS

Tubo-Ovarian Abscess (TOA)

- TOA develops as a result of untreated organisms causing damage and blockage to fallopian tubes with accumulation of bacteria, leukocytes, and fluid within a closed space. Bacteria and inflammation within the tubes extend through the fimbriated end to adjacent ovary, forming a TOA. Compromised perfusion of inner wall of the abscess creates an anaerobic environment in which anaerobes can flourish. Metastatic abscesses can occur by extension of infection to ovaries, bowel, and omentum with adherence of tubal fimbriae to these organs.
- Tubo-ovarian complex (TOC) is an edematous, adherent, infected, thick-walled inflammatory mass with vague margins without a dominant cystic component. The complex is perfused and does not have a devitalized abscess wall or pus in the cavity

- TOAs complicate 15–30% of hospitalized cases of PID.
- Diagnosis
  - Most patients with TOAs are in significant pain and discomfort.
  - Most TOAs are detected through imaging studies (i.e., vaginal ultrasound) and not through physical examination because of extreme patient discomfort and guarding.
  - Suspect in patients with persistent fever despite adequate antibiotics, persistent lower abdominal pain (especially unilateral), or adnexal mass.
  - Transvaginal ultrasound is highly sensitive (90–95%) for diagnosis.
    - TOA appears as a thin-walled, septated, well-demarcated, cystic mass with air-fluid levels.
    - TOC appears as a thick-walled mass with vague margins and no cystic component.
    - TVS can also be used to guide drainage of the abscess.
  - Cultures reveal anaerobic organisms, gram-negative organisms, and polymicrobial infections.
- Treatment
  - 95% of TOCs respond to parenteral triple antibiotic therapy (with ampicillin/gentamicin/clindamicin), but surgical intervention is necessary in up to 25% of the cases.
  - Duration of parenteral antibiotic therapy is not defined clearly. If patients improve clinically and sonographically, then patients can be treated with 10 days of IV antibiotics followed by 10 days of oral antibiotics as an outpatient.
  - Surgical intervention should be considered for an increase in abscess size, persistent fevers, suspected abscess rupture, or lack of clinical improvement in 48–72 hours.
- Surgical options depend on disease severity and include:
  - Transvaginal or transrectal CT or ultrasound-guided percutaneous drainage
  - Laparoscopy or laparotomy with unilateral adnexectomy
  - Total abdominal hysterectomy with bilateral oophorectomy

Fitz-Hugh-Curtis Syndrome (Perihepatitis)
- Affects 1–30% of women with PID
- Characterized by inflammation and adhesion formation between the liver capsule and anterior abdominal wall
- Associated with gonococcal and chlamydial PID
- Clinical presentation of RUQ pain with or without other signs or symptoms of PID
- Possible mild LFT elevation
- The diagnosis is confirmed by laparoscopic visualization of characteristic perihepatic "string-like" adhesions.

LONG-TERM COMPLICATIONS
Infertility
- PID is an established risk factor for infertility.
- The rate of infertility increases with each subsequent episode of PID.
  - After 1 episode, the risk is 8%.
  - After 2 episodes, the risk is 19.5%.
  - After 3 or more episodes, the risk is 40%.
- 30–80% of women with infertility due to tubal occlusion have no prior history of PID.
- Mild to moderate endometritis is not associated with infertility, most likely due to lack of fallopian tube involvement.
- Delay in presentation for PID was shown to increase the risk of infertility and ectopic pregnancy threefold.

Ectopic Pregnancy
Prior episodes of STIs, including chlamydia, gonorrhea, and PID are associated with an increased risk.
Chronic Pelvic Pain (CPP)
- 15% of women in the United States suffer from CPP.
- CPP occurs in 23% of women who develop PID.
- Cause of CPP after PID is uncertain, but may be due to adhesions that result from an inflammatory process.
- It remains controversial if lysis of adhesions alleviates chronic pelvic pain.

REFERENCES

1. Banikarim C, Chacko MR. Pelvic inflammatory disease in adolescents. *Adolesc Med Clin.* 2004;15(2):273–285.
2. Beigi RH, Wiesenfeld HC. Pelvic inflammatory disease: new diagnostic criteria and treatment. *Obstet Gynecol Clin N Am.* 2003;30:777–793.
3. Centers for Disease Control and Prevention: Sexually transmitted diseases treatment guidelines 2002. *MMWR.* 2006;55(No. RR11):56.
4. Epperly ATA, Viera AJ. Pelvic inflammatory disease. *Clin Fam Prac.* 2005;7:(No.1):67–78.
5. Mishell Jr DR, Stenchever MA, Droegemueller W, et al. *Comprehensive Gynecology,* 4th ed. St. Louis, MO: Mosby, 2001.
6. Ness RB, Soper DE, Holley RL, et al. Effectiveness of inpatient and outpatient treatment strategies for women with pelvic inflammatory disease: Results from the pelvic inflammatory disease evaluation and clinical health (peach) randomized trial. *Am J Obstet Gynecol.* 2002;186:5;929–937.
7. Risser WL, Cromwell PF, Bortot AT, et al. Impact of new diagnostic criteria on the prevalence and incidence of pelvic inflammatory disease. *J Pediatr Adolesc Gynecol.* 2004;17:39–44.
8. Ross, J. Pelvic inflammatory disease. *Clin Evid Concise.* 2005;13:463–464.
9. Simms I, Stephenson JM. Pelvic inflammatory disease epidemiology: What do we know and what do we need to know? *Sex Transm Infect.* 2000;76(2):80–87.

CODES
ICD9-CM (2006)
- 615.0 Inflammatory disease, acute
- 615.1 Inflammatory disease, chronic
- 614.0 Salpingitis/oophoritis, acute
- 614.1 Salpingitis/oophoritis, chronic
- 098.0 Acute gonorrhea of lower genitourinary tract
- 099.53 Cervicitis, chlamydial

KEY WORDS
- Pelvic Inflammatory Disease
- Upper Genital Tract Infection/Inflammation
- Salpingitis
- Tubo-ovarian Abscess

PELVIC MASS

Mina J. Guico, MD
Joseph A. Diaz, MD

KEY CLINICAL POINTS

- Pregnancy should be first ruled out in reproductive age women.
- Increased likelihood of malignancy if the following characteristics are present:
  - Complex or solid appearing cyst
  - Presence of ascites
  - Prepubescent or postmenopausal age
- Avoid laparoscopic attempt if suspicious for malignancy to prevent risk of rupture and spilling of malignant cells in the pelvis

 BASICS

DESCRIPTION

- Pelvic masses may be solid or cystic lesions located in the pelvic region.
- Pathology may occur in the adnexal region (contains ovary, fallopian tube, round ligament), uterus, bowel, or retroperitoneum.
- The etiology of pelvic masses differs between reproductive and postmenopausal ages.
- Initial evaluation should always exclude pregnancy in women of reproductive age.

EPIDEMIOLOGY

- Reproductive age women
  - Adnexal masses are less likely to be malignant—incidence 5–18%.
  - Chronic pelvic inflammatory disease (PID) is common in this age group and when left untreated or undertreated may result in tubo-ovarian abscess
  - Physiologic and functional ovarian cysts occur as a normal process of ovulation
  - Uterine fibroids (leiomyoma) may develop in 40% of premenopausal women by age 50
  - A benign ovarian tumor (mature cystic teratoma) is most common in the 2nd and 3rd decades of life and is responsible for 50% of ovarian tumors in the 25–50 year range. It accounts for 90% of germ cell tumors and 25% of all ovarian tumors
- Postmenopausal women
  - The risk of malignancy of adnexal masses is 30–60%.
  - Ovarian CA is the 5th leading cause of death in women, affecting 1 in 70 during their lifetime.
  - Consider metastasis to ovary from other primary malignancies (i.e., breast and GI tract).

RISK FACTORS

- Reproductive age
  - Approximately 46% of patients with tubo-ovarian abscess have history of PID
  - Leiomyoma:
    - It is 3–5 times more common in African American women.
    - Overweight
    - Nulliparity
  - Functional cysts arise from normal physiologic variation due to elevated gonadotropin, but there is increased propensity to form individual follicular cysts in cystic fibrosis patients.

- Postmenopausal women
  - Ovarian cancer:
    - Lifetime risk increased to 5% with family history in one 1st-degree relative, 7% in 2 or more 1st-degree relatives, and 40% with positive hereditary ovarian cancer syndrome.
    - Advancing age, nulliparity, late menopause, and higher socioeconomic status are other risk factors.

PATHOPHYSIOLOGY

- Reproductive age
  - Tubo-ovarian abscess is due to undertreated or untreated PID that result in scarring of tubal fimbria (may affect the ovaries) leading to a collection of polymicrobial pus collection.
  - Follicular cysts are thin-walled, translucent cysts filled with water, clear or straw-colored fluid situated in the ovarian cortex.
  - Mature cystic teratomas are cystic structures containing elements of all three germ cell layers and may contain bone and teeth.
  - Leiomyoma is a benign tumor composed of smooth muscle cells in concentric whorls.
- Postmenopausal women
  - Ovarian cancer may arise from the surface of the ovary (epithelial type, also the most common), egg-producing cells (germ-cell), or from supportive tissue ((stromal type, least common).

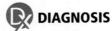 **DIAGNOSIS**

SIGNS AND SYMPTOMS

- Reproductive age
  - Tubo-ovarian abscess typically presents as abdominal/pelvic pain with fever.
  - Functional cysts are frequently asymptomatic, but may cause abdominal pain and pressure if increased size or if cyst ruptures.
  - Mature cystic teratomas are usually asymptomatic unless tumor ruptures or cause torsion presenting as an acute abdomen.
  - Patients with leiomyomas present with back pain, pelvic pain or pressure, menorrhagia, and history of infertility.
- Postmenopausal women
  - Ovarian cancer symptoms are usually vague and when detected, the disease is usually beyond the ovaries. Symptoms may include pelvic heaviness, urinary frequency, dyspepsia, anorexia, and abdominal bloating.

Physical Exam

- Pelvic/bimanual exams are important to distinguish size, location, consistency, and mobility of masses.
- Bladder should be empty during bimanual examination.
- Reproductive age
  - Tubo-ovarian abscess may present as fever, purulent cervical discharge, and cervical motion tenderness.
  - Functional cysts may be palpated, but may rupture during pelvic exam that may cause no pain or transient pelvic pain.
  - Mature cystic teratoma on palpation, has both cystic and solid components with doughy consistency, occurs bilaterally 10–15% of the time

– Patients with leiomyomas present with an enlarged, irregularly shaped uterus, which may be pedunculated arising from the fundus. Their condition may be misdiagnosed as an ovarian mass.
• Postmenopausal women
  – Ovarian cancer may be associated with pleural effusion, abdominal distention with ascites, abdominopelvic mass, and groin adenopathy.

TESTS
Lab
• Quantitative serum β-HCG to rule out pregnancy
• CBC to check for leukocytosis
• CA-125:
  – Increased levels >65 U/mL found in 80% of ovarian cancer cases
  – Approximately 50% sensitivity in stage I and 90% in stage II
  – Lacks specificity needed for screening
  – May be elevated in benign conditions like endometriosis, PID, liver and renal disease

Imaging
• Transvaginal/transabdominal ultrasound:
  – Most valuable diagnostic study in the initial evaluation of pelvic mass
  – Differentiates simple, complex, and solid tumors
  – Postmenopausal ovary twice the size of contralateral ovary; presence of ascites are suspicious for malignancy
• CT Scan:
  – Increased resolution and ability to distinguish subtle differences enable identification of some tumors.
• MRI:
  – Provides detailed evaluation of pelvic anatomy with excellent tissue contrast ability
  – Able to diagnose some benign entities especially endometriosis

DIFFERENTIAL DIAGNOSIS
• Gynecologic
  – Pregnancy
  – PID leading to tubo-ovarian abscess
  – Ectopic pregnancy
  – Polycystic ovarian syndrome
  – Fallopian tube cancer
  – Uterine cancer
  – Functional cyst
  – Benign ovarian cancer
  – Endometriosis
  – Leiomyoma
  – Ovarian cancer
• Non-gynecologic
  – Appendicitis/abscess
  – Diverticulosis
  – Colon cancer
  – Bladder tumor
  – Polycystic kidney disease
  – Retroperitoneal mass

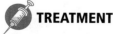 **TREATMENT**

GENERAL MEASURES
• Reproductive age
  – Tubo-ovarian abscess:
    • Broad spectrum intravenous antibiotics

– Functional cysts:
  • Majority will spontaneously be reabsorbed or rupture within 4–8 weeks of the initial diagnosis.
  • Ultrasonography to establish if cyst is simple or complex
  • A simple cyst <10 cm may be followed after 4–8 weeks or 2–3 menstrual cycles. OCPs may be used during this time.
  • If the cyst size is stable or enlarged during follow-up or initial evaluation reveals complex cyst, laparoscopic evaluation or cystectomy is indicated to r/o malignancy.
– Leiomyoma:
  • For symptomatic patients, progesterone (with or without estrogen) danazol or GnRH agonists may be used.
  • Myomectomy may be done to remove tumor alone.
  • Hysterectomy if pregnancy is not desired
– Mature cystic teratoma:
  • Risk of rupture or slow spilling of sebaceous fluid from tumor may present as an acute abdomen.
  • Operative treatment is cystectomy with normal preservation of normal ovarian tissue as much as possible.
• Post-menopausal age
  – Ovarian cancer
    • Annual rectovaginal evaluation, CA-125 determination and transvaginal ultrasound are recommended for high-risk patients.
    • The chance of malignancy increases with age (>50 years old) and size of cyst (>10 cm for premenopausal or >3 cm for postmenopausal women).
    • Simple cyst <3 cm, asymptomatic with normal Pap smears and CA-125 levels may be observed but with serial follow-up with ultrasonography at 3, 6, 9, and 12 months.
    • Cysts >3 cm or solid fixed masses should undergo exploratory surgery.
    • If positive for ovarian cancer, adjuvant chemotherapy follows.

SURGERY
Laparotomy vs. Laparoscopy
• Laparoscopy has the accompanying risk of spilling malignant cells into peritoneal cavity by rupture of ovarian capsule during removal of mass.
• Preoperative criteria for laparoscopy:
  – Age (postmenopausal has increased likelihood of malignancy)
  – Ultrasonographic characteristics including nonadherent smooth and thin-walled cysts, absence of papillae, or internal echoes.

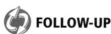 **FOLLOW-UP**

COMPLICATIONS
• Reproductive age
  – Tubo-ovarian abscess:
    • Increased likelihood of infertility and ectopic pregnancy
  – Functional cyst:
    • Recurrence after laparoscopy may be 2%.
    • Higher recurrence up to 40% for simple drainage
    • Rupture of corpus luteum cyst may cause slight to severe bleeding.
    • Rarely, adnexal torsion may occur in 1% of cases of theca lutein cysts.
  – Mature cystic teratoma:
    • May undergo malignant transformation in 1–2%, usually over age 40
    • May be associated with thyrotoxicosis, carcinoid syndrome, and auto-immune hemolytic anemia

- Rupture of contents in peritoneal cavity is the most serious complication, occurring in 0.7–4.6% of the patients.
  – Leiomyoma:
  - Degeneration occurs when there is decreased blood supply, but has a 0.3–0.7% chance for malignant degeneration.
  - Approximately 1 in 4 women eventually undergo hysterectomy after myomectomy due to recurrence.
- Post-menopausal age
  – Ovarian cancer:
  - Outcomes are poor with 5-year survival rates for all stages of only 35%.

REFERENCES

1. Morgan A. Adnexal mass evaluation in the emergency department. *Emerg Clinf North Am*. 2001;19:799–816.
2. Stenchever M. Differential diagnosis of major gynecologic problems by age groups: Vaginal bleeding, pelvic pain, pelvic mass. In: Stenchever M, ed. Comprehensive Gynecology. 4th ed. St. Louis, MO; Mosby, 2001:665–713.
3. Williams R, Elam G. Gynecology. In: Rakel, ed. Textbook of Family Practice. 6th ed. Philadelphia, PA; W.B. Saunders Company, 2002;679–681.
4. Droegemueller W. Infections of the upper genital tract: Endometritis, acute and chronic salpingitis. 4th ed. In: Stenchever M, ed. Comprehensive Gynecology. St. Louis, MO; Mosby, 2001;726–727.
5. Hernandez E, Miyazawa K. The pelvic mass, patient's ages and pathologic findings. *J Reprod Med*. 1988;33:361–364.
6. Koonings PP, Campbell K, Mishell DR Jr, et al. Relative frequency of primary ovarian neoplasms: A ten year review. *Obstet Gynecol*. 1989;74:921–926.
7. Killackey MA, Neuwirth RS. Evaluation and management of pelvic mass: A review of 540 cases. *Obstet Gynecol*. 1988;71:319–322.

CODES
ICD9-CM
789.3

KEY WORDS

- Adnexal Mass
- Adnexal Pain
- Amenorrhea
- Pregnancy
- Physiologic Cysts
- Ovarian Cancer
- CA-125

PELVIC ORGAN PROLAPSE

Vivian W. Sung, MD, MPH

KEY CLINICAL POINTS

- Pelvic organ prolapse is a common, distressing, and disabling condition affecting up to 30% of women of all ages.
- Pelvic organ prolapse may have a significant impact on a patient's quality of life and body image.

 BASICS

DESCRIPTION

Pelvic organ prolapse occurs when the normal supports of the pelvic organs fail, allowing the pelvic organs to "prolapse" into the vagina.

EPIDEMIOLOGY

- In general, it is difficult to study given the long latency period.
- The prevalence of pelvic organ prolapse increases with age; therefore, the changing demographics of the population will result in more affected women.
- The direct cost of surgery for prolapse is estimated to be greater than $1 billion per year.
- Lifetime risk for undergoing surgery for prolapse or incontinence is 11% in the United States.

Incidence

- Anterior vaginal prolapse ("bladder prolapse", "cystocoele"): 9.3 cases per 100 women per year
- Posterior vaginal prolapse ("rectocoele"): 5.7 cases per 100 women per year
- Uterine prolapse: 1.5 cases per 100 women per year

Prevalence

- Anterior vaginal prolapse: 34.3%
- Posterior vaginal prolapse: 18.3%
- Uterine prolapse: 14.2%

RISK FACTORS

- Predisposing factors (congenital)
  - Neurologic, connective tissue, musculoskeletal
  - Genetic
- Inciting factors (acquired)
  - Vaginal delivery
  - Pelvic surgery
  - Neurologic injury
- Promoting factors
  - Obesity
  - Smoking
  - Chronic straining, constipation
  - Frequent heavy lifting
- Decompensating factors
  - Aging
  - Menopause
  - Neuropathy, myopathy
  - Debilitation
  - Medication

PATHOPHYSIOLOGY

Weakening or injury of pelvic supportive structures (connective tissue, pelvic floor muscles, nerves) result in prolapse of pelvic organs

ETIOLOGY

- Childbirth
  - Labor and delivery may result in direct damage to connective tissue supports and muscles (disruption)
  - Indirect damage may result in injury to nerves and muscles (ischemia, compression, stretching)
    - Pudendal nerve latency has been shown to be prolonged after delivery, although this recovers over time
- Connective tissue disorders
  - Ehlers-Danlos
- Pelvic neuropathy
  - Chronic constipation, straining, vaginal childbirth may cause chronic stretching and injury to pudendal nerve
- Congenital disorders
  - Spina bifida
  - Bladder exstrophy
- Postoperative effects
  - Pelvic surgery may disrupt innervation to pelvic supportive tissues
- Obesity
- Chronic cough
- Smoking

ASSOCIATED CONDITIONS

- Urinary incontinence
- Fecal incontinence
- Depression

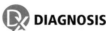 DIAGNOSIS

SIGNS AND SYMPTOMS

- Vaginal bulge
  - Patients may describe as "sitting on a bulge, golf ball, tennis ball" or "something dropped"
- Vaginal pressure
- Erosions or ulcerations of cervix and vaginal epithelium from prolonged prolapse
- Pelvic pain
- Urinary symptoms
  - Poor stream
  - Urinary hesitancy
  - Straining to void
  - Incomplete emptying
  - Recurrent urinary tract infections
  - Need to reduce bulge digitally to void ("splinting")
- Defecatory symptoms
  - Constipation
  - Incomplete evacuation
  - Need to reduce bulge digitally to initiate or finish bowel movement
- Sexual dysfunction
  - Uncomfortable during sexual relations
  - Avoidance of sexual relations due to altered body image and embarrassment

History

- Severity of symptoms
  - How long?
  - How bothersome?
- Exacerbating factors
  - Lifting, straining
  - Time of day

- Symptom type
  - Bulging
  - Pelvic pressure
  - Discomfort
  - Urinary symptoms
  - Defecatory symptoms
- Coexisting pelvic floor disorders
  - Urinary incontinence
  - Urinary tract infections
  - Fecal incontinence
- Impact on quality of life
  - Actual versus desired activity level
  - Psychosocial impact
  - Sexual function impact
- Prior therapies
  - Physical therapy, Kegel exercises
  - Pessary trial
  - Prior surgeries

Physical Exam
- Pelvic examination
  - Examination of pelvic support and all vaginal areas should be done with patient resting and with patient straining with Valsalva maneuver.
  - Examination of each compartment with split speculum on straining
    - Cervix or vaginal cuff
    - Anterior vaginal wall
    - Posterior vaginal wall
    - Genital hiatus (length of vaginal opening)
    - Perineal body
  - Vulvar or vaginal atrophy
  - Cough stress test to r/o stress incontinence
  - Bimanual exam
  - Recto-vaginal exam
    - Poor sphincter tone
    - Anal sphincter defect
- Neurologic examination
  - Anal wink reflex
  - Pelvic muscle strength
  - Sensation

TESTS
- Urodynamic evaluation if significant prolapse to rule out associated stress incontinence
- Post-void residual

Lab
Urine culture to rule out infection

Imaging
- Usually not necessary
- Defecogram if defecatory symptoms not consistent with exam findings
  - Radiologic study in which barium contrast is introduced into the rectum and radiologic images are taken.
  - Produces anatomic depiction of changes that occur in the rectum and anal canal during defecation and movement of the pelvic floor.
- Dynamic MRI of the pelvis is performed during rest and with Valsalva to evaluate pelvic prolapse (predominantly for research purposes or if symptoms not consistent with exam findings).

DIFFERENTIAL DIAGNOSIS
- Rectal prolapse
- Pelvic mass

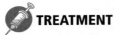 **TREATMENT**

GENERAL MEASURES
- Treatment goal is to minimize the impact of condition or achieve a cure.
- Treatment strategy depends on the severity of the symptoms, degree of bother, associated pelvic floor conditions, prior surgery, and the patient's willingness to accept the risks and success rates of different interventions, as well as the patient's general health and activity level.

Observation
- Patient is not bothered by findings and prolapse is mild or moderate
- Patient is not bothered, but prolapse is severe
  - Recommend following up every 3 months to reassess the risks and benefits of observation

Nonsurgical Management
- Pelvic floor exercises
  - Utility for prolapse is uncertain
  - Essentially no adverse effects
- Pessary
  - Large variety available
  - Acceptability to patient an issue
  - Correct fit includes following:
    - Symptom resolution
    - Patient should not feel pessary nor be uncomfortable
    - Will stay in place even with Valsalva or other straining
  - Initial follow-up 2–3 weeks
  - Patients may be taught self-care of ring pessary, but other types require office visits approximately every 1–3 months for continued care
  - At follow-up visits:
    - Pessary is removed and inspected
    - Vaginal walls are inspected for evidence of abrasions or ulcerations from pessary (may need a different size)
    - Vaginal atrophy or erosions treated with topical estrogen cream
    - Vaginal discharge (may be treated with Trimo-San gel, Milex Products, Chicago, Il)
    - Bacterial vaginosis (may be treated with metronidazole)
  - Patients who will not follow-up are not candidates for pessaries as prolonged neglect may result in the pessary becoming impacted in the vagina or erosion of pessary into bladder or rectum.
  - Successful in patients where a good fit can be achieved

SURGERY
Type and extent of repair will depend on precise defects, patient's desires and expectations, associated pelvic floor disorders (incontinence), and the patient's age, medical status, and comorbidities.
- Obliterative
  - Closure of vagina
  - Short operative time
  - Regional or local anesthesia
  - No desire for future sexual intercourse
  - Decrease in peri-operative morbidity for older women compared to reconstructive procedures
- Reconstructive
  - Compartment-specific repair depending on what is prolapsed and causing symptoms

- *Apical prolapse* requires re-suspending the vaginal apex to nearby pelvic ligaments (uterosacral or sacrospinous), muscles (ileococcygeus), or the sacrum (sacral colpopexy).
- Includes vaginal, abdominal, laparoscopic approaches
- *Anterior vaginal prolapse* requires a cystocele repair (vaginal approach) or paravaginal defect repair (abdominal or laparoscopic approach).
- *Posterior vaginal prolapse* requires a rectocele repair (vaginal approach).

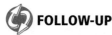 **FOLLOW-UP**

Issues for Referral
- Unsuccessful conservative management
- Visible prolapse (beyond hymen)
- Significant symptoms
- Recurrent urinary tract infections

PROGNOSIS
Prognosis is variable depending on type of repair.

COMPLICATIONS
Severe prolapse left untreated may result in urinary retention, frequent urinary tract infections, pyelonephritis, vaginal ulcerations, erosions, and infections.

REFERENCES

1. Weber AM, Richter HE. Pelvic organ prolapse. *Obstet Gynecol*. 2005;106:615–634.
2. Hendrix SL, Clark A, Nygaard I, et al. Pelvic organ prolapse in the Women's Health Initiative: Gravity and gravidity. *Am J Obstet Gynecol*. 2002;186:1160–1166.
3. Olsen AL, Smith VJ, Bergstrom JO, et al. Epidemiology of surgically managed pelvic organ prolapse and urinary incontinence. *Obstet Gynecol*. 1997;89:501–506.
4. Subak LL, Waetjen LE, van den Eeden S, et al. Cost of pelvic organ prolapse surgery in the United States. *Obstet Gynecol*. 2001;98:646–651.
5. Walters MD, Karram MM, eds. Urogynecology and Reconstructive Pelvic Surgery. 2nd ed. St. Louis: Mosby, Inc.; 1999.

ADDITIONAL READING

Swift SE. The distribution of pelvic organ support in a population of female subjects seen for routine gynecologic health care. *Am J Obstet Gynecol*. 183;277–285.
Luber KM, Boero S, Choe JY. The demographics of pelvic floor disorders: Current observations and future projections. *Am J Obstet Gynecol*. 2001;184:1496–1503.
Bent AE, Ostergard DR, Cundiff GW, Swift SE, eds. Urogynecology and Pelvic Floor Dysfunction. 5th ed. Philadelphia: Lippincott Williams & Wilkins; 2003.

CODES
ICD9-CM
- 618.00 Cystocele
- 618.2 Uterovaginal prolapse, incomplete
- 618.3 Uterovaginal prolapse, complete
- 618.4 Rectocele
- 618.5 Vaginal eversion post hysterectomy
- 618.8 Vaginal outlet relaxation
- 728.87 Levator muscle weakness
- 625.6 Stress urinary incontinence
- 788.31 Urge incontinence

KEY WORDS

- Pelvic Organ Prolapse
- Pessary
- Quality of Life
- Uterine Prolapse
- Cystocele
- Rectocele
- Urinary Incontinence
- Fecal Incontinence

PERIPARTUM CARDIOMYOPATHY

Margaret A. Miller, MD

KEY CLINICAL POINTS

- Peripartum cardiomyopathy occurs in last month of pregnancy or first 5 months postpartum.
- Left ventricular function normalizes within 6 months in 50% of patients.
- Patients with persistent LV dysfunction have the highest rate of death with a subsequent pregnancy and should be strongly advised against pregnancy in the future.
- Patients with (PPCM) are at increased risk of thrombosis.

 BASICS

DESCRIPTION
- Peripartum cardiomyopathy is a dilated cardiomyopathy that is unique to pregnancy.
- Occurs in last month of pregnancy or first 5 months postpartum
- High index of suspicion necessary as symptoms of early heart failure may be attributed to normal pregnancy
- May recur in subsequent pregnancy

EPIDEMIOLOGY
Incidence
- True incidence is unknown
- Incidence varies greatly by region
  - Occurs 1/15,000 in US
  - Occurs 1/6,000 in Japan
  - Occurs 1/100 in South Africa

RISK FACTORS
- Advanced maternal age
- Multiparity
- Multiple gestation
- African descent
- Hypertension
- Preeclampsia

Genetics
A few cases of familial peripartum cardiomyopathy have been reported.

ETIOLOGY
- The cause of peripartum cardiomyopathy is unknown but may be multifactorial.
- Possible contributing factors include:
  - Abnormal immune response to pregnancy
  - Myocarditis
  - Maladaptive response to the hemodynamic stress of pregnancy
  - Stress activated cytokines

ASSOCIATED CONDITIONS
- Thromboembolism: Women with PPCM are at increased risk of thrombosis
- Arrhythmia

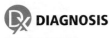 DIAGNOSIS

PRE-HOSPITAL
- Most patients with PPCM are young and have no comorbid cardiopulmonary conditions.
- They may appear clinically well, even with significant LV dysfunction.

- Many of the symptoms of early heart failure such as palpitations, dyspnea, and edema occur in normal pregnancy
- High index of suspicion required for prompt diagnosis.

Diagnostic Criteria
National Heart, Lung and Blood Institute and Office of Rare Diseases (NIH) definition:
- Development of cardiac failure in last month of pregnancy or within five months of delivery
- Absence of a identifiable cause for cardiac failure (i.e., valvular heart disease, ischemia, pericardial disease)
- Absence of recognizable heart disease prior to pregnancy
- LV dysfunction demonstrated by classic echocardiographic criteria

SIGNS AND SYMPTOMS
History
- Onset of symptoms after 36 weeks gestation or in first 5 months after delivery. Symptoms include:
  - Dyspnea
  - Cough
  - Orthopnea
  - Paroxysmal nocturnal dyspnea
  - Fatigue
  - Palpitations
  - Hemoptysis
  - Chest pain
  - Abdominal pain
- No previous history of heart disease
- Family history of cardiomyopathy
- Assessment of NYHA functional class

Physical Exam
- Height and weight
- BP may be normal or elevated
- Tachycardia
- Elevated jugular venous pressure
- Third heart sound
- Pulmonary rales
- Peripheral edema
- Ascites
- Cardiomegaly
- Hepatomegaly
- Arrhythmias

TESTS
Lab
- Initial lab evaluation of all patients presenting with new onset heart failure should include
  - CBC, urinalysis, electrolytes (including calcium and magnesium), BUN, creatinine, fasting glucose, lipid profile, liver function tests and TSH
- Lab testing for other causes of dilated cardiomyopathy is reasonable if there is clinical suspicion.
- Brain Natriuretic Peptide (BNP)
  - Levels likely increase due to normal volume expansion in pregnancy
  - Has not been validated for use in pregnancy
- EKG
  - May reveal LVH, LBBB, left or right atrial enlargement
  - Signs of ischemic heart disease should be assessed.

Imaging
- CXR findings will be the same as the nonpregnant population.
- Echocardiogram shows depressed left ventricular ejection fraction (LVEF), decreased fractional shortening and increased left ventricular end-diastolic dimension.
- There are no echocardiographic features that distinguish PPCM from other forms of dilated cardiomyopathy.

Diagnostic Procedures/Surgery
Endomyocardial biopsy is not routinely recommended due to low diagnostic yield.

Pathological Findings
No clear pathognomonic findings on endomyocardial biopsy

DIFFERENTIAL DIAGNOSIS
- Cardiogenic pulmonary edema due to previously undiagnosed cardiomyopathy or valvular heart disease
  - Unlike PPCM, symptoms would most likely present at 28–30 weeks, coinciding with peak blood volume in pregnancy
- Noncardiogenic pulmonary edema occurs in pregnancy in association with
  - Infection (especially pyelonephritis)
  - Preeclampsia
  - Use of tocolytics or excessive IV fluids
- Pulmonary hypertension may present with progressive dyspnea and signs of right-sided heart failure.

 ## TREATMENT

INITIAL STABILIZATION
- For acute decompensation
  - Oxygenation to keep PaO2 >95%
  - Diuresis
  - Treat hypertension
- Fetal monitoring

GENERAL MEASURES
As with other forms of heart failure, important components of treatment include:
- Restriction of sodium intake
- Diuresis
- Afterload reduction
- Beta-blockers

Diet
Sodium restriction

Activity
- May be limited by symptoms
- Bedrest should not be recommended
- NYHA functional class is an important predictor of prognosis

IV Fluids
Should be avoided

 ## MEDICATION (DRUGS)

First Line
- Diuretics
  - Loop diuretics are safe in pregnancy and breastfeeding.
- Hydralazine
  - First choice drug for afterload reduction during pregnancy
- Beta-blockers
  - No role in acute treatment
  - Use in the postpartum period for patients who continue to have symptoms and LV dysfunction despite >2 weeks of standard heart failure therapy

Second Line
- ACE-inhibitors
  - Contraindicated in pregnancy.
  - Drug of first choice postpartum
  - Switch from hydralazine to ACE-I postpartum
  - Safe in breastfeeding except use with caution if very premature infant
  - Best data for benefit in long term survival
- Digoxin
  - May be used safely in pregnancy for symptom control
  - Little benefit in the acute setting
- Immunosuppressive therapy
  - Limited data on benefit

 ## FOLLOW-UP

DISPOSITION
Admission Criteria
- Evidence of active heart failure
- Hypoxia—O$_2$ saturation <95%
- Arrhythmia
- Embolism

Issues for Referral
Refer to cardiologist for help with management of LV dysfunction and monitoring with serial echocardiography

PROGNOSIS
- Mortality
  - In United States, mortality estimates range from 25–50%.
  - Black women are 6.4 times more likely to die from PPCM than white women.
  - Most deaths occur in first 3 months postpartum and are due to progressive heart failure, arrhythmias, and thromboembolic events.
- Left ventricular function
  - Severity of LV dysfunction at presentation is the most important determinant of prognosis
  - LVEF normalizes within 6 months in 50%
  - <10% have progressively worsening LVEF and ultimately require heart transplant
  - Remainder of patients may continue to have some degree of LV dysfunction
  - Risk in subsequent pregnancy varies according to recovery of LV function

ALERT
Recommendations for subsequent pregnancy
- All patients with previous PPCM should undergo echocardiography
  - If results are normal should perform dobutamine stress echocardiography
  - Patients with normal results on echocardiogram but decreased reserve on stress testing should be warned that they may not tolerate the hemodynamic stress associated with pregnancy.
- Patients who have persistent LV dysfunction have highest rate of death with a subsequent pregnancy and should be strongly advised against pregnancy in the future.
- Patients with full recovery can be told that the mortality rate is low, but chance of worsening LV function may be as high as 35%.

COMPLICATIONS
- Thrombosis
  - Patients with PPCM are at an increased risk of thrombosis

– No definitive evidence regarding when or how to initiate anticoagulation for patients with PPCM or heart failure in general
– Given hypercoagulable state of pregnancy, reasonable to consider anticoagulation in
  • Patients with LVEF <35%
  • Patients with thrombus on echocardiogram
  • Atrial fibrillation
  • History of a previous embolic event
• Arrhythmias
  – Supraventricular arrhythmias most common
  – Treatment is the same as in the nonpregnant population

PATIENT MONITORING

Monitoring in labor and delivery
• Excess catecholamines associated with labor may precipitate arrhythmia
• Maternal cardiac monitoring recommended during labor
• Adequate pain management important and consideration should be given to early epidural
• Right heart catheter
  – Controversial for monitoring in labor and delivery
  – Risks and benefits should be considered as in the non pregnant population
  – Highest risk period for worsening heart failure is postpartum period due to fluid shifts occurring in the first few postpartum days.
  – Strict attention to fluid management required.

REFERENCES

1. Elkayam U, Tummala P, Kalpana R. Maternal and fetal outcomes of subsequent pregnancies in women with peripartum cardiomyopathy. *NEJM*. 2001;24:1567–1571.
2. Pearson G, Veille JC, Rahimtoola S. Peripartum Cardiomyopathy. National heart, lung and blood institute and office of rare diseases (National Institute of Health) Workshop recommendations and review. *JAMA*. 2000;282:1183–1188.
3. Tidswell M. Peripartum Cardiomyopathy. *Crit Care Clin*. 2004;20:777–788.
4. The task force on the management of cardiovascular diseases during pregnancy of the European Society of Cardiology. Expert consensus document on management of cardiovascular diseases during pregnancy. *Eur Heart J*. 2003;24:761–781.
5. Whitehead S, Berg C, Chang J. Pregnancy-related mortality due to cardiomyopathy: United States, 1991–1997. *Obstet Gynecol*. 2003;102:1326–1331.

ADDITIONAL READING

Lee R, et al., eds. Medical Care of the Pregnant Patient. Philadelphia: American College of Physician; 2000.

CODES
ICD9-CM
674.5 Peripartum cardiomyopathy

KEY WORDS

• Cardiomyopathy
• Shortness of Breath
• Dyspnea on Exertion
• Lower Extremity Edema
• Pregnancy

POLYCYSTIC OVARIAN SYNDROME (PCOS)

Michelle A. Stozek Anvar, MD

KEY CLINICAL POINTS

- It is important to diagnose polycystic ovary syndrome (PCOS) so that patients can be monitored for the metabolic and physical effects that are associated with this syndrome.
- PCOS is a risk factor for the early development of type 2 diabetes.

 BASICS

DESCRIPTION
- PCOS is a heterogeneous disorder with symptoms that generally begin at or just prior to puberty.
- In 1935, Stein and Leventhal described a group of women with obesity, hisuitism, amenorrhea, and polycystic ovaries.
- Since that time, attempts have been made to more definitively classify this disorder.
- In 2003, an international consensus group defined PCOS as 2 of following 3 conditions:
  - Androgen excess
  - Polycystic ovaries
  - Oligo- or amenorrhea
- Other causes of these symptoms need to be ruled out to make the diagnosis.

GENERAL PREVENTION
This syndrome may have a genetic component but symptoms can in part be controlled by maintaining a normal weight.

EPIDEMIOLOGY
Incidence
Usually begins around menarche, but may occur earlier or later especially when associated with weight gain.

Prevalence
Prevalence is estimated to be 5–10% of female population.

Genetics
There may be a genetic tendency as rates vary among ethnic groups; multiple genes have been associated with the syndrome.

PATHOPHYSIOLOGY
The pathophysiology of PCOS is complex and still unclear, but seems to involve a genetic predisposition and possibly environmental factors that affect gonadotropin levels.

ASSOCIATED CONDITIONS
- Diagnosis of this syndrome confers a risk of developing the following:
  - Diabetes
    - Approximately 30–40% of the patients have impaired glucose tolerance.
    - Approximately 10% of the patients have diabetes by the 4th decade.
  - Hypertension
  - Cardiovascular disease
  - Sleep apnea
  - Hyperlipidemia/dyslipidemia
  - Endometrial hyperplasia and carcinoma
- Obesity: At least 30% of the patients with PCOS are obese.

 DIAGNOSIS

- Several sets of criteria have been established over the years.
- According to a 2003 International Consensus group (European Society of Human Reproductive Medicine /American Society of Reproductive Medicine):
  - Must exclude other causes of irregular menses and androgen excess (hyperprolactinemia, congenital adrenal hyperplasia, Cushing syndrome, androgen secreting neoplasm, acromegaly)
  - Two of the following:
    - Oligo-ovulation or anovulation
    - Elevated androgens or clinical manifestation of androgen excess (hirsultism, acne, alopecia)
    - Polycystic ovaries
      ○ Not needed for diagnosis
      ○ Presence alone not enough for diagnosis
  - Need to exclude other endocrine causes such as: Congenital adrenal hyperplasia and androgen secreting tumors.
    - Concerning features include: Late or rapid onset of symptoms, virilization (frontal balding, severe acne, deepening of voice, clitoromegaly), onset well after puberty.
- The 1990 NIH Consensus Criteria:
  - Oligo- or anovulation
  - Evidence of hyperandrogenism
  - Exclusion of other causes

SIGNS AND SYMPTOMS
History
Screen for the following:
- Oligomenorrhea or amenorrhea
- Male pattern hair growth
- Acne
- Infertility
- Sleep apnea
- Weight gain

Physical Exam
PCOS is associated with the following:
- Obesity
- Hypertension
- Hirsutism (in particular hair on chin, upper lip, around nipples, and on lower abdomen)
- Male pattern balding or alopecia
- Acanthosis nigricans
- Acne

TESTS
Lab
- Serum androgens
  - Free and total testosterone
  - Serum DHEA
- LH and LH:FSH ratio
  - Used frequently in the past
  - >2:1 ratio consistent with PCOS
  - May not be sensitive for diagnosis of PCOS as levels of these hormones vary over the course of the menstrual cycle

- Fasting blood glucose and consider an oral glucose tolerance test
  - Rule out diabetes/impaired glucose tolerance
- Fasting lipid panel including total cholesterol, LDL, HDL, and triglycerides

Imaging
- Pelvic ultrasound
  - Not required for diagnosis
  - Can identify ovarian cysts and rule out other pathology
  - Polycystic ovaries
    - Generally have > 10 small cysts
    - The presence of cystic ovaries alone is not enough to validate the diagnosis.

DIFFERENTIAL DIAGNOSIS
It is important to consider and rule out the following:
- Hyperprolactinemia
- Congenital adrenal hyperplasia
- Cushing's syndrome
- Androgen secreting neoplasm
- Acromegaly

TREATMENT

Treatment is based on screening for associated problems and management of the clinical disease characteristics.

GENERAL MEASURES
- Oligomenorrhea and amenorrhea
  - Return to normal menstrual cycles may be achieved with weight loss
  - Endometrial biopsy and/or gynecology referral are indicated in patients with amenorrhea, because they are at risk for endometrial cancer.
- Hyperandrogenism
  - Mechanical removal, such as waxing and electrolysis, can be effective.
- Insulin resistance and impaired glucose tolerance
  - The American Diabetes Association considers PCOS a risk factor that requires regular diabetic screening.
  - It is not clear if an oral glucose tolerance test should be performed to detect further patients with impaired glucose tolerance.
  - Weight loss and aerobic exercise is important
- Obesity
  - A healthy lifestyle should be encouraged and even mild weight loss can help with menstrual symptoms.
  - Use of metformin has been associated with modest weight loss.

Diet
A healthy diet to maintain a normal weight is an important component of treatment.

MEDICATIONS

First Line
- Oligomenorrhea and amenorrhea
  - Hormonal methods
    - Combined hormonal methods
      - Oral contraceptive pills
    - Periodic progesterone withdrawal bleeding

- Metformin
  - Addresses hyperinsulinemia
  - May also help patient return to a normal menstrual cycle
  - Only FDA approved for treatment of diabetes
- Hyperandrogenism: Several possible medications to address these symptoms
  - Hormonal methods
    - Combined estrogen-progesterone methods containing norgestimate, desogestrel, and particularly drospirenone can limit androgen levels.
  - Spironolactone 100–200 mg daily
    - Has an anti-androgen effect in these doses
    - Can be used in combination with oral contraceptives
- Insulin resistance and impaired glucose tolerance:
  - Biguanides and *thiazolidinediones* decrease insulin resistance and may also improve ovulation and fertility, hirsutism, and acne.
- Obesity
  - Metformin has been associated with modest weight loss.

FOLLOW-UP

Issues for Referral
- A gynecologic or endocrine referral may be indicated if the diagnosis is not clear or if there are other endocrine diagnoses that explain the symoptomatology.
- Patients with concern for endometrial abnormalities should be referred for further evaluation.
  - Endometrial biopsy and/or gynecology referral are indicated in patients with amenorrhea as they are at risk for endometrial cancer.
- Fertility may be an issue that requires referral to a gynecologist or reproductive endocrinologist.

PROGNOSIS
Dependent on management of symptoms and monitoring of associated symptoms.

COMPLICATIONS
- Patients with PCOS may have an increased cardiac risk secondary to their risk of diabetes, obesity, hypertension, and dyslipidemia.
- Obstetrical/gynecological complications include infertility, menstrual abnormalities, and endometrial hyperplasia secondary to chronic anovulation.
- Patients are also at risk for sleep apnea.

PATIENT MONITORING
Monitor for the following:
- Diabetes/impaired glucose tolerance
- Lipid abnormalities
- Obesity
- Menstrual abnormalities
- Sleep apnea

Pregnancy Considerations
- There is an increased rate of early miscarriage of unclear etiology.
- Irregular ovulation may result in delayed time until conception.
- Weight loss is the 1st line of therapy. If not successful, referral to a gynecologist for use of clomiphene and possibly metformin may be indicated.
- Metformin is class B in and the *thiazolidinediones* are class C in pregnancy.

REFERENCES

1. Apridonidze T, Essah PA, Iuorno MJ, et al. Prevalence and characteristics of the metabolic syndrome in women with polycystic ovary syndrome. *J Clin Endocrinol Metab*. 2005;90:1929–1935.
2. Assis R, Woods K, Reyna R, et al. The prevalence and incidence of polycystic ovary syndrome in an unselected population. *J Clin Endocrinol Metab*. 2004;89:2745–2749.
3. Ehrmann DA. Medical progress: Polycystic ovary syndrome. *N Engl J Med*. 2005;352:1223–1236.
4. Ehrmann DA, Barnes RB, Rosenfield RL, et al. Prevalence of impaired glucose tolerance and diabetes in women with polycystic ovary syndrome. *Diabetes Care*. 1999;22:141–146.
5. Fogel RB, Malhotra A, Pillar G, et al. Increased prevalence of obstructive sleep apnea syndrome in obese women with polycystic ovary syndrome. *J Clin Endocrinol Metab*. 2001;86:1175–1180.
6. Harborne L, Fleming R, Lyall H, et al. Descriptive review of the evidence for the use of metformin in polycystic ovary syndrome. *Lancet*. 2003;361:1894–1901.
7. Moghetti P, Castello R, Negri C, et al. Metformin effects on clinical features, endocrine and metabolic profiles, and insulin sensitivity in polycystic ovary syndrome: A randomized, double-blind, placebo-controlled 6-month trial, followed by open, long-term clinical evaluation. *J Clin Endocrinol Metab*. 2000;85:139–146.
8. Pasquali R, Vicennati V, Calzoni F, et al. Effect of long-term treatment with metformin added to hypocaloric diet on body composition, fat distribution, and androgen and insulin levels in abdominally obese women with and without the polycystic ovary syndrome. *J Clin Endocrinol Metab*. 2000;85: 2767–2774.
9. The Rotterdam ESHRE/ASRM-sponsored PCOS Consensus Workshop Group. Revised 2003 consensus on diagnostic criteria and long-term health risks related to polycystic ovary syndrome. *Fertil Steril*. 2004;81:19–25.

ADDITIONAL READING

Ehrmann DA. Medical progress: Polycystic ovary syndrome. *N Engl J Med*. 2005;352:1223–1236.
Polycystic ovary syndrome. In: Larsen PR, ed. Williams Textbook of Endocrinology. 10th ed. Saunders, 2002;627–637.

CODES
ICD9-CM
256.4 Stein Leventhal syndrome

KEY WORDS

- Polycystic Ovary Syndrome
- Stein Leventhal Syndrome
- Oligomenorrhea

POSTPARTUM DEPRESSION

Neeta Jain, MD

KEY CLINICAL POINTS

- Postpartum Blues is a self-limited disorder involving mild depressive symptoms which typically remits 2 weeks after delivery.
- Postpartum Depression (PPD) affects up to 10–20% of mothers.
- Postpartum Psychosis requires hospitalization as there is a high risk for child neglect, infanticide, and maternal suicide.

 BASICS

DESCRIPTION

- DSM-IV-TR defines postpartum depression as the onset of depression symptoms within the first 4 weeks following parturition.
- In clinical practice, however, it is not uncommon to consider the postpartum as the period up to 12 months following delivery.

GENERAL PREVENTION

- Women are more likely to seek help from their primary care physician or obstetricians rather than mental health professionals.
- It is important to ask about their mood, feelings toward their child and refer to mental health professional for further evaluation.
- Administer the Edinburgh Postnatal Depression Scale (EPDS), a self-report 10-item scale that is specific for postpartum depression.

EPIDEMIOLOGY

- **Postpartum Blues**
  - Not considered a psychiatric disorder
  - Estimated to occur in 50–85% of women within 1st week after delivery
- **Postpartum Depression**
  - Prevalence range from 10–20%
  - Is common within 6–12 weeks after parturition
- **Postpartum Psychosis**
  - Occurs in approximately 1 in 500–1,000 live births
  - Usually presents within 48–72 hours
  - Although 75% of cases begin within first 2 weeks, risk remains high up to 6 months after delivery.

Incidence
Ranges from 7.8% over 6 weeks to 14% by 12 weeks

Prevalence
Reported prevalence rates of PPD vary depending on the defined period.
- 8.2–23% from 6–16 weeks

RISK FACTORS

- **Risk Factors for Postpartum Blues and Postpartum Depression**
  - History of Premenstrual Dysphoric Disorder
  - Previous history of depression or PPD
  - Family history of depression
  - Depression during pregnancy
  - Stressful negative life events
  - Unplanned pregnancy
  - Inadequate social support
- **Risk Factors for Postpartum Psychosis**
  - History of bipolar disorder
  - Previous postpartum psychosis
  - Primiparity

ETIOLOGY
Unclear etiology
- Numerous theories implicate the hypothalamic-pituitary-gonadal axis with inconclusive data.
- Current hypothesis is that some women have an inherent neuroendocrine sensitivity to psychological, environmental, and physiologic factors, which is triggered by the onset of menarche, increasing their risk to mood dysregulation during their reproductive years.

ASSOCIATED CONDITIONS
Thyroid dysfunction
- In the 6 months following delivery, women experience thyroid dysfunction at rates of up to 10%.

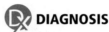 **DIAGNOSIS**

History
- **Postpartum Blues**
  - Usually presents 4 or 5 days to first 2 weeks after delivery
  - Considered to be a "normal" physiologic response to the hormonal events of childbirth
  - Symptoms include labile mood, tearfulness, anxious mood, irritability, elation, poor concentration, insomnia, hypersensitivity
  - Symptoms are typically self-remitting but 20% of women can develop depressive symptoms
- **Postpartum Depression**
  - Usually presents within 6–12 weeks to 1st year after delivery
  - Resembles major depressive episode
  - Sleep disturbance, particularly inability to return to sleep after feeding baby or when infant is asleep
  - Labile mood with prominent anxiety and irritability
  - Overanxious, overwhelmed, or unable to take care of baby
  - Feelings of inadequacy or failure as a mother
  - History of frequent calls or visits about own health or baby's without objective reasoning and inability to be reassured
  - Distressing intrusive thoughts with or without compulsions
  - Suicidal or homicidal ideation
- **Postpartum Psychosis**
- Usually presents within the first 48–72 hours after delivery
  - Delusional beliefs, often pertaining to the baby (infant is possessed or has special powers) or self
  - Hyperviligance about the baby
  - Insomnia and psychomotor hyperkinesias
  - Perplexed, confused, or disoriented
  - Impaired cognition or delirium-like symptoms with waxing and waning course
  - Visual, auditory, olfactory, or tactile hallucinations

TESTS
- Medical work-up should be initiated to rule out organic etiologies, such as
  - Thyroid abnormalities
  - Sheehan's syndrome
  - Pregnancy-related autoimmune disorders
  - Intracranial mass
- Studies that implemented screening protocols have reported increased rates of detection.
  - Use of the Edinburgh Postnatal Depression Scale (EPDS) can aid in early detection.
  - The scale may be obtained on the internet: http://www.patient.co.uk/showdoc/40002172

Lab
- TSH
- Toxicology screen
- CBC

Imaging
Consider MRI if suspicion of intracranial mass or Sheehan's syndrome

DIFFERENTIAL DIAGNOSIS
- Thyroid abnormalities
- Sheehan's syndrome
- Pregnancy-related autoimmune disorders
- Intracranial mass
- Illicit drug use

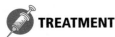 **TREATMENT**

Most successful treatment strategies are multifactorial, including
- Education
- Psychotherapy
- Group support
- Referrals to self-help and national organizations
- Involvement of spouse and/or family members
- Psychopharmacological management, if appropriate

GENERAL MEASURES
- **Postpartum Blues**
  - Women generally respond to education, support and reassurance that symptoms typically remit within 2 weeks after delivery.
- **Postpartum Depression**
  - Women with mild to moderate depression usually are responsive to reduction of psychological stressors, mobilization of family/partner support, individual, or group therapy and self-help groups.
  - Women with severe depressive symptoms or functional impairment in their daily life should discuss antidepressant medication use with their clinician.
    - Decision to use medications should take into consideration whether the patient is breast-feeding.
    - Hospitalization if suicidal
    - Electroconvulsive therapy (ECT)
- **Postpartum Psychosis**
  - Psychiatric hospitalization is almost always indicated as risk for neglect of the child, infanticide, and suicide is high.
    - Mood stabilizers
    - Neuroleptics
    - Antidepressants
    - Benzodiazepines
    - ECT

Complementary and Alternative Medicine
Light therapy and Omega-3 fatty acids are promising alternatives.

 MEDICATION (DRUGS)

- Patients should be informed about limitations on current data (small sample size, case studies, and imperfect FDA categories).
- No medication should be used without discussing risks and benefits with both patient and her partner.
- Little is known in terms of risks of long-term neurobehavioral sequelae after exposure to psychotropic medications in a developing brain versus the risk of untreated depression for the patient and infant.

First Line
- Sertraline: Starting dose 25 mg daily
- Nortriptyline: Starting dose 25 mg daily

Second Line
Fluoxetine: Starting dose 10 mg daily

ALERT
For breastfeeding mothers:
- FDA has not approved any antidepressant for use during lactation.
- Psychotropic medications are excreted in breast milk.
- Nursing mothers should be prescribed the minimum dosage to achieve a symptom reduction.
- Taking medication immediately after breast-feeding minimizes the amount present in milk and maximizes clearance before the next feeding.
- Short-acting agents are preferable to long-acting agents.
- Bottle-feeding supplementation is encouraged to minimize drug exposure.
- Assessment by pediatrician should be made to establish baseline behavior, sleep, and feeding patterns.
- Infant drug clearance increases from nearly 33% of mother's weight-adjusted clearance to 100% by 6 months of age.
- For premature infants, liver enzymes are immature and drug clearance is slow; psychiatric medication levels may accumulate and adversely affect the infant.
- Paroxetine exposure in utero has been associated with neonatal withdrawal symptoms that persisted 10 days after birth.

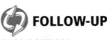 **FOLLOW-UP**

DISPOSITION
Admission Criteria
- Psychosis
- Inability to care for self or infant

Issues for Referral
- Assessment by pediatrician should be made to establish baseline behavior, sleep, and feeding patterns prior to initiation of psychotropic medications.
- Nursing mothers should be referred to mental health providers and closely monitored by the physician.

PROGNOSIS
- Prompt detection and treatment for these women is imperative in the overall impact on the mother-infant dyad.
- Untreated depression has consistently shown adverse outcomes in social, emotional, and behavioral development in children of depressed mothers.
- The longer duration of untreated symptoms in women may prolong total recovery once treatment is undertaken.

COMPLICATIONS
Recurrence
- Women with prior history of postpartum depression have a 50% recurrence with each subsequent delivery.
- A previous history of depression is associated with a 25% risk of depression after delivery.
- A previous postpartum psychosis is associated with 20–50% risk of relapse following subsequent deliveries.
- Women with a history of bipolar disorder and postpartum psychosis have a 50% risk of relapse with each successive delivery.

REFERENCES

1. Bloch M, Daly RC, Rubinow DR. Endocrine factors in the etiology of postpartum depression. *Comp Psych*. 2003;44:234–246.
2. Born L, Zinga D, Steiner M. Challenges in identifying and diagnosing postpartum disorders. *Primary Psychiatry*. 2004;11(3):29–36.
3. Burt VK, Hendrick VC, eds. Concise Guide to Women's Mental Health. 2nd Ed. Washington: American Psychaitric Publishing; 2001.
4. Corral MK, Kostaras D. Bright light therapy's effect on postpartum depression. *Am J Psych*. 2000;157:303–304.
5. Cox JL, Holden JM, Sagovsky R. Detection of postnatal depression: development of the 10-item Edinburgh postnatal depression scale. *Br J Psych*. 1987;150:782–786.
6. Flynn HA. Epidemiology and phenomenology of Postpartum Mood Disorders. *Psych Annals*. 2005;35:544–551.
7. Haddad PM, Pal BR, Wieck A, et al. Neonatal symptoms following maternal paroxetine treatment: Serotonin toxicity or paroxetine discontinuation syndrome? *J Psychopharmcol*. 2005;19:554–557.

8. Helland IB, Smith L, Saugstad OD, et al. Maternal supplementation with very long chain n-3 fatty acids during pregnancy and lactation augments children's IQ at 4 years of age. *Pediatrics*. 2003;111:e39–44.

MISCELLANEOUS

- Postpartum Support international: www.postpartum.net
- Drug Registries: www.fda.gov/wome

CODES
ICD9-CM
- 311 Depressive disorder NOS
- 296.2 Major depressive disorder, single episode
- 298.0 Depressive type psychosis

KEY WORDS

- Postpartum Depression
- Depression
- Pregnancy

PREGNANCY, ASTHMA

Jill Newstead-Angel, MD
Ghada Bourjeily, MD

KEY CLINICAL POINTS

- The main goals for asthma in pregnancy are the same as asthma in the general population. They include adequate asthma control and prevention of exacerbations and hospitalizations.
- "It is safer for pregnant women with asthma to be treated with asthma medications than for them to have asthma symptoms and exacerbations. . . Inadequate control of asthma is a greater risk to the fetus than asthma medications are".

 ## BASICS

DEFINITION
- Same as asthma in the nonpregnant patient
- Chronic inflammatory disease of the airway characterized by:
  - Reversible airway obstruction and heightened airway reactivity

EPIDEMIOLOGY
Asthma affects between 3.7% and 8.4% of pregnant women and is the most common chronic respiratory disease affecting pregnant women.
- There is an increasing prevalence of asthma in women of childbearing age.
- Approximately 1/3 of asthmatics improve during pregnancy, 1/3 stay the same, and 1/3 get worse.

RISK FACTORS
Risk factors for asthma are the same as for the general population. (See Asthma chapter.) Gastroesophageal reflux disease and nasal congestion are more common in pregnancy and may be associated with worsening symptoms of asthma.
Risk factors for asthma exacerbations during pregnancy are:
- Function of baseline asthma severity as defined by classification based on recommendations of NAEPP working group on asthma in pregnancy.
- Frequency of asthma exacerbations are lower in patients whose asthma remains mild throughout pregnancy.
- Patients on daily asthma medications should be considered to have functionally moderate asthma.
- Patients on regular oral steroids should be classified as functionally severe.
- Asthma exacerbations are most frequent between weeks 17–36 gestational age with an improvement in symptoms in the last month of pregnancy.
- The better the control, regardless of baseline severity, the better the outcome.

PATHOPHYSIOLOGY
- Same as in the nonpregnant patient however there are some physiological changes that occur to the respiratory system during pregnancy.
- Hormonally mediated increase in minute ventilation during pregnancy with increase in tidal volume. Respiratory rate is relatively unchanged.
- Arterial blood gas shows a compensated respiratory alkalosis with a normal $PaCO_2$ in pregnancy being 28–32 mmHg; pH 7.40–7.45.
- Increase in pH secondary to respiratory alkalosis is blunted by an increase in renal excretion of bicarbonate
- Mild increase in PaO_2 up to 110 mmHg

- Structural changes to chest wall result in decrease in functional residual capacity. Otherwise, pulmonary function tests are relatively unchanged in pregnancy.

ASSOCIATED CONDITIONS
- Rhinitis
- Sinusitis
- GERD

 ## DIAGNOSIS

Same as in the nonpregnant patients

SIGNS AND SYMPTOMS
History
- Same as in the nonpregnant patient
- Additional questions to ask:
  - Relation of asthma symptoms to gastroesophageal reflux disease, rhinitis, sinusitis
- Identify patients at risk for fatal asthma:
  - History of intubations
  - Frequent emergency room visits
  - Previous history of hospitalization or intensive care admission for exacerbation

Physical Exam
Same as in the nonpregnant patient however remember to examine patient either seated or if supine with a lateral tilt to the pelvis to prevent compression of IVC by uterus and therefore, a reduction in venous return.

TESTS
Lab
Blood gas: Pregnant women have a compensated respiratory alkalosis so an increase in $PaCO_2$ may mean impending respiratory failure.

Imaging
Radiological procedures may be needed to rule out diseases that either exacerbate asthma such as pneumonia or those that may mimic asthma such as pulmonary emboli. Ionizing radiation exposure to less than 5 rads during pregnancy is not thought to increase the risk for congenital malformations, growth restriction or miscarriage.
- Chest x-ray: <0.005 rads
- Chest CT: <0.03 rads
- V/Q scan: <0.06 rads

Diagnostic Procedures/Surgery
Pulmonary functions tests:
- Reversible obstructive pattern

DIFFERENTIAL DIAGNOSIS
The differential diagnosis of acute asthma during pregnancy should include other conditions that may complicate pregnancy such as:
- Pulmonary edema
- Amniotic fluid embolism
- Pulmonary embolism
- Cardiomyopathy
- Dyspnea of pregnancy
- Gastroesophageal reflux disease
- Post nasal drip

- Worsening rhinitis
- Foreign body/upper airway obstruction

TREATMENT

PRE-HOSPITAL

The treatment goal for the pregnant asthma patient is to provide optimal therapy to maintain control of asthma for maternal health and quality of life as well as for normal fetal maturation. Please refer to Table 1 for severity classification.

- Asthma management during pregnancy:
  - Assessment and monitoring of asthma including objective measures of pulmonary function on a monthly basis
  - Control of factors contributing to asthma severity
  - Patient education
  - Stepwise approach to pharmacological therapy

ASTHMA EXACERBATION

- Assess severity:
  - Can patient speak in full sentences
  - Accessory muscle use and suprasternal retractions suggest severe exacerbation
  - Note presence of fetal activity
  - Measure peak expiratory flow: A value less than 50% of personal best or predicted suggest severe exacerbation
- Prevention of maternal hypoxia, hypercarbia, reversal of bronchospasm and prevention of exhaustion are important.
  - Remember that a $PaCO_2$ of 35 mmHg or greater in the mother may imply impending respiratory failure. Fetal hypoxemia and acidosis can occur even though maternal hypoxemia is absent.
  - Oxygen supplementation should be given to maintain adequate O_2 saturation to help prevent fetal hypoxemia.
  - Fluid status should be assessed carefully and IV fluid hydration administered as necessary to help with placental perfusion.

Initial treatment:

- Short acting inhaled beta$_2$-agonist: Up to 3 treatments of 2–4 puffs by MDI at 20 minute intervals or a single nebulizer treatment.
- Ipratropium bromide (500 μg) may be administered concomitantly in severe cases.
- Systemic steroids should be given to patients who show no improvement with the initial bronchodilator treatment in either symptoms or the peak flows and to those with a moderate or severe exacerbation.
- The decision to hospitalize the patient or discharge home is based on response to treatment in the first 4 hours in the emergency room.

MEDICATION (DRUGS)

Stepwise approach for managing asthma based on NAEPP guidelines 2004 update

- Mild intermittent asthma:
  - Short acting bronchodilators, particularly short-acting inhaled beta$_2$-agonists, recommended as quick relief medication for treating symptoms as needed. Albuterol is the preferred agent as it has the most safety data related to use in pregnancy
- Mild persistent asthma:
  - Daily low dose inhaled corticosteroid
  - Budesonide is the preferred inhaled steroid as it has been studied and found the mothers that used Budesonide during

pregnancy had no adverse outcomes. Beclomethasone has also been used safely in pregnancy however if requiring high doses of inhaled steroids, there is more data with Budesonide in higher doses and pregnancy.
  - No data indicate that other inhaled corticosteroids are unsafe during pregnancy therefore inhaled corticosteroids (other than Budesonide) may be continued during pregnancy if these agents were used prior to the pregnancy.
- Moderate persistent asthma:
  - Combination of low dose inhaled corticosteroid and long acting beta$_2$-agonist, or increase the dose of the inhaled steroid to a medium dose range
  - Long acting beta agonists have similar pharmacologic and toxicologic profiles as the short acting beta agonists therefore should have a safety profile similar to Albuterol
  - Salmeterol has been around longer than Formoterol (the 2 long acting beta agonists) therefore would be the agent of choice
- Severe persistent asthma:
  - Increase the dose of inhaled corticosteroid to the high dose range.
  - If this is insufficient, addition of oral steroid may be necessary.
  - Although oral corticosteroids may have some risk during pregnancy, the benefit of treating a severe exacerbation with steroids by far outweigh the risks associated with the medication.

First Line

Budesonide and albuterol have the most safety data associated with their use during pregnancy.

Second Line

Cromolyn, leukotriene receptor antagonists (LRA) and theophylline are alternatives but not preferred treatments.

MANAGEMENT OF ACUTE ASTHMA DURING LABOR AND DELIVERY

All regularly scheduled medications should be continued during labor and delivery

- Patients who were treated with systemic steroids chronically or with numerous short courses of steroids during the pregnancy should be given stress doses of steroids every 8 hours until 24 hours postpartum starting from the onset of labor.
- Avoid morphine and meperidine as they may cause histamine release.
- If tocolytic therapy is considered for preterm labor, avoid Indomethacin as it may induce bronchospasm in aspirin sensitive asthmatics. Systemic beta agonists should be avoided as the systemic plus inhaled beta agonists may cause significant adverse effects.

Discharge Criteria

- Adequate treatment of exacerbation; control of symptoms with a return to near baseline pulmonary function tests
- Close medical follow up
- Prior to discharge, review asthma education with patients as well as have an asthma exacerbation plan outlined with the patient.

PROGNOSIS

More severe asthma in the preconception period tends to worsen during pregnancy.

COMPLICATIONS

- There is an association with increasing asthma severity and symptoms and decreased fetal growth.

- If using oral steroids during pregnancy monitor for gestational diabetes, preeclampsia, and intrauterine growth restriction.

PATIENT MONITORING

- Monthly evaluations of asthma history and pulmonary function are recommended.
- At initial visit, baseline spirometry should be performed and should be monitored at follow up outpatient visits.
- Patients are advised to monitor their peak flows at home and taught to use them as part of an outpatient asthma care plan.
- Patients should monitor fetal activity. It is recommended that serial fetal ultrasounds starting at 32 weeks be considered for patients with sub optimally controlled or moderate to severe asthma.

REFERENCES

1. Bracken MB, Triche EW, Belanger K, et al. Asthma symptoms, severity, and drug therapy: A prospective study of effects on 2205 pregnancies. *Obstet Gynecol*. 2003;104:739–752.
2. Hanania N, Belfort M. Acute asthma in pregnancy. *Crit Care Med*. 2005;33(suppl):S319–S324.
3. Kwon HL, Belanger K, Bracken MB. Asthma prevalence among pregnant and child bearing-aged women in the United States: Estimates from national health surveys. *Ann Epidemiol*. 2003;13:317–324.
4. NAEPP Expert Panel Report. Managing asthma during pregnancy: recommendations for pharmacologic treatment 2004 update. *J Allergy Clin Immunol*. 2005;115:34–46.
5. Norjavaara E, Gerhardsson de Verdier M. Normal pregnancy outcomes in a population-based study including 2968 pregnant women exposed to budesonide. *J Allergy Clin Immunol*. 2003;111:736–741.
6. Schatz M, Dombrowski MP, Wise R, et al. Asthma morbidity during pregnancy can be predicted by severity classification. *J Allergy Clin Immunol*. 2003;112:283–288.
7. Schatz M. Interrelationships between asthma and pregnancy: A literature review. *J Allergy Clin Immunol*. 1999;103(suppl): S330–S336.

ADDITIONAL READING

Murphy VE, Gibson PG, Clifton VL. Asthma during pregnancy: Mechanisms and treatment implications. *Eur Resp J*. 2005;25:731–750.
Cousins L. Fetal oxygenation, assessment of fetal wellbeing, and obstetric management of the pregnant patient with asthma. *J Allergy Clin Immunol*. 1999;103(suppl):S343–S349.

CODES

ICD9-CM

- 493.00 Asthma, unspecified
- 646.93 Antepartum

KEY WORDS

- Asthma
- Pregnancy

PREGNANCY, CHOLESTASIS

Sumona Saha, MD
Silvia D. Degli-Esposti, MD

KEY CLINICAL POINTS

- Disorder of 2nd and 3rd trimesters of pregnancy
- Prompt diagnosis and treatment improves maternal symptoms and fetal outcomes
- Likely to recur with subsequent pregnancies

 BASICS

DESCRIPTION

- Typically a benign cholestatic disorder in the mother
- Associated with fetal complications
  - Meconium staining
  - Preterm delivery
  - Intrapartum fetal distress
  - Intrauterine fetal demise
- Resolves promptly after delivery

GENERAL PREVENTION

- Ursodeoxycholic acid (UDCA) to modify bile acid pool and decrease distribution of bile acids in fetal circulation
- Delivery when fetal maturity has been achieved to avoid late fetal death

EPIDEMIOLOGY

- Cases reported from all over the world, however, significant geographic variations exist in incidence and prevalence
- Occurs in women of all ages

Incidence

- Incidence varies by country and ethnicity
  - Rare in North America, Asia, and Australia
  - Highest incidence reported in Chile-Bolivia (6–27% of births)
    - Native Araucanian Indians of Chile most affected
  - Second highest incidence reported in Sweden (2% of births)
- Incidence also varies by season
  - Highest rates reported in November

Prevalence

- Less than 1% in North America, UK, Asia, and Australia
- 1–1.5% in Scandinavia
- 15.6% in Chile-Bolivia
  - Prevalence may be decreasing in Chile for unclear reasons

RISK FACTORS

- Multiparity
- Advanced maternal age
- Twin gestation
- Personal history of cholestasis on oral contraceptives
- Family history of cholestasis of pregnancy

Genetics

- Genetic predisposition suggested by high incidence of disease in certain ethnic groups
- No specific genetic abnormality yet identified
  - Multi Drug Resistance 3 gene (MDR3) has been implicated
    - MDR3 codes for canalicular phospholipid transporter involved in biliary excretion of phospholipids
    - Heterozygosity for MDR3 gene defect may predispose women to disease development

PATHOPHYSIOLOGY

Defect in biliary excretion of steroid metabolites may result in saturation of hepatic transporters and injure the canalicular membrane leading to cholestasis

ETIOLOGY

- Likely multifactorial
  - Environmental factors
    - Low serum selenium levels in affected women may account for geographic and seasonal variation
  - Estrogen effects
    - Estrogen known to produce cholestasis in animal models
    - Affected women may have exaggerated response to the high levels of estrogen during pregnancy
  - Progesterone effects
    - Affected women have elevated levels of progesterone metabolites which may saturate hepatic transport systems
    - Exogenous progesterone given to delay premature delivery found to trigger disease development
  - Genetic defects

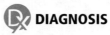 **DIAGNOSIS**

PRE-HOSPITAL

Diagnosis relies on clinical history, including the timing of gestation, and laboratory studies

SIGNS AND SYMPTOMS

- Primary symptom is severe pruritus
  - Mostly involves hands and feet
    - May extend to trunk, extremities, eyelids and rarely the oral cavity
  - Worse at night
    - Can cause sleep deprivation leading to psychological distress
- Jaundice
  - Occurs in only 10–20% of cases
  - Develops after onset of pruritus
- Nausea/vomiting
- Steatorrhea
  - May be subclinical
- Anorexia
- Poor weight gain

History

- Inquire about nature of pruritus
  - Time of onset
    - Usually begins during the second or third trimesters but cases have been reported in first trimester
  - Distribution
  - Intolerability
    - Has been associated with suicidal ideation
- Obtain family history
- Obtain medication history

Physical Exam

- Generally benign
- Skin exam
  - May see evidence of excoriation
  - Jaundice, if present, is mild

TESTS

Mainly non-invasive testing to make diagnosis

Lab
- Most sensitive abnormality is elevated fasting serum bile acids
  - May be elevated 10–25 fold in affected women
    - Risk of fetal complications highest when bile acids are $\geq$40 μmol/L
  - Conjugated bile acids, especially cholic acid, are elevated
    - Elevated serum cholic acid can predict disease development
- Bilirubin usually normal
  - If elevated, usually does not exceed 6 times the upper limit of normal (ULN)
- Transaminases elevated
  - May be 2–10 times above the ULN
- Alkaline phosphatase levels difficult to interpret
  - Physiologically increased due to placental production to 2–3 times above the ULN
- GGT normal or modestly elevated
- Prothrombin time normal or elevated
  - If elevated, due to vitamin K deficiency rather than hepatic dysfunction

Imaging
Not helpful in making diagnosis

Diagnostic Procedures/Surgery
Liver biopsy rarely necessary for diagnosis

Pathologic Findings
- Bland cholestasis
  - Bile plugs in hepatocytes and canaliculi without surrounding inflammation
  - No signs of biliary obstruction
  - Occurs predominantly in centrilobular regions
- Portal tracts normal

DIFFERENTIAL DIAGNOSIS
- Viral hepatitis
  - Consider when transaminases >1000 units
- Biliary obstruction
- Primary biliary cirrhosis
- Primary sclerosing cholangitis
- Drug-induced hepatotoxicity
- Benign recurrent intrahepatic cholestasis

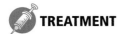 TREATMENT

PRE-HOSPITAL
Goals of treatment are improvement of maternal symptoms and fetal outcomes

INITIAL STABILIZATION
- Evaluate for fetal distress and fetal lung maturity
  - Nonstress test
  - Amniocentesis

GENERAL MEASURES
- Manage aggressively to decrease poor fetal outcomes
  - Close fetal surveillance
  - Medication to lower bile acids
  - Delivery after fetal lung maturity
- Delivery is curative
  - Timing of delivery depends on severity of maternal symptoms, gestational age and presence of fetal distress
    - Patients should be delivered by 38 weeks, or if cholestasis is severe by 36 weeks if fetal lung maturity can be achieved

Diet
No specific dietary recommendations

Activity
As tolerated

Nursing
- Fetal monitoring
- Supportive care

SPECIAL THERAPY
- Obstetric management
  - Must be prepared to terminate pregnancy in severe cases to prevent intrauterine death
    - Can give antenatal steroids to promote fetal lung maturity

IV Fluids
- May be mild to moderately dehydrated due to associated nausea and vomiting
  - Administer normal saline as needed

Complementary and Alternative Medicine
- S-adenosyl methionine (SAMe)
  - Has been shown in some studies to decrease pruritus, bile acids level, and aminotransferase levels
  - More studies needed

 MEDICATION (DRUGS)

Several medications have been used to treat pruritus with no significant improvement in biochemical profile or fetal outcome (e.g., antihistamines, benzodiazepines, phenobarbital)

First Line
- Ursodeoxycholic acid (UDCA)
  - Modifies bile acid pool and displaces toxic bile acids from hepatic membranes
  - Recommended dose is 15/mg/kg/day divided in 2 doses
  - FDA category B

Second Line
- Cholestyramine
  - Binds bile acids in the intestine and increases bile acid excretion in feces
  - Improves pruritus but does not improve biochemical profile or fetal outcome
  - Prolonged use can cause vitamin K malabsorption and worsen coagulopathy
  - Recommended dose is 8–16 g/day
  - FDA category C
- Hydroxyzine
  - Antihistamine that helps relieving itching
  - Recommended dose is 25–50 mg/day
  - FDA category C

SURGERY
- Cesarean section
  - Recommended in cases of fetal distress, heavy meconium staining of amniotic fluid

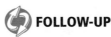 FOLLOW-UP

DISPOSITION
Management usually in outpatient setting

Admission Criteria
- Fetal distress requiring emergent delivery
- Maternal coagulopathy requiring administration of IV vitamin K or fresh frozen plasma

Discharge Criteria
- Maternal symptoms resolved
- Fetal stability
- Successful delivery

Issues for Referral
- Bilirubin or transaminases elevated above expected range
  - Refer to gastroenterology to evaluate for other causes of LFT abnormalities in pregnancy

PROGNOSIS
- No long term sequelae
  - Symptoms and lab abnormalities resolve 1–2 weeks after delivery
- Recurrence common in subsequent pregnancies (40–60%)

COMPLICATIONS
- Postpartum hemorrhage
  - Due to malabsorption of fat soluble vitamins especially when cholestyramine used
    - Give prophylactic vitamin K to all patients
- Cholelithiasis
  - 2.7 fold risk of postpartum gallstone formation in primiparous women

PATIENT MONITORING
- Monitor patient every 2–4 weeks
  - Assess severity of symptoms
  - Follow fasting serum bile acid levels
  - Assess psychological well being
    - Be aware that suicide has been reported in severe cases
- Monitor fetus weekly especially near term
  - Weekly nonstress test (NST)

REFERENCES

1. Riely CA, Bacq Y. Intrahepatic cholestasis of pregnancy. *Clin Liver Dis*. 2004;8:167–176.
2. Sandhu BS, Sanyal AJ. Pregnancy and liver disease. *Gastroenterol Clin N Am*. 2003;32:407–436.
3. Benjaminov FS, Heathcote J. Liver disease in pregnancy. *Am J Gastroenterol*. 2004;99:2479–2488.
4. Glantz A, Marschall H-U, Mattson L-A. Intrahepatic cholestasis of pregnancy: Relationships between bile acid levels and fetal complication rates. *Hepatology*. 2004;40:467–474.
5. Doshi S, Zucker SD. Liver emergencies during pregnancy. *Gastroenterol Clin N Am*. 2003;32:1213–1227.
6. Wakim-Fleming J, Zein NN. The liver in pregnancy: Disease vs benign changes. *Cleveland Clinic Journal of Med*. 2005;72:713–727.

ADDITIONAL READING

Riely CA, Davila R. Pregnancy related hepatic and gastrointestinal disorders. In: *Feldman: Sleisenger & Fordtran's Gastrointestinal and Live Diseaser*, 7th ed. St. Louis: Saunders, 2002; 1448–1449.

CODES
ICD9-CM
- 646.7 Liver disorders in pregnancy
- 656.3 Fetal distress affecting management of mother
- 666.0 Third stage post-partum hemorrhage

KEY WORDS
- Pruritus
- Bile Acids
- Preterm Labor
- Intrauterine Fetal Demise

PREGNANCY, CHRONIC HYPERTENSION

Raymond O. Powrie, MD

KEY CLINICAL POINTS

- Most women with chronic hypertension in pregnancy can expect good pregnancy outcomes.
- The main risk of chronic hypertension in pregnancy is that of superimposed preeclampsia.
- Methyldopa and labetalol are the preferred agents for treatment of chronic hypertension in pregnancy.
- Opinion varies as to whether the target blood pressure for hypertension control in pregnancy is <160/100 or <140/90. Both approaches are acceptable.

 BASICS

DESCRIPTION

- Hypertension is the most common medical problem seen in pregnancy.
- Its management requires familiarity with:
  - Treatment goals
  - Preferred agents
  - Screening for superimposed preeclampsia
- An important general guideline for the diagnosis and management of hypertension in pregnancy is as follows:
  - Hypertension occurring prior to 20 weeks gestation is almost certainly chronic hypertension.
  - Elevations in blood pressure that occur after 20 weeks gestation should raise suspicion of the diagnosis of preeclampsia.

GENERAL PREVENTION

Although there is little research in this area, strategies to prevent chronic hypertension in nonpregnant patients are likely also effective in pregnant patients.

- Exercise
- An appropriate diet
- Maintaining an ideal, but pregnancy-appropriate weight

EPIDEMIOLOGY

Incidence

Chronic hypertension complicates 5% of pregnancies.

RISK FACTORS

- Unchanged from the nonpregnant population.
- Chronic hypertension is more common among older women, the obese, and African Americans.

Genetics

Chronic hypertension is believed to be polygenic in origin with penetrence being greatly affected by lifestyle.

PATHOPHYSIOLOGY

The pathophysiology of chronic hypertension in pregnancy is unchanged from that in nonpregnant patients.

ALERT

Blood pressure typically decreases in the 1st 2 trimesters of pregnancy by 10–15 mmHg.

- Therefore, many women with chronic hypertension may have improvement of their BP early in pregnancy only to see it rise again in the 3rd trimester.

ETIOLOGY

- The etiology of chronic hypertension is heterogeneous and remains poorly described.

- Consider secondary causes of hypertension in all patients with new onset or difficult to control hypertension:
  - Endocrine causes
    - Diabetes, thyroid and parathyroid disease, pheochromocytoma, hyperaldosteronism
  - Renal causes
    - Intrinsic renal disease
    - Renovascular disease
  - Medications/drug use
  - Alcohol
  - Coarctation of the aorta
  - Sleep apnea

ASSOCIATED CONDITIONS

Approximately 20% of the patients with chronic hypertension will develop superimposed preeclampsia.

 DIAGNOSIS

PRE-HOSPITAL

Chronic hypertension in pregnancy that is not severe and is not associated with superimposed preeclampsia is managed as an outpatient.

SIGNS AND SYMPTOMS

- Chronic hypertension is defined as blood pressures >140/90 and is generally asymptomatic.
  - Because blood pressure normally decreases in the 1st 2 trimesters by 10–15 mmHg, a blood pressure >130/80 in the 2nd trimester is suggestive of underlying chronic hypertension being masked by pregnancy.
- Blood pressure should be measured manually with an appropriate sized cuff with the patient in the sitting position and the brachial artery at the level of the heart.

History

Evaluate patient for evidence of:

- Secondary causes of hypertension, particularly if the diagnosis is new (see Hypertension chapter)
  - Renovascular hypertension is the most common secondary cause in this age group.
  - Pheochromocytoma is the most dangerous.
- Superimposed preeclampsia in all patients >20 weeks gestation (i.e., headache, visual phenomena, epigastric or right upper quadrant pain)

Physical Exam

Evaluate patient for evidence of:

- Secondary causes of hypertension in patients not previously identified as having chronic hypertension
- Superimposed preeclampsia in all patients >20 weeks gestation (i.e., worsening hypertension, retinal vasospasm, evidence of pulmonary edema, epigastric tenderness, clonus)

ALERT

Evidence of preeclampsia should lead to a prompt referral to an obstetric provider as preeclampsia is a complex disorder with both maternal and fetal complications.

TESTS

Lab

- Initial evaluation of chronic hypertension in pregnancy should include a work-up of secondary causes of hypertension:
  - CBC, Potassium, Creatinine, Urinalysis, Calcium, TSH, EKG

- Many providers also obtain "baseline preeclampsia labs" during the 1st 1/2 of pregnancy for comparison later in the pregnancy should blood pressure begin to rise.
  - CBC, Creatinine, uric acid, AST and a 24-hour urine for protein

Imaging
Women with chronic hypertension in pregnancy
- Should receive an early ultrasound to confirm dating
- Often undergo additional fetal testing in the 3rd trimester to evaluate fetal well being:
  - Serial ultrasounds for growth and
  - Regular fetal "non stress tests" or biophysical profiles
  - Measurement of umbilical artery flow

DIFFERENTIAL DIAGNOSIS
- Improper blood pressure measurement technique
- Secondary hypertension (see Etiology)
- White coat hypertension
- Preeclampsia

 ## TREATMENT

PRE-HOSPITAL
Chronic hypertension in pregnancy is managed as an outpatient unless severe, symptomatic, or there is evidence for superimposed preeclampsia.

GENERAL MEASURES
- All experts agree that BP >160/100 due to chronic hypertension in pregnancy warrants treatment with antihypertensive medications.
- Some experts advocate treatment for BP >140/90, whereas others would not treat until the BP is >160/100 unless "target organ" damage present. No evidence exists that treatment of BP <160/100 confers a short-term benefit to the mother or fetus.
- Patients with BP >170–180/105–110 (opinions differ as to the exact number) require
  - Urgent evaluation for "target organ" damage
  - Urgent treatment of blood pressure
  - Gestational age appropriate assessment of fetal well being
- BP <170–180/105–110 but >160/100 also requires medical treatment, but not necessarily immediate lowering if mother is asymptomatic and fetus has reassuring fetal testing.
- BP >140/90
  - Requires consideration of preeclampsia if occurring after 20 weeks gestation
  - Does not necessarily require medication
  - Some experts treat all BP >140/90 in pregnancy whereas others treat BP >160/100.
- On every encounter after 20 weeks gestation, women should be evaluated for signs and symptoms of preeclampsia.
  - Particularly true if BP >140/90.
  - If any signs or symptoms of preeclampsia are identified, laboratory testing for preeclampsia should be obtained.
  - Evidence of preeclampsia will generally necessitate admission to hospital.

Diet
- Research has not demonstrated any benefits of dietary restrictions on the management of hypertension in pregnancy.
- A diet rich in whole grains, fruits and vegetables, and low in fats and sodium is advisable for pregnant and nonpregnant women with hypertension.

Activity
- Patients with mild to moderate hypertension in pregnancy and no evidence of preeclampsia can maintain normal activity.
- Rising blood pressure in the 3rd trimester can be a harbinger of preeclampsia and often is managed by having the patient limit activity and stop working outside the home.

Complementary and Alternative Medicine
No alternative or complementary medications have been shown to affect outcomes related to hypertension in pregnancy.

 ## MEDICATION (DRUGS)

- It is important for clinicians to note that one option for treatment of chronic hypertension in pregnancy is to discontinue medication and only treat if BP rises above 160/100. Because BP often decreases in the 1st 2 trimesters, many women do well with this option.
- The only antihypertensive agents that are known to be harmful to the developing fetus are ACE inhibitors and ARBs. However, published data about the other available agents are limited.

First Line
If treatment with medication is deemed desirable:
- Labetalol (starting at 100 mg b.i.d. to a maximum of 800 mg q8h)
- Methyldopa (250 mg b.i.d. to a maximum of 3,000 mg given t.i.d. to q.i.d.)
  - The best safety data are available for these 2 agents; therefore, they are the preferred antihypertensive agents in pregnancy.

Second Line
- Nifedipine, pindolol, and acebutolol are all reasonable second line choices.
- Other agents, such as HCTZ, other calcium channel blockers (aside from nifedipine), clonidine, and prazosin, are not known to be harmful in pregnancy but should be considered 3rd line agents.
- ACE inhibitors and likely angiotensin receptor blockers (ARBs) are toxic to the fetus, and should be stopped prior to conception.

SURGERY
- There is no role for surgery in the treatment of primary hypertension in pregnancy.
- Chronic hypertension is not an indication for cesarean delivery.
- Surgical treatment for secondary causes of hypertension such as thyrotoxicois, hyperparathyroidism, and pheochromocytoma can and should be carried out in pregnancy when indicated.

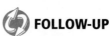 ## FOLLOW-UP

DISPOSITION
Breast-feeding
- Patients with hypertension may breastfeed.
- No antihypertensive agents are known to be harmful for breast-feeding, but sparse data about the safety of the agents in breast-feeding exists.
- Methyldopa, labetalol, nifedipine, acebutalol, HCTZ, enalapril, captopril and metoprolol are all approved by the American Academy of Pediatrics for use in breast-feeding.
- Atenolol and propanolol are concentrated in breast milk and should probably be avoided in breast-feeding mothers.

Admission Criteria

Pregnant women with chronic hypertension should generally be admitted to the hospital if their BP is >170/105 or if there is clinical or laboratory evidence of preeclampsia.

Discharge Criteria

- Chronic hypertension can be managed as an outpatient if preeclampsia has been confidently ruled out and blood pressure is <160/100.
- Patients with suspected superimposed preeclampsia should generally be managed as an inpatient until delivery.

Issues for Referral

- Chronic hypertension in pregnancy should be comanaged with an obstetrician experienced with this condition or a maternal fetal medicine specialist.
- Secondary causes of hypertension in pregnancy should also be referred to the relevant specialist.

PROGNOSIS

- Prognosis is excellent for women with mild to moderate hypertension in pregnancy as long as they do not develop superimposed preeclampsia.
- Uncontrolled severe hypertension represents a risk both to mother and fetus.

COMPLICATIONS

- Chronic hypertension is associated with a slight increased risk of placental abruption, miscarriage, and intrauterine fetal demise.
- Approximately 20% of women with chronic hypertension will develop superimposed preeclampsia and may develop any of the complications associated with the disorder (see Preeclampsia chapter).

PATIENT MONITORING

- Monitor BP every month for the first 32 weeks of pregnancy, every 2 weeks until 36 weeks, and then every week.
- Each visit after 20 weeks gestation should include a history and physical looking for evidence of superimposed preeclampsia.

- Obstetric providers will often do additional weekly fetal testing after 32–34 weeks.

REFERENCES

1. Magee LA, Abdullah S. The safety of antihypertensives for treatment of pregnancy hypertension. *Expert Opin Drug Saf*. 2004;3:25–38.
2. Roberts JM, Pearson G, Cutler J, et al. NHLBI Working Group on Research on Hypertension during Pregnancy. Summary of the NHLBI Working Group on Research on Hypertension during Pregnancy. *Hypertension*. 2003;41:437–445.
3. Sibai BM. Diagnosis and management of gestational hypertension and preeclampsia. *Obstet Gynecol*. 2003;102:181–192.

CODES

ICD9-CM

- 642.0 Benign essential hypertension complicating pregnancy, childbirth, and the puerperium
- 642.3 Transient hypertension of pregnancy
- 642.4 Mild or unspecified preeclampsia
- 642.5 Severe preeclampsia
- 642.6 Eclampsia
- 642.7 Preeclampsia or eclampsia superimposed on preexisting hypertension
- 642.9 Unspecified hypertension complicating pregnancy, childbirth, or the puerperium

KEY WORDS

- Hypertension
- Pregnancy
- Preeclampsia

PREGNANCY, DERMATOSES

Mohsin K. Malik, MD
Lynn E. Iler, MD

KEY CLINICAL POINTS

- 6 major dermatoses of pregnancy
  - Herpes gestationis
  - Pruritic urticarial papules and plaques of pregnancy (PUPPP)
  - Prurigo of pregnancy
  - Pruritic folliculitis of pregnancy
  - Pustular psoriasis of pregnancy
  - Intrahepatic cholestasis of pregnancy
- All tend to resolve in weeks to months postpartum
- Herpes gestationis, pustular psoriasis of pregnancy, and intrahepatic cholestasis of pregnancy are associated with increased maternal and fetal risk.

 BASICS

DESCRIPTION

There are 6 major dermatoses that are unique to pregnancy and all tend to resolve in the postpartum period.

- Herpes gestationis (pemphigoid gestationis)
  - Presents with blisters
  - Resembles bullous pemphigoid clinically and histologically
  - Onset typically in 2nd or 3rd trimester
  - Increased risk to mother and fetus
- PUPPP, prurigo of pregnancy, and pruritic folliculitis of pregnancy
  - All pruritic eruptions on trunk and extremities
  - Etiology unknown; some authors consider different manifestations of same disease
  - All typically begin in 2nd or 3rd trimester
  - No increased risk to mother or fetus
- Pustular psoriasis of pregnancy (impetigo herpetiformis)
  - Resembles pustular psoriasis clinically
  - Onset typically in 3rd trimester
  - Increased risk to mother and fetus
- Intrahepatic cholestasis of pregnancy
  - Characterized by severe pruritus in absence of significant skin findings, though excoriations and jaundice may be present
  - Diagnosis made by serum elevated bile acids in addition to pruritus
  - Onset typically in 2nd or 3rd trimester
  - Increased risk to mother and fetus

EPIDEMIOLOGY

Prevalence

- Herpes gestationis: 1 in 50,000 pregnancies
- PUPPP: 1 in 160–300 pregnancies
- Prurigo of pregnancy: 1 in 300–450 pregnancies
- Pruritic folliculitis of pregnancy: Rare, incidence unknown
- Pustular psoriasis of pregnancy: Rare, incidence unknown
- Intrahepatic cholestasis of pregnancy: 1 in 150–1,300 pregnancies

RISK FACTORS

- PUPPP
  - Primigravida status
  - Multiple gestation pregnancy
- Intrahepatic cholestasis of pregnancy
  - Family history
  - Personal history of hepatitis C
  - Multiple gestation pregnancy

Genetics

- Herpes gestationis more common in
  - Individuals with HLA-DR3, HLA-DR4, or both
  - Whites
- Intrahepatic cholestasis of pregnancy
  - Associated with HLA-B8 and HLA-BW16

ETIOLOGY

- Herpes gestationis: Autoimmune disorder closely related to bullous pemphigoid
- Autoantibodies are directed against bullous pemphigoid antigen 2, a 180-kd protein found in the basement membrane zone.
- PUPPP: Unknown etiology
  - Abdominal distention may cause damage to connective tissue and thereby trigger an inflammatory response.
  - Hormonal or autoimmune causes are not consistently implicated in pathology.
- Prurigo of pregnancy: Unknown etiology, may result from physiological pruritus in women with atopic tendencies
- Pruritic folliculitis of pregnancy: Unknown
- Pustular psoriasis of pregnancy: Unknown
  - Debate exists as to whether it is a form of pustular psoriasis or a separate entity.
  - Generally no personal or family history of psoriasis
- Intrahepatic cholestasis of pregnancy: Likely combination of hormonal and environmental factors in genetically predisposed women
  - Estrogens and progesterones interfere with hepatic bile acid secretion.

ASSOCIATED CONDITIONS

- Herpes gestationis is associated with autoimmune disease, especially Graves' disease.
- Prurigo of pregnancy is associated with a family history of intrahepatic cholestasis of pregnancy.

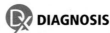 **DIAGNOSIS**

SIGNS AND SYMPTOMS

History

In general, the physician should inquire about:

- Gestational age
- Parity
- Dermatoses in previous pregnancies
- Family history of dermatoses in pregnancy
- Personal or family history of autoimmune disease including
  - Blistering diseases
  - Connective tissue disease

Physical Exam

- Herpes gestationis
  - Pruritic, erythematosus, or urticarial plaques that develop into tense vesicles or bullae
  - Begins periumbilically, sparing striae, and progress to the abdomen and thighs
  - May become generalized, but face and mucous membranes generally spared
- PUPPP
  - Begins as pruritus that occurs within abdominal striae (striae gravidum)

- Erythematous/urticarial papules and plaques then develop within abdominal striae
- Eruption spreads to buttocks, medial thigh, breasts, and arms over course of days
- Face and periumbilical skin spared
- Lesions coalesce into larger plaques, giving heterogenous and polymorphous overall appearance
- Despite pruritus, excoriations generally absent
- Prurigo of pregnancy
  - Grouped, erythematous papules and nodules on extensor aspects of extremities and often on the abdomen
  - Can be excoriated or crusted
- Pruritic folliculitis of pregnancy
  - Follicular papules and pustules on the abdomen and, less commonly, limbs
  - Can become generalized
  - Similar in appearance to steroid acne
- Pustular psoriasis of pregnancy
  - Begins with erythematous plaques that have pustular margins
  - Plaques expand outward and leave eroded and crusted centers
  - Concentric rings of erythema and pustules may result
  - Early lesions are on inner thigh, intertriginous areas of groin, and axillae
  - Lesions expand with pustules remaining on leading edge, outward to trunk/extremities
  - Some have painful mucous membrane erosions
  - Constitutional symptoms common (fever, chills, malaise, nausea, vomiting, diarrhea)
- Intrahepatic cholestasis of pregnancy
  - Generalized pruritus during 3rd trimester is the hallmark
  - Pruritus may be worse at night
  - Jaundice occurs in about 20%
  - Excoriations may be present, but there are no primary skin lesions

ALERT
Pruritic folliculitis of pregnancy, prurigo of pregnancy, and PUPPP can be difficult to differentiate clinically.

TESTS
- PUPPP
  - No specific tests required, but biopsy may differentiate from herpes gestationis
- Prurigo of pregnancy: No specific tests

Lab
- Pustular psoriasis of pregnancy
  - Elevated leukocyte count
  - Elevated erythrocyte sedimentation rate
  - Hypocalcemia
  - Hypoalbuminemia
- Intrahepatic cholestasis of pregnancy
  - Elevated bile acids required for diagnosis
    - Predominant elevation in cholic acid
    - Postprandial cholic acid level is highly sensitive
    - Risk of fetal complications increases with fasting bile acids $>40 \mu$mol/L
  - Elevated LFTs: Particularly alkaline phosphatase
  - Elevated cholesterol, triglycerides, phospholipids
  - Rule out other causes of hepatic dysfunction
    - HAV, HBV, HCV
    - No history of hepatotoxic drugs
  - Monitor prothrombin time

- Pruritic folliculitis of pregnancy:
  - Cultures can help differentiate from folliculitis

Diagnostic Procedures/Surgery
Biopsy required for diagnosis of
- Herpes gestationis
- PUPPP: Mainly to differentiate from Herpes gestationis

Pathologic Findings
Herpes gestationis
- Histology shows the subepidermal vesicle with mixed inflammatory infiltrate.
- Direct immunofluorescence shows a linear deposition of C3, and sometimes IgG, at the basement membrane zone of lesional and perilesional skin.
- Indirect immunofluorescence has a low sensitivity, but shows antibasement membrane zone antibodies.

DIFFERENTIAL DIAGNOSIS
- Infectious causes
- Drug reactions
- Autoimmune disease
  - Bullous pemphigoid and other blistering skin diseases
  - Connective tissue disease

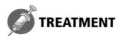

TREATMENT

SPECIAL THERAPY
In one study, breast-feeding reduced the duration of herpes gestationis.

MEDICATION (DRUGS)

- Herpes gestationis
  - Mild cases
    - Topical steroids
    - Antihistamines for pruritus (diphenhydramine, hydroxyzine)
  - Most cases require systemic steroids.
    - Prednisone: 20–40 mg daily and tapering up or down based on disease activity
  - Severe cases may require other immunosuppressive agents or LHRH analogue (goserelin).
- PUPPP
  - Usually only requires symptomatic relief
    - Topical corticosteroids
    - Antihistamines for pruritus
    - Systemic corticosteroids for severe, intractable pruritus
- Prurigo of pregnancy
  - Usually only requires symptomatic relief
    - Topical corticosteroids
    - Antihistamines for pruritus
- Pruritic folliculitis of pregnancy
  - Treatment is not well described, but symptomatic control with topical steroids and antihistamines appears effective
- Pustular psoriasis of pregnancy
  - Warrants treatment with systemic steroids given the increased maternal and fetal risk
  - Prednisone: 15–40 mg per day with increasing doses if insufficient clinical response
  - Treatment of hypocalcemia and hypoalbuminemia, as needed

- Intrahepatic cholestasis of pregnancy
  - Delivery by 36–38 weeks generally indicated depending on severity of cholestasis
  - Antipruritics are usually ineffective
  - Emollients for mild cases
  - Optimal medical therapy not established, but choices include: epomediol, silymarin, Phenobarbital, dexamethasone, activated charcoal, S-adenosyl-L-methionine, Ultraviolet B light
  - For severe cases, anion exchange resins: Cholestyramine, ursodeoxycholic acid

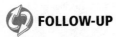 **FOLLOW-UP**

Issues for Referral
Clarification of diagnosis by dermatologist and management by obstetrician

PROGNOSIS
- Herpes gestationis
  - Postpartum exacerbation is common.
  - It generally resolves spontaneously over weeks to months postpartum.
  - It often recurs in subsequent pregnancies.
  - Recurrences tend to begin earlier and to be more severe in each subsequent pregnancy.
  - Some cases flare with oral contraceptive use.
  - Mild placental insufficiency places fetus at risk for preterm delivery, low birth weight
  - Small number of newborns born to mothers with herpes gestationis develop a bullous eruption, which resolves spontaneously over several weeks
- PUPPP
  - Self-limited and generally resolves in the days to weeks postpartum
  - Recurrence in subsequent pregnancies rare
  - No known increased risk to mother or fetus
- Prurigo of pregnancy
  - Generally resolves in the early postpartum period, but rarely may persist for months
  - Often recurs in subsequent pregnancies
  - No increased maternal or fetal risk
- Pruritic folliculitis of pregnancy
  - Resolves in several weeks postpartum
  - Some reports of low fetal birth weight or premature delivery, but generally not considered to increase maternal or fetal risk
- Pustular psoriasis of pregnancy
  - Rapid resolution postpartum
  - Recurs in subsequent pregnancies
  - Recurrences tend to begin earlier and to be more severe in each subsequent pregnancy.

- It increases the risk of maternal mortality, but there is a markedly better prognosis with systemic corticosteroids.
- Placental insufficiency or stillbirth can occur even when the disease is controlled with steroids.
- Intrahepatic cholestasis of pregnancy
  - Pruritus resolves several days postpartum.
  - Recurrence in subsequent pregnancies in about 1/2 of patients
  - Increased rates of fetal distress, preterm delivery, stillbirth, and meconium-stained amniotic fluid
  - Vitamin K absorption may be impaired, leading to increased prothrombin time, uterine and intracranial hemorrhage

REFERENCES

1. Ahmadi S, Powell FC. Pruritic urticarial papules and plaques of pregnancy: Current status. *Australas J Dermatol*. 2005;46:53–58.
2. Chaidemenos G, Lefaki I, Tsakiri A, et al. Impetigo herpetiformis: Menstrual exacerbations for 7 years postpartum. *J Eur Acad Dermatol Venereol*. 2005;19:466–469.
3. Engineer L, Bhol K, Ahmed AR. Pemphigoid gestationis: A review. *Am J Obstet Gynecol*. 2000;183:483–491.
4. Glantz A, Marschall HU, Mattsson LA. Intrahepatic cholestasis of pregnancy: Relationships between bile acid levels and fetal complication rates. *Hepatology*. 2004;40:467–474.
5. Henson TH, Tuli M, Bushore D, et al. Recurrent pustular rash in a pregnant woman. *Arch Dermatol*. 2000;136:1055–1060.
6. Kroumpouzos G, Cohen LM. Pruritic folliculitis of pregnancy. *J Am Acad Dermatol*. 2000;43:132–134.
7. Kroumpouzos G, Cohen LM. Dermatoses of pregnancy. *J Am Acad Dermatol*. 2001;45:1–19; quiz 19–22.
8. Kroumpouzos G, Cohen LM. Specific dermatoses of pregnancy: An evidence-based systematic review. *Am J Obstet Gynecol*. 2003;188:1083–1092.

CODES
ICD9-CM
- 646.8 Herpes gestationis
- 698.9 PUPPP, prurigo of pregnancy, pruritic folliculitis of pregnancy, intrahepatic cholestasis of pregnancy (unspecified pruritic disorder)
- 696.1 Pustular psoriasis of pregnancy

KEY WORDS

- Pregnancy
- Pruritus
- Jaundice
- Rash

PREGNANCY, HEADACHES

Niharika Mehta, MD
Lucia Larson, MD

KEY CLINICAL POINTS

- Headaches are common in pregnancy.
  - Common etiologies (migraine, tension) prevail
  - Benign conditions are often undertreated.
- Certain unusual causes of headache deserve particular consideration in pregnancy and postpartum period.
  - Consider preeclampsia in the differential diagnosis after 20 weeks gestation
- CT and MRI are safe to perform in pregnancy when indicated.

 ## BASICS

DESCRIPTION

- Headaches account for 1/3 of neurological problems in pregnancy, with migraine and tension headaches being the commonest causes.
- Certain causes of headache, otherwise considered rare in non-pregnant population, deserve special consideration in pregnancy.

GENERAL PREVENTION

- Reduce sleep deprivation
- Stress reduction
- Dietary modification (see Diet)
- Avoidance of other known triggers

EPIDEMIOLOGY

Prevalence

- Headache as a symptom is reported by more than 80% women of childbearing age.
- During pregnancy, headaches are most common in the first trimester.
- Migraine headaches
  - Tend to improve in pregnancy in most patients
  - However, up to 25% of patients will experience no improvement in pregnancy
  - Some women may experience the first attack of migraine during pregnancy
  - May recur or occur for the first time in the postpartum period in up to 40% women

RISK FACTORS

Several factors may contribute towards increased tendency for headaches in pregnancy.

- Sleep deprivation
- Stress
- Hormonal changes
- Discontinuation of caffeine

PATHOPHYSIOLOGY

- Migraine headaches have been linked to falls in estrogen levels, which may explain in part their improvement in pregnancy and worsening postpartum.
- Tension headaches are thought to be due to muscle contraction and are often related to periods of stress.

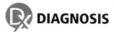 ## DIAGNOSIS

SIGNS AND SYMPTOMS

Certain features in a patient with headache warrant further work up:

- Systemic signs (fever, weight loss, h/o HIV or malignancy)
- Neurologic symptoms or signs
- Onset: Sudden, abrupt, new onset
- Older patient: New onset progressive headache
- Previous headache history: Change in frequency, severity, or clinical features

History

Certain clues in history may suggest specific causes.

- Tension
  - Daily headaches
  - Related to stress
  - Squeezing in nature
  - Worse in afternoon
- Migraine
  - Severe
  - Throbbing
  - Unilateral
  - Worse with activity
  - Sensitivity to light/sound
  - Nausea, vomiting
- Preeclampsia
  - >20 weeks gestation
  - Associated visual disturbance
  - Nausea, vomiting
  - Epigastric pain
- Pseudotumor cerebri
  - Retro-orbital headache
  - Worse when supine
  - Obesity, particularly rapid weight gain
  - Diplopia
- Space occupying lesion
  - Focal headache
  - Associated with seizures
  - Visual field defects (pituitary tumors)
- Infectious causes
  - Fever
  - Photophobia
  - Vomiting
  - Neck stiffness (meningitis)
  - Sinus tenderness, facial pain (sinusitis)
- Non CNS causes
  - Hyperthyroidism
  - Sleep apnea
- SAH
  - Sudden, severe headache
  - Neurologic signs
  - Collapse
  - Sentinel headache

- Cerebral vein thrombosis (CVT)
  - Postpartum period
  - After miscarriage
  - History of thrombophilia
  - Subacute or sudden onset headache
  - 30–60% have neurologic signs, may be transient

Physical Exam
- Physical exam in most patients with tension, migraine or cluster headache is normal.
- Following features may be present with infection, tumor, bleed, thrombosis or preeclampsia.
  - Fever
  - Neck stiffness
  - Neurologic signs
  - Papilledema
  - Epigastric/RUQ tenderness (in preeclampsia)
  - Hypertension (Preeclampsia, CNS event)
  - Nasal mucosal and sinus congestion is common in pregnancy
    - Caution as overdiagnoses of chronic sinusitis common

TESTS
Lab
- Preeclampsia
  - Elevated creatinine (Normal for pregnancy ≤0.8 mg/dl)
  - Elevated liver enzymes
  - Thrombocytopenia
  - Hemoconcentration
  - Elevated uric acid (Normal for pregnancy ≤4.5 mg/dl)
  - Proteinuria
    - Gold standard is 24-hour urine collection
    - Accuracy of protein:creatinine ratio in pregnancy has not been established.
- Thyroid function tests, urine toxicology screen, sleep studies can be ordered as indicated by history and physical.

Imaging
Both CT (with and without contrast) and MRI are safe to perform in pregnancy.
- Indications for imaging in pregnancy are same as in non-pregnant patients.
- Avoid use of gadolinium unless the benefit of the additional information gained outweighs the unknown risk of its use.
- MRV is the test of choice for suspected cerebral vein thrombosis.
- MRA is useful to identify aneurysms and arteriovenous malformations.

Diagnostic Procedures/Surgery
- Lumbar puncture indicated for suspected
  - Meningitis
    - Aseptic meningitis picture possible in CVT
    - Pregnant women are at increased risk of listeriosis.
      - Maternal listeriosis is associated with fetal demise.
  - Intracerebral bleed
  - Pseudotumor cerebri
- Visual field testing may be indicated in
  - Pituitary tumors
  - Pseudotumor cerebri

DIFFERENTIAL DIAGNOSIS
- Differential in pregnancy is essential same as non pregnant.
- Particular consideration should be given to:
  - Preeclampsia
  - AVM/Aneurysms
    - Typically asymptomatic in nonpregnant women
    - However, with expansion of blood volume during pregnancy, may increase in size and cause headaches.

- The risk for initial rupture of AVM is highest in the second trimester and during labor and delivery.
- The risk for rupture of aneurysm increases with each trimester of pregnancy and decreases in the postpartum period.
  - Cerebral vein thrombosis and stroke

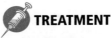 ## TREATMENT

GENERAL MEASURES
- Reassurance that migraine and tension headaches are benign and do not have adverse effects on fetus often helpful
- Stress management
- Improve sleep deprivation if possible

Diet
- Certain foods such as nuts, chocolate, and cheeses may trigger migraine headaches and are best avoided.
- Caffeine withdrawal: 150–300 mg of caffeine intake per day is acceptable in pregnancy.

Complementary and Alternative Therapies
- Magnesium 400–800 mg daily has shown some benefit as migraine prophylaxis and is safe in pregnancy.
- No evidence exists regarding safety of herbal remedies such as feverfew, butterbur in pregnancy.
- Vitamin supplements (riboflavin, coenzyme Q10, and hydroxocobalamin) have not been studied in pregnancy.
- Acupuncture, chiropractic, and massage may be helpful (see Migraine Headache chapter).

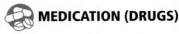 ## MEDICATION (DRUGS)

- Tension headaches in pregnancy are best managed with acetaminophen, heat, massage, and rest.
- Migraine headache
  - Abortive therapy:
    - Combination of acetaminophen 1 gm, antiemetic, and a caffeinated beverage
    - Antiemetics which are safe in pregnancy: Metoclopramide, Compazine, promethazine
    - Magnesium sulfate 1g IV is useful for acute treatment of migraine in nonpregnant patients and can be safely used in pregnancy.
    - Avoid triptans, NSAIDs
    - Codeine, meperidine are safe in pregnancy
  - Prophylaxis:
    - Amitriptyline, nortriptyline, beta blockers such as metoprolol or pindolol, low dose aspirin (81 mg)
    - Avoid propranolol and atenolol because of association with intrauterine growth restriction
- Preeclampsia
  - If suspected as cause of headache, delivery (either by induction or cesarean section) may be appropriate.
  - Magnesium sulfate IV may be added for seizure prophylaxis.
- CVT
  - Warrants full anticoagulation for at least 6–12 months.
    - During pregnancy, heparin (unfractionated or low molecular weight) is the only option.
    - Coumadin is contraindicated in pregnancy.

ALERT
Several medications can be used for treatment of headaches. Use in pregnancy of some medications based upon risk is described below.

First Line
Medications with acceptable risk (safest):
- Acetaminophen, metoclopramide, prochlorperazine, promethazine, codeine, meperidine, morphine, oxycodone, methadone, prednisone, amitriptyline, beta blockers (see above for exceptions)
  - Avoid use of narcotics for prolonged periods and at high doses at term.

Second Line
Moderate risk (less safety data available):
- Calcium channel blockers
- NSAIDs
  - Occasional use in first 2 trimesters may be safe but contraindicated in 3rd trimester.
- Selective Serotonin Reuptake Inhibitors

ALERT
High or unknown risk (Avoid use in pregnancy)
- Aspirin 325 mg dose
  - ASA 81 mg daily has been shown to be safe in pregnancy
- Acetaminophen with butalbital
- Ergotamine
- Triptans
- Valproic acid
- Phenobarbital
- Although newer antiepileptic medications are FDA category C, the lack of adequate safety data precludes their use in pregnancy for this indication.

SURGERY
Surgical management is appropriate if indicated for treatment of AVM, aneurysm, or intracerebral tumors or bleeds.

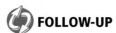 **FOLLOW-UP**

Admission Criteria
- Similar to non-pregnant
- Admission for suspected preeclampsia is appropriate

Issues for Referral
Consider neurology referral for:
- Atypical headache or uncertain diagnosis
- Associated neurologic signs/symptoms
- Treatment failure

PROGNOSIS
Prognosis for successful pregnancy outcome is excellent with most common causes of headache.
- Preeclampsia, listeriosis, massive intracranial bleed or stroke may be associated with poor fetal outcome.

REFERENCES

1. Lee E, et al. Medical Care of the Pregnant Patient. Philadelphia: American College of Physicians; 2000.
2. Loder E, Martin VT. Headache: ACP Key Diseases Series. Philadelphia: American College of Physicians; 2004.
3. Nelson-Piercy C. Handbook of Obstetric Medicine. St. Louis: Mosby-Year Book:1997.
4. Scharff L, Marcus DA, Turk DC. Headache during pregnancy and in the postpartum: A prospective study. *Headache.* 1997;37:203–210.
5. Von Wald T, Walling AD. Headache during pregnancy. *Obstet Gynecol Surv.* 2002;57:179–185.

CODES
ICD9-CM
- 784.0 Headache
- 307.81 Tension headache
- 346.1 Common migraine
- 348.2 Benign intracranial hypertension (Pseudotumor cerebri)
- 642.5 Severe pre-eclampsia
- 642.4 Mild or unspecified pre-eclampsia
- 671.5 Other phlebitis and thrombosis (cerebral venous thrombosis)

KEY WORDS
- Headache
- Migraine Headache
- Pregnancy
- Pseudotumor Cerebri
- Cerebral Vein Thrombosis
- Preeclampsia

PREGNANCY, HYPEREMESIS

Colleen R. Kelly, MD
Silvia D. Degli-Esposti, MD

KEY CLINICAL POINTS

- Occurs in 0.3–1.5% of live births
- Pharmacologic therapy is beneficial for severe or protracted symptoms.
- Though the prognosis is generally good, severe, untreated disease may result in significant maternal and fetal morbidity.

 BASICS

DESCRIPTION

Hyperemesis gravidarum is a condition of severe nausea and vomiting during pregnancy leading to fluid, electrolyte and acid-base imbalance, nutritional deficiency and weight loss.

- Ketonuria and weight loss of greater than 5% of pre-pregnancy body weight distinguish hyperemesis from normal nausea and vomiting of pregnancy.
    - The symptoms often require hospitalization.

GENERAL PREVENTION

- There is no prevention.
- Early intervention can improve symptoms and may decrease hospitalizations.

EPIDEMIOLOGY

- More common in Western populations
- Hyperemesis patients are more likely to be younger and nonwhite.
- They are less likely to be Hispanic or married.
- Average 1.3 hospital admissions per patient with hyperemesis

Incidence

Hyperemesis gravidarum occurs in 0.3–1.5% of all live births.

Prevalence

- Nausea and vomiting occur in up to 80% of pregnant women.
    - Usually improves by 16 weeks gestation
- In up to 20% of patients, symptoms persist throughout pregnancy.

RISK FACTORS

- Primigravida
- Family history of hyperemesis in the patient's mother
- History of hyperemesis in previous pregnancy
- Multiple gestation
- Gestational trophoblastic disease
- Certain fetal anomalies
    - Trisomy 21, hydrops fetalis
- Helicobacter pylori infection

Genetics

Family history of hyperemesis is not uncommon suggesting underlying genetic predisposition.

ETIOLOGY

- Exact cause is unknown
- Hormones of pregnancy including β-HCG and estrogen are felt to play a key role by directly causing or lowering the threshold for nausea and vomiting.
    - Symptoms are most severe at the time of peak HCG levels.
    - High estrogen levels slow intestinal transit time and gastric emptying.

ASSOCIATED CONDITIONS

- Gastroesophageal reflux
- Depression
- Suppression of TSH/mild hyperthyroidism

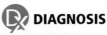 **DIAGNOSIS**

SIGNS AND SYMPTOMS

Hyperemesis is a clinical diagnosis. Delineating hyperemesis from nausea and vomiting of pregnancy can be difficult. The proposed criteria are most widely accepted:

- Intractable nausea and vomiting with:
    - Ketonuria
    - Loss of >5% of prepregnancy body weight

History

- History of hyperemesis in prior pregnancy or in the patient's mother
- Onset of nausea and vomiting in the 1st trimester, usually starting at 4–5 weeks gestation
    - Vomiting that begins after 12 weeks gestation should not immediately be attributed to nausea and vomiting of pregnancy.
- Patients often report ptyalism (excessive saliva) and spitting.
- Assess for gastroesophageal reflux symptoms (retrosternal discomfort and heartburn) as this may precipitate nausea and vomiting.
- Pregnancy-unique quantification of emesis and nausea (PUQE) scoring system can be administered at each visit.
    - 3-question survey that measures the severity of nausea and vomiting
        - Includes number of daily vomiting episodes, length of nausea per day in hours, and number of retching episodes per day

Physical Exam

- Weight
    - Assess for weight loss (>5%) or inadequate weight gain
- Signs of volume depletion
    - Tachycardia
    - Postural hypotension
    - Dry oral mucosa
- Muscle wasting and weakness
- Thyroid examination
    - Assess for goiter or thyroid nodule

TESTS

Lab

- Urinalysis
    - Assess for ketones or infection
- Electrolytes and renal function
    - Severe hyponatremia is a reported complication.
    - Hypokalemia common
- Prealbumin
- TSH
    - Exclude acute thyrotoxicosis
        - The alpha subunit of β-HCG is identical to TSH and interacts with the TSH receptor leading to reduced production of TSH.
        - Free T4 may be slightly elevated, though these patients are clinically euthyroid.

- Helicobacter pylori serology
  - A few studies have shown an association with H. pylori and there are case reports of symptom improvement after eradication.
- Liver function tests
  - Abnormal in up to 50% of patients hospitalized with hyperemesis
    - Mild elevation in transaminases is most common (ALT > AST)

Imaging
Ultrasound (abdominal and pelvic):
- Exclude gallbladder disease, multiple gestation and hydatidiform mole

DIFFERENTIAL DIAGNOSIS
- Nausea and vomiting of pregnancy
- Acute thyroiditis
- Eating disorders
- Biliary tract disease
- Hepatitis
- Gastroesophageal reflux disease

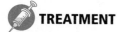 **TREATMENT**

INITIAL STABILIZATION
- Correct fluid and electrolyte imbalance
- Patients at risk for Wernicke encephalopathy should be treated with thiamine replacement.
  - Avoid dextrose-containing fluids.

GENERAL MEASURES
Goals:
- Maintain fluid and electrolyte balance.
- Maintain adequate caloric intake.
- Control nausea and vomiting.

Diet
- Hyperemesis diet should be recommended.
  - Eat small portions frequently.
  - Avoid an empty stomach, which may aggravate nausea.
  - Separate solids and liquids.
  - Eat primarily high carbohydrate foods.
  - Avoid fatty foods, dairy and high fiber foods.
  - Limit spicy or highly seasoned foods.
- Vitamin supplementation
  - Prenatal vitamins containing iron may aggravate symptoms.
  - Patients may substitute noniron formulations or children's chewable vitamins, which may be better tolerated.

Activity
- Patients should be encouraged to maintain usual activity.
- In severe cases, patients may require time away from work.

IV Fluids
- IV fluid and electrolyte replacement should be initiated on hospitalized patients.
  - Avoid dextrose containing fluids, which may precipitate Wernicke encephalopathy.
- Patients with severe symptoms and recurrent hospitalizations should be considered for outpatient intravenous therapy.
  - Maintaining adequate hydration improves nausea.
  - Can be administered through a visiting nurse or patients may be taught to self-administer fluids and intravenous medications
- Iatrogenic complications may occur.

- Hypercoagulability of pregnancy and dehydration from hyperemesis results in high risk of thrombosis.
  - Infection or thrombosis of indwelling catheters used for long-term fluid replacement or TPN occurs in up to 50%.
- Peripheral access is preferable.

Complementary and Alternative Medicine
- Behavioral therapy
  - Patients who are depressed or experiencing anticipatory nausea and vomiting may benefit.
- Ginger
- Vitamin B6/Pyridoxine
- Acupressure
  - Wrist bands marketed for treatment of motion sickness are available over the counter and may help some patients.

 MEDICATION (DRUGS)

There is often anxiety and reluctance to prescribe antiemetic agents in pregnancy, but extensive data shows lack of teratogenesis and good fetal safety data with the following medications:

First Line
Patients who vomit pills may need to be treated with suppositories or intravenous formulations.
- Phenothiazines
  - Chlorpromazine and prochlorperazine
- Antihistamines
  - Promethazine and cyclizine
- Prokinetic drugs
  - Metoclopramide and domperidone
- Acid suppression
  - H2 Blockers
    - Ranitidine, famotidine

Second Line
- Antiemetics
  - HT3 receptor antagonists
    - Ondanzetron: Widespread, off label use
- Acid suppression
  - Proton pump inhibitors
    - Rabeprazole, esomeprazole, pantoprazole, lansoprazole all pregnancy category B
- Corticosteroids have been used
  - Discordant results in randomized controlled trials
    - Should be considered unproven and used only as a last resort

SURGERY
- In cases of severe protein-calorie malnutrition, a duodenal or jejunal feeding tube placement may be necessary.
- A catheter for venous access may be placed in patients requiring prolonged intravenous therapy or TPN.

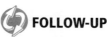 **FOLLOW-UP**

DISPOSITION
Most women can continue to eat and drink enough to be treated as outpatients.

Admission Criteria
Any woman who is ketotic and unable to maintain hydration should be hospitalized.

Discharge Criteria
Patient should be tolerating enough oral intake to maintain hydration or plans for outpatient intravenous therapy should be in place.

Issues for Referral
- Referral to a dietician for discussion of hyperemesis diet
- Initiation of tube feeds or parenteral nutrition should be done in conjunction with a nutritionist.
- Severe or complicated cases may be referred to a gastroenterologist or maternal fetal medicine specialist.

PROGNOSIS
- Mild to moderate nausea and vomiting in pregnancy is not associated with adverse fetal outcomes.
- In most patients with hyperemesis, pregnancy outcome is favorable.
  - Symptoms generally abate as the pregnancy progresses and resolve in most by 18 weeks gestation.
  - When weight loss >5% infants may be born earlier, weigh less, and may be small for gestational age.

COMPLICATIONS
- Wernicke encephalopathy
- Mallory-Weiss tears of the esophagus
- Low infant birth weight
- Maternal or fetal death
- Severe depression
- Termination of pregnancy

PATIENT MONITORING
Patients with severe hyperemesis should be seen weekly with longer duration between visits as symptoms abate.
- Weight should be assessed at each visit.
- Periodic monitoring of prealbumin and electrolytes is advisable.

REFERENCES

1. Abell T, Riely C. Hyperemesis gravidarum. *Gastrointestinal Clin North Am*. 1992;21:835–849.
2. Bailit JL. Hyperemesis gravidarium: Epidemiologic findings from a large cohort. *Am J Obstet Gynecol*. 2005;193(3 pt 1): 811–814.
3. Goodwin TM. Hyperemesis gravidarum. *Clin Obstet Gynecol*. 1998;41:597–605.
4. Kazerooni T, Taallom M, Ghaderi AA. Helicobacter pylori seropositivity in patients with hyperemesis gravidarum. *Int J Gynaecol Obstet*. 2002;79:217–220.
5. Koren G, Boskovic R, Hard M, et al. Motherisk-PUQE (pregnancy-unique quantification of emesis and nausea) scoring system for nausea and vomiting of pregnancy. *Am J Obstet Gynecol*. 2002;186:228–231.
6. Verberg MFG, Gillot DJ, Al-Fardan N, et al. Hyperemesis gravidarum, a literature review. *Human Reproduction Update*. 2005;11:527–539.

ADDITIONAL READING

Funai, Edmund F. Hyperemesis gravidarum. UpToDate. www.uptodate.com.
Findings from the First international Conference on Nausea and Vomiting in Pregnancy. http://www.nvp-volumes.org/.

CODES
ICD9-CM
- 643 Excessive vomiting in pregnancy
- 643.0 Mild hyperemesis gravidarum
- 643.1 Hyperemesis gravidarum with metabolic disturbance

KEY WORDS
- Hyperemesis Gravidarum
- Nausea and Vomiting in Pregnancy (NVP)

PREGNANCY, HYPERTHYROIDISM

Elvis Pagan, MD
Raymond O. Powrie, MD

KEY CLINICAL POINTS

- The diagnosis of hyperthyroidism in pregnancy is complicated by:
  - Overlap of hyperdynamic symptoms frequently seen in normal pregnancies
  - Pregnancy-related changes in thyroid function testing
- Untreated hyperthyroidism has been associated with adverse fetal outcomes.
  - Antithyroid medications and beta blockers are the mainstay of treatment of Grave disease in pregnancy.
  - It is necessary to balance controlling maternal symptoms and limiting the antithyroid effect on the fetus.
  - Radioactive iodine is contraindicated in pregnancy, because it may result in fetal thyroid ablation.

 BASICS

DESCRIPTION
- Hyperthyroidism is a common endocrine disorder encountered in pregnancy.
- Adverse maternal outcomes of poorly controlled hyperthyroidism include:
  - Congestive heart failure
  - Thyroid storm
  - Preeclampsia
- Potential adverse fetal outcomes include miscarriage, IUGR, and stillbirth.

GENERAL PREVENTION
Screening for thyroid disease is outlined in the Pregnancy and Hypothyroidism chapters.

EPIDEMIOLOGY
- Predominance: Female > Male (7:1)
- It typically occurs prior to age 50 with the peak incidence between 20–40 years of age.
- Asian and white populations are more likely to develop hyperthyroidism than other races.

Incidence
Lifetime incidence in women is approximately 2%.

Prevalence
Hyperthyroidism will complicate 1–2 of every 1,000 pregnancies.

RISK FACTORS
- Prior history of hyperthyroidism or autoimmune thyroid disease
- Family history of hyperthyroidism
- Other autoimmune disorders (particularly those seen with polyglandular autoimmune syndrome, type II) such as:
  - Type I diabetes
  - Addison's disease
  - Pernicious anemia
  - Celiac disease
  - Primary biliary cirrhosis
- Tobacco use

Genetics
- Increased frequency of Graves' disease is seen in those with HLA-B8 and HLA-D3 antigens.
- There is a 20% concordance in monozygotic twins.

PATHOPHYSIOLOGY
- Similar to the nonpregnant population
- In pregnancy, human chorionic gonadotropin (hCG) may stimulate the thyroid gland.
  - The hCG molecule shares an alpha subunit common to TSH and, therefore, has some TSH-like activity.
  - Molar pregnancy or gestational trophoblastic neoplasm, a state in which hCG is often excessively elevated, may manifest itself as severe hyperthyroidism.

ETIOLOGY
- Graves' disease is the leading cause of hyperthyroidism, accounting for approximately 95% of hyperthyroidism seen in pregnancy.
- Other causes are similar to that seen in nonpregnant patients with the following exceptions:
  - Transient gestational thyrotoxicosis
    - A condition characterized by hyperthyroidism in the 1st trimester and usually coexists with hyperemesis
    - Not likely a disorder per se, but a result of excessive thyroidal stimulation from hCG
  - Trophoblastic disease as discussed earlier
  - Postpartum thyroiditis
    - A condition that may result in transient hyperthyroidism postpartum, much like subacute (de Quervain) thyroiditis
    - Typically the initial hyperthyroid state goes unnoticed only to manifest itself as hypothyroidism in the period that follows.

ASSOCIATED CONDITIONS
- Hyperemesis gravidarum
- Trophoblastic disease or hydatidiform mole
- Preeclampsia
- Hypertension

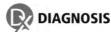 **DIAGNOSIS**

PRE-HOSPITAL
Management of hyperthyroidism in pregnancy is typically done on an outpatient basis.

SIGNS AND SYMPTOMS
Clinical presentation is similar to nonpregnant patients with the following exceptions:
- Weight loss may not be dramatic given the tendency for weight to increase with pregnancy.
- Maternal presentation is further complicated by the fact that many signs and symptoms of hyperthyroidism are also seen in normal pregnancy, such as:
  - Heat intolerance
  - Irritability
  - Emotional lability
  - Moist, warm skin
  - Hyperreflexia
  - Increased pulse rate

TESTS
Lab
- Thyroid function tests (TFTs) remain the mainstay of diagnosing hyperthyroidism in pregnancy, however there are changes in

thyroid function during pregnancy that may be misinterpreted for a hyperthyroid state:
  - Increase in serum total thyroxine (T4) and triiodothyronine (T3)
    - Caused by increased production of serum thyroxine-binding globulin (TBG) secondary to stimulatory effects of estrogen
  - TSH is slightly suppressed in the 1st trimester.
  - Free T4 and T3 are mildly increased but typically remain within the normal range.
- Abnormal TSH levels should be investigated further with free thyroid hormone levels.
- Thyroid stimulating immunoglobulins (TSI)
  - Obtain TSI levels if Graves' disease is suggested by clinical presentation or by TFT abnormalities
  - TSI levels are important in assessing the likelihood for development of Fetal Graves' Syndrome (see Complications)

Imaging
Radioactive iodine uptake (RAUI) test
- Contraindicated in pregnancy as the iodine can be taken up by the fetal thyroid and result in fetal thyroid ablation
- Fetal thyroid development begins typically at about 10 weeks gestation.
- If RAIU is inadvertently conducted prior to 10 weeks gestation, pregnant patients should be counseled that there is a high likelihood for normal fetal thyroid development.

Pathological Findings
Unchanged from non pregnant patients. See Hyperthyroidism chapter.

DIFFERENTIAL DIAGNOSIS
- Anxiety
- Tachyarrhythmias
- Trophoblastic disease
- Pheochromocytoma
- Transient gestational thyrotoxicosis

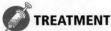 **TREATMENT**

PRE-CONCEPTION
- Patients with a history of hyperthyroidism should be told to plan conception at a time of documented euthyroidism.
- Both hyperthyroidism and hypothyroidism have been implicated in adverse fetal outcomes.
- Patients who are planning to become pregnant who have recently had radioactive iodine thyroid ablation should consider deferring pregnancy for at least 6 months given the long half-life of these agents and their potential to affect fetal thyroid development.

INITIAL STABILIZATION
- Hyperthyroidism in pregnancy is typically evaluated and treated on an outpatient basis.
- The following considerations should be made, however, in addressing more concerning features of this disease:
  - Hyperemesis
    - May coexist with hyperthyroidism
    - Assess volume status
    - IV fluids if indicated
  - Symptomatic patients
    - Beta blockers and antithyroid drugs (ATDs) can be used in pregnant patients with significant symptoms.
  - Heart failure from uncontrolled hyperthyroidism
    - The incidence may be increased in pregnant patients compared to nonpregnant patients.

- Management, however, does not differ between the 2 groups.
  - Thyroid storm
    - Should be managed similarly to nonpregnant patients with the following modifications:
      o Fetal monitoring
      o If steroids are indicated, use steroids that cross the placenta less readily (i.e., prednisone or methylprednisolone).

GENERAL MEASURES
The overall goal is to keep the patient at the higher end of the euthyroid state throughout pregnancy with the lowest possible dose of ATDs.

Diet
- Increased caloric intake may be necessary to offset the caloric deficit that occurs from a hypermetabolic state of pregnancy.
- Decreased sodium intake is advocated if hyperthyroidism is complicated by hypertension.

Radiotherapy
Radioactive iodine ablation is contraindicated in pregnancy as it can result in fetal thyroid ablation.

 MEDICATION (DRUGS)

- PTU and Methimazole may cross the placenta, cause suppression of the fetal thyroid, and result in fetal hypothyroidism or in fetal goiter.
- If used appropriately, however, ATDs do not appear to result in an adverse fetal outcome.

First Line
Polythiouracil (PTU)
- Preferred ATD in pregnancy
- Use lowest dose possible to control maternal symptoms as may suppress fetal thyroid.
  - Start with 50 mg PO t.i.d.
  - Limit dose if possible to <300 mg per day
  - Aim for free T4 levels in the upper limit of the normal range.
    - Mild maternal hyperthyroidism is preferred over hypothyroidism.

Second Line
Methimazole (Tapazole)
- Concern of increased fetal risk of scalp defects (aplasia cutis)
  - This association is weak if existent
- May be used if the patient is allergic or intolerant of PTU
- Use lowest possible dose
  - Start with 10 mg PO per day
  - Limit dose if possible to <20 mg per day

SURGERY
- Surgery may be indicated in those patients with severe hyperthyroidism not responsive to or intolerant of antithyroid drugs.
- If surgery is necessary, it is preferable to perform surgery in the 2nd trimester when the risk of miscarriage or preterm labor may be less.

 FOLLOW-UP

DISPOSITION
- Breast-feeding
  - Medications
  - PTU, Methimazole, and beta-blockers other than atenolol are generally safe.

– Approximately 20–30% of the serum levels of atenolol is transmitted to breast milk.
- Radioactive Iodine
  – Postpartum women receiving radioactive iodine for either therapeutic or diagnostic reasons should delay breast-feeding.
  – Timing of the resumption of breast-feeding depends on iodine formulation and dose.
  – Technecium-99m Petechnetate and I-123 are the preferred agents for thyroid scans in patients wishing to breast-feed.
    • Patients are typically counseled to pump and discard their breast milk for 24 hours.
  – I-131 is agent typically used in ablation
    • Given the long half-life (8 days) and large dose used for ablation, breast-feeding should be deferred for several months.
    • Treatment is generally delayed until after the infant has been weaned.

Admission Criteria
- Typically managed in an outpatient setting
- Admission is reserved for patients presenting with thyroid storm, heart failure, or for fetal indications.

Issues for Referral
- To obstetrician to evaluate for fetal goiter and neonatal hyperthyroidism
- To endocrinologist:
  – Confusing or fluctuating TFTs
  – Persistent symptoms despite ATD treatment
  – Severe presenting symptoms, such as thyroid storm or heart failure
  – Patient with palpable thyroid nodule(s)
- To surgery if medical treatment unsuccessful

PROGNOSIS
- Most maternal and fetal complications occur in patients with untreated hyperthyroidism.
- Graves' disease typically improves in the 3rd trimester, but may flare up postpartum.

COMPLICATIONS
- Maternal complications:
  – Preeclampsia
  – Congestive heart failure
  – Arrhythmia
  – Thyroid storm
- Fetal complications:
  – Miscarriage
  – IUGR or small-for-gestational age
  – Prematurity
  – Placental abruption
  – Stillbirth

– Congenital malformations?
– Neonatal or fetal Graves' hyperthyroidism
  • Increased risk in mothers with untreated Graves' disease and with high TSI levels (>300%)
  • May occur in asymptomatic mothers who have been treated for Graves' disease in the past as persistent circulating TSI antibodies may cross the placenta.

PATIENT MONITORING
- Monitor TSH and free T4 every 4 weeks.
- Adjust ATD dose to keep the free T4 level in the high-normal to slightly elevated range.
- Frequent monitoring is necessary as many women decrease or stop their ATDs later in pregnancy.
- ATD requirements often increase postpartum as Graves' disease may flare during this period.
- Fetal monitoring with serial ultrasounds to assess tachycardia, goiter, growth and hydropic changes may be necessary.

REFERENCES

1. Davis LE, Lucas MJ, Hankins GD, et al. Thyrotoxicosis complicating pregnancy. *Am J Obste Gynecol*. 1989;160: 63–70.
2. Lao T. Thyroid disorders in pregnancy. *Curr Opin Obstet Gynecol*. 2005;17:123–127.
3. Mestman JH. Hyperthyroidism in pregnancy. *Best Pract Res Clin Endocrinol Metab*. 2004;18:267–288.
4. Yang K, Burrow G. Thyroid disease In: Lee RV, et al, eds. Medical Care of the Pregnant Patient. Philadelphia: American College of Physicians; 2000:276–283.

CODES
ICD9-CM
- 242.0 Graves' disease
- 242.1 Toxic uninodular goiter
- 242.1 Toxic nodular goiter, unspecified
- 242.8 Thyrotoxicosis of other specified origin
- 242.9 Thyrotoxicosis without mention of goiter
- 775.3 Neonatal thyrotoxicosis
- 643.0 Hyperemesis gravidarum

KEY WORDS
- Graves' Disease
- Postpartum Thyroiditis
- Thyroid Storm
- Hyperemesis
- Neonatal Graves' Disease
- Pregnancy

PREGNANCY, HYPOTHYROIDISM

Elvis Pagan, MD
Raymond O. Powrie, MD

KEY CLINICAL POINTS

- Untreated hypothyroidism during pregnancy may result in adverse fetal outcome and has been linked to impaired intellectual development in children.
- Diagnosis of hypothyroidism in pregnancy is complicated by the difficulty in distinguishing signs and symptoms suggestive of hypothyroidism from normal pregnancy.
- Postpartum thyroiditis is a disorder that is unique to pregnancy whereby postpartum hypothyroidism may result from an autoimmune mediated destruction of the thyroid gland.

 BASICS

DESCRIPTION

- Complex hormonal and metabolic changes occur during pregnancy that affect thyroid function and result in increased thyroid hormone demand and production.
- Increased production of thyroid hormone may be compromised in those pregnant women with preexisting hypothyroidism.
- Maintaining a euthymic state is particularly important in pregnancy as maternal thyroid hormone deficiency has been associated with adverse fetal outcomes and impaired intellectual development in children.

GENERAL PREVENTION

- There are no current recommendations for universal screening of all women before or during pregnancy.
- The Endocrine Society, however, recommends screening with TSH in women belonging to high risk groups or with symptoms suggestive of hypothyroidism.
  - Screening should occur, preferably, prior to pregnancy or in early gestation.
  - High risk groups in which screening should be considered are noted in the risk factors section of this chapter.

EPIDEMIOLOGY

- Thyroid disease is common in women and is seen 5–10 times more commonly in women than in men.
- Primary hypothyroidism is most likely to manifest itself between the ages of 40–60 but is often seen in women of childbearing years.

Prevalence

- 1–2% of women who become pregnant are already receiving thyroxine therapy for hypothyroidism.
- 2% of women may enter pregnancy with subclinical, undiagnosed hypothyroidism.
- Postpartum thyroiditis affects approximately 5–9% of women in the postpartum period.

RISK FACTORS

- Women already on thyroxine or with a history of hypothyroidism
- History of postpartum thyroiditis
- Those who have type I diabetes or other autoimmune disorders
- Family history of autoimmune thyroiditis or other autoimmune disease
- Past history of neck irradiation, thyroid ablation, or thyroidectomy

Genetics

- The disease clusters in families with concordance rate approaching 40–50% in monozygotic twins.

- HLA-DR3 and HLA-DR4 have been linked to Hashimoto's disease
- HLA-DR5 has been linked to postpartum thyroiditis

PATHOPHYSIOLOGY

- Similar to the nonpregnant population
- Most common cause of primary hypothyroidism in women of childbearing age is immune-mediated destruction of the thyroid gland.

ETIOLOGY

- Hashimoto's thyroiditis
  - Main cause of hypothyroidism in pregnancy (as is the case outside of pregnancy)
  - May also flare postpartum like many other autoimmune diseases
- Otherwise, causes of hypothyroidism during pregnancy are the same as those outside of pregnancy with the following exceptions:
  - Iodine deficiency
    - Rare cause of hypothyroidism in the United States both during and outside of pregnancy
    - Incidence in both United States and third world countries is believed to increase during pregnancy due to increased urinary iodine secretion and fetal uptake of iodine.
  - Postpartum thyroiditis
    - Can also contribute to hypothyroidism
    - Autoimmune mediated inflammation of the thyroid resulting initially in hyperthyroidism, which may go undiagnosed, followed by a self-limited period of hypothyroidism
    - Features of hypothyroidism typically present no sooner than 3 months postpartum, with peak incidence at about 5 months postpartum.

ASSOCIATED CONDITIONS

- Other autoimmune disorders
  - Diabetes mellitus
  - Idiopathic adrenal insufficiency
  - Hypoparathyroidism
  - Myasthenia Gravis
  - Vitiligo
- Possible increased risk of preeclampsia

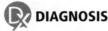 DIAGNOSIS

PRE-HOSPITAL

Management of hypothyroidism in pregnancy is typically done on an outpatient basis.

SIGNS AND SYMPTOMS

History

- Clinical presentation is similar to nonpregnant patients.
- However, presentation is complicated by the fact that many signs and symptoms of hypothyroidism are also seen in normal pregnancy, such as:
  - Fatigue or lethargy
  - Constipation
  - Muscle cramps and arthralgias
  - Carpal tunnel syndrome
  - Weight gain
  - Dry skin
  - Puffiness/edema

Physical Exam
- Thyroid gland may be mildly enlarged with normal pregnancy although this should not be notable on palpation.
- Mild goiter may be seen during pregnancy in regions where iodine intake is low.
- Significant thyroid growth in pregnancy should prompt further evaluation.
- Other exam findings suggestive of hypothyroidism are similar in pregnancy to that seen in nonpregnant patients.

TESTS
Lab
- Thyroid function tests remain the mainstay of diagnosing hypothyroidism in pregnancy.
- However, there are major changes in thyroid function during pregnancy that may make interpretation of these results difficult:
  - Serum thyroxine-binding globulin (TBG)
    - Production increases due to estrogen effect
    - Leads to an increase in both serum total thyroxine (T4) and triiodothyronine (T3)
  - TBG excess in pregnancy results in a low T3-resin uptake.
  - Serum TSH
    - Transiently low in the first trimester
    - Therefore, borderline high TSH during this time in pregnancy may actually represent a hypothyroid state.
  - Free T4 and T3
    - Mildly increased but typically remain within the normal range
    - Free T4 index is also still accurate.
- Screening for hypothyroidism should still be initiated by checking TSH.
  - If the TSH is abnormal or suspicion remains for hypothyroidism, then free T4 index should be checked.
  - Checking antithyroid peroxidase antibodies and/or antithyroglobulin antibodies may also be helpful in diagnosing autoimmune thyroiditis such as Hashimoto's or postpartum thyroiditis.

ALERT
- Mothers treated for Graves' disease with thyroid ablation in the past may still have circulating thyroid antibodies which may cross the placenta and result in neonatal Graves' disease.
- These mothers should have thyroid stimulating immunoglobulins checked as high titers have been implicated in increasing the risk of neonatal Graves' disease.

Pathological Findings
Unchanged from the non pregnant patient. See Hypothyroidism chapter.

DIFFERENTIAL DIAGNOSIS
- Anxiety
- Depression
  - Postpartum thyroiditis may be confused with postpartum depression
- Systemic diseases
  - CHF
  - Nephrotic Syndrome
  - Hepatic failure

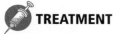 TREATMENT

PRE-HOSPITAL
- Patients who have documented hypothyroidism should be told to plan conception at a time of documented euthyroidism.

- Consideration should be made to increasing the dose of levothyroxine at the time of conception even prior to initial evaluation and laboratory testing.
- This recommendation stems from increased thyroxine requirements noted to occur as early as the 5th week of gestation as well as the importance of thyroid hormone on fetal brain development, a process which is important in early gestation.
- This should be considered particularly in those patients who have had thyroid ablation or total thyroidectomy as they are the least able to increase thyroid hormone production.

GENERAL MEASURES
Restore euthyroid state.

Diet
If constipation is a significant symptom, would recommend high fiber diet

Activity
As tolerated

ALERT
- Breast feeding is safe in mothers on levothyroxine.
- Small amount of this drug is excreted into breast milk but at too low of a concentration to cause neonatal concerns.
- Infants with congenital hypothyroidism may actually benefit from the low level of thyroxine found in the breast milk of mothers on levothyroxine.

Complementary and Alternative Medicine
Use of unregulated thyroid replacement is not recommended in pregnancy because of the critical nature of supplying the exact thyroid dose in these patients.

 MEDICATION (DRUGS)

Levothyroxine (Synthroid, Levothroid)
- Dose
  - Starting dose 50–100 kg/day
  - Increase by 25 kg/day every 4–6 weeks until TSH normalizes.
- Patients should stay on the same brand of medication throughout pregnancy to avoid agent specific variation in bio-availability.
- Transplacental transfer of levothyroxine negligible and has not been associated with birth defects but may be auspiciously increased in fetuses with hypothyroidism.
- Significant possible interactions
  - Prenatal vitamins and ferrous sulfate may decrease the absorption of levothyroxine when taken together.
  - Patients should be counseled to take these medications at separate times during the day.

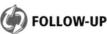 FOLLOW-UP

Admission Criteria
- Typically managed in an outpatient setting.
- Admission criteria same for pregnant patients, particularly if presenting with myxedema coma.
- Management during labor is unchanged except the need for neonatal testing in mothers treated with thyroid ablation for Graves' disease in the past.

Issues for Referral
- If neonatal Graves' disease is confirmed or suspected, then referral to maternal fetal medicine (MFM) or neonatology may be warranted.

- Reason to refer to endocrinologist:
  - Confusing or fluctuating TFTs
  - Hypothyroidism persisting despite increasing levothyroxine dosing
  - Central hypothyroidism implicated as cause of hypothyroidism
  - Patient presents with myxedema coma
  - Thyroid nodule palpated on exam

ALERT
New thyroid nodules in pregnancy should be aggressively investigated because of the high incidence of malignancy.

PROGNOSIS
- Thyroid hormone requirements typically increase with pregnancy and may increase by as much as 50%.
- Hypothyroid patients with poor reserve may not be able to generate the amount of thyroid hormone necessary for maternal and fetal well-being without further supplementation.
- Incidence of fetal complications that result from hypothyroidism is minimized in adequately treated, euthymic mothers.

COMPLICATIONS
- Most women with untreated hypothyroidism will not be able to conceive as hypothyroidism can cause anovulation.
- Complications to mother are similar to those outside of pregnancy except for an increased risk of preeclampsia.
- The added concern of hypothyroidism in pregnancy is the impact this disease may have on the fetus.
- Potential fetal complications include the following:
  - Spontaneous abortion
  - Fetal loss
  - Low birth weight
  - Neuropsychological impairment
  - Congenital hypothyroidism
  - Congenital anomalies

PATIENT MONITORING
- Check TFTs 6–8 weeks after conception.
- Check TFTs at least once every trimester.
- Some clinicians may monitor TFTs more frequently, as often as monthly, particularly following an adjustment in levothyroxine dose or if there have been significant TFT fluctuations.

- Many experts aim to keep the TSH in midrange of normal as hyperthyroidism may also result in adverse fetal outcomes.

REFERENCES

1. Alexander E, Marqusee E, Lawrence J, et al. Timing and magnitude of increases in Levothyroxine requirements during pregnancy in women with hypothyroidism. *N Engl J Med.* 2004;351:241–249.
2. Brent GA. Maternal thyroid function: interpretation of thyroid function tests in pregnancy. *Clin Obstet Gynecol.* 1997;40:3–15.
3. Haddow J, Palomaki GE, Allan WC, et al. Maternal thyroid deficiency during pregnancy and subsequent neuropsychological development of the child. *N Engl J Med.* 1999;341:549–555.
4. Mazzaferrri EL. Evaluation and management of common thyroid disorders in women. *Am J Obstet Gynecol.* 1997;176:507–514.
5. Montoro, MN. Management of hypothyroidism during pregnancy. *Clin Obstet Gynecol.* 1997;40:65–80.

CODES
ICD9-CM
- 244 Acquired hypothyroidism
- 244.0 Postsurgical hypothyroidism
- 244.1 Other postablative hypothyroidism
- 244.2 Iodine hypothyroidism
- 244.3 Other iatrogenic hypothyroidism
- 244.8 Other specified acquired hypothyroidism
- 244.9 Unspecified hypothyroidism
- 243 Congenital hypothyroidism

KEY WORDS
- Autoimmune Thyroiditis
- Myxedema
- Postpartum Thyroiditis
- Graves' Disease
- Pregnancy

PREGNANCY, ACUTE FATTY LIVER OF

Sumona Saha, MD
Silvia D. Degli-Esposti, MD

KEY CLINICAL POINTS

- Disorder of 3rd trimester of pregnancy
- Rare and potentially fatal
- Early recognition and prompt delivery improves maternal and fetal outcomes

 BASICS

DESCRIPTION
- Can progress to fulminant liver failure and eventual maternal and fetal death
  - Maternal mortality rate 18%
  - Fetal mortality rate up to 45%
- May exist on continuum with pre-eclampsia and hemolysis, elevated liver enzymes, and low platelets (HELLP) syndrome
- Associated with inherited defect in fatty acid oxidation in mother and fetus

GENERAL PREVENTION
- Delivery when fetal maturity has been achieved to avoid progression to fulminant liver failure and late fetal demise

EPIDEMIOLOGY
- Rare disease
- Worldwide distribution
  - No specific geographic or ethnic clusterings
- Occurs mostly in the 3rd decade of life

Incidence
- 1 in 10,000–15,000 deliveries

Prevalence
RISK FACTORS
- Primiparity
- Multiple gestation
- Male fetus

Genetics
- Of the affected women, 10–20% have a mutation in the long-chain 3-hydroxyacyl-coenzyme A dehydrogenase (LCHAD).
  - The mitochondrial enzyme is involved in the break down of the long-chain fatty acids in the liver.
  - The deficiency leads to the accumulation of long-chain fatty acids.

PATHOPHYSIOLOGY
- Precise mechanism unknown, but may involve LCHAD deficiency in mother and fetus
  - LCHAD deficiency may be partial in mother and full in fetus
- Proposed mechanism
  - Fetus homozygous for LCHAD mutation is unable to oxidize long-chain fatty acids
  - Fatty acids then enter maternal circulation via placenta
  - Mothers heterozygous for LCHAD mutation cannot cope with increased load of fatty acids leading to accumulation in liver

ETIOLOGY
- Genetic defect in fatty acid oxidation may cause accumulation of triglycerides within hepatocytes and lead to hepatic dysfunction and failure

ASSOCIATED CONDITIONS
- Pre-eclampsia
  - Seen in 50% of patients
  - Can be difficult to distinguish between the two entities

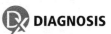 **DIAGNOSIS**

PRE-HOSPITAL
- Pregnancy is generally progressing normally until disease occurs

SIGNS AND SYMPTOMS
- Initial manifestations
  - Nausea/vomiting
  - Right upper quadrant or epigastric pain
  - Malaise
  - Anorexia
- Jaundice is usually not present until 1–2 weeks after the onset of symptoms.
- Pruritus is rare and should prompt investigation into other causes.

History
- Inquire about symptoms
  - Be aware that initial symptoms are nonspecific
- Time of onset
  - Usually occurs between 30–38 weeks, however, has been reported as early as 26 weeks and immediately postpartum

Physical Exam
- Usually benign in early disease
  - Liver edge rarely palpable
- Late disease findings consistent with fulminant liver failure
  - Encephalopathy
  - Asterixis
  - Ascites

TESTS
- Liver biopsy is gold standard for diagnosis, however, is rarely done
- Lab abnormalities more specific to fatty liver of pregnancy (e.g., hypoglycemia, prolonged PT and PTT) help to distinguish this disease from pre-eclampsia and HELLP

Lab
- Leukocytosis
- Transaminases elevated
  - Usually <1,000
- Direct hyperbilirubinemia
  - Usually 5–15 mg/dL
- Alkaline phosphatase elevated
- Hyperuricemia
- Hyperammonemia
- Hypoglycemia
- PT and PTT prolonged
- Fibrinogen low
- Antithrombin III levels low
- Thrombocytopenia
  - Abnormalities in coagulation profile disproportionately more severe than thrombocytopenia

Imaging
- Ultrasound, CT, and MRI not useful in making diagnosis although findings may suggest fatty liver

Diagnostic Procedures/Surgery
- Liver biopsy rarely done, but is helpful diagnostically
  - Coagulation abnormalities in mother may increase procedure-related morbidity
  - Can be done percutaneously or via transjugular approach after hepatic hematoma or rupture has been ruled out by CT or MRI

Pathological Findings
- Hallmark finding is microvesicular steatosis
  - Most prominent in central zone
  - Periportal hepatocytes spared
  - Hepatic architecture intact
- Oil red-O or Sudan III stain on frozen tissue confirms diagnosis
  - Special stains for fat
  - Useful as microvesicular changes may be inconspicuous

DIFFERENTIAL DIAGNOSIS
- Pre-eclampsia involving the liver
- HELLP syndrome
- Pancreatitis
- Fulminant viral hepatitis
  - Hepatitis A, B, C, delta, and E
  - HSV
- Autoimmune hepatitis
- Drug-induced injury
  - Tetracycline
  - Valproic acid
- Hepatic hematoma or rupture

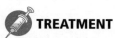 **TREATMENT**

PRE-HOSPITAL
- Maintain high index of suspicion in patient with elevated LFTs in 3rd trimester

INITIAL STABILIZATION
- Assess degree of hepatic dysfunction
  - Check PT/PTT, fibrinogen, platelet count

GENERAL MEASURES
- Patients require maximal monitoring, expeditious delivery, and aggressive supportive care.
  - May need ICU level care
- Management requires multidisciplinary team (i.e., obstetrics and gynecology, gastroenterology, transplant hepatology, critical care medicine).
- Be aware that clinical deterioration can be precipitous.

Diet
- Low sodium (2 gm) if ascites present

Activity
- As tolerated

Nursing
- Fetal monitoring
- Strict monitoring of input and output
- Frequent neurological checks to monitor for encephalopathy in advanced cases

SPECIAL THERAPY
- Aggressive supportive care as needed
  - Transfusion of blood products
  - Hemodialysis

- Mechanical ventilation
- Antibiotics

IV Fluids
- Infusion of concentrated glucose (5% or 10% dextrose) in patients with hypoglycemia

Complementary and Alternative Medicine
- None recommended

 MEDICATION (DRUGS)

Used to treat associated morbidities until disease course reverses
- Proton pump inhibitors
  - To treat reflux esophagitis due to intense vomiting
- Lactulose
  - To treat encephalopathy
- Magnesium or benzodiazepines
  - To treat seizures if present
- 1-deamino-8-d-vasopressin (DDAVP)
  - To treat diabetes insipidus

SURGERY
- Liver transplantation
  - Occasionally required in patients who deteriorate or do not improve after delivery

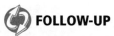 **FOLLOW-UP**

DISPOSITION
Suspected diagnosis requires prompt admission.

Admission Criteria
- Unexplained severe right upper quadrant or epigastric pain
- Elevated liver function tests in the 3rd trimester
- Acute renal failure
- Coagulopathy
- Fetal distress

Discharge Criteria
- Delivery of fetus
- Normalization of PT
- Decrease in bilirubin, transaminases
- Stabilization of renal function
- Ability to tolerate oral diet

Issues for Referral
- Fulminant liver failure despite delivery and aggressive supportive care
  - Refer to liver transplant center
- Screen all infants of affected mothers for LCHAD deficiency.
  - Refer to genetic counselor

PROGNOSIS
- Delivery usually curative
  - Survivors have no long-term sequelae.
  - Most survivors improve 1–4 weeks after delivery.
- Rare to progress after delivery
- Can recur in subsequent pregnancies
- The infant may have LCHAD deficiency.
  - At risk for nonketotic hypoglycemia with associated coma if early dietary interventions not made

COMPLICATIONS
- Maternal complications
  - Encephalopathy
  - Seizures

- Cerebral edema
- Gastrointestinal hemorrhage
- Renal failure
- Hypoglycemia
- Infection
- Disseminated intravascular coagulation
  • Placental infarcts
  • Postpartum hemorrhage
• Fetal complications
- Asphyxiation
- Intrauterine demise

PATIENT MONITORING
• Monitor in ICU given risk for rapid deterioration
• Place on continuous fetal monitor

REFERENCES

1. Benjaminov FS, Heathcote J. Liver disease in pregnancy. *Am J Gastroenterol*. 2004;99:2479–2488.
2. Doshi S, Zucker SD. Liver emergencies in pregnancy. *Gastroenterol Clin N Am*. 2003:32:1213–1227.
3. Sandhu BS, Sanyal AJ. Pregnancy and liver disease. *Gastroenterol Clin N Am*. 2003:32:407–436.
4. Steingrub JS. Pregnancy-associated severe liver dysfunction. *Crit Care Clin*. 2004:20:763–774.
5. Tan ACITL, van Krieken JHJM, Peters WHM, et al. Acute fatty liver in pregnancy. *Netherlands J Med*. 2002;60:370–373.
6. Wakim-Fleming J, Zein NN. The liver in pregnancy: Disease vs benign changes. *Cleveland Clinic J Med*. 2005;72:713–721.

ADDITIONAL READING

Riely CA, Davila R. Pregnancy-related hepatic and gastrointestinal disorders. In: Feldman, ed. Sleisenger & Fordtran's Gastrointestinal and Liver Disease. 7th ed. WB Saunders; 2002:1148–1454.

CODES
ICD9-CM
• 646.7 Liver disorders in pregnancy
• 643.2 Late vomiting in pregnancy
• 666.0 Third stage post-partum hemorrhage

KEY WORDS

• Abnormal Liver Function Tests
• Fulminant Liver Failure

PREGNANCY, POSTPARTUM CARE

Cristina Pacheco, MD
Melissa Nothnagle, MD

KEY CLINICAL POINTS

- The postpartum period is a time of significant emotional and physical adjustment.
- The following issues deserve special attention at the postpartum office visit:
  - Breastfeeding
  - Postpartum depression
  - Sexuality and contraception
  - Medical complications
    - Persistent bleeding
    - Endometritis
    - Urinary incontinence
    - Thyroid disease
- Some women may benefit from postpartum visits earlier than 6 weeks, especially breastfeeding women, adolescents, and those at high risk for postpartum depression.

 ## BASICS

DESCRIPTION
- Includes the first 6 weeks after delivery
- A key time period for healing of the mother, growth and development of the infant, and initiation of the bond between them

GENERAL PREVENTION
- Many providers see patients at 2 weeks postpartum to assess infant feeding, maternal mood, and adjustment to parenting.
- Routine office visit at 6 weeks postpartum

EPIDEMIOLOGY
Prevalence
Prevalence of symptoms in the postpartum period:
- Pain 15–62%
- Urinary incontinence 11%
- Fatigue 70%
- Depression 20%
- Sexual problems 18%

RISK FACTORS
For postpartum depression:
- Previous history of mood disorders
- Lack of supportive partner/family
- Stressful home environment

ASSOCIATED CONDITIONS
- Postpartum depression
- Endometritis
- Mastitis
- Urinary incontinence
- Venous thromboembolism
- Hyper/hypothyroidism

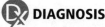 ## DIAGNOSIS

SIGNS AND SYMPTOMS
- Depressed mood or excessive anxiety, especially regarding infant care, suggests depression.
- Excessive fatigue may be a sign of depression, anemia, or thyroid disease.

- Swollen, warm, or tender areas in breasts suggest mastitis.
- Endometritis produces fever and lower abdominal pain and may be associated with malodorous vaginal discharge.
- Prolonged vaginal bleeding may be associated with retained products of conception, infection, or bleeding disorders.

History
- Assess adjustment to motherhood
- Screen for depression
- Breastfeeding history
  - Frequency and duration of feedings
  - Nipple problems
  - Signs of mastitis
- Vaginal lochia
  - Postpartum vaginal discharge, containing blood, mucus, and placental tissue
  - Lochia typically continue for 4–6 weeks after childbirth.
- Sexual history
  - Resumption of sexual activity
  - Dyspareunia
  - Libido
- Contraceptive method
  - Assess satisfaction and adherence
- Urinary incontinence
- Hemorrhoids

Physical Exam
- General: Fatigue, pallor
- Breasts: Engorgement, warmth, tenderness; chafing, irritation, bleeding of nipples
- Cardiovascular: Heart rate, murmur
- Abdomen: Uterine fundus should be non-tender, firm and below umbilicus (or non-palpable).
- Extremities: Edema, varicosities
- Genitourinary: Excessive edema, discharge, healing of lacerations, hemorrhoids

TESTS
No testing required if normal history and physical exam and uncomplicated pregnancy and delivery.

Lab
- Hemoglobin, hematocrit and TSH if excessive fatigue
- TSH if signs of hyper- or hypothyroidism
- Fasting blood glucose if history of gestational diabetes

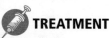 ## TREATMENT

GENERAL MEASURES
- Promote breastfeeding with education and behavioral interventions (see Breastfeeding chapter).
- Offer Rubella immunization if mother not immune
- Contraception
  - Contraceptive counseling should take place prenatally
  - Adherence/satisfaction should be reassessed postpartum
  - Contraceptive options
    - Lactational amenorrhea
      - Effective if exclusive on-demand breastfeeding, amenorrhea, and less than 6 months postpartum

- Barrier methods
  - o Diaphragm and cervical cap must be re-fitted at 6 week postpartum visit.
- Progestin-only methods (progestin-only oral contraceptives, DMPA)
  - o Best hormonal contraceptive for breastfeeding women
  - o Start at 6 weeks postpartum (earlier initiation is acceptable if high risk for unintended pregnancy)
- Estrogen-containing contraceptives (combination oral contraceptives, contraceptive patch, contraceptive ring)
  - o Delay initiation until 4 weeks postpartum because of increased risk of venous thromboembolism
  - o Estrogen may interfere with lactation; delay initiation until 6 weeks postpartum and breastfeeding is well-established (or use progestin only method)
- Intrauterine device (IUD)
  - o Both copper IUD and progestin-releasing IUD are safe in breastfeeding.
  - o Due to slightly higher expulsion rates with immediate postpartum insertion, most U.S. providers insert IUDs at 4–6 weeks postpartum.

MEDICATION (DRUGS)

- NSAIDs are the treatment of choice for postpartum pain relief and are safe for breast-feeding women.
- Continue prenatal vitamins while breast-feeding.

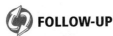

FOLLOW-UP

Issues for Referral

- Refer to lactation specialist to assist with breast-feeding difficulties.
- Gynecologic referral for suspected retained products of conception or trauma to the uterus, vagina, cervix, or other structures.
- Refer to urologist or gynecologist for severe or persistent urinary incontinence.
- Psychiatric referral or hospitalization may be indicated for severe postpartum depression or psychosis.

PROGNOSIS

- The majority of women have an excellent prognosis during the postpartum period.
- Some women may benefit from postpartum visits earlier than 6 weeks, especially breastfeeding women, adolescents, and those at high risk for postpartum depression.

REFERENCES

1. Bowes WA, Katz VL. Postpartum care. In: Gabbe SG, Niebyl JR, Simpson JL, eds. Obstetrics: Normal and Problem Pregnancies. 4th ed. New York: Churchill Livingstone; 2002:702–708.
2. Blenning CE, Paladine H. An approach to the postpartum office visit. *Am Fam Physician*. 2005;72:2491–2496.
3. Brown S. Maternal health after childbirth: Results of an Australian Population Based Survey. *Br J Obstet Gyn*. 1998;105:156–161.
4. Epperson CN. Postpartum major depression: Detection and treatment. *American Family Physician*. 1999;59:2247–2254, 2259–2260.
5. Up to Date. Overview of post partum care. 2005. Accessed: October 15, 2005. www.uptodol.com.

CODES
ICD9-CM
- V24.2 Routine Postpartum care
- V24.1 Supervision of lactation
- 670 Major puerperal infection
- 671 Venous complications of pregnancy and puerperium
- 675 Mastitis or breast abscess
- 676 Breast engorgement, cracked nipple, breastfeeding problems

KEY WORDS

- Postpartum Care
- Puerperium
- Breast-feeding
- Postpartum Depression
- Endometritis
- Mastitis

PREGNANCY, PREECLAMPSIA

Raymond O. Powrie, MD

KEY CLINICAL POINTS

- Preeclampsia complicates 5% of all pregnancies and up to 10% of 1st pregnancies.
- Preeclampsia generally occurs close to term and resolves after delivery. However, it can occur anytime after 20 weeks gestation.
- Fetal complications of preeclampsia include: preterm delivery, intrauterine growth restriction, placental abruption and intrauterine fetal demise.
- Maternal complications of preeclampsia include: Severe hypertension, stroke, pulmonary edema, renal insufficiency, hepatic failure, DIC, seizure, and death.
- Suspected or confirmed preeclampsia requires the involvement of an obstetrician.

 ## BASICS

DESCRIPTION
Preeclampsia is a disorder that is unique to pregnancy.

GENERAL PREVENTION
- No effective strategy has been definitively proven to prevent preeclampsia.
- Some evidence exists that ASA 81 mg/day started at 12 weeks gestation may decrease risk but experts disagree on validity of these findings.

EPIDEMIOLOGY
Incidence
Preeclampsia complicates 5% of pregnancies.

RISK FACTORS
- Maternal: Age <18 or >35 years, chronic hypertension, renal disease, 1st pregnancy, primipaternity, thrombophilias, SLE, obesity and insulin resistance.
- Fetal: Multiple gestation, fetal hydrops, molar pregnancy, triploidy.

Genetics
The genetic basis of preeclampsia remains undefined but risk is increased for
- Patients with a family history
- Pregnancies fathered by men who have previously fathered a preeclamptic pregnancy
- Patients with inherited thrombophilias

PATHOPHYSIOLOGY
Preeclampsia is characterized by an abnormal vascular response to the formation of the placenta that is associated with:
- Increased systemic vascular resistance
- Enhanced platelet aggregation
- Activation of the coagulation system
- Endothelial-cell dysfunction

ETIOLOGY
Remains one of medicine's great mysteries. It appears to develop in 3 distinct phases
- First, the preeclamptic mother's endometrium has a maladaptive immune response to the invading trophoblast, leading to inadequate or 'superficial' placentation.
- Second, this inadequate placentation is complicated later in pregnancy by alterations in angiogenic growth factors and increased placental 'debris' in the maternal circulation.
- Third, these changes lead to a maternal inflammatory response, the features and severity of which in any given patient are

probably modulated by maternal endothelial and cardiovascular health. In women less able to tolerate the endothelial stress from inadequate placentation, the maternal preeclamptic syndrome becomes manifest.

ASSOCIATED CONDITIONS
See Risk Factors.

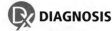 ## DIAGNOSIS

PRE-HOSPITAL
Screening for evidence of preeclampsia is part of every prenatal visit after 20 weeks gestation.

SIGNS AND SYMPTOMS
History
Patients with preeclampsia may be asymptomatic but can present with
- Headache
- Visual scintillations or scotoma
- Epigastric pain
- Excessive weight gain or profound edema

Physical Exam
- Blood pressure >140/90
- Epigastric or hepatic tenderness
- Clonus
- Facial edema
- Retinal vasospasm on fundoscopic exam
- Findings of pulmonary edema

TESTS
Lab
- Abnormal CBC
  - Thrombocytopenia
  - Hemoconcentration (Hgb >12 g/dL at term) or less commonly, a hemolytic anemia
- Elevated creatinine (>0.8 mg/dL in pregnancy)
- Uric acid (>5 mg/dL in pregnancy)
- Elevated AST
- Proteinuria on urinalysis or 24 hour urine (>300 mg/24 hour)

Imaging
- Women at high risk for preeclampsia generally receive an early ultrasound to establish pregnancy dating which may help guide decisions about early delivery later in pregnancy.
- Obstetricians will often obtain regular assessments of fetal well-being in the 3rd trimester (non stress tests, biophysical profiles and serial ultrasounds for fetal growth) in patients with suspected preeclampsia and in those at high risk for the condition.

Pathologic Findings
- When specimens are available, affected maternal organs can show evidence of edema, infarction, and hemorrhage.
- Affected kidneys may have a characteristic lesion called 'glomerular endotheliosis.'
- Placenta may be smaller than expected and/or show evidence of infarction, thrombosis, or abruption.
- Fetus/neonate may be small for gestational age.

DIFFERENTIAL DIAGNOSIS
- Worsening of established or previously unidentified chronic hypertension in third trimester (see Pregnancy, Chronic Hypertension chapter)

- 'HELLP' syndrome
  - A severe variant of preeclampsia characterized by **h**emolysis, **e**levated **l**iver enzymes and **l**ow **p**latelets
- Primary renal disease
- SLE
- HUS/TTP
- Acute fatty liver of pregnancy

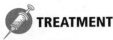 **TREATMENT**

PRE-HOSPITAL
- Patients with suspected preeclampsia should be urgently evaluated by an obstetrical provider.
- Patients with moderate or severe hypertension (>160/100), epigastric pain, persistent headache, and visual phenomena after 20 weeks gestation should generally be sent to an obstetrical emergency room.

GENERAL MEASURES
- Patients with symptoms, signs, or laboratory features of preeclampsia warrant the following interventions:
  - Immediate, careful review for other symptoms, signs, and laboratory features of preeclampsia.
  - Treatment of hypertension
    - Evaluate for secondary causes in all patients with new onset of hypertension in whom the diagnosis of preeclampsia is not clear
    - Evaluate for target organ damage
  - Obstetrician to obtain evaluation of fetal well-being that is appropriate for gestational age.
- Patients with preeclampsia should be delivered unless prolonging the pregnancy benefits the fetus (prematurity) or there is uncertainty about the diagnosis.
- Patients with preeclampsia typically placed on bed rest with bathroom privileges to improve placental perfusion although benefits not proven.

Diet
- No established role prevention/management
- Avoid excessive sodium and fluids.

IV Fluids
- Patients with preeclampsia are prone to pulmonary edema and should be kept euvolemic.

Complementary and Alternative Medicine
No alternative or complementary medications (including calcium, fish oils and antioxidants) have been shown to affect outcomes.

 MEDICATION (DRUGS)

First Line
- Seizure/Eclampsia
  - Intravenous magnesium
    - Shown to prevent seizures in preeclampsia
    - May decrease maternal mortality
    - Therefore should be given to all women who are being delivered for preeclampsia.
- HTN
  - BP >170–180/105–110 (opinions vary as to exact number) requires emergent treatment
    - IV labetalol
    - IV hydralazine
    - PO short acting nifedipine

- BP <170–180/105–110 but >160/100 require treatment but do not need immediate lowering if mother is asymptomatic and fetus has reassuring fetal testing. Initiation of an oral agent is appropriate for these patients.
    - Labetalol
    - Methyldopa
    - Nifedipine
  - BP <160/100 in the setting of preeclampsia does not necessarily require medical treatment if mother is asymptomatic.
- Prematurity
  - Mothers between 24– 34 weeks gestation should be given 48 hours of betamethasone or equivalent to decrease neonatal complications of prematurity.

Second Line
- Seizures
  - Treat acute seizures with IV lorazepam followed by loading with magnesium.
  - Persistent seizures on magnesium may be treated with phenytoin.
- HTN
  - IV nitroprusside or nitroglycerine if first line agents have failed.

SURGERY
Patients with preeclampsia may be delivered vaginally. The indications for cesarean delivery remain fetal and obstetrical.

 FOLLOW-UP

DISPOSITION
Breastfeeding
- Patients delivered for preeclampsia may breastfeed.
- No antihypertensive agents are definitely known to be harmful for breastfeeding.
  - Magnesium, methyldopa, labetalol, HCTZ, nifedipine, acebutolol, enalapril, captopril, and metoprolol approved by American Academy of Pediatrics for use in breastfeeding
  - Atenolol and propanolol are concentrated in breast milk and should probably be avoided

Admission Criteria
- Patients with suspected or documented preeclampsia generally managed as inpatients.
- The decision to manage preeclampsia as an outpatient should be approached warily and made by an obstetric provider only.

Discharge Criteria
- Patients admitted for suspected preeclampsia can be discharged once preeclampsia has been confidently ruled out and BP remains <160/100.
- Patients with documented preeclampsia generally managed in the hospital until delivery.
- Once delivered, patients can be discharged once symptoms and signs have resolved and preeclampsia labs are normalizing.
  - Start antihypertensive therapy in patients with BP >160/100 (according to some experts) or BP >140/90 (according to others). No evidence exists that treatment of blood pressures <160/100 in pregnancy is of short term benefit to mother or fetus.
  - Magnesium can be discontinued once the patient begins her postpartum diuresis (generally 24–48 hours postpartum).

Issues for Referral
- To obstetrical provider for suspected and established preeclampsia

- To maternal fetal medicine and neonatology for preeclampsia occurring before 34 weeks gestation to help guide management decisions and counsel patients.
- Consider involvement of ICU physicians for pulmonary edema, CVA, hepatic or renal failure.
- To hematology for brisk hemolysis or severe thrombocytopenia as may require plasmapheresis for possibility of HUS/TTP.

PROGNOSIS

- Most patients with preeclampsia do well and improve 24–48 hours postpartum.
- Patients presenting with epigastric pain, hemolysis, elevated liver enzymes, and/or low platelets have a more worrisome course and are sometimes treated with high dose dexamethasone in addition to delivery.
- Preeclampsia (particularly occurring before 34 weeks gestation) increases lifetime risk of cardiovascular disease.
  - Heart healthy lifestyle should be encouraged.

COMPLICATIONS

- Fetal complications: preterm delivery, intrauterine growth restriction, placental abruption and intrauterine fetal demise.
- Maternal complications: severe hypertension, stroke, pulmonary edema, renal insufficiency, hepatic failure, DIC, seizure and death.
- Blood pressure elevations may persist and require treatment for up to 3 months postpartum.
- Seizures may occur up to 7 days postpartum

PATIENT MONITORING

- In asymptomatic patients not being delivered:
  - Monitor BP several times a day
  - Preeclampsia blood work (CBC, Cr, Uric acid, AST, urinalysis) q3d and with any change in status.
- Symptomatic patients are usually delivered.
  - BP measurement, testing of fetal well being, and preeclampsia blood work often carried out several times a day in these patients.
- Postpartum patients with preeclampsia may still have seizures for up to 7 days and blood pressure may be affected for up to 3 months.
  - Monitor blood pressure regularly in the weeks following delivery until it normalizes.
  - Medication regimen may need frequent readjustments while the effects of preeclampsia gradually dissipate.

REFERENCES

1. Magee LA, Abdullah S. The safety of antihypertensives for treatment of pregnancy hypertension. *Expert Opin Drug Saf*. 2004;3:25–38.
2. Roberts JM, Cooper DW. Pathogenesis and genetics of pre-eclampsia. *Lancet*. 2001;357:53–56.
3. Sibai BM. Diagnosis and management of gestational hypertension and preeclampsia. *Obstet Gynecol*. 2003;102:181–192.
4. Sibai B, Dekker G, Kuperminc M. Pre-eclampsia. *Lancet*. 2005;365:785–799.

ADDITIONAL READING

Duley L, Henderson-Smart DJ, Knight M, et al. Antiplatelet agents for preventing pre-eclampsia and its complications. Cochrane Database Syst Rev. 2004;(1):CD004659.
Duley L. Evidence and practice: The magnesium sulphate story. *Best Pract Res Clin Obstet Gynaecol*. 2005;19:57–74.

CODES
ICD9-CM

- 642.0 Benign essential hypertension complicating pregnancy, childbirth, and the puerperium
- 642.3 Transient hypertension of pregnancy
- 642.4 Mild or unspecified preeclampsia
- 642.5 Severe preeclampsia
- 642.6 Eclampsia
- 642.7 Preeclampsia or eclampsia superimposed on pre-existing hypertension
- 642.9 Unspecified hypertension complicating pregnancy, childbirth, or the puerperium

KEY WORDS

- Hypertension
- Preeclampsia
- Eclampsia
- Pregnancy

PREGNANCY, PRENATAL CARE

Eric A. Wright, DO
Melissa Nothnagle, MD

KEY CLINICAL POINTS

- Preconception care is an important part of prenatal care and permits early identification of modifiable risk factors.
- Women who receive prenatal care early in pregnancy have better outcomes than women who receive late or no prenatal care.
- Prenatal care should be initiated in the first trimester in order to establish pregnancy dating and detect high-risk conditions requiring referral.

 ## BASICS

DESCRIPTION
- Quality prenatal care includes a thorough history of maternal medical risk factors, family history, and psychosocial issues.
- There is limited evidence as to the optimum number of prenatal visits.
  - The average number of prenatal visits in developed countries is 7–11.
  - Frequency of visits should be based on the initial risk assessment.
- Usual schedule of United States prenatal visits:
  - Monthly beginning with preconception care until 30–32 weeks
  - Every 2 weeks until 36 weeks gestation, then weekly until delivery.

GENERAL PREVENTION
- General age-appropriate preventive care
- Prevention of neural tube defects
  - Folic acid supplementation at least 1 month prior to conception
- Genetic risk factor screening
  - Offer disease-specific carrier screening to couples from ethnic groups at high risk for cystic fibrosis, Tay-Sachs disease, thalassemias, and sickle cell disease.
  - Offer genetic counseling for couples with family history of genetic disorders.
- Infectious disease screening and prevention
  - Assess immunity to rubella and varicella.
    - Offer immunization and advise postponing conception for 3 months if status is non-immune.
  - Screen for HIV, hepatitis B, syphilis
    - Immunization for hepatitis B can be given at any time during pregnancy.
  - Counsel on exposure to CMV, parvovirus B19, and toxoplasmosis
  - Offer influenza vaccination to all women who expect to deliver during flu season.
- Management of chronic conditions
  - Hypertension
    - Avoid ACE-Is, ARBs, thiazide type diuretics
  - Diabetes mellitus
    - Optimize control prior to conception (normal HgbA1C).
    - Transition to insulin if using oral hypoglycemics
    - HMG CoA reductase inhibitors (statins) are contraindicated in pregnancy.
    - Folic acid supplementation 1 mg per day
  - Epilepsy
    - Optimize control prior to conception.

- Folic acid supplementation 1 mg per day
- Offer genetic counseling
  - DVT/hypercoagulable state
    - Transition to heparin if using warfarin
  - Depression/anxiety
    - Avoid benzodiazepines
    - Counsel women on risks/benefits of SSRIs in pregnancy based on latest available research findings.
    - Monitor closely for postpartum depression.
- Lifestyle/environment
  - Assess tobacco, alcohol, or drug use/dependence and provide counseling and assistance with cessation efforts.
  - Screen for domestic violence.
  - Screen for nutritional deficiencies.
  - Recommend regular moderate exercise.
  - Screen for environmental toxin exposure at work and in the home.
- If a preconception visit has not taken place, the above interventions should be done at the initial prenatal visits.

EPIDEMIOLOGY
Prevalence
- Approximately 85% of the women in the United States receive early prenatal care (starting in the 1st trimester).
- Approximately 3.5% of the women in the United States receive late or no prenatal care.

RISK FACTORS
Groups at higher risk for late or no prenatal care include African-American women, teenagers, poor women, and women who use drugs.

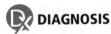 ## DIAGNOSIS

The diagnosis of pregnancy is confirmed with urine or serum beta human chorionic gonadotropin measurements.

SIGNS AND SYMPTOMS
History
- At every prenatal visit
  - Nausea or vomiting
  - Vaginal bleeding
  - Abdominal pain
  - Fetal movement
    - Usually noted by 20 weeks
- 1st Trimester
  - Establish EDD (estimated delivery date) as early as possible, based on first day of LMP. Ultrasound to establish EDD if dates by LMP and clinical exam do not agree within 2 weeks or patient presents after first trimester
  - Assess adjustment to pregnancy, social support
- 2nd Trimester
  - Symptoms of preterm labor
- 3rd Trimester
  - Symptoms of preeclampsia

Physical Exam
- Complete physical exam at initial visit including pelvic exam to assess uterine size.
- At every visit:
  - Weight

– Blood pressure
– Fundal height (beginning at 20 weeks)
  • If fundal height 4 cm greater or less than gestational age in weeks, obtain ultrasound to assess fetal growth and amniotic fluid volume.
– Fetal heart rate (beginning at 12 weeks gestation)
– Abdominal palpation for fetal position (beginning at 32–36 weeks gestation)
  • If nonvertex presentation at ≥36 weeks, offer external cephalic version if indicated.

TESTS
Lab
• At every prenatal visit:
  – Urinalysis for protein and glucose
• Preconception or early prenatal labs:
  – Rh and ABO type and antibody screen
  – Hemoglobin and hematocrit
  – Hepatitis B surface antigen
  – Hepatitis C antibody testing for women with risk factors
  – HIV antibody screen
  – Syphilis, chlamydia, gonorrhea
  – Rubella antibody screen
  – Pap smear if not done in past year
  – Hemoglobin electrophoresis for women in high risk ethnic groups
  – Urine culture to screen for asymptomatic bacteriuria (at least once early in gestation)
    • Defined as > 100,000 colonies of a single pathogen
    • Risk of pyelonephritis ~30% in women with untreated bacteriuria in pregnancy
    • Treat with antibiotic regimen and repeat culture after treatment to document cure
  – Offer screening for trisomies 21 and 18 and neural tube defects with maternal serum markers at 15–20 weeks gestation (optimal timing is 16–18 weeks)
    • Diagnostic procedures such as level II ultrasound, amniocentesis, or chorionic villous sampling should be offered to high risk mothers or those with an abnormal screening test.
• Mid-gestational and 3rd trimester labs
  – Gestational diabetes (GDM) screening with 1 hour nonfasting 50 g oral glucose challenge at 24–28 weeks
    • GDM screening not routinely required in Caucasian women younger than 25 with normal prepregnant weight and no family or personal history of diabetes
  – Hemoglobin/hematocrit at 24–28 weeks
  – Syphilis and HIV screening at 24–28 weeks in at-risk women
  – Vagino-rectal swab for Group B Strep (GBS) at 35–37 weeks

Imaging
• Routine ultrasound for purposes other than gestational age evaluation when indicated has not been shown to improve outcomes.
• Ultrasonography at 10–14 weeks can measure nuchal translucency to screen for trisomy 21.
• Exposure to ionizing radiation through imaging studies (X-ray, CT) has the most potential for harm to the fetus in the first 10–14 weeks of pregnancy.
  – Ionizing radiation should generally be avoided but not withheld if benefits to mother's health outweigh potential risks to fetus.
  – The cumulative upper limit of radiation exposure needed to harm fetus is approximately 5 rads.
  – Estimated pelvic radiation exposure for common tests:

• Chest x-ray: 0.00007 rads
• Abdominal x-ray: 0.245 rads
• Chest CT: 0.100 rads

 ## TREATMENT
GENERAL MEASURES
Diet
• Caloric requirements increase by 340–450 kcal/day in 2nd and 3rd trimesters.
• Recommended weight gain for women with a normal prepregnant BMI is 25–35 pounds total.
• Caffeine consumption should not exceed 150–300 mg per day.
• Unpasteurized dairy products, soft cheeses, raw eggs, and undercooked meats should be avoided due to risk of bacterial or parasitic contamination.
• Fish high in mercury should be avoided.

Activity
• Daily moderate exercise should be encouraged unless an obstetrical contraindication is present (e.g., preterm labor, preeclampsia).
• Activities that involve risk of falls or abdominal trauma should be avoided.
• Sexual intercourse is not contraindicated during pregnancy.
• To reduce risk of toxoplasmosis infection, pregnant women should avoid contact with cat litter and should wear gloves and wash hands after gardening.

 ## MEDICATION (DRUGS)
• Folic acid
  – Start 1 month prior to conception and continue through first 3 months pregnancy
  – For low risk women: 400 mcg per day
  – For women with diabetes or epilepsy: 1 mg per day
  – For women with a previous fetus/infant with a neural tube defect: 4 mg per day
• Prenatal vitamins should include 400 mcg folic acid and 30 mg elemental iron.
  – Additional iron supplementation (60–120 mg/day) is recommended for women with hemoglobin less than 10–11 mg/dL due to iron deficiency.
• Few drugs have established as safe for use during pregnancy. Limit use of prescription and over-the-counter medicines in pregnancy to situations in which the benefits outweigh potential risks.

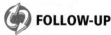 ## FOLLOW-UP
DISPOSITION
Admission Criteria
Pregnant women should be referred to the hospital for evaluation if they experience any of the following:
• Signs/symptoms of labor (contractions, vaginal bleeding, leakage of fluid) prior to 37 weeks
• Serious medical complications (e.g., hyperemesis gravidarum, pyelonephritis, poorly controlled diabetes)
• Minor trauma after viability (24 weeks)
• Signs and symptoms of preeclampsia (BP > 140/90, proteinuria, hyperreflexia, headache, visual changes, right upper quadrant pain, nausea, edema)

Issues for Referral

- Primary care physicians whose scope of practice does not include prenatal care should refer women to a prenatal care provider at the time of pregnancy diagnosis.
- Referral to a qualified provider should be made whenever a high-risk condition is identified that is beyond the scope of practice of the primary prenatal care provider.

PATIENT MONITORING

Post-term pregnancy

- After 41 weeks gestation, assess fetal well-being using nonstress testing and amniotic fluid index.
- Offer induction of labor after 41 weeks gestation.

REFERENCES

1. Brundage SC. Preconception health care. *Am Fam Physician*. 2002;65:2507–2514.
2. Hayashi RH, et al. Guidelines for clinical care: Prenatal care. University of Michigan health system, revision July 2004. Available at: http://cme.med.umich.edu/iCME/prenatal04/guideline.asp.
3. Kirkham C, Harris S, Grzybowski S. Evidence-based prenatal care: Part I. General prenatal care and counseling issues. *Am Fam Physician*. 2005;71:1307–1316.
4. Kirkham C, Harris S, Grzybowski S. Evidence-based prenatal care: Part II. Third-trimester care and prevention of infectious diseases. *Am Fam Physician*. 2005;71:1555–1560.
5. National Collaborating Center for Women's and Children's Health. Antenatal care: Routine care for the healthy pregnant woman. Available at: http://www.rcog.org.uk/resources/Public/pdf/Antenatal'Care.pdf.
6. Toppenber KS, Hill DA, Miller DP. Safety of radiographic imaging during pregnancy. *Am Fam Physician*. 1999;59:1813–1818.

CODES
ICD9-CM

- V22.1 Supervision, other normal pregnancy
- V22.2 Pregnancy

KEY WORDS

- Preconception Care
- Prenatal Care
- Pregnancy

PREGNANCY, SEIZURE DISORDER

Lucia Larson, MD

KEY CLINICAL POINTS

- Epilepsy is not a contraindication to pregnancy. Over 90% of women with seizure disorders have successful pregnancies with healthy babies.
- The management goal for epileptic pregnant women is seizure control. The benefits of antiepileptic drugs (AEDs) outweigh the risk of seizures during pregnancy.
- AED monotherapy is associated with significantly fewer congenital anomalies than polytherapy.
- Consider eclampsia as a cause of seizure during pregnancy.

 BASICS

DESCRIPTION

- Seizures are a common neurologic complication of pregnancy.
- Though seizures and AEDs may adversely affect pregnancy outcome, the vast majority of gravid women with seizures will have successful pregnancies and healthy babies.
- Not all seizures occurring in pregnancy are secondary to eclampsia, but it must be strongly considered as a possible cause.

EPIDEMIOLOGY
Incidence

- In the United States, approximately 1 million women of childbearing age have epilepsy.
- Approximately 20,000 babies in the United States are born to women with epilepsy each year.

RISK FACTORS
Risk factors which may compromise seizure control during pregnancy include:

- Noncompliance often out of fear for taking a teratogenic drug during pregnancy
- Nausea and vomiting
- Sleep deprivation
- Stress
- Hormonal factors
- Decreased drug levels secondary to pregnancy physiology

PATHOPHYSIOLOGY

- Most women will not have a change in seizure frequency in pregnancy.
- However, the following physiologic changes in pregnancy may contribute to the increased frequency experienced by some women.
  - Decreased GI absorption
  - Nausea and vomiting of pregnancy, with or without hyperemesis
  - Increased hepatic metabolism
  - Increased glomerular filtration rate
  - Changes in protein binding

ETIOLOGY
Eclampsia must be considered in any pregnant woman who develops a seizure. However, seizures may have the same etiologies in pregnancy as in nonpregnant patients.

ASSOCIATED CONDITIONS

- Congenital anomalies associated with AEDs: Neural tube defects, craniofacial and cardiac anomalies
- Associated obstetric conditions (particularly poorly controlled) include: Miscarriage, intrauterine fetal demise, placental abruption, and intrauterine growth restriction.

 DIAGNOSIS

- The diagnostic evaluation of seizure disorders in pregnancy is similar to that in nonpregnant patients.
- However, eclampsia needs to be ruled out.

SIGNS AND SYMPTOMS

- Pregnant women with seizure disorders present in the same manner as nonpregnant women.
- Additional signs and symptoms to suggest eclampsia include:
  - Headache, visual symptoms
  - Epigastric or abdominal pain
  - Significant edema especially if involving hands and face

History

- Obtain history regarding the seizure disorder and note the following:
  - Type of seizure
    - Tonic-clonic seizures are associated with fetal hypoxia and acidosis but the significance of nonconvulsive seizures are less clear.
  - Frequency of seizures, including elapsed time since last seizure
  - Precipitants of seizure
  - Medication history
- Obtain pregnancy history
  - Determine gestational age
  - Note outcome of previous pregnancies, including the presence of congenital anomalies in other offspring.

Physical Exam
Note features suggestive of eclampsia or other causes of seizures in nonpregnant patients.

- Vital signs including presence of HTN or fever
- Funduscopic exam noting papilledema
- RUQ or epigastric tenderness suggests preeclampsia/eclampsia
- Significant hand or facial edema is suggestive of preeclampsia/eclampsia.
- Focal findings on complete neurologic exam suggest a CNS lesion.

TESTS
Lab

- Laboratories supportive of eclampsia include
  - Abnormal renal function
    - Proteinuria
    - Elevated creatinine (Normal for pregnancy = 0.5–0.8 mg/dL)
    - Elevated uric acid (Normal in pregnancy <4.5)
  - Thrombocytopenia
  - Elevated Hgb (suggesting hemoconcentration)
  - Decreased Hgb (suggesting hemolysis)
  - Elevated AST, ALT
- To evaluate acute seizures in pregnancy obtain
  - Electrolytes, calcium, magnesium
  - Glucose
  - CBC
  - Creatinine
  - Oxygen saturation or ABG

Imaging
- Head CT
  - Fetal radiation dose is approximately 0.01 rads.
  - According to the National Council on Radiation Protection and Measurements, the acceptable total fetal radiation dose during pregnancy = 5 rads.
- MRI
  - Can be safely obtained during pregnancy, particularly after the 1st trimester
  - Gadolinium should be withheld unless the additional information provided from its use outweighs its unknown risk in pregnancy.

Diagnostic Procedures/Surgery
EEGs are safe to perform in pregnancy.

DIFFERENTIAL DIAGNOSIS
Rule out eclampsia in any pregnant woman presenting with a seizure.

TREATMENT

PRE-HOSPITAL
- AEDs are teratogenic, but despite this, the goal of treatment for seizure disorders in pregnant women is to prevent seizures.
- Prepregnancy counseling is instrumental in ensuring the best pregnancy outcome possible.
- Therapy should be optimized at least 6 months prior to a planned pregnancy.
- Seizures in pregnancy are associated with hypoxia and acidosis, which are not well tolerated by a fetus.
- Trauma and aspiration are other complications of seizures which may also have adverse maternal and fetal effects.
- According to the guidelines of the American Academy of Neurology, discontinuation of AEDs could be considered >6 months prior to a planned pregnancy if all the following criteria satisfied:
  - Seizure free for 2–5 years
  - Single seizure type
  - Normal neurologic exam and normal intelligence
  - EEG that has normalized with treatment
- Monotherapy is associated with a significantly lower risk for adverse fetal effects than polytherapy.
  - The particular combination of phenytoin, phenobarbital, and valproic acid is associated with congenital anomalies in 58%.
- Valproic acid has the highest risk of the AEDs for malformations especially when used in doses exceeding 1,100 mg/day.

GENERAL MEASURES
- The same general measures used to treat nonpregnant patients should be administered to pregnant women with acute seizures.
- Supplemental oxygen should be administered to keep oxygen saturation greater than 95%.
- Position the pregnant patient on her left side or with the right hip elevated to prevent obstruction of the inferior vena cava by the gravid uterus.
- Pregnant women have an increased risk for aspiration so early intubation by the most experienced personnel is prudent when there is concern for a compromised airway.
- In addition, fetal evaluation should be done by the obstetrician.

MEDICATION (DRUGS)

- Pregnant women with acute nonclamptic seizures should be treated similarly to nonpregnant patients.
  - Benzodiazepines may be safely used.
  - Phenytoin and phenobarbital can be safely used to prevent recurrent nonclamptic seizures.
  - IV magnesium should be used to prevent recurrent seizures associated with eclampsia.

First Line
- AEDs as a group are teratogenic.
  - Phenytoin, carbamazepine, valproic acid, and phenobarbital are commonly used in pregnancy, but also associated with neural tube defects, craniofacial and cardiac abnormalities.
  - Valproic acid is associated with the highest risk for neural tube defects (1–2%) with an overall incidence of major congenital malformations of 8.6–16.7%.
- Folic acid: ≥4 mg PO daily is recommended to decrease neural tube defects
- Vitamin K: 10 mg PO daily should be given to women beginning at 36 weeks gestation until the end of pregnancy to help prevent hemorrhagic disease of the newborn.
  - Neonate should be given 1 mg Vitamin K intramuscularly at birth.

Second Line
- Newer agents such as levetiracetam, oxcarbazepine, gabapentin, and lamotrigine cannot be recommended above older agents given limited data in human pregnancy.
- Of the newer agents, best data for lamotrigine
  - There was a 2.9% major malformation rate among 414 pregnancies noted in a voluntary registry by the manufacturer.

FOLLOW-UP

- Pregnant women need to be monitored for effectiveness of their medication and for adverse effects associated with AEDs.
- Most women need increased doses of AED during pregnancy.
- Free drug levels should be obtained whenever possible because total levels may be misleading secondary to changes in protein binding.
- Routine screening with maternal serum alpha-fetoprotein at 16–18 weeks and Level II ultrasounds done at 18–20 weeks can help to identify congenital anomalies before birth.
- Monitor AED levels for 8 weeks postpartum
  - After delivery, the dose of AED should be decreased to halfway between pre-pregnancy and pregnancy doses for 2 weeks.
  - At that time, the pre-pregnancy dose can generally be resumed.
- Breastfeeding should be encouraged but neonates should be monitored for sedation and difficulty feeding.
- In addition to the usual safety issues (such as avoidance of driving), women with seizure disorders should be counseled on several issues regarding the care of their newborns so that their babies are safe if a seizure occurs.
  - The neonate should be given sponge baths instead of being placed in a bathtub.
  - Diapers should be changed on the floor rather than on a changing table.
  - Try to have others carry a baby up stairs.

DISPOSITION

Admission Criteria

Pregnant women with new onset seizures should be admitted to evaluate for eclampsia.

Discharge Criteria

Women without eclampsia who have controlled seizures and reassuring fetal testing may be discharged with outpatient follow-up.

Issues for Referral

- Obstetricians should be involved to help evaluate for eclampsia, to identify congenital anomalies, and to monitor fetal well-being.
- A neurologist should be consulted if any uncertainty about the cause of noneclamptic seizures and about which AED is most appropriate.
- Pregnant women with epilepsy should be entered in a registry regardless of whether they take medications.
  - (888) 233-2334 (Federal antiepileptic drug pregnancy registry)
  - www.aedpregnancyregistry.org

PROGNOSIS

- The majority of women who have treated seizure disorders have successful pregnancies with healthy babies.
- The better controlled a woman's seizures are prior to pregnancy, the more likely they will be controlled during pregnancy.
- Women with seizure disorders are NOT more likely to develop preeclampsia/eclampsia.

COMPLICATIONS

- Congenital anomalies associated with AEDs are primarily neural tube defects, craniofacial, and cardiac anomalies.
- Other complications in the offspring include dysmorphisms and postnatal developmental delay.
- Obstetric complications associated with seizure disorders (particularly poorly controlled) include miscarriage, intrauterine fetal demise, placental abruption, and intrauterine growth restriction.

PATIENT MONITORING

Many experts recommend monitoring *free* drug levels every month during pregnancy and postpartum.

REFERENCES

1. Jeha LE, Morris HH. Optimizing outcomes in pregnant women with epilepsy. *Cleve Clin J Med*. 2005;72:938–945.
2. Tomson T, Battino D. Teratogenicity of antiepileptic drugs: State of the art. *Curr Opin in Neurol*. 2005;18:135–140.
3. Vajda F, Lander C, O'Brien T, et al. Australian pregnancy registry of women taking anitepileptic drugs. A summary update report from the Austrailian Pregnancy Registry. *Epilepsia*. 2004;45:1455.

ADDITIONAL READING

Adab N, Tudur SC, et al. Common antiepileptic drugs in pregnancy in women with epilepsy (Cochrane review) In: Editor names, eds. The Cochrane Library. Chichester, UK: John Wiley and Sons, Ltd.; 2004.

Crawford P. Best practice guidelines for the management of women with epilepsy. *Epilepsia*. 2005;46:117–124.

Lee E, et al. Medical Care of the Pregnant Patient. Philadelphia, PA: American College of Physicians; 2000.

Nelson-Piercy C. Handbook of Obstetric Medicine. St Louis, MO: Mosby-Year Book, Inc.; 1997.

 MISCELLANEOUS

- Resources for both clinicians and patients include:
  - www.efa.org (The Epilepsy Foundation)
  - www.otispregnancy.org (Web site for the Organization of Teratology Information Services)

CODES

ICD9-CM

- 780.39 Seizure, NOS
- 646.93 Pregnancy, antepartum
- 646.91 Pregnancy, postpartum
- 642.63 Eclampsia, antepartum
- 642.61 Eclampsia, postpartum
- 345.91 Seizure w/status

KEY WORDS

- Seizure Disorder
- Pregnancy
- Eclampsia and Preeclampsia
- Grand Mal Seizure
- Tonic-Clonic Seizure
- Epilepsy

PREGNANCY, SUBSTANCE ABUSE

Neeta Jain, MD

KEY CLINICAL POINTS

- Substance abusers are seen from all socioeconomic strata, ages, and races.
- No amount of alcohol during pregnancy is reported as safe; 20–25% of pregnant women smoke or drink alcohol
- Risk of substance abuse relapse high in postpartum period

 BASICS

DESCRIPTION
- In a pregnant patient, hazardous substance use is comprised of illicit drug use, tobacco, and alcohol.
- Such substance use is associated with increased negative obstetrical and perinatal outcome.
- Substance abusers are seen from all socioeconomic strata, ages, and races.

GENERAL PREVENTION
- Pregnancy provides a unique opportunity for medical intervention.
- For many women, motivation to modify behavior is high at this time.
- However, risk for relapse is high in the postpartum period.

EPIDEMIOLOGY
- 20–25% of pregnant women smoke or drink alcohol.
- 3% of pregnant women use an illicit substance
- In a survey among women aged 15–44 years:
  - Approximately 90% of women drank alcohol
  - 44% smoked marijuana
  - 14% smoked cocaine.
- Each year, 200,000 offspring are exposed to illicit substances in utero, and 800,000 offspring are exposed in utero to alcohol.

Incidence
- Estimates of the incidence of prenatal substance abuse differ remarkably, from 375,000 infants exposed to 625,000 exposed annually.
- The incidence of fetal alcohol syndrome (FAS) is 1–2 live births per 1,000. The rates of fetal alcohol effects (FAE) are approximately 3–5 live births per 1,000.

Prevalence
- Underestimated prevalence rates are common since women are reluctant to admit substance use.
- Nicotine is approximately 20–30%.
- Alcohol is approximately 14–15%.

RISK FACTORS
- Less than 20 years of age
- Less than a high school education
- Nonwhite
- Single

ETIOLOGY
There may be an underlying psychiatric disorder such as depression, anxiety, bipolar disorder, schizophrenia

ASSOCIATED CONDITIONS
- **Nicotine**
  - Not an illicit drug but its use has been associated with
    - Spontaneous abortion
    - Placental abruption
    - Premature rupture of membranes (PROM)

- Intrauterine growth retardation (IUGR)
- Preterm delivery
- **Alcohol**
  - No quantity of use has been reportedly safe in pregnancy.
  - The term fetal alcohol spectrum disorder encompasses a broad spectrum of adverse outcomes in infants exposed to alcohol during pregnancy.
  - The effects span a spectrum of severity from Alcohol Related Effects (ARE) to Fetal Alcohol Syndrome (FAS).
    - The diagnosis of FAS comprises four criteria, all of which must be present:
      o Structural: Shortened palpebral fissures, thin upper lip, flattened philtrum, flat midface, micrognathia, epicanthal folds, low nasal bridge.
      o Growth: Retardation in height and weight below 95th percentile
      o Cognition: Mild to moderate mental retardation (MR)
      o Behavioral: Poor coordination, hypotonia, irritability, attentional deficits in childhood
  - Main characteristics of FAE include:
    - Congenital anomalies, malformations, and dysplasias
    - Alcohol-related neurodevelopmental disorder (ARND): delayed motor and speech, hearing impairments, information processing difficulties, math and short-term memory deficits, behavioral problems, and mild to moderate MR
- Cannabis
  - Most commonly used illicit substance taken in pregnancy
  - Offspring of heavy users (6 joints daily) had smaller head circumferences at all ages
- **CNS Stimulants** (cocaine, methamphetamine, methylphenidate, antiobesity meds) cause maternal vasoconstriction and hypertension increasing obstetrical complications:
  - Spontaneous abortions
  - Preterm labor
  - Abruption placenta
  - Meconium staining
  - Intrauterine growth retardation (IUGR)
- **Opioids** increased risk of obstetrical complications such as
  - IUGR
  - PROM
  - Abruption placenta
  - Pregnancy-induced hypertension
  - Meconium staining
  - Maternal and neonatal infection
  - Stillbirth
- In patients with intravenous drug use
  - Endocarditis
  - Skin abscess
  - Sexually transmitted diseases if involved with sex for drugs

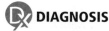 **DIAGNOSIS**

SIGNS AND SYMPTOMS
- **Cocaine:** Ingesting large amounts of cocaine can intensify the user's high, but can also lead to
  - Bizarre, erratic, and violent behavior
  - Tremors, vertigo, muscle twitches
  - Irritability, anxiety, paranoia, and restlessness
- **Heroin:** Initial rush associated with

- Warm flushing of skin
- Dry mouth
- Heavy feeling in the user's arms and legs
- Nausea, vomiting, and severe itching
- Following the initial effects, the user will be drowsy for several hours with clouded mental function
- **Withdrawal Syndromes in Neonates** are associated with use of cocaine and opioids.
  - Cocaine withdrawal
    - Neonates exposed to cocaine in pregnancy may experience symptoms on postnatal days 2–3.
    - Symptoms include jitteriness, hyperactive moro, excessive sucking, hypertonia, abnormal EEG and seizures, hyperreflexia, sleep disturbance and poor habituation.
  - Heroin or opioid-related withdrawal
    - Symptoms occur in 30–80% of exposed neonates, within 3–12 hours post delivery for heroin and 48–52 hours post maternal dose for methadone.
    - Associated symptoms include increased irritability, disorganized sleep, high pitch, hypertonia, tremors, seizures, poor feeding, diarrhea, dehydration, diaphoresis, nasal stuffiness, fever, temperature instability.

History

- A history of past and present substance use should be obtained in a nonjudgmental manner.
- There is no simple screen tool for identifying drug abusers. Signs and symptoms suggestive of a high-risk substance user consists of:
  - Late initiation of prenatal care
  - Multiple missed prenatal visits
  - Impaired work performance
- T-ACE is a screening question specific to identifying risk-drinking (alcohol intake sufficient to potentially damage the embryo/fetus) in pregnancy:
  - How many drinks does it take for you to feel high (tolerance)?
  - Do you feel annoyed by people complaining about your drinking?
  - Have you ever felt the need to cut down on your drinking?
  - Have you ever had a drink first thing in the morning (eye-opener)?
- A score of 2 is assigned to the Tolerance question and a score of 1 to all the others.
- Score ≥2 is considered positive for risk-drinking, indicating need to pursue history consumption in greater detail.
- If all 4 questions are answered positively, there is a 62.7% likelihood of risk-drinking.

Physical Exam

- Cocaine:
  - Constricted blood vessels
  - Dilated pupils
  - Increased temperature, heart rate, and blood pressure
  - Track marks if intravenous use
  - Tremors, muscle twitching
  - Bizarre erratic behavior, paranoia
- Heroin
  - Constricted pupils
  - Track marks if intravenous use
  - Stupor, obtundation
  - Bradycardia
  - Respiratory suppression

TESTS

All pregnant women should be screened for use of illicit substances.

Lab

- Maternal urine is the best choice for marijuana, cocaine, and opioids.
- Informed consent should be obtained prior to testing.

DIFFERENTIAL DIAGNOSIS

- Thyroid disorders
- Psychiatric disorders
  - Depression
  - Psychosis
  - Anxiety

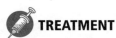 **TREATMENT**

PRE-HOSPITAL

- In managing pregnant patients with chemical dependence or abuse, interplay of different treatment modalities is most effective.
- Supportive psychotherapy includes individual counseling, group therapy, and self-help groups such as Alcoholic Anonymous, Narcotic Anonymous.
- Behavioral treatment: pregnant women who have received smoking cessation intervention had a 70% improvement in abstaining.

INITIAL STABILIZATION

Opioid-dependent pregnant women may require inpatient detoxification or referral to a methadone maintenance program.

GENERAL MEASURES

Women who continue to use illicit substances, alcohol, or receive >20 mg methadone per day should be discouraged from breastfeeding.

 MEDICATION (DRUGS)

Pharmacological management may be an option and should be referred to a specialist

 FOLLOW-UP

The obstetrical provider is critical for screening, counseling, and initiating referral to specialized treatment

Issues for Referral

Management of intoxication or withdrawal symptoms may require referral to inpatient medical unit.

PROGNOSIS

- High risk of relapse is common after delivery.
- Professionals working with this population must tackle many issues associated with substance use: poverty, poor parenting skills, lack of education or job training, child abuse, physical or sexual abuse, poor support, and risk of sexual transmitted disease.

REFERENCES

1. Bolnick JM, Rayburn WF. Substance use disorders in women: Special considerations during pregnancy. *Obstet Gynecol Clin N Am*. 2003;30:545–558.
2. Burt VK, Hendrick VC, eds. Concise Guide to Women's Mental Health, 2nd ed. Washington: American Psychaitric Publishing; 2001.

3. Chang G. Substance use in pregnancy. Available at: http://www.utdol.com/application/topic.asp?file=maternal/5807&type=A&selectedTitle=2~99. Accessed October 4, 2005.
4. Curet LB, His AC. Drug abuse in pregnancy. *Clin Obstet Gyn*. 2002;45:73–88.
5. Ebrahim SH, Gfroerer J. Pregnancy-related substance use in the United States during 1996–1998. *Obstet Gynecol*. 2003;101:374.

CODES
ICD9-CM
- V65.42 Counseling on substance use and abuse
- V22 Pregnancy
- 305.2 Cannabis abuse
- 305.5 Opioid abuse
- 305.0 Alcohol abuse
- 305.6 Cocaine abuse
- 305.1 Tobacco dependence

KEY WORDS
- Pregnancy
- Substance Abuse
- Alcohol Use
- Drug Use
- Cocaine
- Heroin
- Tobacco Use

PREGNANCY, THE COMMON COLD

Raymond O. Powrie, MD

KEY CLINICAL POINTS

- Most common cold remedies are not particularly effective in changing the course or symptomatology of the common cold and should not be routinely recommended in or out of pregnancy.
- If patients are insistent about options for symptomatic relief, acetaminophen, pseudoephedrine, oxymetalozine nasal spray, and chlorpheniramine are the agents for which the best pregnancy safety data exists.

 BASICS

DESCRIPTION

- Upper respiratory infections (URIs) represent the most common reason for doctor visits.
- Pregnant women are likely at a similar risk for URIs as the general population.

GENERAL PREVENTION

- Regular hand washing and avoidance of infected individuals remains the best defense against the common cold.
- Pregnant women should receive the influenza vaccine to decrease incidence and severity of influenza during pregnancy.

EPIDEMIOLOGY
Incidence
Although largely unstudied, there is no reason to believe that the incidence, risk factors, and pathophysiology of the common cold is different in pregnancy than what is reported for the general population.

RISK FACTORS
Risk factors for the common cold are likely unchanged in pregnancy.

PATHOPHYSIOLOGY
The pathophysiology of the common cold, while largely unstudied in pregnancy, is likely to be unchanged in pregnant patients.

ETIOLOGY

- The pathogens most frequently associated with common cold symptoms are the rhinoviruses, coronaviruses, and the respiratory syncytial virus.
- Causes of URI likely do not differ from those described in nonpregnant women.

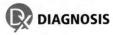 DIAGNOSIS

PRE-HOSPITAL
URIs are generally managed as an outpatient.

SIGNS AND SYMPTOMS
There is no evidence that the signs and symptoms of upper respiratory infections in pregnancy differ from that seen in the non pregnant population.

History
- The common cold generally lasts from 3–7 days but may persist for up to 2 weeks in 25% of patients.
- Symptoms of the common cold are unchanged from the non-pregnant population:
  - Rhinitis
  - Nasal congestion
  - Rhinorrhea
  - Sneezing
  - Sore throat
  - Cough
- Typically not 1 of these symptoms predominating

Physical Exam
The physical exam is usually normal.

TESTS
Lab
Laboratory evaluation is rarely necessary in the management of the URI.
- If a CBC is obtained the provider should be aware that a mild leukocytosis with a normal differential is normal in pregnancy.

Imaging
Although almost never necessary in the diagnosis and management of the common cold, a chest x-ray, sinus x-ray and/or CT scan of the sinuses can all be safely done in pregnancy in the rare circumstances that they will be clinically indicated.

DIFFERENTIAL DIAGNOSIS
- Acute sinusitis
  - This diagnosis should generally be reserved for those patients with URIs whose symptoms persist without improvement (or worsen) beyond 7 days who also have maxillary tooth or facial pain (particularly if unilateral), tenderness over the maxillary sinus, and/or purulent nasal secretions.
- Pharyngitis (viral or bacterial)
- Bronchitis
- Influenza
  - May be more common and more severe in pregnant patients
- Pneumonia
  - The absence of tachypnea, fever, and crackles on lung auscultation strongly suggest that pneumonia is not present in patients presenting with cough and sputum.
- Pregnancy rhinitis
  - Presents as nasal congestion with clear nasal discharge
  - Found in 22% of women in 3rd trimester
  - Usually requires no treatment but may be responsive to pseudoephedrine, nasal ipratropium, and/or nasal steroids.
- Allergic rhinitis

 TREATMENT

GENERAL MEASURES
- The common cold is self-limited and does not require treatment.
- Treatment is for management of symptoms only and patients should be clearly informed that medication will not affect the course or duration of the illness.
- Treatment, other than the use of antipyretics to bring down significant fever, is not likely to confer any benefit to embryo or fetus.
- Only those agents with a strong track record of safety in pregnancy should therefore be used for this indication in pregnancy.
- Maternal fever should be treated with cooling and acetaminophen because of the remote possibility that maternal pyrexia in the first trimester may increase the risk of congenital anomalies.

- Rest and fluids are routinely recommended for all patients suffering from the common cold.

ALERT
Avoid unnecessary and/or ineffective cold remedies in pregnancy.

Diet
No role for diet has been proven for the management of the common cold in or out of pregnancy.

Complementary and Alternative Medicine
No alternative or complementary medications have been shown to affect outcomes related to the common cold.
- Echinacea
  - Limited data suggests may be "safe" in pregnancy, but the nonpregnant data suggests it is ineffective.
- Vitamin C
  - Supraphysiologic doses of have been associated with neonatal scurvy in case reports and should be avoided.
  - Possibility of such effects cautions against use of supraphysiologic doses of any nutritional supplement in pregnancy.
- Zinc
  - Similarly, excess in pregnancy may increase the risk of congenital anomalies.

 MEDICATION (DRUGS)

First Line
- Antibiotics
  - Despite their widespread use and individual patients' strongly stated preferences, no study has shown any benefit of treatment with antibiotics for uncomplicated upper respiratory tract infections. This is true even if the nasal discharge is purulent.
- The following agents are all generally considered to be justifiable for the symptomatic treatment of the common cold in pregnancy for those patients who feel medication is necessary:
  - Acetaminophen 325–1000 mg every 4–6 hours to a maximum of 3000 mg/day.
  - Pseudoephedrine
    - Probably safe throughout pregnancy but some experts suggest avoidance in 1st trimester
  - Chlorpheniramine and Diphenhydramine
    - Avoid in setting of preterm labor
  - Ipratropium 0.06% nasal spray 2 sprays each nostril 3 or 4 times daily
  - Cromolyn powder/spray intranasally q2h during day on days 1 and 2 and then q.i.d. on days 3–7
  - Short term use of dextromethorphan, codeine, hydrocodone
- The following common cold treatments have limited or concerning human pregnancy data and should be avoided for this indication in pregnancy:
  - NSAIDs and ASA
  - Ephedrine
  - Phenylephrine
- Although commonly used, human data about safety of newer antihistamines cetirizine, fexofenadine, and loratadine (and their limited efficacy for the common cold) make their use for this indication in pregnancy inappropriate.
- Guaifenesin
  - Use in pregnancy is probably justifiable
  - Some experts avoid its use in the 1st trimester because of possible increased incidence of inguinal hernias in one study.

 FOLLOW-UP

DISPOSITION
Breastfeeding
- Patients with the common cold who are nursing should be encouraged to breastfeed as breast milk may help confer some passive immunity to their baby.
- Symptomatic treatment of common cold symptoms during breast feeding can be done with:
  - Acetaminophen
  - Cromolyn sodium powder/spray
  - Nasal ipratropium
  - Antihistamines, such as loratadine and fexofenadine (both approved by the American Academy of Pediatricians [AAP]), and probably cetirizine and diphenhydramine (although these may cause infant drowsiness)
  - Pseudoephedrine (approved by AAP although some data suggests it but may decrease or even "dry up" breast milk production)
  - Dextromethorphan, codeine, and guaifenesin (although the lack of efficacy of the latter agent makes its use not advisable despite its probable safety)
  - Ibuprofen
  - Phenylephrine (limited data but probably safe)
- Agents which should be avoided because of either concerning or limited data with respect to breast feeding safety include:
  - ASA
  - Ephedrine

Admission Criteria
The common cold is almost universally managed as an outpatient.

Issues for Referral
Common cold symptoms persisting beyond 2 weeks may require a referral to an otolaryngologist if the etiology does not become clear after careful consideration of the full differential diagnosis.

PROGNOSIS
Symptoms generally resolve within 7–10 days of onset. Again, a longer course warrants consideration of the full differential diagnosis.

COMPLICATIONS
- URIs are responsible for up to 40% of asthma exacerbations.
- URIs are complicated by acute bacterial sinusitis in up to 2.5% of cases.
  - Acute sinusitis may be more likely to complicate the common cold in pregnancy due to pregnancy related hyperemia and congestion of the upper airway.

REFERENCES

1. Briggs GG, Freeman RK, Yaffe SJ. Drugs in Pregnancy and Lactation: A Reference Guide to Fetal and Neonatal Risk 6th ed. Philadelphia: Lippincott Williams & Wilkins; 2002.
2. Gilbert C, Mazzotta P, Loebstein R, et al. Fetal safety of drugs used in the treatment of allergic rhinitis: A critical review. *Drug Saf*. 2005;28(8):707–719.
3. Powrie RO. Drugs in pregnancy: Respiratory disease. *Best Pract Res Clin Obstet Gynaecol*. 2001;15(6):913–936.
4. REPROTOX [database online]. Reproductive Toxicology Center, Columbia Hospital for Women Medical Center, Washington DC. Accessed February 26, 2006.
5. TW Hale. Medications and Mother's Milk, 10th ed. Amarillo, Texas: Pharmasoft Medical Publishing; 2002.

ADDITIONAL READING

Incaudo GA. Diagnosis and treatment of allergic rhinitis and sinusitis during pregnancy and lactation. *Clin Rev Allergy Immunol*. 2004 ;27(2):159–177.

Smith MB, Feldman W. Over-the-counter cold medications. A critical review of clinical trials between 1950 and 1991. *JAMA*. 1993;269:2258.

CODES
ICD9-CM
- 460 Acute nasopharyngitis (common cold)
- 461 Acute sinusitis
- 466 Acute bronchitis
- 472.0 Chronic rhinitis
- 477.0–477.9 Allergic rhinitis

KEY WORDS

- Upper Respiratory Infections
- Common Cold
- Bronchitis
- Sinusitis
- Pregnancy

PREGNANCY, TUBERCULOSIS

Elvis Pagan, MD
Ghada Bourjeily, MD
Iris L. Tong, MD

KEY CLINICAL POINTS

- Active, untreated tuberculosis (TB) may cause adverse fetal outcomes and, therefore, should be treated during pregnancy.
- Latent TB should be treated in pregnant women with high risk of reactivation
  - Treatment of latent TB can be deferred until after pregnancy in lower risk patients
- Anti-tuberculous drugs do not appear to adversely affect the fetus.
  - Pyrazinamide, however, is not often used in pregnancy because of limited safety data.
- There may be an increased risk of TB drug-induced hepatoxicity in pregnancy.
  - LFTs should be monitored with treatment.

 BASICS

DESCRIPTION

- Tuberculosis is a contagious disease caused by *Mycobacterium tuberculosis*. Typically, disease is manifested in the lungs.
- Primary TB infection:
  - Recent exposure to organism that progresses to clinical disease.
  - Approximately 20% of inoculated individuals will develop primary TB.
- Latent TB infection (LTBI):
  - Exposure to TB without clinical illness, but inactive TB organisms persist in the body.
  - Patients will have positive tuberculin skin test with CXR that is negative for active disease.
  - Patients are asymptomatic, but have a 10–15% lifetime risk of progression to clinical disease, or "reactivation", if not treated.
- Reactivation TB:
  - LTBI which progresses to clinical disease
  - May occur months to years after initial infection
- Pleural TB:
  - Occurs as a result of delayed hypersensitivity to the tuberculous bacilli.
  - Usually presents as an acute febrile illness
  - Should be differentiated from tuberculous empyema characterized by purulent fluid and a high load of tuberculous bacilli.
- Extrapulmonary TB
  - 20% of all cases of TB in small study on pregnant patients in Chandigarh, India
  - Most often involves (in order of decreasing frequency): Genitourinary system, lymph nodes, skeletal system, CNS, pericardium

GENERAL PREVENTION
Proper precautions when in contact with active TB patients

EPIDEMIOLOGY
- Predominance: Female = Male
- Rates vary by race:

- Highest rates are in Asians and Pacific Islanders.
- Among foreign born, non-Hispanic blacks had the highest rate in 2003
- 10× more likely in Asians, Pacific Islanders
- 8× more likely in non-Hispanic blacks
- 5× more likely in Hispanics, Native Americans

Incidence
- Number of cases per year declining in the United States:
- Incidence now at 5 new cases/100,000
  - The number of cases of TB among those born in the United States is declining.
  - The number of cases among the foreign-born population is unchanged.
- New cases largely due to Asian immigrants, as Asian countries, particularly China and India, have the highest incidence worldwide.

Prevalence
In the United States, 15 million people are estimated to be currently infected with TB.

RISK FACTORS
- Environment
  - Foreign-born
  - Homeless
  - Correctional institute
  - Health care workers
- Immunocompromised
  - HIV is the greatest known risk factor
  - Diabetes
  - Organ transplant patients
  - Immunosuppressive agents (steroids, chemotherapeutic drugs, TNF inhibitors)
  - Malignancy
  - Chronic renal failure
  - Low body weight
  - Intestinal bypass or gastrectomy
  - Intravenous (IV) drug use or alcoholism
- Pregnancy does not appear to be a risk factor.
- The CDC recommends screening all patients with any identifiable risk factor with Tuberculin skin testing on a yearly basis.

PATHOPHYSIOLOGY
Tuberculosis is predominantly acquired by inhaling airborne droplets from an infected individual who has expelled the organism by coughing, sneezing, talking, or singing.

ETIOLOGY
Infection is caused by the organism *Mycobacterium tuberculosis*. Defining characteristics of this bacterium include:
- Acid fast bacillus (AFB)
- Aerobic
- Slow growing

ASSOCIATED CONDITIONS
- HIV
- Immunosuppression

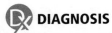 **DIAGNOSIS**

SIGNS AND SYMPTOMS
History
- Primary TB
  - Often asymptomatic
  - Fever most common symptom
  - Pleuritic chest pain
  - Cough
  - Fatigue
  - Arthralgias
  - Pharyngitis
- Reactivation TB
  - Usually begins insidiously
  - Cough ($1/2$–$2/3$), initially nonproductive
  - Fever ($1/2$)
  - Night sweats ($1/2$)
  - Chest pain ($1/3$)
  - Dyspnea ($1/3$)
  - Hemoptysis (less than $1/4$)

Physical Exam
- Fever
- Rales on lung exam
- Adenopathy
- Bone tenderness
- Abdominal tenderness
- Meningeal signs or altered mental status

TESTS
Tuberculin skin testing with purified protein derivative (PPD)
- >5 mm induration, considered positive if:
  - HIV-positive
  - Recent contact with active TB patients
  - Fibrotic changes on chest radiographs consistent with prior TB
- >10 mm induration, considered positive if:
- Organ transplants/other immunosuppression receiving the equivalent of 15 mg/day of prednisone for ≥ 1 month
  - Foreign-born
  - Homeless
  - Correctional institute
  - Health care workers
  - Diabetes
  - Organ transplant patients
  - Other immunosuppressive agents
  - Malignancy
  - Chronic renal failure
  - Low body weight
  - Intestinal bypass or gastrectomy
  - IV drug use or alcoholism
- >15 mm induration, positive if no risk factors

ALERT
Bacille calmette guerin (BCG) vaccination
- BCG is usually given in endemic areas to prevent disseminated TB in children.
- Receiving BCG in the past is a marker for prior inhabitance of an endemic area.
- Does not affect PPD testing and, thus, does not change criteria for positive PPD
- Positive PPD readings in patients who have received BCG are TRUE positives.

- Diagnosing active TB may be based on clinical response to therapy. A microscopic diagnosis is preferable:
  - Micro smear and culture
  - Nucleic acid amplification assays
  - PPD not helpful in diagnosing active disease

Lab
- Abnormal lab findings may include:
  - Anemia
  - Leukocytosis or leukopenia
  - Hyponatremia (SIADH)
  - Hypoalbuminemia
- For lung disease
  - Sputum sample for AFB and culture
    - Also necessary to determine infectivity
    - Expectorated sputum preferred
    - Highest yield is on morning sputum
    - 3 samples on separate days still recommended, although some studies suggest 2 will detect 95% of the cases.
    - Induced sputum may be necessary if unable to obtain an expectorated sputum sample
  - Bronchoscopy
    - Does not offer significant increase in sensitivity with smear or culture versus induced sputum
    - May be helpful to identify alternate diagnoses

Imaging
- Chest X-ray findings in Primary TB
  - Hilar adenopathy (65%)
  - Pleural effusion (33%)
  - Pulmonary infiltrates (25%)
    - Usually in lower lobes
    - Right sided lung disease more common
- Chest X-ray finding in reactivation TB
  - Typically apical involvement
  - Infiltrates may also be found in superior segments of lower lobes
  - Cavities (20% +)
  - Atypical presentation (20%)
    - Hilar adenopathy
    - Infiltrates in lower lung zones
    - Pleural effusions
    - Solitary nodules

Diagnostic Procedures/Surgery
- For lymphadenopathy
  - Fine needle aspiration
  - Lymph node biopsy
- For suspected meningitis
  - Lumbar puncture

Pathologic Findings
Caseating granulomas on histology

DIFFERENTIAL DIAGNOSIS
- Pulmonary TB: Pneumonia (bacterial or fungal), sarcoid, malignancy

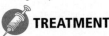 **TREATMENT**

GENERAL MEASURES
- Isolation of infectious patients
  - Patients should be considered infectious if:
    - Coughing
    - Undergoing cough-inducing procedures
    - Sputum smears positive for AFB
    - CXR findings suggestive of active disease

- Not receiving therapy
- Just started therapy (<2 weeks)
- Poor clinical response to therapy
- Patients no longer considered infectious when
  - On adequate treatment
  - Significant clinical response to therapy
  - 3 consecutive negative sputum smears
- Patients with extrapulmonary TB are usually not at risk for infecting others.

 MEDICATION (DRUGS)

First Line
- Latent TB infection
  - Isoniazid (INH): 300 mg every day × 9 months with pyridoxine 50 mg every day to decrease the risk of neuropathy associated with INH
  - Pregnant women at high risk for reactivation should be treated, even in the first trimester.
    - High risk for reactivation: HIV, DM, immunosuppression, close contact with active TB patients, and recent converters
  - For lower risk patients, can defer treatment 3–6 months after pregnancy to avoid risk of hepatoxicity from INH
- Active pulmonary or extrapulmonary TB
  - In general, treatment should include a 4-drug regimen initially with or without directly observed therapy (DOT) for 6 months depending on regional drug sensitivity.
  - Regimen options for nonpregnant populations (all for total of 26 weeks):
    - Daily INH, rifampin (RIF), ethambutol (EMB) or streptomycin (SM), and pyrazinamide (PZA) for 8 weeks, then INH and RIF for 18 weeks
  - Can be given daily or 3×/week DOT
    - Daily INH, RIF, EMB or SM, and PZA × 2 weeks, then 2×/week × 6 weeks (DOT), then INH and RIF 2×/week (DOT) × 18 weeks
    - INH, RIF, EMB or SM, and PZA 3×/week (DOT) × 26 weeks
  - Regimen for pregnant patients
    - Duration of treatment extended to 9 months
    - Daily INH, RIF, and EMB for 8 weeks then INH/RIF daily OR biweekly for 7 months
    - Regimen excludes PZA because of lack of safety data in pregnancy. No teratogenicity due to PZA, however, has been identified. PZA may be necessary in HIV + or in areas with high rates of multidrug resistant TB.

 FOLLOW-UP

DISPOSITION
- No suggestion that TB complicates the course of pregnancy or delivery
- The fetus may be at risk if maternal disease is active and untreated.
- Increased incidence of fetal complications have been suggested in some studies:
  - Prematurity
  - Small-for gestational age
  - Miscarriages
  - Preeclampsia

Issues for Referral
Given complexity of treating TB in pregnancy, referral to a specialist experienced in treating TB is necessary.

PROGNOSIS
Multiple studies demonstrate that with appropriate TB treatment, the prognosis is the same in nonpregnant and pregnant women.

COMPLICATIONS
- Reactivation of Latent TB infection
  - HIV-seronegative: 10–15% lifetime risk
  - HIV-seropositive: 7–10% annual risk
- Congenital TB
  - Rare (329 cases reported worldwide)
  - High mortality
  - Predominantly seen in women with miliary TB, or with involvement of the endometrium or placenta
  - Patients with active disease, particularly if extrapulmonary, should have the placenta evaluated for *Mycobacterium Tuberculosis*.
- Neonatal TB
  - Acquisition by neonate is possible particularly if mother has active disease at time of delivery
  - A period of separation from mother is recommended if mother is infectious
  - INH prophylaxis is considered in neonates of mothers with active disease
- INH Hepatitis
  - Occurs in 0.1–1% of patients taking INH
  - Mild INH toxicity (AST<100 and asymptomatic) occurs in 10–20% of patients
  - INH hepatitis is typically symptomatic: Nausea, vomiting, anorexia, abdominal pain, jaundice, malaise
  - INH is continued unless patient with symptomatic hepatitis or AST >5X ULN
  - A retrospective study demonstrated that pregnant women are 4× more likely to develop INH hepatitis than nonpregnant women.

ALERT
Breast-feeding
- Patients with active, untreated TB should not breast-feed.
- All anti-TB medications are considered safe in breast-feeding.
- If a mother is on INH, she should continue taking pyridoxine 50 mg PO every day.
- Conservative groups recommend neonatal screening for hepatitis and neuropathy while the mother is on these medications.

PATIENT MONITORING
- Based on limited data, there is a concern that pregnant patients are more likely to develop severe TB drug-induced hepatitis.
- Check LFTs monthly during pregnancy and several months postpartum while the patient is on medications.

REFERENCES

1. Brodie D, Schluger NW. The diagnosis of tuberculosis. *Clin Chest Med*. 2005;26:246–271.
2. Division of Tuberculosis Elimination. Tuberculosis and Pregnancy, Center for Disease Control Fact Sheet, April 2005.
3. Franks AL, Binkin NJ, Snider DE Jr, et al. Isoniazid hepatitis among pregnancy and postpartum Hispanic patients. *Public Health Rep*. 1989;104(2):151–155.
4. Jana N, Vasishta K, Saha SC, et al. Obstetrical outcomes among women with extrapulmonary tuberculosis. *N Engl J Med*. 1999;341(9):645–649.
5. Laibl VR, Sheffield JS. Tuberculosis in pregnancy. *Clin Perinatol*. 2005;32(3):239–747.

6. MMWR Morbidity and Mortality Weekly Report. 2006;55(11):305–308.

7. Schneider E, Moore M, Castro KG. Epidemiology of tuberculosis in the United States. *Clin Chest Med*. 2005;26(2):183–195.

8. Smith KC. Congential tuberculosis: A rare manifestation of a common infection. *Curr Opin Infect Dis*. 2002;15(3):269–274.

CODES
ICD9-CM
- 011.9 Pulmonary tuberculosis, unspecified
- 771.2 Congenital tuberculosis
- 795.5 Positive PPD

KEY WORDS
- Pregnancy
- Tuberculosis
- Latent TB Infection
- PPD

PREGNANCY, VAGINAL BLEEDING

Michael P. Plevyak, MD
Sudeep K. Aulakh, MD

KEY CLINICAL POINTS

- 1st trimester bleeding:
  - Complicates at least 20% of pregnancies
  - Bleeding not always followed by spontaneous abortion (SAB) but has increased risk of SAB
  - <10% with vaginal bleeding and fetal heart activity abort
- Late 2nd or 3rd trimester bleeding
  - Seen in 3–4% of pregnancies
  - Most common cause is placental abruption or placenta previa
  - Bleeding may be life threatening

 BASICS

DESCRIPTION

- 1st trimester bleeding
  - Caused by
    - Implantation bleed
    - Spontaneous abortion (SAB)
    - Ectopic pregnancy (EP)
    - Molar pregnancy
    - Genital tract pathology
  - Bleeding not always followed by SAB
    - <10% with vaginal bleeding and fetal heart activity abort
  - Increased risk of SAB, preterm delivery, placental abruption, fetal growth restriction, and preterm membrane rupture (if heavy)
- Spontaneous abortion is the loss of an intrauterine pregnancy (IUP) before 20 weeks
  - Threatened abortion: Vaginal bleeding with a closed cervix, +/– cramping
  - Inevitable abortion: Heavier bleeding with cramping and dilated cervix
  - Incomplete abortion: Passage of some but not all of the pregnancy through the cervix
  - Complete abortion: Expulsion of entire uterine contents
  - Missed abortion: Embryonic death with retention of pregnancy, +/– bleeding
  - Septic abortion: Infection usually following induced abortion or procedure (e.g., amniocentesis); also with incomplete abortion
- Ectopic pregnancy: Implantation at a site other than the uterine cavity (>95% in fallopian tube)
- Late 2nd or 3rd trimester bleeding
- Placental abruption:
  - Premature separation of placenta
  - Associated with contractions and tender uterus
- Placenta previa:
  - Placental tissue lying near or covering os
  - Painless bleeding
- Most common cause is placental abruption or placenta previa
- Uncommon causes: Uterine rupture, vasa previa, genital laceration, genital cancer, bleeding disorder
- Bleeding may be life threatening

Incidence

- 1st trimester bleeding: Occurring in at least 20% of pregnancies
  - Spontaneous abortion:
    - 10–15% of recognized pregnancies
    - 80% occur by 12 weeks
  - Ectopic pregnancy: 19/1000 pregnancies

- Late 2nd or 3rd trimester bleeding:
  - seen in 3–4% of pregnancies
  - Placental abruption: 8/1000 births
  - Placenta previa: 5/1000 births

RISK FACTORS

- Spontaneous abortion: Advancing maternal age, prior miscarriage, tobacco or alcohol use, moderate/high caffeine consumption
- Ectopic pregnancy: Prior tubal surgery, prior ectopic pregnancy, tubal pathology, in utero DES exposure, prior genital infections, multiple sexual partners, infertility, intrauterine device, tobacco use
- Placental abruption: Trauma, prior abruption, thrombophilia, hypertension, multiple gestation, increasing parity, rapid uterine decompression, tobacco, cocaine use, preterm membrane rupture
- Placenta previa: Maternal age, increasing parity, multiple gestation, prior cesarean deliveries (CD) and curettages, tobacco use

ETIOLOGY

- Spontaneous abortion:
  - 1/3 are anembryonic at <8 weeks
  - Chromosomal abnormalities comprise ~50%
  - Also: Uterine anomaly, maternal infection or endocrinopathy, teratogens, thrombophilia, diagnostic procedures, autoimmune disease
- Ectopic pregnancy:
  - 90% result from impaired tubal function, particularly chronic salpingitis
  - Nearly 10% have Salpingitis isthmica nodosa
    - Consists of ≥1 diverticula of tubal epithelium in isthmic region of fallopian tube
- Placental abruption:
  - Majority due to chronic vascular pathology at maternal-fetal interface with placental separation the end-stage event
  - Trauma, cocaine use, or rapid decompression cause minority
- Placenta previa:
  - Increased placental surface area, reduced oxygen delivery, or endometrial scarring promote placental implantation over os

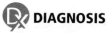 **DIAGNOSIS**

SIGNS AND SYMPTOMS

- Spontaneous abortion:
  - Amenorrhea followed by vaginal bleeding and variable low midline abdominal pain
- Ectopic pregnancy:
  - Amenorrhea followed by vaginal bleeding and abdominal pain
  - Pain: Often unilateral, may radiate to shoulder
  - Lightheadedness or shock if ruptured ectopic
  - 50% asymptomatic before tubal rupture
- Placental abruption:
  - Majority with vaginal bleeding and abdominal pain, may have uterine contractions (often frequent, prolonged or tetanic)
  - Bleeding absent in 20% (concealed abruption)
  - Chronic/persistent bleeding +/– pain is common

- Placenta previa:
  - Painless vaginal bleeding in 70–80%
  - Bleeding with contractions in 10–20%
  - Incidental diagnosis or asymptomatic in 10%

Physical Exam
- Spontaneous abortion:
  - Enlarged uterus, abdominal tenderness
  - No vaginal/cervical lesion or trauma
  - Cervix may be opened or closed
- Ectopic pregnancy:
  - Abdominal, cervical, or adnexal tenderness
  - Pelvic mass, enlarged uterus
  - Orthostatic changes
- Placental abruption:
  - Enlarged, tender and/or rigid uterus
  - Absence of vaginal/cervical pathology
- Placenta previa:
  - Enlarged, nontender uterus
  - Absence of vaginal/cervical pathology

TESTS
Lab
- 1st trimester bleeding:
  - Single serum β-HCG level:
    - Confirms pregnancy
    - Does not separate normal from abnormal pregnancy
    - Useful if above 1500–2000 IU/L as gestational sac seen at these levels with transvaginal ultrasound (TVUS)
  - Serial quantitative serum β-HCG:
    - Normal pregnancy: Level doubles every 2 days
    - An increase of $\leq$50% in a 48-hour period is associated with a nonviable pregnancy
    - Spontaneous abortion: Prolonged doubling time or decreasing levels
    - Ectopic pregnancy: Prolonged doubling time; rarely with β-HCG >50,000 IU/L
  - Other tests (e.g., progesterone) less useful
- Late–2nd or 3rd trimester bleeding:
  - Serum/ urine β-HCG to confirm pregnancy
  - Complete blood count
  - Coagulation studies if suspect abruption
    - Fibrinogen <200 mg/dL and platelets <100,000/μL with severe abruption

Imaging
Ultrasound (US) is critical in determining cause of vaginal bleeding in any trimester
- 1st trimester TVUS:
  - Normal intrauterine pregnancy (IUP):
    - Gestational sac seen when β-HCG >1500–2000 IU/L or by 5 weeks gestation
    - Yolk sac seen by 5th week or mean gestational sac diameter (MSD) >8 mm
    - Fetal cardiac activity at 5.5–6 weeks and with crown-rump length (CRL) >5 mm
  - Spontaneous/missed abortion:
    - Absent yolk sac at MSD $\geq$8 mm
    - Absent fetal pole at MSD $\geq$16 mm
    - Absent fetal heart activity with CRL >5 mm
  - Ectopic pregnancy
    - If β-HCG <1500 and TVUS negative for IUP, then repeat both in 2–3 days.
    - If β-HCG does not double and TVUS still negative, non-viable pregnancy is present.

- Absence of IUP with β-HCG >1500–2000 IU/L highly suggestive, especially if complex adnexal mass also present
- Extrauterine gestational sac is diagnostic but seen in <50% of cases
- Fluid in cul de sac not specific; also seen with ruptured/hemorrhagic ovarian cyst
- 2nd/3rd trimester abdominal/TV US:
  - Placental abruption
    - Detects ~50% of cases
    - Primarily used to rule out placenta previa
  - Placenta previa
    - Seen in 5–15% of second trimester scans with >90% resolving by 37 weeks
    - TVUS is gold standard for diagnosis
    - Safe and detects over 99% of cases

Diagnostic Procedures/Surgery
- 1st trimester bleeding
  - Serial serum β-HCG and US usually diagnostic
  - Uterine dilation and curettage (D + C):
    - Presence of chorionic villi excludes EP
    - Limited diagnostic tool: high false negative rate (20%); may disrupt normal pregnancy
    - If β-HCG level does not decline by 15% 8–12 hours after curettage, then suspect EP
  - Laparoscopy is rarely required to diagnose EP
- Late 2nd or 3rd trimester bleeding
  - Rarely need more than history, physical and US to make diagnosis
  - Biopsy suspicious lesions

DIFFERENTIAL DIAGNOSIS
- 1st trimester bleeding
  - Physiologic/implantation bleeding
  - Spontaneous abortion
  - Ectopic pregnancy
  - Gestational trophoblastic disease
  - Genital tract trauma, neoplasm, or infection
- Late 2nd or 3rd trimester bleeding
  - Labor
  - Placental abruption
  - Placenta previa
  - Vasa previa
  - Genital tract trauma, neoplasm or infection
  - Bleeding disorder
  - Uterine rupture

 TREATMENT

PRE-HOSPITAL
If bleeding is profuse, may need to alert:
- Blood bank
- Operating room and anesthesia (D&C, CD)
- Labor and delivery for fetal monitoring
- ICU if hypovolemic shock, coagulopathy

INITIAL STABILIZATION
- With mild bleeding:
  - Obtain IV access and US
  - Continuously monitor fetus if beyond 23 weeks
- With profuse bleeding:
  - Monitor vital signs, urine output and blood loss
  - Establish large bore IV × 2
  - Consider red blood cell transfusion or crystalloid infusion to maintain blood pressure and urine output

– Platelets, cryoprecipitate and/or fresh frozen plasma for abruption complicated by DIC
– CBC, coagulation profile, β-HCG level
– Continuously monitor fetus if beyond 23 weeks

GENERAL MEASURES

- 1st trimester bleeding:
  – Spontaneous abortion: Unless abortion is inevitable or bleeding is profuse, expectant management is recommended until
    • Symptoms resolve
    • Nonviable pregnancy is diagnosed or
    • Patient progresses to inevitable abortion
  – Expectant management of missed, inevitable, or incomplete abortion successful in about 80%, but may take $\geq$2 weeks
  – Antibiotics and prompt uterine evacuation for septic abortion
- Ectopic pregnancy: Expectant management, medical or surgical therapy (See Ectopic Pregnancy chapter)
- Late-2nd or 3rd trimester bleeding: Assess degree of bleeding, fetal gestational age, and status
  – Delivery is generally indicated for persistent profuse bleeding regardless of gestational age or for compromised maternal/fetal status
  – Conservative management successful in most
  – Antenatal corticosteroids for fetal lung maturation between 24–34 weeks gestation
  – Tocolytics if maternal/fetal status is stable

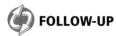

MEDICATION (DRUGS)

- Spontaneous abortion (missed or inevitable):
  – Misoprostol (not FDA approved): 600–800 mcg per vagina, repeated in 24 hours if necessary, successful in 70–90%
  – Doxycycline 100 mg PO q12h × 2 doses lowers rate of postprocedure infection
- Ectopic pregnancy (see Ectopic Pregnancy)
- Anti-D Immune globulin, 300 mcg IM, in any trimester if bleeding, Rh negative, and unsensitized

SURGERY

- Spontaneous abortion:
  – D + C for profuse bleeding, septic abortion, definitive treatment
- Ectopic pregnancy: Surgery indicated for:
  – Ruptured ectopic pregnancy, especially if hemodynamically unstable
  – Cannot comply with medical therapy posttreatment monitoring
  – Desires definitive therapy
  – High risk for medical therapy failure
- Placental abruption:
  – CD for profuse bleeding or nonreassuring fetal status
  – Vaginal delivery is possible and preferable with coagulopathy, especially with fetal demise
- Placenta previa: CD is only option for delivery

FOLLOW-UP

Issues for Referral
Refer to Ob-Gyn for any bleeding in pregnancy

COMPLICATIONS

- Spontaneous abortion
  – Septic abortion comprises 1–2% of obstetric cases of sepsis
- Ectopic pregnancy
  – Leading cause of maternal death in first trimester ($\sim$10% of cases)
  – Decreased live birth rate ($\sim$50%) after EP
- Placental abruption
  – Fetal demise seen in up to 15% of abruptions
  – Coagulopathy in 10–20% with fetal demise
  – Increased rate of fetal growth restriction and prematurity
- Placenta previa
  – Maternal mortality is <1%
  – Perinatal mortality <10% (mostly from prematurity)
  – Placenta accreta in 5% without prior CD; 25% with 1 prior CD and $\sim$50% with $\geq$2 prior CD
    • Cesarean hysterectomy in $\sim$2/3 patients
- Recurrence rate
  – Spontaneous abortion
    • 14–21% after 1 prior SAB, 24–29% after 2 SAB, and 31–33% after 3
    • Prior live birth decreases recurrence risk
  – Ectopic pregnancy
    • 15% after 1 EP, 30% after 2
    • Rates comparable after medical or surgical management
  – Placental abruption
    • 5–15% after 1 abruption, 25% after 2
    • Second abruption with fetal demise in 7%
  – Placenta previa: 4–8%

REFERENCES

1. Clark SL. Placenta previa and abruptio placentae. In: Creasy RK, Resnik R, Iams JD, ed. Maternal-Fetal Medicine: Principles and Practice, 5th ed. Philadelphia: Saunders; 2004:707–722.
2. Coppola PT, Coppola M. Vaginal bleeding in the first 20 weeks of pregnancy. *Emerg Med Clin North Am.* 2003;21:667–677.
3. Dogra V, Paspulati RM, Bhatt S. First trimester bleeding evaluation. *Ultrasound Q.* 2005;21:69–85.
4. Simpson JL. Fetal wastage. In: Gabbe SG, Niebyl JR, Simpson JL, ed. Obstetrics: Normal and Problem Pregnancies, 4th ed. Philadelphia: Churchill Livingstone; 2002;729–753.
5. Tulandi T, Sammour A. Evidence-based management of ectopic pregnancy. *Curr Opin Obstet Gynecol.* 2000;12:289–292.

CODES
ICD9-CM
- 634.0 Spontaneous abortion
- 633.0 Ectopic pregnancy
- 641.2 Premature separation of placenta
- 641.1 Placenta previa

KEY WORDS

- Pregnancy
- Vaginal Bleeding
- Antenatal Hemorrhage
- Miscarriage
- Pregnancy Loss
- Abruptio Placentae
- Placenta Accreta

PREGNANCY, VENOUS THROMBOEMBOLISM

Margaret A. Miller, MD

KEY CLINICAL POINTS

- Pregnancy is associated with an increased risk of thrombosis.
- Pulmonary embolism is the leading cause of maternal mortality in the United States.
- Pregnant women should be aggressively investigated when they present with clinical symptoms that are suspicious for DVT or PE.
- Pregnant women at increased risk for DVT or PE should receive prophylactic anticoagulation throughout pregnancy.

 BASICS

EPIDEMIOLOGY
- Venous thromboembolism is up to 10 times more common in pregnancy.
- Thrombosis occurs with equal frequency in each trimester.
- Approximately 80–90% of DVT in pregnancy occurs in the left leg.
- The daily risk of thrombosis in the 6-week postpartum period is 4 times greater than during pregnancy.
- Unusual sites of thrombosis such as ovarian vein thrombosis, cerebral vein thrombosis, and subclavian vein thrombosis occur more frequently in pregnancy.

Incidence
- In antenatal period: 5–12 per 10,000
- Postpartum: 3–7 per 10,000

RISK FACTORS
- Established risk factors
  - Thrombophilia
  - Family history of thrombosis
  - Previous thromboembolism
  - Previous superficial phlebitis
  - Cesarean section
- Possible risk factors
  - Prolonged bed rest
  - Maternal age
  - Parity
  - Tobacco use
  - Preeclampsia

PATHOPHYSIOLOGY
Factors that contribute to the increased risk for thrombosis in pregnancy include:
- Stasis due to hormonal and mechanical factors
- Hypercoagulability due to increase in clotting factors and decrease in fibrinolysis
- Vascular damage caused by delivery contributes to increased risk postpartum

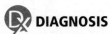 **DIAGNOSIS**

SIGNS AND SYMPTOMS
History
- DVT
  - Peripheral edema is common in pregnancy, but is usually symmetric.
  - Pt most often presents with lower extremity pain, swelling, and discoloration.
  - Majority of DVTs in pregnancy occur in the LLE

- Pelvic vein thrombosis may present with abdominal, flank or back pain, often in the setting of postpartum endometritis.
- Pulmonary embolism
  - Baseline HR increases by 10–20 bpm in normal pregnancy.
  - Respiratory rate is not increased in pregnancy. Although minute ventilation is increased leading to a respiratory alkalosis, this is achieved primarily through an increase in tidal volume and not respiratory rate.
  - Dyspnea and palpitations are common in normal pregnancy, tachypnea is not.
  - Chest pain and hemoptysis should alert clinician to possible pathology.
  - Young patients with no comorbid lung disease may present with only minor symptoms and normal appearing ABG in the presence of significant PE.

TESTS
Lab
- D-dimer levels change throughout normal gestation and the threshold for an abnormal result has not been clearly established in pregnancy. D-dimer should not be used exclusively to rule out PE.
- ABG results change in pregnancy.
  - PaO_2 is increased in pregnancy. Average PaO_2 is 100.
  - $PaCo_2$ is decreased to 28–32 in normal pregnancy.

Imaging
- Ultrasound
  - Imaging procedure of choice for suspected DVT in pregnancy
- Venograms
  - Gold standard for diagnosis of DVT
  - Consider risks (anaphylaxis, contrast-induced renal dysfunction, radiation exposure to fetus)
- MRI
  - May be needed if pelvic thrombosis suspected and ultrasound negative
- Ventilation/perfusion scan
  - Test of choice to rule out PE in pregnancy
  - Significantly fewer nondiagnostic results in pregnant population, perhaps because of lower incidence of underlying lung disease
- CT angiography
  - Not well validated in pregnancy
  - May be associated with significant radiation exposure to breast tissue
  - Use only if V/Q scan unavailable

Diagnostic Procedures/Surgery
Angiography
- Gold standard test for PE
- Necessary in patients with nondiagnostic V/Q scan and high clinical suspicion
- Brachial route associated with less radiation exposure than femoral route

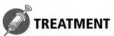 **TREATMENT**

Management of women on long-term anticoagulation in pregnancy
- Women on long-term anticoagulation should be counseled about the risks of teratogenicity associated with coumadin and appropriate birth control should be discussed.

- In women who desire pregnancy, warfarin should be switched to prophylactic doses UFH or LMWH as soon as birth control is discontinued.
- Warfarin is safe in breastfeeding and patients may be restarted on warfarin immediately after delivery

Treatment of Acute VTE in Pregnancy

- Adjusted dose LMWH throughout pregnancy OR
- IV heparin to maintain PTT in therapeutic range for 5 days followed by adjusted dose subcutaneous UFH or LMWH for the remainder of pregnancy
- Duration of treatment should be at least 6 months of full-dose anticoagulation.
- If patient still pregnant after 6 months full-dose treatment, subsequent treatment in pregnancy is controversial. At least prophylactic doses should be continued until 6 weeks postpartum, with some clinicians choosing to continue full-dose.
- Anticoagulation should be continued for 6 weeks postpartum.

Prevention of VTE in Pregnancy

- Approach to prevention of VTE in pregnancy varies with severity of risk
- Recommendations range from clinical surveillance in low risk patients to therapeutic dose unfractionated heparin (UFH) or low molecular weight heparin (LMWH) in high risk patients.
- Although data is limited, the following recommendations may be used to guide therapy:
- Recommend antepartum clinical surveillance with postpartum prophylactic UFH or LMWH
  - Single VTE associated with a transient risk factor, but consider prophylaxis
  - Thrombophilia with no history of VTE or poor obstetric outcome, but consider prophylaxis
    - Prophylactic dose UFH or LMWH
      - Recommend for:
    - Single idiopathic episode of VTE
    - Single VTE associated with a thrombophilia
  - Consider for:
    - No history of VTE, but history of antithrombin-3 deficiency, prothrombin gene heterozygosity/homozygosity, or factor V leiden
    - No history of VTE or poor obstetric outcome, but history of APA. Add low-dose aspirin (81 mg) in such patients
    - Single episode of VTE associated with transient risk if prior VTE in pregnancy or estrogen-related (OCPs) or if other significant risk factors (obesity, strong family history)
- Recommend therapeutic dose UFH or LMWH
  - Multiple episodes of VTE
  - Antiphospholipid antibody (APA) syndrome
  - Patients on long-term anticoagulation

Management of women with mechanical heart valves

- Anticoagulation must be continued throughout pregnancy to reduce risk of thrombosis and embolism.
- Data insufficient to make definitive recommendations
- Warfarin is associated with the lowest risk of thrombosis and systemic embolization, but can lead to embryopathy and neonatal hemorrhage.

Three options are reasonable:
- Adjusted dose LMWH
- Aggressive adjusted-dose UFH
- UFH or LMWH until the 13th week, change to warfarin until 32–36 weeks, then restart UFH or LMWH

Management of anticoagulation in labor and delivery

- For patients on full-dose anticoagulation, most obstetricians opt to schedule a planned induction or cesarean section.

Anticoagulation is stopped 24 hours prior to delivery and restarted 6–24 hours postpartum.

- If labor and delivery occurs within 1 month of acute thrombosis, IV heparin should be initiated and discontinued 4–6 hours prior to the anticipated delivery. In addition, consideration should be given to placement of a temporary IVC filter while the patient is off anticoagulation.
- For patients on prophylactic UFH, advise them to stop UFH 24 hours prior to planned delivery or at first sign of labor.
- Epidural or spinal anesthesia is contraindicated in women who have had a dose of LMWH within the prior 12–24 hours because of the risk of epidural hematoma.
- For this reason, consider changing LMWH to UFH at 36 weeks gestation to allow full options for pain management in labor.

 MEDICATION (DRUGS)

Dosing

- Prophylactic dose heparins
  - UFH: 5,000 sq b.i.d. in 1st trimester, 7,500 u sq b.i.d. in 2nd trimester, 10,000 u sq b.i.d. in 3rd trimester
  - LMWH: Enoxaparin 30 mg per day or b.i.d. in first trimester, 40 mg per day or b.i.d. after 28 weeks OR
  - Dalteparin: 5,000 u sq per day or b.i.d.
- Adjusted-dose heparins
  - UFH: Sq q12 hours to keep mid-interval PTT in therapeutic range
  - LMWH: Weight-adjusted full treatment doses; twice daily doses preferable as half-life is shorter in pregnancy
- Warfarin
  - For postpartum prophylaxis, adjust the dose to target INR of 2–3.
  - For mechanical heart valves, adjust the dose to target INR of 3–4.
- Aspirin
  - Prophylactic use in pregnancy = 81 mg per day

Maternal Complications

- Bleeding
  - Occurs in 2% of pregnant women treated with UFH, very uncommon with LMWH
- Heparin induced thrombocytopenia (HIT)
  - Incidence may be less in pregnant populations, but monitoring still required (see below).
- Osteoporosis
  - Long-term UFH therapy is associated with an increased risk of osteoporosis. The risk may be less with LMWH.

Fetal Complications

- Warfarin
  - Associated with congenital malformations, especially with exposure at 6–12 weeks gestation
  - May be associated with neurodevelopmental problems in children exposed in the 2nd or 3rd trimester
  - Cause anticoagulant effect in fetus, increasing risk of bleeding in the neonate at time of delivery
- UFH and LMWH
  - Neither drug crosses the placenta, so there is no potential for fetal teratogenicity or bleeding.
- Aspirin
  - Full-dose (325 mg) associated with birth defects and bleeding and should not be used in pregnancy
  - Low-dose (81 mg) safe in pregnancy

SURGERY

- Consider use of thrombolytics/thrombectomy in pregnant women with massive PE and hemodynamic instability
- Data is limited, but no reports of teratogenicity associated with thrombolytics
- Major risk in pregnancy is maternal hemorrhage

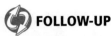 **FOLLOW-UP**

COMPLICATIONS

- Pregnant women with acute VTE have a high rate of subsequent post-thrombotic syndrome and chronic deep venous insufficiency.
- Use of graduated compression stockings may reduce this risk.

PATIENT MONITORING

- Clinical vigilance and aggressive investigation for symptoms suspicious for DVT or PE
- Platelet monitoring for patients on UFH or LMWH

REFERENCES

1. Bates S, Greer I, Hirsh J, et al. Use of antithrombotic agents during pregnancy. The seventh ACCP conference on antithrombotic and thrombolytic therapy. *Chest.* 2004;126:627S–644S.
2. Brill-Edwards P, Ginsberg JS, Gent M, et al. Safety of withholding heparin in pregnant women with a history of venous thromboembolism. Recurrence of Clot in this Pregnancy Study Group. *N Engl J Med.* 2000;343;1439–1444.
3. Chan WS, Ray JG, Murray S, et al. Suspected pulmonary embolism in pregnancy: clinical presentation, results of lung scanning, and subsequent maternal and pediatric outcomes. *Arch Intern Med.* 2002:162:1170–1175.
4. Ray JG, Chan WS. Deep vein thrombosis during pregnancy and the puerperium: A meta-analysis of the period of risk and the leg of presentation. *Obstet Gynecol Surv.* 1999;54:265–271.
5. Rodgers MA, Walker MC, Wells PS. Diagnosis and treatment of venous thromboembolism in pregnancy. *Best Pract Res Clin Haematol.* 2003;16:279–296.

ADDITIONAL READING

Lee R, Rosene-Montella K, Barbour L, Garner P, Keely E, eds. Medical Care of the Pregnant Patient. Philadelphia: ACP-ASIM; 2000.

CODES
ICD9-CM

- 671.9 Thrombosis pregnancy
- 671.3 Deep vein
- 671.2 Superficial vein
- 673.2 Pulmonary embolism in pregnancy

KEY WORDS

- Deep Venous Thrombosis (DVT)
- Lower Extremity Edema
- Hypercoagulable State
- Pulmonary Embolism

PREGNANCY, UTI

Lucia Larson, MD
Niharika Mehta, MD

KEY CLINICAL POINTS

- Physiologic changes in pregnancy predispose gravidas to asymptomatic bacteriuria, cystitis, and pyelonephritis.
- Asymptomatic bacteriuria (ASB)
- Affects approximately 5–10% of all pregnancies
- If untreated, is associated with pyelonephritis in 20–30% of women.
- Acute pyelonephritis or untreated UTI is associated with obstetric, maternal and neonatal complications.

 BASICS

DESCRIPTION
UTI in pregnancy can be categorized as
- Asymptomatic bacteriuria
- Defined as bacterial colonization of the urinary tract $>10^5$ bacteria/ml in the absence of symptoms
- Acute cystitis
- Acute pyelonephritis

GENERAL PREVENTION
- The Infectious Disease Society of America recommends universal screening for bacteriuria in pregnant women.
    - Obtain urine culture at least once in early pregnancy.

EPIDEMIOLOGY
Incidence
- Bacterial infections of the urine can occur in 17–20% of pregnancies.
- Untreated ASB is associated with pyelonephritis in 20–30% pregnant women.

RISK FACTORS
- UTI before pregnancy
- Sexual intercourse
- Increasing age and parity
- Lower socioeconomic class
- Sickle cell hemoglobinopathy
- Diabetes mellitus
- Urinary tract malformations
- AIDS
- Steroid therapy

PATHOPHYSIOLOGY
- The normal physiological changes in pregnancy predispose gravid women to urinary tract infections.
    - Changes in the urinary collecting system lead to urinary stasis.
        - Progesterone induces smooth muscle dilatation in the ureters.
        - There is ureteral compression from the gravid uterus or iliac vessels.
    - Changes in urine composition result in a desirable culture medium for pathogens.
        - Aminoaciduria
        - Glycosuria
        - pH changes

ETIOLOGY
- *Escherichia coli* is the causative organism in 70–90% cases but any organism of the GI/GU track may be identified.

- *Klebsiella pneumoniae* and *Proteus* species may play a role in recurrent infection.
- When group B streptococci cause UTI, it is associated with vaginal colonization and increased risk for neonatal infection.

ASSOCIATED CONDITIONS
Pregnant women with UTI may have associated
- Preterm labor
- Pulmonary edema occurs in up to 8% pregnant women with pyelonephritis
- More common in women with preterm labor who are on a β-agonist for tocolysis

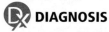 DIAGNOSIS

SIGNS AND SYMPTOMS
Diagnosis of symptomatic UTI is usually clinical.

History
- Symptoms of cystitis:
    - Frequency
    - Urgency
    - Dysuria
    - Hematuria
    - Lower abdominal pain
    - Absence of systemic illness
    - Preterm labor
- Symptoms of pyelonephritis:
    - Flank pain
    - Fever
    - Shaking chills
    - Nausea
    - Vomiting
    - Less often, features of cystitis
    - Preterm labor

Physical Exam
- ASB
    - Normal physical exam
- Cystitis
    - Absence of fever
    - Suprapubic tenderness
- Pyelonephritis
    - Costovertebral angle tenderness
    - Abdominal tenderness
    - Fever
    - Hypotension

TESTS
Lab
- For ASB and cystitis
    - Pyuria on urinalysis
    - Positive urine culture
- For Pyelonephritis
    - Pyuria on urinalysis
    - Positive urine culture
    - CBC
        - Leukocytosis
        - Anemia
        - Thrombocytopenia
    - Chemistry
        - Elevated creatinine (Normal for pregnancy 0.5–0.8 mg/dl)

- Hypokalemia
- Elevated LDH (secondary to endotoxin mediated hemolysis)
  - Blood cultures
    - Pathogens isolated from blood rarely differ from those in corresponding urine but may be helpful.
    - Obtain blood cultures if complicated by sepsis, respiratory distress or temperature of at least 39°C.
    - Positive blood cultures require 2 weeks of IV antibiotic treatment

Imaging
- Renal ultrasound:
  - Obtain only if unresponsive to initial treatment
  - US should be read by an experienced radiologist because the baseline physiologic changes of pregnancy will show a dilated collecting system and suggest hydronephrosis.
  - The presence of a ureteral jet argues against obstruction.
- CXR if pulmonary symptoms or hypoxia present.

Diagnostic Procedures/Surgery
Further diagnostic procedures or surgery is generally not indicated unless complications with abscess or obstructing renal stones develop.

DIFFERENTIAL DIAGNOSIS
- Occasionally, other causes of abdominal pain and fever in a pregnant woman can be confused with UTI and pyelonephritis.
- These would include the following:
  - Appendicitis
  - Cholecystitis
  - Inflammatory bowel disease
  - Lower lobe pneumonia
  - Chorioamnionitis

 TREATMENT

PRE-HOSPITAL
- Unlike in the nonpregnant patient, asymptomatic bacteria are treated in pregnancy to prevent maternal and fetal morbidity.
- Untreated ASB is associated with pyelonephritis in up to a third of patients.
  - With treatment the risk of pyelonephritis is reduced by 75%.
  - The number needed to treat to prevent 1 case of pyelonephritis is 7.
  - The treatment of acute cystitis and ASB is similar.
  - A 3–7 day course of antibiotics is recommended with many experts preferring the 7 day course despite a lack of clear data to support this.

GENERAL MEASURES
Early aggressive treatment of pyelonephritis is important in preventing complications.

ALERT
- Current standard of care for treatment of pyelonephritis in pregnancy includes hospitalization and parenteral antibiotics.
  - Most patients respond within 72 hours, after which oral therapy based on culture and sensitivity results can be instituted.
  - Continue oral antibiotics to complete a 2-week course.
- Maintain adequate hydration while monitoring fluid intake and output carefully.
- Given the risk for pulmonary edema, monitor closely for the development of pulmonary symptoms including checking pulse oximetry with vital signs.

- Involve the obstetrician for monitoring of fetal well-being and for the development of preterm labor.

Activity
As tolerated but bed rest may be recommended by the obstetrician if preterm labor is present.

Nursing
Requires expertise in routine fetal heart rate monitoring

IV Fluids
Normal saline at 150–200 cc/hour or at a rate felt to provide adequate hydration in an individual patient but monitor for pulmonary edema.

Complementary and Alternative Therapies
- Cranberry juice consumption may be associated with fewer recurrent UTIs in nonpregnant patients.
- It can be considered for use in pregnant women as well.

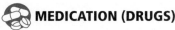 MEDICATION (DRUGS)

- Penicillins, cephalosporins, and aminoglycosides can be safely used in pregnancy.
- Fluoroquinolones should be avoided for this indication in pregnancy.
- ASB and cystitis
  - 3- or 7-day course of antibiotics recommended
  - Suggested antibiotic regimens in pregnancy and lactation include:
    - Amoxicillin 500 mg t.i.d.
    - Ampicillin 250 to 500 mg q.i.d.
    - Cefalexin 250 mg q.i.d.
    - Nitrofurantoin SR 100 mg b.i.d.
    - Sulfisoxazole 500 mg q.i.d.
    - Amoxicillin-clavulanic acid 250–500 mg t.i.d.
- Pyelonephritis
  - Hospitalization
  - IV antibiotics initially, then switch to oral antibiotics to complete 2-week course
  - Suggested antibiotic regimens in pregnancy and lactation include:
    - Ampicillin 2 g IV q6h/Gentamycin 2 mg/kg load then 1.7 mg/kg in 3 divided doses (once daily dosing of gentamicin has not been adequately studied in pregnancy).
    - Ampicillin-sulbactam 3g IV q6h
    - Ceftriaxone 1 g IV/IM daily
    - Piperacillin 4 g IV q6h

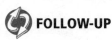 FOLLOW-UP

- For ASB and cystitis:
  - Obtain urine culture for "test of cure" 1 week after completing treatment.
    - If negative, screen monthly with urine cultures
    - If positive, treat and follow urine culture one week after completion of treatment
    - If bacteriuria persists after a second treatment, prophylactic antibiotic for duration of pregnancy is indicated.
- For pyelonephritis
  - Suppressive therapy for the duration of pregnancy is recommended after a single episode of pyelonephritis as the recurrence risk of pyelonephritis in the same pregnancy is 25%.

– Suggested antibiotic regimens for prophylaxis in pregnancy include:
  - Nitrofurantoin 100 mg per day
  - Cephalexin 250 mg per day
  - Ampicillin 250 mg per day

Admission Criteria
All pregnant patients with suspected pyelonephritis should be admitted because of the risk of preterm labor and pulmonary edema.

Discharge Criteria
Most patients can be discharged after they have been afebrile for 24 hours and there are no active obstetrical or pulmonary concerns.

Issues for Referral
- Recurrent UTI in the presence of calculi or urinary tract anomalies warrants a Urology referral.
- Pregnant women with pyelonephritis should be followed by an obstetrician.

PROGNOSIS
UTI can recur before delivery in 15–20% of pregnant patients.
- Non-pharmacologic measures which may help to prevent recurrence include:
- Increasing fluid intake
- Emptying bladder after sexual intercourse
- Double voiding (to ensure no residual urine in bladder)
- Cleaning perineum "front to back" after defecation to minimize risk of bowel organisms colonizing the urethra

COMPLICATIONS
- Preterm delivery is associated with pyelonephritis in 6–50% of pregnant women.
- Pulmonary edema occurs in up to 8% of gravidas with pyelonephritis.
- Sepsis
- Recurrent infection or failure to clear infection.

PATIENT MONITORING
- ASB or cystitis
  - Document "test of cure" by urine culture one week after treatment
- Pyelonephritis
  - Monitor monthly urine cultures in patients with a history of pyelonephritis during pregnancy.
  - Treat with prophylactic antibiotics for the duration of pregnancy

REFERENCES

1. Gilstrap LC, Cunninghamm FG, Whalley PJ. Acute pyelonephritis in pregnancy: An anterospective study. *Obstet Gynecol*. 1981;57:409–413.
2. Nicole LE, Bradely S, et al. Infectious Diseases Society of America guidelines for the diagnosis and treatment of asymptomatic bacteriuria in adults. *Clin Infect Dis*. 2005;40(5):643–654.
3. Vazques JC, Villar J. Treatments for symptomatic urinary tract infections during pregnancy (Review). *The Cochrane Database of Systematic Reviews*. 2003;(4):CD002256.
4. Velasco M, Martinez JA, Moreno-Martinez A, et al. Blood cultures for women with uncomplicated pyelonephritis: Are they necessary? *Clin Infect Dis*. 2003;37:1127–1130.
5. Wing DA. Pyelonephritis. *Clin Obstet Gynecol*. 1998;41:515–526.

ADDITIONAL READING

Lee E, et al. *Medical Care of the Pregnant Patient*. Philadelphia: American College of Physicians; 2000.
Nelson-Piercy C. *Handbook of Obstetric Medicine*. St. Louis: Mosby-Year Book; 1997.

CODES
ICD9-CM
- 599.0 UTI
- 590.10 Pyelonephritis without lesion
- 590.11 Pyelonephritis with lesion
- 646.91 Unspecified complication of pregnancy, postpartum
- 646.93 Unspecified complication of pregnancy, antepartum
- 646.53 Bacteriuria in pregnancy, antepartum
- 646.54 Bacteriuria in pregnancy, postpartum

KEY WORDS
- Pregnancy
- UTI
- Asymptomatic Bacteriuria
- Cystitis
- Pyelonephritis
- Fever
- Flank Pain
- Dysuria Preterm Labor
- Pulmonary Edema

PREMENSTRUAL MOOD DISORDER

Carolyn J. O'Connor, MD

KEY CLINICAL POINTS

- Premenstrual syndrome (PMS) and premenstrual dysphoric disorder (PMDD) are a spectrum of premenstrual mood disorders.
- PMDD is a severe form of PMS encompassing emotional and physical symptoms that affects the patients' usual level of functioning and requires treatment.
- The emotional and physical symptoms have a cyclic recurrence during the luteal phase of menstrual cycle (2 weeks prior to onset of menstrual cycle).

 BASICS

DESCRIPTION

- PMS includes a constellation of emotional and physical symptoms that tend not to affect level of functioning.
- PMDD is characterized by behavioral symptoms of marked mood swings, depression, extreme fatigue, irritability, tension, increased appetite, and cravings.
- Physical symptoms include: Abdominal bloating, breast tenderness and headache.
- PMDD is a diagnosis used to indicate severe PMS associated with deterioration in functioning that occurs exclusively during the luteal phase of the menstrual cycle and requires treatment.

GENERAL PREVENTION

- Avoidance of caffeine and alcohol
- Nutritious diet, low in saturated fats and sweets
- Daily exercise regimen of at least 30 minutes

EPIDEMIOLOGY

- Premenstrual symptoms usually begin when women are in their 20s.
- Women often do not present for treatment until symptoms have been present for at least 10 years and have progressed.
- Symptoms begin with the luteal phase of the menstrual cycle when estrogen and progesterone levels begin to fall. Symptoms improve approximately 3 days into menses.

Prevalence

- Up to 80% of women experience PMS symptoms
- Only 3–8% meet diagnostic criteria for PMDD
- Prevalence of PMDD does not appear to be dependent on socioeconomic, cultural, or ethnic differences

RISK FACTORS

- Age: Late 30s to early 40s
- Personal history of major mood disorder
- Family history of mood disorder
- Premenstrual depression
- Premenstrual mood disorder
- Past history of sexual abuse
- Past, present, or current domestic violence

Genetics

Controversial, but may play a role as concordance rate is 2 times higher in monozygotic versus dizygotic twins.

PATHOPHYSIOLOGY

- Results from the interaction of cyclic changes in ovarian steroids with central neurotransmitters.
- Serotonin is most implicated neurotransmitter

- Others implicated include: GABA, beta-endorphins, and the autonomic nervous system
- Patients with PMS have lower levels of serum serotonin when compared to controls
- Symptoms of PMS are ameliorated by serotonin agonists and aggravated by depletion of serotonin precursors (tryptophan)

ETIOLOGY

- Unknown, complex, and multifactorial
- Changes in hormone levels likely affect centrally acting neurotransmitters
- May be a deficiency in prostaglandins related to an inability to convert linoleic acid to prostaglandin precursors

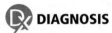 **DIAGNOSIS**

- Comprehensive assessment of symptoms with patient's daily ratings of symptoms for at least 2 consecutive menstrual cycles during luteal phase
- Based on symptoms, severity, timing, and exclusion of other diagnoses
- Symptoms emerge in the second 1/2 of the menstrual period and subside shortly after the onset of menstruation.
- Significant interference with work/school and social activities/relationships
- Most commonly used diagnostic criteria are from the American Psychiatric Association (DSM-IV) criteria for PMDD and the University of San Diego (UCSD) criteria for PMS.
  - DSM-IV criteria for PMDD:
    - May be superimposed on other psychiatric disorders provided it is not merely an exacerbation of that disorder
  - UCSD criteria:
    - Can only be met in the presence of physical and affective symptoms and in the absence of a concomitant psychiatric disorder

SIGNS AND SYMPTOMS

- DSM-IV criteria: At least 5 symptoms, including 1 of the first 4:
  - Depressed mood
  - Anxiety, tension
  - Labile mood
  - Irritability, anger
  - Decreased interest in usual activities
  - Difficulty concentrating
  - Fatigue, tiredness
  - Appetite changes (overeating/cravings)
  - Hypersomnia/insomnia
  - Feeling out of control/overwhelmed
  - Physical symptoms: Breast tenderness, bloating, HA, joint/muscle pain
- UCSD criteria: At least 1 of 6 behavioral symptoms:
  - Fatigue, irritability, depression, expressed anger, poor concentration, and social withdrawal
- At least 1 of 4 somatic symptoms
  - Breast tenderness, abdominal bloating, headache, and swollen extremities
- Most common scales used for assessment of symptoms:
  - COPE (calendar of premenstrual symptoms) women rate the daily severity of 10 physical symptoms and 12 behavioral symptoms based on a 4-point Lickert scale.
  - PAF (premenstrual assessment form)

- MDQ (moos menstrual distress questionnaire)
- The concurrent validity of PAF with other psychometric inventories is not as well established as with COPE.

History
- Obtaining a record of symptoms, including severity and timing that correlates with the luteal phase of the menstrual cycle
- Regularity of menstrual cycle
- Family history of PMS and PMDD
- Personal history of mood disorders

Physical Exam
Normal

TESTS
Lab
Role is limited in screening for other medical disorders in differential diagnosis
- CBC, chemistry profile, TSH
- Consider FSH

Imaging
None

Diagnostic Procedures/Surgery
None

DIFFERENTIAL DIAGNOSIS
- Anemia
- Hypothyroidism
- Hyperthyroidism
- Depression
- Anxiety disorder
- Panic disorder
- Bipolar affective disorder
- Hyperprolactinemia
- Personality disorder
- Chronic fatigue syndrome
- Drug or alcohol abuse
- SLE
  - Also consider disorders of the adrenal system, CVD, eating disorders when appropriate

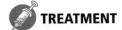

TREATMENT

GENERAL MEASURES
Reserve pharmacologic therapy for patients who meet strict criteria for PMS or PMDD

Diet
- Limit caffeine, alcohol, and sodium intake
- Increase consumption of complex carbohydrates
  - No RCT to support this

Activity
Aerobic activity at least 30 minutes at least 3 times a week

No RCT to support this but does alleviate symptoms of depression

Dietary Supplementation
Data is insufficient
- Vitamin B6 50–100 mg/day
  - Meta-analysis of studies show in above doses there may be a reduction in physical and depressive symptoms. No good quality RCT. Doses of 200 mg/day or greater are associated with peripheral neuropathy.
- Calcium carbonate 1,200 mg/day during luteal phase
  - One RCT reported reduction in physical and emotional symptoms.

- Magnesium 200 mg–360 mg/day
  - Conflicting studies on benefit
- Evening primrose oil, vitamin A, vitamin E
  - No good studies to support use. Vitamin E has been shown to be affective with mastalgia.

Complementary and Alternative Therapies
Cognitive—behavioral therapy and relaxation therapy
Studies regarding the efficacy have been inconsistent.

MEDICATION (DRUGS)

- SSRIs
  - Several RCT have shown that many SSRIs are superior to placebo.
  - Continuous dosing or dosing only during the luteal phase may be equally effective.
    - Fluoxetine: 10–20 mg/day
    - Sertraline: 50–150 mg/day
    - Paroxetine: 10–30 mg/day
    - Paroxetine CR: 12.5–25 mg/day
    - Citalopram: 20–40 mg/day
    - Fluvoxamine: 25–50 mg/day
    - Venlafaxine: 75–150 mg/day (SNRI)
- Anxiolytics
  - Alprazolam: Titrate to 1 to 2 mg/day. Reduces depression, irritability and anxiety. Limited by an abuse potential
  - Buspirone: Up to 60 mg/day
- Oral contraceptives
  - Do not reliably improve mood but can help with physical symptoms
- Ovulation suppression
  - GnRH agonist: Leuprolide 3.75 mg IM every month or 11.25 mg IM every 3 months
  - Danazol: Androgenic effects limit use
  - Medroxyprogesterone acetate
- Diuretics: Spironolactone 25–100 mg/day during luteal phase improves bloating and weight gain
  - RCT show effectiveness with bloating symptoms and weight gain. Some studies show some improvement in emotional symptoms.
- Herbal preparations
  - Gingko, kava, St. John's wort, and evening primrose oil have not been studied adequately.
  - Chaste berry fruit (vitex agnus castus): 20 mg/day
    - More effective than placebo in placebo-controlled trials.

First Line
- Initial treatment should be non-pharmacological and geared toward lifestyle changes.
- For mild to moderate symptoms first approach includes:
  - Diet, exercise, OTCs such as NSAIDs for physical symptoms
  - Recommend calcium 1,200 mg/day
  - Consider:
    - Addition of magnesium (up to 360 mg/day)
    - Vitamin B6 (not to exceed 200 mg/day)
    - OCPs for cramps and abdominal bloating
    - Spironolactone for bloating and breast tenderness

Second Line
For more severe symptoms the drug of choice:
- SSRIs:
  - Should be given an adequate trial of 2 months before initiating another SSRI for treatment failure
- Anxiolytics
  - Try buspirone first as no addictive potential

- GNRH agonist treatment
  - After above have failed

SURGERY

- A hysterectomy with bilateral oophorectomy is curative as demonstrated in RCT.
- A hysterectomy alone has some benefit, but more studies are needed.
- Data very limited on endometrial ablation and laparoscopic bilateral oophorectomy
- Indications for surgery
  - For recalcitrant cases in which previous therapies have been adequately pursued but failed
  - Patients should be evaluated by a psychiatrist to preclude other psychiatric comorbidities.
  - Patient should have completed the possibility of child bearing.
  - Should be a last resort as surgery alone carries the risk for morbidity and mortality

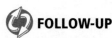 **FOLLOW-UP**

Patients should record symptoms during 2 consecutive menstrual cycles.

- Ascertain diagnosis and begin treatment based on symptom complexity.
- Re-evaluate therapy in 2 months.
- If stable, monitor patient every 4–6 months.
- Continue effective treatment for at least 9–12 months.

Issues for Referral

Consider psychiatric referral

- Treatment ineffective
- Mood symptoms associated with suicidal ideation
- Mood symptoms associated with inability to function despite treatment

PROGNOSIS

- Symptoms improve rapidly with treatment
- Symptoms predictably recur upon cessation of treatment except after oophorectomy

COMPLICATIONS

- Side effects of medical treatment
- Recurrence of symptoms upon cessation of treatment
- Treatment failures

REFERENCES

1. Dell DL. Premenstrual syndrome, premenstrual dysphoric disorder, and premenstrual exacerbation of another disorder. *Clin Obstet Gynecol*. 2004;47:568–575.
2. Dickerson L. Practical therapuetics. Premenstrual syndrome. *Am Fam Physician*. 2003;67:1743–1752.
3. Grady-Weliky TA. Clinical practice. Premenstrual dysphoric disorder. *N Engl J Med*. 2003;348:433–438.
4. Johnson S. Premenstrual syndrome, premenstrual dysphoric disorder, and beyond: A clinical primer for practitioners. *Obstet Gynecol*. 2004;104:845–859.
5. Ling FW. Recognizing and treating premenstrual dysphoric disorder in the obstetric, gynecologic, and primary care practices. *J Clin Psychiatry*. 2000;61:9–16.
6. Premenstrual dysphoric disorder. In: Diagnostic and Statistical Manual of Mental Disorders, 4th ed. Washington, DC: American Psychiatric Association; 2004:771–774.

CODES

ICD9-CM

- 625.4 PMDD
- 625.4 PMS

KEY WORDS

- Premenstrual Dysphoric Disorder
- Premenstrual Syndrome
- Late Luteal Phase Dysphoric Disorder
- Depression
- Anxiety

PREVENTATIVE HEALTH

Catherine Malone Smitas, MD

KEY CLINICAL POINTS

Preventative Health encompasses early detection and prevention of disease
- An ideal screening test is inexpensive, sensitive, and detects a disease in which early treatment improves outcome.
- Primary prevention is disease reduction through vaccination, lifestyle modification, and medications.

SCREENING

The U.S. Preventive Services Task Force (*USPSTF*) is the leading agency reviewing evidence-based data and offering prevention guidelines. Recommendations are based on the quality of the available evidence, and the risks and benefits of each test. Table 1 summarizes *USPSTF* screening guidelines, as well as the guidelines of other professional organizations if they differ.

VACCINATION

The following is a list of recommended vaccines in adults. For patients who were not vaccinated as adults, refer to the Center for Disease Control (CDC) website. (www.cdc.gov)
- **Tetanus, diphtheria (Td)**
  - Every 10 years
- **Measles:**
  - Some adults should get a "booster":
    - Persons exposed to measles
    - College students
    - Health care workers
    - Those who are traveling outside of the United States
  - **Do not give to**
    - Pregnant patients
    - Those with HIV who are severely immunosuppressed
- **Varicella**
  - 2 doses, 1–2 months apart
  - All women who do not have evidence of Varicella immunity
  - **Do not vaccinate pregnant women** or those who might become pregnant in the month following vaccination
- **Influenza**
  - Administered yearly
  - Age 50 and over
  - Patient with chronic disease
    - Pulmonary
    - Cardiovascular
    - Renal
    - Diabetes
    - Immunosuppressive conditions
  - Health Care workers
- **Streptococcus Pneumoniae**
  - Administered 1 or 2 times
  - Patients 65 years and older
  - Patients with chronic disorders
    - Pulmonary
    - Cardiovascular
    - Diabetes
    - Renal disease
    - Functional or surgical asplenia
  - High risk patients and those who received first vaccine under age 65 should get a "booster" 5 years later.
- **Hepatitis A**
  - 2 doses, 6–12 months apart

- Patients with chronic liver disease or risk factors for hepatitis
- **Hepatitis B**
  - 3 doses at 0, 1–2, and 4–6 months
    - Hemodialysis patients
    - Health care workers
    - Patients with risk factors for sexually transmitted diseases
- **Meningococcal Vaccine**
  - Single dose
    - Surgical or functional asplenia
    - College students
    - Military recruits
    - Laboratory workers

SUPPLEMENTS, DIET, AND EXERCISE

- **Aspirin**: Recommended by The American College of Cardiology (*ACC*) and *USPSTF* for primary prevention in patients with a greater than 3% risk of coronary disease over 5 years. Optimal dose is not known. USPSTF recommends 75 mg or more per day.
- **Calcium:** 1,000 mg/day in women under age 50, 1,200 mg/day in women 50 and older
- **Vitamin D**: 400 IU/day in young and middle aged women, 800 IU/day
- **Folic Acid**: 0.4 mg/day, women of childbearing age to prevent neural tube defects
- **Physical Activity:**
  - *ACC* recommends 30 minutes of exercise most days of the week for the primary prevention of hypertension, obesity, coronary artery disease and diabetes.
  - *The American Association of Clinical Endocrinologists (ACCE)* recommends weight bearing exercise for the prevention of osteoporosis.
- **Balanced Diet:** A balanced diet low in saturated fats and cholesterol, advocated by *ACC, American Diabetes Association (ADA), ACCE.*

REFERENCES

1. AACE Osteoporosis Task Force. American Association of Clinical Endocrinologists Medical Guidelines for Clinical Practice for the Prevention and Treatment of Postmenopausal Osteoporosis: 2001 Edition, With Selected Updates for 2003. *Endo Prac.* 2003;19:544–564.
2. ACIP. Recommended Adult Immunization Schedule–United States, October 2005–Sept 2006. *MMWR.* 2005;54.
3. American Cancer Society. www.cancer.org.
4. Bond J. for the Practice Parameters Committee for the American College of Gastroenterology. Polyp Guideline: Diagnosis, Treatment, and Surveillance for Patients with Colorectal Polyps. *AJG.* 2000;95:3053–3063.
5. Mosca L, Appel LJ, Benjamin EJ, et al. Evidence-Based Guidelines for Cardiovascular Disease Prevention in Women. *JACC.* 2004;43:900–921.
6. National Cholesterol Education Program. Detection, Evaluation, and Treatment of High Blood Cholesterol in Adults (Adult Treatment Panel III). *NIH.* 2001;01-3670.
7. US Department of Health and Human Services. The Seventh Report of the Joint National Committee on Prevention, Detection, Evaluation, and Treatment of High Blood Pressure. *NIH.* 2004;04-5230.

Table 1

Condition	Screening Recommendations (USPSTF)	Other Recommendations
Alcohol Abuse	• All patients, but optimal interval of screening unknown • Screen for "risky" drinking (>3 drinks at one time or >7 per week) and "harmful" drinking (drinking with adverse consequence or dependence)	
Breast Cancer	**Mammogram** • Start at age 40, every 1–2 years • Age when screening stops depends on co-morbidities **Clinical Breast Exam/Self Breast Exam** • *USPSTF* finds insufficient evidence to recommend clinical breast exam or self breast exam as adjuvant screening	*American Cancer Society:* • Mammogram every 1–2 years starting age 40 • Clinical breast exam every 3 years in women age 20–40 and then yearly over age 40. • Breast self exam as an "option," but not an alternative

Cervical Cancer	**Papanicolaou Smear**
	• All women who are sexually active until age 65
	• Yearly until age 30 then every 2–3 years if patient has had 3 consecutive normal tests
	• Liquid-based cytology tests are more sensitive but also more costly and are only cost-effective if screening interval is increased to every 3 years
	• Patients who have had a total hysterectomy for benign disease should *not* be screened
		American Cancer Society:
		• One of the following options:
		  – Yearly screening with conventional test until age 30, then every 2 years
		  – Every 2 years using liquid-based test
		  – One of the above options until age 30, then every 3 years with liquid test plus HPV PCR
		• Continue screening until age 70 in women who have not been routinely screened
		• Screen women with HIV, history of DES exposure, or immunosuppression annually, regardless of age

Chlamydia	Yearly in all sexually active women until age 25 and those with risk factors older than 25	

Colorectal Cancer	• Begin screening at age 50
	• Patients with a family history of colon cancer before age 60 in a first degree relative should begin screening at an earlier age
	• **Average-risk patients** –Screening options based on patient preference, risk factors, and complication rates
	  – Annual fecal occult blood testing (FOBT); if positive, colonoscopy
	  – Flexible sigmoidoscopy
	  – FOBT plus sigmoidoscopy
	  – Colonoscopy
	  – Double contrast barium enema alone is inferior option
	• **High-risk patients:** Colonoscopy is preferred method
	• Stop screening at age 80 or based on estimated mortality from co-morbid conditions
		American Cancer Society:
		• Offers the following choices:
		  – FOBT annually
		  – Flexible sigmoidoscopy every 5 years
		  – Annual FOBT *plus* sigmoidoscopy every 5 years
		  – Double-contrast barium enema every 5 years
		  – Colonoscopy every 10 years
		American College of Gastroenterology:
		• Colonoscopy is the preferred screening test
		• In patients whom colonoscopy can not be completed, a double contrast barium enema with flexible sigmoidoscopy should be performed

Depression	All women, interval is unclear	
Diabetes	**Fasting Blood Sugar** (≥126) • All patients with hypertension or hypercholesterolemia • *USPSTF* found insufficient evidence to evaluate screening asymptomatic patients without risk factors • Fasting blood sugar is the most reliable, least expensive test • Another option is the 2-hour post-load plasma glucose	*American Diabetes Association:* • Screen all persons age 45 or older every 3 years • Patients with risk factors – family history, obesity, hypertension, should be screened at an earlier age and at more frequent intervals
HIV	• Screen patients with risk factors • All pregnant women regardless of risk factors	
Hypertension	• All patients over age 18 with office sphygmomanometer • Patients should have blood pressure checked at least twice, 2 weeks apart before being diagnosed with hypertension	*Joint National Committee 7:* • Check blood pressure every 2 years if normotensive and • More frequently if blood pressure elevated
Hypercholest-erolemia	**Serum Total Cholesterol and HDL** • Only check LDL and triglycerides if risk factors or abnormal total cholesterol • Start at age 45 if no risk factors • If risk factors, start at age 20 • Stop at age 75 unless has risk factors *and* is healthy	*American Association of Clinical Endocrinologists:* • Screen all patients every 5 years beginning at age 20 • If risk factors, screen more frequently *National Cholesterol Education Program (ATP III):* • Check *complete* fasting lipid panel (total cholesterol, LDL, HDL, triglycerides) every 5 years starting at age 20
Obesity	**Body Mass Index** • Each visit	*American College of Cardiology:* • Goal BMI 18–24

Osteoporosis	**Dual-energy X-ray Absorptiometry**
	• Women beginning at age 65
	• Start at age 60 if with risk factors
	• Low weight (<70 kg) is greatest risk factor
	• All women with a non-traumatic fracture regardless of age
	• Interval unknown, but at least 2 years between tests
		American Association of Clinical Endocrinologists
		• Post menopausal women should be screened if:
		  – Age <65 but weigh <127 lbs
		  – Family history of osteoporotic fracture
		  – Consider hip protectors in patients who have fallen or are at risk for falling

Syphilis	Screen those with risk factors using RPR or VDRL, and if positive FTA-ABS or TP-PA as confirmatory test	
Tobacco Use	Screen at every interaction	

8. US Preventative Services Task Force. The Guide to Clinical Preventive Services 2005. *AHRQ*. 2005;05-0570.

CODES
ICD9-CM
- V70 General medical exam
- V72.31 Routine gynecologic exam
- V65.3 Dietary surveillance and counseling

KEY WORDS
- Prevention
- Screening
- Vaccination
- Cancer

PSEUDOTUMOR CEREBRI (PTC)

Bismruta Misra, MD, MPH

KEY CLINICAL POINTS

- PTC is a diagnosis of exclusion.
- PTC is a preventable cause of blindness.
- High index of suspicion in:
  - Obese young women complaining of chronic daily headaches and normal neuro exam except for papilledema
  - Recent treatment with retinoic acid, tetracycline for acne

BASICS

DESCRIPTION
- Increased intracranial pressure (ICP) without a space-occupying lesion and with normal cerebrospinal fluid analysis
- When secondary cause not discovered, known as Idiopathic intracranial hypertension
- Also known as benign intracranial hypertension

GENERAL PREVENTION
- Maintaining a normal body mass index is the best way to prevent onset of PTC
- Avoiding medications that are associated with developing PTC

EPIDEMIOLOGY
Incidence
- 1/100,000 in general population
  - 4/100,000 women age 15–44
  - 19/100,000 women ages 20–44 who are more than 20% ideal body weight
  - Rarely occurs in patients over age 45

RISK FACTORS
Weight gain and obesity

Genetics
No known genetic association

PATHOPHYSIOLOGY
Pathogenesis still uncertain but proposed mechanisms involve:
- Increased CSF production
- Decreased CSF absorption
- Elevated cerebral venous pressure

ETIOLOGY
- Magnetic resonance venography demonstrates that those with increased venous sinus pressure have decreased CSF absorption.
- Central obesity may raise intra-abdominal filling pressure causing increased cardiac filling pressure, which impedes venous return from the brain and thereby causes increased ICP.
- Known pharmacologic association between increased levels of serotonin and norepinephrine and decreased CSF production
- One hypothesis is that low levels may account for increased CSF pressure and explain high incidence of depression, anxiety, and obesity in patients with PTC

ASSOCIATED CONDITIONS
- Medications: Amiodarone, anabolic steroids, cyclosporine, indomethacin, growth hormone, leuprorelin (LH-RH analogue), levothyroxine, lithium, naladixic acid, oral contraceptives, penicillin, retinoic acid compounds (accutane, trans-retinoic acid) steroids (use and withdrawal), sulfa antibiotics, tetracyclines, vitamin A

- Endocrine disorders: Adrenal insufficiency, hypo- and hyperparathyroidism, hypo- and hyperthyroidism, obesity, menarche, pregnancy, polycystic ovary syndrome
- Nutritional disorders: Hyper and hypovitaminosis A, hyperalimentation in nutritional deficiency
- Obstruction to venous drainage: Cerebral venous thrombosis (hypercoagulable states, antiphospholipd antibody syndrome, polycythemia), mastoiditis, superior vena cava syndrome, increased right heart pressure
- Hematologic/oncologic: Iron deficiency anemia, sickle cell anemia, pernicious anemia, gastrointestinal hemorrhage, cryofibronogenemia, antiphospholipid antibody syndrome, carcinomatous and lymphomatous meningitis
- Rheumatologic disorders: Systemic lupus erythematosis, Bechet's disease, sarcoidosis
- Infectious: Lyme disease, infectious mononucleosis, HIV infection, after childhood varicella
- Other: Head trauma, neprhotic syndrome, obstructive sleep apnea, Paget's disease, Turner syndrome, uremia

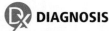 DIAGNOSIS

PRE-HOSPITAL
PTC is a diagnosis of exclusion.

SIGNS AND SYMPTOMS
- Headache: Most common complaint. Daily, retro-ocular, worsening with eye movement, recumbent position, and straining
- Transient visual obscurations: Brief episodes of monocular or binocular visual loss lasting seconds
- Pulsatile tinnitus: Noises described as whooshing or heartbeat sound either unilateral or bilateral
- Diplopia: Horizontal and binocular due to pseudo sixth nerve palsy
- Visual loss: May be initial presenting symptom, either blurred vision, tunnel vision, severe PTC can result in complete blindness
- Other: Neck stiffness, facial palsy, arthralgias, depression, radicular pain

History
- Recent weight gain
- New medications
- Underlying medical conditions (see associated condition list)

Physical Exam
- Papilledema: Almost all cases of PTC, usually bilateral
- 6th nerve palsy: 10% to 20% of PTC cases
- Reduced visual fields: Enlarged "blind spot," constricted visual fields

TESTS
Lab
- Cerebrospinal fluid analysis
  - Elevated opening pressure >250 mm of water
  - Normal cell count, glucose, and protein
- Other: Hypercoagulable workup if suspicious for venous sinus thrombosis

Imaging
Magnetic Resonance Imaging (MRI)
- Must do prior to lumbar puncture to rule out space occupying lesion and ventriculomegaly

- Flattening of posterior sclera: 80%
- Empty sella: 70% of PTC cases
- Magnetic resonance venography to evaluate for cerebral venous thrombosis (especially in those who are taking oral contraceptives, post-partum, known coagulopathy

Diagnostic Procedures/Surgery
Lumbar puncture
- Measure opening pressure in lateral decubitus position with legs relaxed. Pressures taken in sitting or prone (i.e., under fluoroscopy) are not valid.
- For optimal CSF flow: 18G–20G spinal needle
- CSF should be analyzed for glucose, protein, cell count, bacterial, fungal, mycobacterium, and cytology.

DIFFERENTIAL DIAGNOSIS
Any condition that causes an increased ICP should be in the differential diagnosis and ruled out prior to diagnosing PTC.
- Head injury
- Cerebral hemorrhage: Subdural, epidural, intracranial
- Meningitis/encephalitis
- Brain mass: Tumor, abscess
- Hydrocephalus
- Hypernatremia

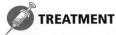 ## TREATMENT

INITIAL STABILIZATION
If an underlying associated condition is found, treatment of the condition is important:
- Continuous positive airway pressure for those with obstructive sleep apnea
- Anticoagulation for those with hypercoagulable state
Treatment based on level of symptoms and visual function
- Mild to moderate papilledema
  - With and without Headache:
    - Weight loss and low salt diet
    - If no improvement then consider acetazolamide and/or furosemide
- Moderate papilledema
  - Start acetazolamide
- If continued visual deterioration:
  - Increase dose
  - Intermittent Lumbar punctures or continuous lumbar drainage
- Severe papilledema
  - High dose acetazolamide, lumbar punctures, continuous drainage
  - If worsens: Surgical options may need to be entertained

GENERAL MEASURES
Diet
Weight loss using low salt diet and exercise is the mainstay of treatment for obese patients with PTC.

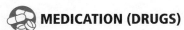 ## MEDICATION (DRUGS)

First Line
- Acetazolamide: 1–4 g daily in divided doses
  - Reduces CSF production by carbonic anhydrase inhibition

Second Line
- Furosemide: 40–120 mg daily in divided doses, works by decreasing CSF volume

- Sprinolactone/triamtereine:
  - Used in patients allergic to sulfa
- Topiramate: 100–400 mg day, antiepileptic
  - Useful for headache prevention and has a desirable side effect of weight loss
- Corticosteroids: Used only for short-term use
  - Can rapidly decrease ICP if medication is tapered, rebound intracranial hypertension can occur
- Medications used in the treatment of migraines can help the headaches associated with PTC
  - Can cause undesirable side effects (e.g., tricyclic antidepressants can cause weight gain, calcium channel blockers can cause peripheral edema)
  - Should be used with caution

SURGERY
- Repeated lumbar punctures are sometimes necessary if medical treatment unsuccessful with goal to keep opening pressure <200 mm H_2O
- Optic nerve sheath decompression:
  - Involves fenestrating the sheath of an edematous optic nerve
  - Treatment of choice for
    - Those with severe papilledema with extension into macula
    - Those whose vision is deteriorating despite optimal medical management
- Cerebrospinal fluid shunting
  - Lumboperitoneal shunting preferred over ventricular shunting (because ventricles are not enlarged in PTC)
    - Associated with 50% failure rate
    - May require multiple revisions
- Bariatric surgery is not helpful in the acute setting, but may be an option for the long-term management of morbidly obese patients.

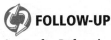 ## FOLLOW-UP

Issues for Referral
PTC is best managed with a team approach involving a primary care physician, neurologist, neuro-ophthalmologist, and neurosurgeon.

PROGNOSIS
Visual acuity is usually restored and preserved with early treatment.

COMPLICATIONS
- Recurrence:
  - Recurrence in almost 40% of the patients with PTC, but not while the patients are being treated
  - Visual loss is the outcome if PTC is not treated.

PATIENT MONITORING
Current recommendations include follow-up exams including neuro-opthamologic testing every 6–12 months for 5 years after the diagnosis, because of the high reoccurrence rate, especially once treatment is completed.

Pregnancy Considerations
- Occurrence of PTC in pregnancy is similar to nonpregnant women.
- PTC can develop or worsen in pregnancy.
- There is no increased risk of fetal loss with PTC.
- Acetazolamide is a class C medication that has been shown to be teratogenic in animal studies and safe to use after 20 weeks gestation.

REFERENCES

1. Friedman D. Pseudotumor cerebri. *Neurol Clin*. 2004;22:99–131.
2. Disturbances of cerebrospinal fluid and its circulation including hydrocephalus, pseudotumor, and low-pressure syndromes. In: Ropper A, Brown R, eds. *Adams and Victors' Principles of Neurology*. McGraw-Hill; 2005.
3. Kessler A, Hadayer A, Goldhammer Y, et al. Idiopathic intracranial hypertension. *Neurol*. 2004;63:1737–1739.
4. Radhakrishnan K, Ahlskog JE, Garrity JA, et al. Idiopathic intracranial hypertension. *Mayo Clin Proc*. 1994;69: 169–180.

CODES
ICD9-CM
348.2 Pseudotumor cerebri

KEY WORDS

- Idiopathic Intracranial Hypertension
- Benign Intracranial Hypertension
- Increased Intracranial Pressure
- Headache
- Papilledema
- Obesity
- Acetazolamide

RAYNAUD'S PHENOMENON

Rebecca A. Griffith, MD

KEY CLINICAL POINTS

- The diagnosis of Raynaud's phenomenon can be confirmed by the presence of reversible episodes of peripheral vasospasm characterized by the classic "white, blue, and red" color changes of the affected digits.
- Raynaud's phenomenon symptoms may occur in isolation (primary disease) or in association with an underlying rheumatologic disorder (secondary disease).
- Most patients with Raynaud's phenomenon can be treated with conservative management. Drug treatment with calcium channel blockers or other vasodilators is reserved for those with severe pain or impact on daily routines, as well as the rare patient with digital gangrene or ulceration.

DESCRIPTION

- Raynaud's phenomenon is a disorder characterized by episodes of vasospasm of the fingers and toes in response to cold exposure or stress.
- A classic episode consists of vasoconstriction causing pallor, followed by cyanosis, and often subsequent reactive hyperemia.
- The disorder is divided into primary Raynaud's phenomenon if the patient has no known underlying disorder, and secondary Raynaud's phenomenon if an underlying disease, such as scleroderma or systemic lupus erythematosis (SLE), is identified.

EPIDEMIOLOGY

Raynaud's phenomenon occurs worldwide.

- Primary Raynaud's phenomenon is most common and accounts for the majority of the cases diagnosed by primary care physicians. It is usually diagnosed in:
  - Female > Male (2:1)
  - Teens or 20s, with median age of onset of 14
  - Familial predisposition
- Secondary Raynaud's phenomenon is often diagnosed after age 40, but may predate the diagnosis of systemic illness by up to 2 years or longer.

Prevalence

The prevalence of Raynaud's phenomenon follows a geographic distribution related to differences in climate:

- Overall prevalence of primary Raynaud's phenomenon is 10%.
  - Mild climates: Prevalence in women and men reported to be 4.7–5.7% and 3.2–4.3%, respectively
  - Colder climates: Prevalence rises to 20% in women and 13% in men
- Secondary Raynaud's phenomenon prevalence data are incomplete, however, it may occur in:
  - Systemic sclerosis patients: Up to 90%
  - SLE patients: 10–40%
  - Primary Sjögren's syndrome patients: 33%
  - Dermatomyositis/polymyositis patients: 20%
  - Rheumatoid arthritis patients: 10–20%

RISK FACTORS

- Living in cold climate
- Female gender
- Family history
  - Raynaud's phenomenon present in up to 30% of 1st-degree relatives

PATHOPHYSIOLOGY

The pathophysiology of triphasic color changes is as follows:

- Vasoconstriction of digital vessels produces pallor

- Deoxygenation of static venous blood causes cyanosis
- Reactive hyperemia leads to erythema

ETIOLOGY

Although the etiology of Raynaud's phenomenon is largely unknown, it is likely mediated by the following mechanisms:

- Neurogenic:
  - Initially thought that increased vasoconstrictor response in reaction to cold stimuli caused by hyper-reactivity of parasympathetic nervous system
  - Also a role for central sympathetic system
- Blood vessel endothelium:
  - Most important cellular element
  - Demonstrates abnormal responses to both endothelium-dependent (sole mechanism in secondary Raynaud's) and endothelium-independent induced vasodilatation
  - Damaged endothelium may also affect clotting system and other blood elements
- Inflammatory and immune system
  - Involves tumor necrosis factor, T cells, lymphokines, and immune complex deposition
  - Seen in severe cases associated with connective tissue disorders, but also in other subsets

ASSOCIATED CONDITIONS

Secondary Raynaud's phenomenon is by definition associated with other disorders

- Rheumatologic diseases
  - Diagnosed in almost all patients with systemic sclerosis
  - SLE, RA (10–15%), Sjögren's syndrome, MCTD
- Mechanical injury
  - Vibration (hand arm vibration syndrome)
  - Frostbite, occupational cold exposure
- Vasospastic diseases
  - Migraines
  - Prinzmetal or atypical angina
  - Pulmonary hypertension
- Infections
  - Chronic liver disease, Parvovirus B19, *H. pylori*
- Medication
  - Chemotherapeutic agents
  - Interferon
  - Ergots
  - Of note: β-blockers have been reported to cause Raynaud's phenomenon, but this association has not been confirmed in well-designed studies.

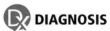 DIAGNOSIS

SIGNS AND SYMPTOMS

Symptoms occur in patients with exposure to cold temperatures or in times of stress and have classically been described as "white, blue, red" changes.

- Initially, affected areas may be pale or blanched (white) in appearance
- More commonly seen is cyanosis (blueness) of the skin limited to the involved digits
- Episode ends with painful hyperemia causing redness of the digits
- Attack may begin in 1 or more digits but usually spreads to symmetrically involve digits of both hands

- Most commonly involves the fingers, however can involve toes, ears, nose, nipples

History
Patients should be questioned to ascertain the nature of the attacks and to rule out an underlying cause or associated disorder.
- Diagnosis is dependent on:
  - History of sensitivity to the cold
  - Episodic, sharply demarcated areas of pallor and/or cyanosis affecting distal digits
- To classify as primary or secondary, the physician should determine whether symptoms of an underlying disorder is present.
  - For rheumatologic diseases:
    - Fever, myalgias, arthritis, dry mucous membranes, rashes, cardiopulmonary abnormalities
  - History of mechanical injury, use of vibratory tools
  - Medication history
- Raynaud's symptoms precipitated by changes in position could be more indicative of thoracic outlet syndrome.
- Important to assess smoking status as nicotine can exacerbate vasospasm

Physical Exam
- Primary Raynaud's phenomenon
  - Normal aside from findings in involved areas during an attack
  - No tissue necrosis, ulceration, or gangrene
  - Normal nail-fold capillaries
- Secondary Raynaud's phenomenon
  - The exam will demonstrate findings consistent with the underlying disease.
  - Digital ulcerations and gangrene can be seen in severe cases, particularly in association with immune-mediated diseases.
  - Nail-fold capillaries will be abnormal.

TESTS
Lab
- If a patient has history and physical exam consistent with primary Raynaud's phenomenon, specifically including normal nail-fold capillaries and no digital lesions, no further studies needed
- Patients with signs or symptoms suggestive of underlying disease in the absence or presence of abnormal nail-fold capillaries should have additional work-up undertaken including:
  - Complete blood count
  - General chemistry profile
  - Urinalysis
  - Other tests may be indicated based on suspected or known underlying disease
    - Antinuclear antibodies
    - Rheumatoid factor
    - Disease-specific auto-antibodies such as, anticentromere, antismith, antiribonucleoprotein
    - C3 and C4 complement levels
  - If the above tests are unrevealing, the following tests should be done:
    - Thyroid function tests
    - Serum protein electrophoresis
    - Cryoglobulins

Imaging
The diagnosis of Raynaud's phenomenon is clinical; however, imaging can help to distinguish primary from secondary and to rule out other disorders included in the differential diagnosis.

- Capillaroscopy is the examination of nail-fold capillaries under magnification.
  - It can be performed with an ophthalmoscope set at a high diopter, 10–40.
  - A drop of mineral oil or immersion oil at base of the fingernail can help to visualize the capillaries.
  - Normal capillaries may be difficult to see, but will appear as orderly loops.
  - Abnormal capillaries are enlarged, tortuous, and can demonstrate the characteristic "dropout" of scleroderma.
- History of asymmetric or single-digit attacks, and patients with findings of vascular abnormalities (absent pulses, asymmetric blood pressure) or critical ischemia should have further diagnostic evaluation including:
  - Arterial Doppler ultrasonography
  - Angiography if indicated

DIFFERENTIAL DIAGNOSIS
- Neuropathic conditions
  - Carpal tunnel syndrome
  - Ulnar nerve palsy
- Vascular disorders
  - Thromboangiitis obliterans (Buerger disease)
    - More common in men, lower extremities and presents with claudication symptoms
  - Atherosclerosis with small vessel occlusion
    - More common in men, not symmetric
  - Thoracic outlet syndrome
  - Vasculitis
- Cryoglobulinemia, hyperviscosity states, antiphospholipid antibody syndrome can also cause cyanotic digits

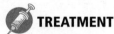 **TREATMENT**

GENERAL MEASURES
Conservative management is recommended for all patients with Raynaud's phenomenon
- Dress warmly, including gloves, stockings, hat
- Avoid sudden cold exposure or stress
- Avoid vasoconstrictive agents, including nicotine, ergots, sympathomimetic drugs

Complementary and Alternative Therapies
Biofeedback and relaxation techniques have not shown clear benefit in reducing attacks.

 MEDICATION (DRUGS)

Medication may be used in patients for whom conservative therapy does not control symptoms or in whom symptoms are severe enough to impact activities of daily life, work, or social life.

First Line
Calcium-channel blockers:
- Most widely used agents
- Nifedipine best studied and has been shown to decrease frequency and severity of attacks as compared to placebo
  - Dose: Sustained release nifedipine 30–120 mg/day or Amlodipine 5–20 mg/day orally
  - Side effects: Edema, tachycardia, constipation, orthostatic hypotension

Second Line
- Prazosin found to be more effective than placebo, but less well tolerated than calcium-channel blockers

- Dose: Prazosin 1–5 mg twice daily
- Side effects: Dizziness, palpitations, syncope, postural hypotension
- Losartan shown to be more effective than nifedipine in patients with scleroderma
  - Dose: Losartan 25–100 mg/day orally
  - Side effects: Dizziness, headache, fatigue
- Fluoxetine shown to improve symptoms in one study
  - Dose: 20–40 mg/day orally
  - Side effects: Insomnia, nausea, diarrhea, tremors
- Other vasodilators
  - Many used but not well-studied
  - Nitroglycerin often used in combination with calcium-channel blocker but may take up to 3 months to show effect
    - $^1/_4$–$^1/_2$ inch of 2% ointment applied topically each day
    - Side effects: Headache, tachycardia, syncope, rash, nausea, rebound hypertension
- Prostaglandins
  - Intravenous therapy not approved for use but likely helpful as shown in multiple trials
    - Iloprost 0.5–2 ng/kg/min IV over 6–24 hours/day for 2–5 days
    - Side effects: Flushing, diarrhea, headache, hypotension, rash
    - Used in patients with critical ischemia and/or digital ulceration
    - May be second-line after calcium-channel blockers for those with severe disease
  - Oral prostaglandin agents are not shown to be effective in reducing symptoms.
  - Data regarding effectiveness of cilostazol, sildenafil, and bosentan not yet available

SURGERY
- Reserved for refractory cases
- Digital sympathectomy is the most common procedure performed, but endoscopic thoracic sympathectomy is also used.
- Results are not as good in scleroderma-associated disease, but may have an important role in patients with Raynaud's symptoms in the feet.

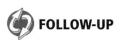 **FOLLOW-UP**

Issues for Referral
Occupational therapy may be helpful.

PROGNOSIS
- Patients with primary Raynaud's phenomenon who do not develop clinical or lab signs of an underlying disease within 2 years of the diagnosis are unlikely to develop a secondary disorder.
- In patients with secondary disease, overall prognosis follows that for the underlying disease.

COMPLICATIONS
- Severe cases can result in digital gangrene and/or ulcerations
- Digital ulcerations are at high risk of infection and should be treated aggressively, even in the absence of the usual markers of infection.
- Digital loss is rare and mainly limited to patients with scleroderma and secondary Raynaud's phenomenon.

REFERENCES
1. Block JA, Sequeira W. Raynaud's phenomenon. *Lancet*. 2001;357:2042–2048.
2. Cush JJ, Kavanaugh A, Stein MC. *Rheumatology, Diagnosis, & Therapeutics*. 2nd ed. Philadelphia: Lippincott Williams & Wilkins; 2005.
3. Hochberg MC, Silman AJ, Smolen JS, et al., eds. *Practical Rheumatology*. 3rd ed. Philadelphia: Mosby; 2004.
4. Tagliarino H, Purdon M, Jamieson B. What is the evaluation and treatment strategy for Raynaud's phenomenon? *J Fam Pract*. 2005;54:553–555.
5. Wigley FM. Raynaud's phenomenon. *N Engl J Med*. 2002;347:1001–1008.

CODES
ICD9-CM
433.0 Raynaud's phenomenon

KEY WORDS
- Vasospasm
- Cold Sensitivity
- Digital Ischemia
- Systemic Sclerosis

RHEUMATOID ARTHRITIS

Lori Lieberman-Maran, MD

KEY CLINICAL POINTS

- Multisystem autoimmune disease
  - Women in 4th and 5th decade
- Symmetric inflammatory arthritis
  - Morning stiffness >1 hour
- Early treatment with DMARDs significantly improves quality of life, morbidity, and disease progression

 BASICS

DESCRIPTION
- Rheumatoid arthritis (RA) is a chronic, multisystem, inflammatory, autoimmune disease.
- Inflammation of the joints can lead to cartilage destruction and inability to function.

EPIDEMIOLOGY
RA is a relatively common autoimmune disease.
- Females > Males (4:1)
  - Bimodal peak age of onset in women between 31–35, then after age 46

Incidence
Annual incidence of 0.2 per 1,000 males and 0.4 per 1,000 females and increases with age.

Prevalence
- Affects 1% of the United States population
  - Worldwide: 0.8% of the adults

RISK FACTORS
The following are associated with a higher incidence of RA, but not necessarily linked to causation.
- Hormonal influence
  - Nulliparity
  - Breast-feeding
- Environmental factors
  - Obesity
  - Tobacco
  - Coffee consumption

Genetics
There are some established genetic risk factors including the presence of:
- HLA-DR4, HLA-DR1
  - Twin studies have heritability of 60%.
  - Siblings have a 2-fold to 4-fold risk of developing RA.

PATHOPHYSIOLOGY
- Immune mediated disease
- CD4+ T cells induce an immune response from unknown endogenous or exogenous antigens.
- Monocytes, macrophages, and fibroblasts are recruited and produce TNF alpha and IL-1 within synovium.
- Matrix metalloproteinases and osteoclasts are then triggered, which results in joint damage.

ETIOLOGY
Unknown
RA is thought to be multifactorial with genetic and environmental factors playing a role.

ASSOCIATED CONDITIONS
There are multiple coexisting conditions associated with RA that impact prognosis. Some important ones to consider include:
- Infection: Incidence doubled in RA
- Osteoporosis: Incidence doubled in RA
- Cardiovascular disease: Accounts for most of the mortality in RA
- Malignancy: Increased 5–8 times over the rate of general population

Pregnancy Considerations
RA goes into remission during pregnancy approximately 75% of the time, but about 80% of women experience a flare postpartum.

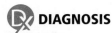 DIAGNOSIS

PRE-HOSPITAL
RA remains a clinical diagnosis, but there are supportive laboratory and radiographic findings.

SIGNS AND SYMPTOMS
Presence of symptoms for at least 6 weeks
- Symmetric, polyarthritis (>3 joints)
- MCPs, PIPs, wrists, elbows, shoulders, cervical spine, hips, knees, ankles, MTPs are affected
- Morning stiffness >1 hour
- Subcutaneous nodules

History
- Gradual onset of joint pain and swelling
- Morning stiffness >1 hour
  - Fatigue
- Inability to perform daily activities

Physical Exam
- Tenderness, warmth, and swelling of joints
- Joint effusions
- Decreased range of motion of affected joints
- Subcutaneous nodules

TESTS
Lab
- Rheumatoid Factor (RF)
  - Present in 60–85% of cases of RA, but specificity is low
  - High titer does have prognostic role and is associated with more severe disease such as erosions, subcutaneous nodules, and extra-articular manifestations
- Antibodies to cyclic citrullinated antigens (CCP)
  - Highest specificity of any antibody: 95%
  - Sensitivity: 50–70%
  - Already present in patients with very early RA and may be associated with more severe disease
- Can also see anemia of chronic disease, elevated platelet count, ESR, and CRP

Imaging
- There are some findings on plain x-ray that are suggestive of RA including:
- Fusiform soft tissue swelling
- Periarticular osteoporosis
- Erosions and cysts
- Loss of joint space

- MRI detects erosions, cysts, and effusions that may not be seen on plain x-ray.

DIFFERENTIAL DIAGNOSIS
Differential diagnosis of a patient with polyarthritis
- Inflammatory disease
  - Psoriatic Arthritis
  - Reactive Arthritis
  - Spondyloarthropathy
  - Crystal arthropathy
  - SLE
  - PMR
- Viral Infection
  - Parvovirus B19
  - Hepatitis B

TREATMENT

INITIAL STABILIZATION
Joint damage occurs early and 30% of patients have radiographic evidence of bony erosions at time of diagnosis, so early intervention is key.
- Goals are remission of symptoms
  - Return of joint function
  - Maintenance therapy

GENERAL MEASURES
There is no cure for RA, but there are several measures available to help improve patient's quality of life using a multidisciplinary approach.

Activity
Most patients with RA can participate in moderate intensity aerobic exercise.

SPECIAL THERAPY
Physical Therapy
There are several modalities that can provide relief.
- Flexibility, range of motion, and aerobic exercise are all useful.
  - Joint protection and energy conservation
  - Splinting of hands or wrists or use of lower extremity orthotics can provide temporary pain relief.

Complementary and Alternative Therapies
Patient education is a proven effective intervention in RA
Local Arthritis Foundation chapter has information

MEDICATION (DRUGS)

3 categories: Nonsteroidal antiinflammatory (NSAIDs), corticosteroids, disease modifying antirheumatic drugs (DMARDs)

First Line
DMARDs
- Should be started within 3 months after onset of symptoms
- Methotrexate (MTX) is considered the first line unless contraindicated
  - Should not be used in patients with underlying liver disease or history of heavy alcohol use
  - Concomitant use of folic acid (1–3 mg/day) significantly decreases side effects
  - Aminotransferase, albumin, and CBC should be monitored every 8 weeks
- Leflunomide: Similar to MTX; long half life
  - Adverse effects include: Myelosuppression and hepatic fibrosis and should monitor CBC, AST, ALT, albumin every 8 weeks

- Sulfasalazine: Safe to use in patients with liver disease
  - Adverse effects include: Myelosuppression; CBC monitored every 2 weeks for first 3 months, then every 3 months
- Hydroxychloroquine: Very well tolerated, effective in mild RA or in combination therapy
  - Adverse effects include: Macular changes therefore patients should have funduscopic examination every year
- Biologic response modifiers: Tumor necrosis factor (TNF) antagonists
  - Etanercept: Soluble TNF-receptor fusion protein
  - Infliximab: Chimeric IgG anti-TNF alpha antibody
  - Adalimumab: Recombinant human IgG monoclonal antibody
  - These drugs appear to be the most effective treatments for RA, but they are costly and have several side effects to consider.
  - Adverse effects of these drugs include: Increased rate of infections, lymphoma, lupus–like autoimmune disease, multiple sclerosis-like demyelinating disease, and worsening of heart failure

Pregnancy Considerations
- MTX is contraindicated in pregnancy: Recommended to discontinue at least 3 months prior to conception
- Leflunomide is contraindicated in pregnancy and should be discontinued 2 years prior to conception, because of its long half-life.
  - The mother can undergo treatment with cholestyramine to bind the drug.

Second Line
- NSAIDs
  - Useful in the first few weeks of symptoms for relief of pain and stiffness
  - Do not slow progression of disease
  - Should be used with DMARD in maintenance therapy
- Corticosteroids
  - Can be used to bridge the effect of DMARD, but should not be used alone
  - All patients should receive supplemental calcium (1–1.5 gm/day) and vitamin D (800 IU/day) while receiving corticosteroids

SURGERY
- There are several surgical procedures for selected patients with severe RA.
- Tenosynovectomy
- Tendon reconstruction
- Joint synovectomy
- Peripheral nerve decompression
- Joint fusion or replacement

 FOLLOW-UP

Patients with RA should be followed frequently to monitor toxicities of medical management and disease progression.

DISPOSITION
Issues for Referral
Referral to a Rheumatologist is crucial so that proper diagnosis is made and early DMARD therapy is initiated within 3 months after the onset of symptoms.

PROGNOSIS
Prognosis has greatly improved with early therapy with DMARDs and newer agents, but there is still significant morbidity associated with RA. Some poor prognostic indicators include:
- Early presence of bony erosions

- Extraarticular features
- Older age at onset,
- Positive RF and anti-CCP antibodies
- Genetic factors such as presence of HLA-DR epitopes
- The long-term prognosis and survival also depends on addressing the coexisting conditions as discussed.

COMPLICATIONS
- Tendon rupture: Most common
- Synovial rupture of knee
- Entrapment neuropathies
- Septic arthritis
- Instability of cervical spine
- Osteoporosis

REFERENCES

1. Choy E, Panayi G. Cytokine pathways and joint inflammation in rheumatoid arthritis. *N Engl J Med*. 2001;344:907–916.
2. Harrison M. Young women with chronic disease: A female perspective on the impact and management of rheumatoid arthritis. *Arthritis Rheum*. 2003;49:846–852.
3. Hochberg M, Silman A, Smolen J, et al., eds. *Rheumatology*. 3rd ed. Edinburgh: Mosby; 2003.
4. O'Dell J. Therapeutic strategies for rheumatoid arthritis. *N Engl J Med*. 2004;350:2591–2602.
5. Olsen N, Stein C. New drugs for rheumatoid arthritis. *N Engl J Med*. 2004;350:2167–2179.

 MISCELLANEOUS

CODES
ICD9-CM
714.0

KEY WORDS

- Rheumatoid Arthritis
- Autoimmune Disease

SCLERODERMA

Mohsin K. Malik, MD
Lynn E. Iler, MD

KEY CLINICAL POINTS

- Scleroderma may be systemic and life-threatening or localized to the skin.
- Treatments are limited and prognosis depends on the degree of involvement.
- An increased risk of malignancy, especially lung cancer, is associated with scleroderma.

 BASICS

DESCRIPTION

- Scleroderma is an autoimmune disease with unknown etiology.
- Scleroderma is a disorder of microvasculature, small arteries, and connective tissue marked by excessive production of extracellular matrix.
- Clinical hallmark of scleroderma is the presence of thickened, sclerotic "bound-down" skin.
- There is a heterogeneous spectrum of disease manifestation, ranging from limited skin involvement to gastrointestinal, pulmonary, renal, cardiac, and other systemic involvement.
  - Gastrointestinal involvement most commonly manifests with esophageal hypomotility, but any part of the GI tract may be involved.
  - Pulmonary involvement includes interstitial lung disease and pulmonary hypertension.
  - Renal involvement has a wide range of severity and includes end-stage renal disease as well as acute-onset renal failure.
  - Cardiac involvement includes myocardial disease, conduction system abnormalities, arrhythmias, and pericardial disease.
- Scleroderma can be divided into localized and systemic forms.
  - Localized scleroderma has skin involvement.
  - Systemic scleroderma further divided into
    - Diffuse cutaneous scleroderma (dcSSc): Rapid onset, multiorgan system involvement
    - Limited cutaneous scleroderma (lcSSc): Gradual onset, prominent vascular involvement +/– CREST (see below)
    - Scleroderma sine scleroderma: Less common, systemic involvement without skin involvement

EPIDEMIOLOGY

- Female > Male (4:1)
  - Among females 35–44, there is a 9:1 female predominance
- Typical onset 30–60 years of age
- The black:white ratio is 1.2:1 overall
  - Among young black women, the black:white ratio is as high as 10:1

Incidence
The incidence rate is 19 per million adults.

Prevalence
- 240 to 270 per million adults
- Prevalence is as high as 400 per million population among females 35–65

RISK FACTORS

- There is a 10-fold to 20-fold higher risk in siblings and 1st-degree relatives of patients with scleroderma.
- Genetics
- Several human leukocyte antigens have been associated with scleroderma. The strongest association is with HLA DRB1*11.

PATHOPHYSIOLOGY

Incompletely understood but involves a sequence of 3 major events:
- Endothelial damage of capillaries and arterioles caused by
  - Antiendothelial antibodies
  - Inappropriate production and response to vasoregulatory molecules
- Immune activation resulting from endothelial damage
  - Leukocyte recruitment and release of growth factors and cytokines
  - Fibroblasts with abnormal phenotype activated
- Increased extracellular matrix deposited by abnormal fibroblasts

ETIOLOGY

Possible contributing factors include:
- Environmental triggers
  - Exposure to silica, vibration, silicone breast implants, or organic solvents has not been consistently implicated.
  - Scleroderma-like syndromes have been reported with exposure to vinyl chloride and rapeseed oil contaminated with aniline and acetanilide.
- Genetics
- Infectious agents, such as cytomegalovirus or borrelia burgdorferi, have been implicated, but not consistently.
- Drugs (bleomycin, cocaine, pentazocine) can cause scleroderma-like syndromes
- Microchimerism (persistence of fetal cells following pregnancy or persistence of maternal cells that cross the placenta) have not been consistently implicated.

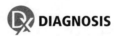 **DIAGNOSIS**

SIGNS AND SYMPTOMS

- Localized scleroderma presents with skin changes only and is not associated with Raynaud's phenomenon.
- Systemic scleroderma classified into 2 main subsets, but can be overlap between the subsets
  - dcSSc
    - Tends to have an abrupt onset of Raynaud's phenomenon along with nonpitting edema of the hands, face, and feet.
    - Constitutional symptoms may be present.
    - Tends to be early involvement of gastrointestinal, renal, and pulmonary systems
  - lcSSc
    - Tends to begin with Raynaud's phenomenon that may be present for years or even decades
    - Over time, there is development of CREST symptoms
      - **C**alcium deposition in the skin (tends to develop later)
      - **R**aynaud's phenomenon persists
      - **E**sophageal dysmotility (tends to develop later)
      - **S**clerodactyly (tends to develop early)
      - **T**elangiectasia (digital and facial, tends to develop early)
    - Pulmonary hypertension usually occurs years after disease onset.
    - Interstitial lung disease and trigeminal neuralgia may also develop later in the disease course.

History
Multiorgan involvement may be present in systemic sclerosis.

SCLERODERMA

- Skin: Pruritus, edema, tightening of skin
- Vascular: Raynaud's phenomenon present in >90%; two-phase color change of fingers/toes in response to cold exposure or emotion
- Gastrointestinal: Dysphagia, gastroesophageal reflux, constipation or alternating constipation/diarrhea, fecal incontinence
- Respiratory: Dry cough, dyspnea, pleuritic chest pain
- Constitutional: Fever, weight loss
- Musculoskeletal: Arthritis, myalgia, limited range of motion

Physical Exam
- Localized scleroderma
  - Morphea
    - Indurated plaques that become white or yellow
    - Erythema may be present at the border ("lilac border")
    - Can be one or several plaques, or may become generalized
  - Linear scleroderma
    - Linear plaque on the face ("en coup de sabre") or extremities, usually solitary
- Systemic sclerosis
  - Skin
    - Sclerosis on fingers, hands, face in lcSSc
    - Sclerosis extends proximally to wrists in dcSSc and can become generalized but usually spares back and buttocks
    - Progressive sclerosis of the face gives an expressionless, mask-like facies
    - Nonpitting edema of hands, feet, or face
    - Flexion contractures
  - Renal: Hypertension
  - Cardiac: Arrhythmia, friction rub

TESTS
Lab
- Antibodies
  - Antinuclear antibodies present in >95%
  - Antitopoisomerase-I (Scl-70) antibody
    - Highly specific for systemic scleroderma
    - More often found in dcSSc than lcSSc
    - Levels correlate with disease severity and activity
  - Anticentromere antibody associated with lcSSc
  - Antinucleolar antibodies (anti–PMScl, anti–U3-RNP, anti–Th/To, anti-RNA-polymerase I and III) have low sensitivity and are of limited use in the diagnosis.
- Screen for renal disease at initial workup
  - Plasma creatinine
  - Urine protein

Imaging
Pulmonary involvement is a major cause of morbidity and mortality and should be evaluated during the initial workup:
- Doppler echocardiography
- Pulmonary function tests, including DLCO
- Chest x-ray (low sensitivity)
- High-resolution CT

Diagnostic Procedures/Surgery
- Punch biopsy of involved skin
- Esophageal involvement is common and can be evaluated using:
  - Barium swallow, esophageal manometry, pH studies
  - Esophagogastroduodenoscopy (EGD) or Esophagoscopy
- Lower gastrointestinal involvement can be evaluated with a barium enema.
- Cardiac:

- ECG (should be part of the initial work-up)
- Echocardiogram

DIFFERENTIAL DIAGNOSIS
- Overlap connective tissue disease or overlap syndrome
  - Systemic lupus erythematosus
  - Dermatomyositis
  - Rheumatoid arthritis
  - Mixed connective tissue disease
- Primary Raynaud's phenomenon
- Myxedema

 ## TREATMENT

GENERAL MEASURES
Nonpharmacologic measures to aid in the control of Raynaud's phenomenon:
- Avoidance of cold
- Use mittens or gloves
- Avoidance of stress
- Avoidance of vasoconstrictors

Physical Therapy
PT/OT for maintaining and improving the range of motion of affected joints

 ## MEDICATION (DRUGS)

- Localized scleroderma (skin involvement)
  - Topical or injected corticosteroids +/– topical calcipotriene
  - UVA Phototherapy can provide benefit in select patients
- Therapy for specific systemic involvement:
  - Raynaud's phenomenon
    - Calcium channel blockers such as nifedipine 30–60 mg daily
    - For severe disease, iloprost 2ng/kg/min IV 8 hours daily for 3 days has been used.
  - Renal disease
    - Angiotensin converting enzyme inhibitors are first-line therapy
    - Calcium channel blockers may be added.
  - Gastrointestinal
    - Proton pump inhibitors for esophageal reflux
    - Promotility agents such as cisapride or erythromycin
- Antifibrotic therapy
  - Penicillamine 125 mg alternate days to 750 mg daily has shown efficacy as a long-term agent in reducing organ system involvement and improving survival.
- Immunomosupressive therapy of limited benefit
  - Corticosteroids: Limited use because of the potential to precipitate renal crisis (acute onset of renal failure)
  - Cyclophosphamide: Efficacy uncertain, but may provide benefit in pulmonary fibrosis when combined with corticosteroids
  - Methotrexate: May provide some improvement in skin disease
  - Cyclosporin: Use limited by nephrotoxicity

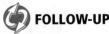 ## FOLLOW-UP

PROGNOSIS
- Localized scleroderma
  - Unpredictable course lasting months to years

– Lesions tend to stabilize after initial presentation and may improve
– Progressive disease has been described
- Systemic scleroderma
  – Mean survival of 11 years from time of diagnosis, but large variations exist
  – Overall survival is 78% at 5 years, 55% at 10 years
  – Female patients have better overall survival than male patients
  – dcSSc has worse prognosis than lcSSc, but difference not as great as previously reported
  – Visceral involvement portends a worse prognosis, especially
    • Renal involvement (impacts short- and long-term survival)
    • Pulmonary hypertension

COMPLICATIONS
- Renal crisis is a leading cause of death.
  – Marked by rapidly progressive renal failure, arterial hypertension, and increased plasma renin activity
  – Occurs in up to 20%, usually in first 4 years
  – Angiotensin converting enzyme inhibitors are the first-line therapy; their use has increased the 9-year survival to nearly 70%.
- Malignancy
  – Increased risk, especially with dcSSc
  – Greatest increase in lung cancer, but breast and bladder also increased

Pregnancy Considerations
- Pregnancy should be managed as high-risk
- Conflicting reports of increased infertility and spontaneous miscarriage associated
- Increased incidence of premature birth and low birth weight

PATIENT MONITORING
- Because of progressive organ system involvement, regular monitoring is warranted based on the individual clinical picture
  – Blood pressure
  – Serum creatinine, urine protein
  – Raynaud's phenomenon
  – ECG
  – Pulmonary function testing
  – High resolution chest CT

- Given increased risk of malignancy, ongoing high index of suspicion for lung cancer
  – Age-appropriate cancer screening

REFERENCES

1. Arnett FC, Cho M, Chatterjee S, et al. Familial occurrence frequencies and relative risks for systemic sclerosis (scleroderma) in three United States cohorts. *Arthritis Rheum*. 2001;44:1359–1362.
2. Hill CL, Nguyen AM, Roder D, et al. Risk of cancer in patients with scleroderma: A population based cohort study. *Ann Rheum Dis*. 2003;62:728–731.
3. Hu PQ, Fertig N, Medsger TA Jr, et al. Correlation of serum anti-DNA topoisomerase I antibody levels with disease severity and activity in systemic sclerosis. *Arthritis Rheum*. 2003;48:1363–1373.
4. Lawrence RC, Helmick CG, Arnett FC, et al. Estimates of the prevalence of arthritis and selected musculoskeletal disorders in the United States. *Arthritis Rheum*. 1998;41:778–799.
5. Mayes MD, Lacey JV Jr, Beebe-Dimmer J, et al. Prevalence, incidence, survival, and disease characteristics of systemic sclerosis in a large US population. *Arthritis Rheum*. 2003;48:2246–2255.
6. Steen VD, Medsger TA Jr. Severe organ involvement in systemic sclerosis with diffuse scleroderma. *Arthritis Rheum*. 2000;43:2437–2444.
7. Steen VD, Oddis CV, Conte CG, et al. Incidence of systemic sclerosis in Allegheny County, Pennsylvania. A twenty-year study of hospital-diagnosed cases, 1963–1982. *Arthritis Rheum*. 1997;40:441–445.

CODES
ICD9-CM
- 701.0 Circumscribed (localized) scleroderma
- 710.1 Systemic sclerosis (scleroderma)

KEY WORDS

- Scleroderma
- Morphea
- Raynaud's Phenomenon
- CREST
- Sclerodactyly

SEXUAL ASSAULT AND ABUSE

Ricardo Restrepo-Guzman, MD
Lidia Trejo, MA

KEY CLINICAL POINTS

- Sexual assault is a common occurrence in the United States.
- It is often associated with subsequent post-traumatic stress disorder (PTSD).
- Physicians face a complex set of medical, psychological, social, and legal issues when treating sexual assault victims and must always consider a multidisciplinary treatment approach.

 ## BASICS

DESCRIPTION

- Sexual assault includes any type of sexual contact, regardless of marital status or sexual orientation, between 2 or more individuals in which 1 of those individuals is involved against his or her will.
- Sexual assault can be verbal, visual, physical, or anything that forces a person to join in unwanted sexual contact or attention.
- The force used by the aggressor can be either physical or nonphysical.
- Sexual assault includes, but is not limited to, stranger assault, acquaintance or date rape, marital rape, and multiple assailants or gang rape.

EPIDEMIOLOGY

Contrary to popular belief, sexual assault does not typically occur between strangers.

Prevalence

According to the National Crime Victimization Survey, conducted by Department of Justice:

- Of the sexually assaulted women: 75% were attacked by husband, partner, friend, or date.
- In United States, a woman is raped every 6 minutes; a woman is battered every 15 seconds.
- Approximately 13–17% of women living in the United States are victims of completed rape; 14% are victims of another form of sexual assault.
- 1 of 5 women has been sexually assaulted by the time she reaches the age of 21.
- Of female victims: 68% are <18 years old
- Only 17% of all known victims seek immediate attention in emergency rooms
  - Hesitation to report assault because it is such a personal and painful experience
  - In 40–60% of sexual assaults, patient does not have visible physical injuries.
  - Lifetime prevalence of PTSD twice as high in women (10.4% versus 5%)
    - Prevalence in women with trauma twice as high than in men (20.4% versus. 8.2%)

ASSOCIATED CONDITIONS

- PTSD
- Psychiatric comorbidity with PTSD: Major depressive disorder and suicidal thoughts, adjustment disorder, other anxiety disorders, substance abuse, sleep disorders, eating disorders, sexual dysfunction, somatization disorders, personality disorder related with childhood sexual abuse
- Sexually transmitted diseases (STDs)

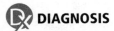 ## DIAGNOSIS

SIGNS AND SYMPTOMS

- PTSD (DSM IV-TR)
  - The person has been exposed to a traumatic event in which both of following are present:
    - Person has experienced, witnessed, or been confronted with event(s) that involve actual or threatened death or serious injury, or a threat to the physical integrity of oneself or others.
    - Person's response involved intense fear, helplessness, or horror. Children may have disorganized or agitated behavior.
  - Re-experiencing symptoms (must have ≥1)
    - Recurrent, intrusive memories of trauma
    - Recurrent, distressing dreams of trauma
    - Sense of reliving the experience (flashbacks)
    - Intense emotional distress at exposure to trauma reminders
    - Physiological response (e.g., increased heart rate or sweating) at exposure to trauma reminders
  - Avoidance and numbing symptoms (Must have 1 of first 2 and 1 other)
    - Efforts to avoid thoughts or feelings related to the trauma
    - Efforts to avoid people, places, or activities related to the trauma
    - Inability to recall important aspects of trauma
    - Decreased interest in activities
    - Detachment from others
    - Restricted range of affect (e.g., unable to have loving feelings)
    - Sense of having a foreshortened future
  - Increased arousal symptoms (must have ≥2)
    - Sleep disturbance
    - Irritability or outbursts of anger
    - Difficulty concentrating
    - Hypervigilance
    - Exaggerated startle response
  - Duration of the disturbance is ≥1 month.
    - Acute: If duration of symptoms is <3 months
    - Chronic: If duration of symptoms ≥3 months
    - Without delay onset: If onset of symptoms at least 6 months after the stressor
  - Disturbance causes clinically significant distress or impairment in social, work, or other important areas of functioning.
- Rape Trauma Syndrome (RTS)
  - Trauma response specific to rape survivor
  - RTS belongs to broader category of PTSD
  - 3 phases that can disrupt physical, social psychological, sexual aspects of victim's life
    - 1. Acute: May last days to weeks after assault
      - Basic response styles usually include 2 types: Expressed and controlled.
      - About 1/2 of rape victims readily demonstrate feelings and will express fear, anger, restlessness, and agitation.
      - The other 1/2 maintain composure and appear calm or subdued; these victims may be shocked or embarrassed.
      - Other symptoms: Revival of other crisis memories/retriggering, anxiety, guilt or self-blame, poor

concentration, confusion, isolation, sleeping or eating disorders
- 2. Reorganization or Denial:
  - May last several weeks or years
  - Victim tries to move to a renewed sense of equilibrium
  - May deny feelings about the rape and be disinterested in talking about it
  - Work to return life back to normal
- 3. Reoccurrence:
  - Feelings from the time of the assault re-emerge and can occur any time after the assault.
  - Feelings can be triggered by many life events, such as puberty, marriage, new sexual relationship, or the birth of a child.
  - Flashbacks, anxiety, anger, depression, and nightmares
- Acute Stress Disorder
  - Characterized by symptoms similar to PTSD
  - Symptoms occur <1 month after exposure, lasts at least 2 days, but not >4 weeks
  - See DSM-IV TR for full diagnostic criteria

TESTS
- Pregnancy test
- Screening for STDs: HIV, chlamydia, syphilis, gonorrhea, trichomonas, hepatitis B and C

 TREATMENT

INITIAL STABILIZATION
- Airway, breathing and circulation
- Basic elements necessary in the care of the victim:
  - Create a safe environment.
  - Place the patient in a quiet and private area.
  - Do not leave the patient alone.
  - Speak quietly and move slowly.
  - Ask permission to perform clinical procedures.
  - Prepare a secure and safe interview setting, which will facilitate the gathering of informed consent, medical/sexual history, and the physical exam.
  - Gather history slowly moving from general to more precise questions.
  - Be aware of retraumatization of and different emotional expressions of trauma in victim
  - Be aware and considerate of the unique situations presented by minority groups: Children, elderly chronically mentally ill, individuals with developmental disabilities, ethnic minorities, lesbian, bisexual and/or transgendered individuals, commercial sex providers, substance abusers, and the homeless.
- Physical examination
  - Only 1 exam to be completed within 72 hours of assault in order for it to be legally valid
  - Can be completed regardless of whether the victim has showered, bathed, douched, changed clothing, brushed teeth, etc.
  - 2 purposes: Medical and forensic
    - Good documentation is essential
    - Document all injuries thoroughly.
    - Physician can make use of writing, diagrams, sketches, body maps, or photographs.
- Collection of evidence
  - Clinicians should be familiar with the requirements in their community.
  - To collect evidence, each state uses a "rape kit."

- Rape kits contain laboratory and exam forms and materials for clinical samples.
- Organized to maintain the chain of evidence
- Anticipate the need to duplicate samples or to perform medical procedures at the same time that the evidence is collected.
- Most states require physician reporting of sexual assault by notifying local police.

SPECIAL THERAPY
- Psychotherapeutic Treatments
  - Psychological debriefing (PD): A single-session, semistructured crisis intervention designed to reduce and prevent unwanted psychological sequelae of traumatic events by promoting emotional processing through the ventilation and normalization of reactions and the preparation for possible future experiences
- Cognitive and Behavioral Treatments:
  - Strongest empirical support for efficacy with PTSD symptoms
  - May be most effective for addressing the avoidance symptom cluster of PTSD
  - Victims can greatly benefit from cognitive therapy, especially in dealing with self-blame, anxiety, and sleep disturbances.
  - Cognitive-behavioral treatments include education regarding the nature of PTSD, exposure and response prevention to memories of trauma, stress inoculation, and challenging cognitions that may be fixed
  - Cognitive processing therapy
    - Variant of cognitive-behavioral therapy specifically designed for treatment of PTSD after sexual assault
    - Focuses on issues of safety, trust, power, control, esteem, and intimacy
    - Attempts to change irrational/faulty beliefs, expectations, appraisals, and attributions
- Eye Movement Desensitization and Reprocessing
  - Patient elicits sequences of large-magnitude, rhythmic saccadic eye movements while holding in mind most salient aspects of traumatic memory
  - Results in a lasting reduction of anxiety
  - Cognitive assessment of memory is changed
  - Frequency of flashbacks, intrusive thoughts, and sleep disturbances decreases
- Group therapy
  - Effects very beneficial for rape victims
  - Many rape crisis centers are based on crisis theory and supportive group psychotherapy.
  - Rely on dissemination of information, active listening, and emotional support.
  - Group sharing of the experience may affect numbness, isolation, fear of isolation, and significantly improve fear and anxiety.
- Hypnosis
  - Victims may find relief of fears, feelings of helplessness, anxiety, and social isolation
  - Feminist self-hypnosis helps to remove false sense of guilt and enables understanding of social context in which assault occurred
- Family/couple therapy
  - Because the reaction of the significant others is often to blame and even to reject the victim, family members can also participate in therapy.
  - Frequent responses by partners and parents are feelings of helplessness, anger, frustration, and homicidal fantasies toward the rapist.

– Beneficial to participate in therapy in order to reorganize and rectify the family's integrity
• Humanistic approach
  – Should be taken across all possible therapies
  – Patient needs understanding, acceptance, and support from the therapist.
  – Client-centered therapy helps the victim express herself, consider different responses, and choose the most appropriate treatment modality.

 ## MEDICATION (DRUGS)

• STD Prophylaxis:
  – Always offer HIV and STD prophylaxis as ~50% do not return for follow-up care.
  – Physicians should be familiar with the local laws regarding the reporting of STDs.
  – Centers for Disease Control (CDC) recommends prophylaxis/treatment for:
    • Chlamydia
      ○ Azithromycin: 1 g PO × single dose
      ○ Do not give to pregnant women.
    • Gonorrhea
      ○ Ceftriaxone: 125–250 mg IM single dose
      ○ May also treat incubating syphilis
    • Trichomoniasis
      ○ Metronidazole: 2 g PO, single dose
      ○ Do not administer to pregnant women.
      ○ Also treats giardia lambia and entamoeba histolytica, which are transmitted anally.
    • Hepatitis B Immunoglobulin (HBIG)
      ○ Can be used as immunization against Hep B and as a postexposure prophylaxis
      ○ A single dose (0.06 mL/kg IM) should be given at the acute care visit.
      ○ More effective within 14 days of exposure
    • HIV: Always test in cases of sexual assault. Repeat testing in 6 months and 1 year (see HIV chapter for medications).
• Pregnancy Prophylaxis
  – Provide counseling for pregnancy prevention
  – Inform victim about risks and interventions
  – Test to rule out a preexisting pregnancy.
  – Levonorgestrel: 0.75 mg PO q12hours × 2 doses
    • Approximately 98% effective if within 24 hours of assault
      ○ Recommended within 72 hours
      ○ Failure rate 1%, with potential teratogenicity in case of pregnancy.
      ○ Common side effect: Nausea/vomiting
• Psychopharmacological treatment for PTSD:
  – Selective serotonin reuptake inhibitor (SSRI): First line treatment. Medications approved by FDA for PTSD:
    • Sertraline (Zoloft):
      ○ Start at 25 mg every morning to improve tolerability.
      ○ Usual daily adult dose 50–200 mg every morning
    • Paroxetine (Paxil):
      ○ Start at 10 mg every morning to improve tolerability
      ○ Usual daily adult dose 10–50 mg every morning

• Other SSRIs could be considered
  ○ Most frequent side effects: Dyskinesia, headache, gastrointestinal discomfort, weakness, sexual dysfunction
– Other antidepressants that may be useful:
  • Selective norepinephrine reuptake inhibitors (SNRIs)
  • Tricyclic antidepressants (TCAs)
  • Monoamino oxidase inhibitor (MAOI)
– Other medications that can be considered with psychiatrist feedback:
  • Second generation antipsychotic
  • Mood stabilizers/anticonvulsants
  • Adrenergic-inhibiting agents
– Benzodiazepines: Not effective for PTSD
  • Should be considered as augmentation in acute phase of illness
  • Use cautiously for hyperarousal

 ## FOLLOW-UP

Issues for Referral
To mental health provider for counseling

REFERENCES

1. American Psychiatric Association. *DSM-IV-TR*, Washington, DC: American Psychiatric Press; 2000.
2. Davidson J, Jobson KO. Psychiatric Annals: Posttraumatic Stress Disorder. 2005;35.
3. Romans SE, Seeman MV. Women's Mental Health: A Life Cycle Approach. *Post-Traumatic Stress Disorder*. 1st ed. Philadelphia: Lippincott; 2006:221–235.
4. Schnicke M, Resick PA. *Cognitive Processing Therapy for Rape Victims: A Treatment Manual*. Newbury Park, CA: Sage Publications; 1993.
5. Solomon SD, Johnson DM. Psychosocial treatment of posttraumatic stress disorder: A practice-friendly review of outcome research. *J Clin Psychol*. 2002;58:947–959.

ADDITIONAL READING

www.rainn.org
www.healthywomen.org
www.4woman.gov
www.ama-assn.org

CODES
ICD9-CM
• E960.1 Rape
• V70.4 Examination for medicolegal reasons
  – V71.6 Assault
  – V71.5 Rape

KEY WORDS

• Sexual Assault
• Sexual Abuse
• Rape
• Post-Traumatic Stress Disorder (PTSD)

SEXUAL DYSFUNCTION

Sybil Cineas, MD
Traci Wolbrink, MD

KEY CLINICAL POINTS

- Female sexual dysfunction (FSD) is highly prevalent.
- Multiple medical, physiological, psychological, and social factors may contribute to FSD.
- Evaluation should focus on identification of illness or factor contributing to FSD.
- Referral to a sexual therapist should be considered especially when there is a history of sexual abuse.

BASICS

DESCRIPTION

- FSD can be defined as disturbance in sexual functioning involving one or multiple phases of the sexual response cycle or pain associated with sexual activity, which results in personal distress.
- The phases of the sexual response cycles have been described in the DSM-IV-TR as desire, excitement, orgasm, and resolution.
- The current classification of sexual dysfunction is based on the first 3 phases of this cycle.
- An international committee convened by the American Foundation of Urological Disease has recommended to revise and to expand the definition of women's sexual dysfunction to include the highly contextual nature of women's sexuality and the tendency of sexual response phases to overlap.
- The current DSM-IV-TR definitions, which do not reflect these recommendations, are used in this chapter.
- FSD includes:
  - Hypoactive sexual desire disorder (HSDD)
  - Sexual aversion disorder
  - Female sexual arousal disorder (FSAD)
  - Female orgasmic disorder (FOD)
- Sexual pain disorders
  - Dyspareunia
  - Vaginismus

Prevalence

The overall prevalence of sexual dysfunction is 43% in women.

- Low sexual desire: 22%
- Arousal problems: 14%
- Sexual pain: 7%

RISK FACTORS

- Neurological disease
  - Stroke
  - Spinal cord injury
  - Parkinsonism
- Genital atrophy
- Genital surgery
- Endocrinopathies
  - Diabetes
  - Hyperprolactinemia
  - Liver and/or renal failure
- Peripheral vascular disease
- Sexual abuse
- Psychological factors, life stressors

- Interpersonal, relationship disorders
- Medications (most common):
  - Selective Serotonin Reuptake Inhibitor (SSRI)
  - Oral contraceptive pills (OCPs)
  - Antihistamines
  - Antihypertensives
  - Anticonvulsants
  - Anticholinergics
  - Drugs of Abuse

PATHOPHYSIOLOGY

- The phases of the sexual response cycle as described in DSM-IV-TR are:
  - Desire: Fantasies about sexual activity and the desire to have sexual activity
  - Excitement: Subjective sense of sexual pleasure and accompanying physiological changes, which consist of pelvic vasocongestion, vaginal lubrication, and expansion and swelling of external genitalia
  - Orgasm: The peaking of sexual pleasure with release of tension and rhythmic contraction of the perineal muscles and contractions of the wall of outer third of vagina.
  - Resolution: Sense of muscular relaxation and general well being
- Disorder of the sexual response may occur at one or more of the phases.
  - Vasculogenic
  - Neurogenic
  - Musculogenic
  - Psychogenic
  - Hormonal alterations may interfere with the phases of the sexual response cycle.

ETIOLOGY

Multiple medical, physiological, psychological, and social factors may contribute to FSD.

ASSOCIATED CONDITIONS

Sexual dysfunction may be associated with mood disorders and anxiety disorders.

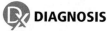 DIAGNOSIS

DSM-IV-TR definitions:

- These disorders may be due to psychological factors or due to combined factors (when a general medical condition or substance use contributes to condition but is not sufficient to account for dysfunction).
- DSM-IV-TR definitions are listed below.
- All disorders cause marked distress or interpersonal difficulty.
- **HSDD**
  - The persistent or recurrent absence of sexual fantasies and desire for sexual activity
- **Sexual Aversion Disorder**
  - Persistent or recurrent aversion to and avoidance of genital sexual contact with a sexual partner
  - May occur with other sexual dysfunction such as dyspareunia
- **FSAD**
  - The persistent or recurrent inability to attain or maintain an adequate response of sexual excitement.

- The response consists of pelvic vasocongestion, vaginal lubrication, and swelling of the external genitalia.
- **FOD**
  - The persistent or recurrent delay in or absence of orgasm following a normal sexual excitement phase.
  - FOD may occur in association with FSAD.
- **Vaginismus**
  - The recurrent or persistent involuntary contractions of the outer third of the vagina as a result of attempted vaginal penetration with penis, finger, tampon, or speculum.
- **Dyspareunia**
  - Genital pain that is associated with sexual intercourse
  - The disturbance is not caused exclusively by lack of lubrication or vaginismus.

SIGNS AND SYMPTOMS
- Low desire/libido
- Avoidance of sexual activity
- Involuntary contraction of outer vagina
- Vaginal dryness
- Fear of genital contact
- Anorgasmia
- Genital pain

History
- Few women volunteer a history of FSD. Ask open questions during the gynecological review of systems such as:
  - "Do you have any sexual concerns that you would like to discuss?"
  - "Are you currently involved in a sexual relationship with men, women, or both?"
  - "Do you have difficulty with desire, genital or subjective arousal, or orgasm?"
- The history should focus on:
  - Past psychosexual development
  - Current social context (relationship quality, sources of stress)
  - Medical factors including medical illness, surgical history, substance use, and medications
- Ask about a history of sexual or psychological abuse.
- When a dysfunction is identified, clarify whether the dysfunction is:
  - Present (lifelong) or acquired
  - Situational (e.g., with certain types of situations, positions or partners) or generalized

Physical Exam
- Physical examination should focus on signs of general illness and endocrinopathies.
- A thorough pelvic examination should be performed.
  - Inspection of external genitalia
  - Speculum exam
  - Bimanual
  - Abdominal exam
  - A rectovaginal exam to rule out endometriosis

TESTS
Lab
Endocrine evaluation for appropriate patients:
- FSH
- LH
- Estradiol
- DHEAS
- Total testosterone, free testosterone
- Prolactin

DIFFERENTIAL DIAGNOSIS
- HSDD
- FSAD
- FOD
- Dyspareunia
- Vaginismus
- Sexual dysfunction due to a general medical condition
- Substance-induced sexual dysfunction
- Major depressive disorder
- HSDD must be distinguished from dysfunction due to hormonal or endocrine abnormalities such as abnormalities in bioavailable testosterone and prolactin, which may be responsible for loss of sexual desire.
- FSAD must be distinguished from dysfunction due to reduction in estrogen levels such as in menopause, atrophic vaginitis, diabetes mellitus, lactation, and pelvic radiotherapy.
- Orgasmic dysfunction is commonly found in women with spinal cord lesions or in those who have had removal of the vulva or vaginal excision and reconstruction. It is also a common complaint in women receiving SSRIs for the treatment of depression.
- Genital pain may be due to insufficient lubrication, UTI, endometriosis, adhesions, atrophic vaginitis, or gastrointestinal conditions.
- Vaginismus may be due to endometriosis or vaginal infection. It may also occur as a result of sexual trauma.

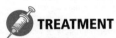

TREATMENT

INITIAL STABILIZATION
- Educate the patient and partner regarding normal anatomy and physiologic response as well as normal physiologic changes that occur with aging and with health problems.
- Encourage open communication between the patient and partner.
- Avoid prescription medications or taper or change medications likely to contribute to FSD.
- Treat underlying medical and psychiatric conditions.

GENERAL MEASURES
- Stop smoking tobacco and drinking alcohol.
- Exercise may improve general sense of well being and body image.

SPECIAL THERAPY
- Psychotherapy for primary sexual disorders both individual and couples therapy.
- A vacuum clitoral device has been approved by the FDA for the treatment of arousal and orgasm disorders.

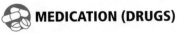

MEDICATION (DRUGS)

- Sildenafil
  - Has been reported to reverse FSD associated with SSRIs
  - Not, however, FDA approved for the treatment of women
- Estrogen replacement therapy may be helpful in postmenopausal women to treat vaginal atrophy and reduce pain with intercourse.
  - Systemic: Conjugated estrogen 0.3 mg every day alone or in combination with medroxyprogesterone 1.5 mg every day if uterus present. Adjust dose based on response
  - Local: Conjugated estrogen cream 0.625 mg/g, 0.5 gm intravaginally for 3 weeks followed by 1–2 times per week for maintenance

– Topical therapy may be preferable as systemic estrogen may increase sex hormone binding globulin (SHBG) and, thereby, reduce bioavailable testosterone, leading to further dysfunction.
– See the Complications section
• Testosterone replacement
– May be helpful in patients with known androgen deficiency from premature ovarian failure or menopausal states.
– A transdermal preparation of 300 mcg/day has been studied in clinical trials.
– Currently, there are no FDA approved preparations for use in women.

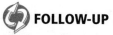 **FOLLOW-UP**

DISPOSITION
• Once a sexual dysfunction is identified upon a clinical visit, it may be necessary for the patient to return at a later time to complete a full sexual assessment.
• A visit with the patient's partner may also be helpful.
• Follow-up will depend on whether a contributing factor or medical illness is identified or treatment is pursued.

Issues for Referral
Indications for referral to a sex therapist:
• Long-standing dysfunction
• Multiple sexual dysfunctions
• Comorbid psychological disorders such as depression, anxiety, substance abuse
• Marital problems
• History of sexual abuse
• Lack of response to pharmacotherapies

COMPLICATIONS
• Testosterone replacement may have associated risks:
– Hepatic disease
– Adverse effect on lipids
– Polycythemia
– Acne
– Alopecia
• Prolonged estrogen/progestin use may increase the risk of CHD, stroke, invasive breast cancer, PE, and DVT in postmenopausal women.
• Estrogen therapy may increase the risk of stroke.

PATIENT MONITORING
Lipid profiles should be measured every 3 months in women receiving testosterone replacement.

REFERENCES
1. American Psychiatric Association. *Diagnostic and Statistical Manual of Mental Disorders*. 4th ed. Washington, DC: American Psychiatric Association; 2000:535–565.
2. Basson R. Women's sexual dysfunction: Revised and expanded definitions. *CMAJ*. 2005;172:1327–1333.
3. Laumann EO, Paik A, Rosen RC. Sexual dysfunction in the United States: Prevalence and predictors. *JAMA*. 1999;281:537–544.
4. Lightner DJ. Female sexual dysfunction. *Mayo Clin Proc*. 2002;77:698–702.
5. Berman JR, Bassuk J. Physiology and pathophysiology of female sexual function and dysfunction. *World J Urol*. 2002;20:111–118.
6. Available at: http://www.femalesexualdysfunctiononline.org.

CODES
ICD9-CM
• 302.71 Female hypoactive sexual desire disorder
• 302.79 Sexual aversion disorder
• 302.72 Female sexual arousal disorder
• 302.73 Female orgasmic disorder
• 302.76 Dyspareunia
• 306.51 Vaginismus
• 625.8 Other female sexual dysfunction

KEY WORDS
• Sexual Desire
• Libido
• Sexual Abuse
• Dyspareunia
• Vaginismus
• Anorgasmia

S

SEXUALLY TRANSMITTED INFECTIONS

Jennifer G. Clarke, MD, MPH

KEY CLINICAL POINTS

This chapter focuses on STIs not discussed elsewhere (herpes, syphilis, chancroid, granuloma inguinale, lymphogronuloma venereum, and human papillomavirus infections) and general approaches to prevention, screening, diagnosis, and treatment.

 BASICS

DESCRIPTION

STIs can be delineated into 4 categories:

- Diseases characterized by ulcerative and nonulcerative lesions: Herpes, syphilis, chancroid, granuloma inguinale, lymphogranuloma venereum, and human papillomavirus infections
- Diseases characterized by cervicitis: *C. trachomatis* and *N. gonorrhoeae*
- Diseases characterized by vaginal discharge: *T. vaginalis*, *C. trachomatis*, and *N. gonorrhoeae* (*G. vaginalis*, *Candida albicans* not STDs)
- Systemic diseases: HIV, hepatitis A, hepatitis B, and hepatitis C

RISK FACTORS

- Sexually active:
  - Oral, anal, or vaginal sexual contact
  - No or inconsistent use of male or female condom
  - Women <25 years
  - Women with new or more than 1 sexual partner
  - History of a prior STI
  - Illicit drug use
- Sexual assault

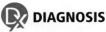 **DIAGNOSIS**

SIGNS AND SYMPTOMS

Herpes

- A recurrent, life-long viral infection
- Genital HSV-2 is more common than HSV-1.
- HSV-2 is more likely than HSV-1 to cause recurrent infections.
- Most persons with HSV-2 have not been diagnosed.
- The virus is often shed in asymptomatic periods.
- Typically painful multiple vesicular or ulcerative lesions.

Syphilis

- Primary: Ulcer or chancre
- Secondary: Rash, lymphadenopathy, and mucocutaneous lesions
- Tertiary: Cardiac, ophthalmic, auditory abnormalities, and gummatous lesions
- Latent syphilis is seroreactivity without clinical evidence of disease
- All should be tested for HIV

Chancroid

- In the United States, 10% coinfected with *T. pallidum* or HSV
- It is a cofactor for HIV transmission.
- Caused by *Haemophilus ducreyi*
- Difficult to culture and no FDA-approved PCR test
- Probable diagnosis if:
  - 1 or more painful genital ulcers
  - No T. pallidum or HSV
- 1/3 have painful ulcer and tender inguinal adenopathy; may also have suppurative inguinal adenopathy.

Granuloma Inguinale

- Caused by intracellular Gram-negative bacterium *Calymmatobacterium granulomatis*
- Rare in the United States
- Painless, progressive ulcerative lesions without regional lymphadenopathy
- The lesions are highly vascular and bleed easily on contact, but may be hypertrophic, necrotic, or sclerotic.

Lymphogranuloma Venereum

- Rare in the United States
- Caused by *C. trachomatis* serovars L1, L2, or L3
- Tender inguinal or femoral lymphadenopathy usually unilateral
- May cause proctocolitis

Genital Warts

- Visible genital warts are usually caused by the human papillomavirus (HPV) types 6 or 11.
- Rarely associated with invasive squamous cell carcinoma
- Usually asymptomatic, but depending on size and location, they can be painful, friable, and pruritic
- Usually ≤10 genital warts and the total wart area is 0.5–1.0 cm

History

- Number of sexual partners
- Type of sexual contact vaginal, oral, or anal
- Condom use
- Associated symptoms: Pelvic pain, vaginal discharge, and fever
- Contraceptive use and possibility of pregnancy

Physical Exam

- Pelvic examination and STI screening
- Skin exam for rashes

TESTS
Lab
Herpes

- Viral culture sensitivity is approximately 50%.
- Sensitivity declines rapidly as lesions heal.
- PCR is not routinely used for genital HSV.
- Antigen detection tests may not distinguish between HSV-1 and HSV-2 and someone may be positive without clinical disease.
- Tzanck preparation is insensitive and not routinely available in all laboratories.
- Serologic testing is only helpful in confirming a prior infection and does not distinguish between anogenital infections and orolabial infections.

Syphilis

- 2 types of tests: Nontreponemal needs confirmation with a treponemal test
- Nontreponemal test antibody titers: Venereal disease research laboratory (VDRL) and rapid plasma reagin (RPR)
- Treponemal tests: Fluorescent treponemal antibody absorbed (FTA-ABS) and *T. palladium* particle agglutination (TP-PA)

Chancroid

Culture for *H. ducreyi* has poor sensitivity and the culture medium not readily available in many labs.

Granuloma Inguinale

- Difficult to culture
- Diagnosis requires visualization of dark staining Donovan bodies on biopsy

- Treatment halts progression of lesions but prolonged treatment may be necessary for reepithelialization

Lymphogranuloma Venereum
Complement fixation titers >=1:64 are consistent with the diagnosis of *Lymphogranuloma Venereum*

Human Papillomavirus Infections
A biopsy may be indicated if the lesions are large or not responsive to therapy.

DIFFERENTIAL DIAGNOSIS
- Genital herpes, syphilis, and chancroid are the most common.
- Non-STD causes include: Vasculitis, Behçet disease, trauma, EBV, and malignancies.

MEDICATION (DRUGS)

Herpes
- Medications do not eradicate the latent virus.
- Treatment regimens differ for the first (F) episode 7–10 days, recurrent (R) episodes 5 days, and suppressive (S) therapy daily.
- Acyclovir (F): 400 mg PO t.i.d.; (R) 800 mg PO b.i.d.; (S) 400 mg PO b.i.d.
- Famciclovir (F): 250 mg PO t.i.d.; (R) 125 mg PO b.i.d.; (S) 250 mg PO b.i.d.
- Valacyclovir (F): 1 g PO b.i.d.; (R) (S) 1 g PO every day

Syphilis
- Benzathine penicillin G 2.4 million units IM in a single dose for primary, secondary, and early latent syphilis
- If penicillin allergy
  - Doxycycline: 100 mg PO b.i.d. 14 days OR
  - Tetracycline: 500 mg PO q.i.d. 14 days
- Late latent syphilis or unknown duration:
  - Benzathine penicillin G 2.4 million units IM every week for 3 weeks
- Penicillin allergy in pregnancy: Patient must be desensitized and treated with penicillin

Chancroid
- Azithromycin: 1 g PO in a single dose
- Ceftriaxone: 250 mg IM in a single dose
- Ciprofloxacin: 500 mg PO b.i.d. for 3 days
- Erythromycin: 500 mg PO t.i.d. for 7 days

Granuloma Inguinale
- Treatment is at least 3 weeks of antibiotics:
  - Doxycycline 100 mg PO b.i.d. OR
  - Trimethoprim-sulfamethoxazole DS PO b.i.d.
- Alternative regimens:
  - Ciprofloxacin 750 mg b.i.d. OR
  - Erythromycin 500 mg q.i.d. OR
  - Azithromycin 1 g every day

Lymphogranuloma Venereum
- Doxycycline 100 mg PO b.i.d. for 21 days
- Alternative regimen:
  - Erythromycin 500 mg q.i.d. for 21 days

Human Papillomavirus Infections
- May resolve without treatment
- Change treatment modality if not improved substantially after 3 provider administered treatments or if not resolved after 6 treatments.
- Treatment may lead to hypo or hyperpigmentation

- Patient-applied:
  - Podofilox 0.5% applied b.i.d. for 3 days then 4 days no therapy for up to 4 cycles
  - Imiquimod 5% cream apply once at night 3 times a week for up to 16 weeks–wash area with soap and water 6–10 hours after treatment
- Provider-administered include: Cryotherapy, Podophyllin resin, Trichloroacetic acid, and surgical removal

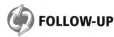

FOLLOW-UP

MANAGEMENT OF SEX PARTNERS

Herpes
- Latex condoms can reduce the risk for genital herpes when infected areas are covered
- May be infectious when asymptomatic
- No prophylactic treatment available

Syphilis
- Follow nontreponemal titers at 6 and 12 months for a 4-fold decrease
- Failure to fall 4-fold by 6 months is probable treatment failure
- Transmission only occurs when mucocutaneous lesions are present
- Sex partners should be treated presumptively if exposed within 90 days preceding the diagnosis of primary, secondary, or early latent syphilis

Chancroid
- Re-examine 3–7 days after treatment
- If no improvement may be a) wrong diagnosis, b) coinfected with another STD, c) patient has HIV, d) treatment not taken, and e) *H. ducreyi* resistant to treatment
- Large ulcers may take >2 weeks to heal
- Sexual partners should be examined and treated if sexually active within 10 days of onset of symptoms

Granuloma Inguinale
Sexual partners within 60 days of symptoms should be examined and offered therapy

Lymphogranuloma Venereum
- Follow until signs and symptoms resolved
- Sexual contacts in the 30 days preceding symptoms should be tested for chlamydial infections and treated

Genital Warts
- Recurrences are most common in the first 3 months following treatment
- Genital warts are not an indication to change the frequency of Pap testing
- Examination of sex partner is not necessary for genital wart management but may be beneficial for education and STD screening

Issues for Referral
If lesions do not improve or increase in size despite therapy then referral for biopsy to rule out malignancy may be necessary.

COMPLICATIONS
Recurrence

REFERENCES

1. Center for Disease Control and Prevention. Sexually transmitted diseases treatment guidelines 2002. *MMWR*. 2002;51:1–80.

CODES
ICD9-CM
- 054.1 Herpes
- 091.0 Syphilis
- 099.0 Chancroid
- 099.2 Granuloma Inguinale
- 099.1 Lymphogranuloma Venereum
- 078.19 Genital Warts

KEY WORDS
- STI
- Genital Ulcers

SJÖGREN'S SYNDROME

Rebecca A. Griffith, MD

KEY CLINICAL POINTS

- Sjögren's syndrome is a chronic, systemic autoimmune inflammatory disorder of the exocrine glands.
- Commonly presents in middle-aged women with the cardinal symptoms of dry eyes and dry mouth.
- Systemic symptoms, such as fatigue, myalgias, and arthralgias, can also be present.
- The mainstay of treatment is avoidance of aggravating factors although lubricating substitutes are useful and immunomodulating agents may be helpful in treating extra-glandular symptoms.

 BASICS

DESCRIPTION

- Sjögren's syndrome is characterized by lymphocytic infiltration of the affected glands, which most often include the salivary and lacrimal glands.
- Classic symptoms include gradual onset of dryness of eyes, mouth, and other body areas (sicca syndrome).
- If the symptoms occur without presence of another autoimmune disorder, it is classified as primary Sjögren's syndrome. When sicca symptoms are present in patients with a preexisting diagnosis of autoimmune disease, it is known as secondary Sjögren's syndrome.

EPIDEMIOLOGY

Primary Sjögren's syndrome is a disease of white women with 2 age peaks.

- 1st peak during 20s and 30s
- 2nd peak at time of menopause
- Apparent association with HLA DR haplotypes

Prevalence

- Estimated prevalence of 0.2–3% of the general population in the United States
  - Female > Male (9:1)
  - Is 1 of the 3 most common autoimmune disorders
- Prevalence of secondary Sjögren's syndrome is reported as:
  - In patients with rheumatoid arthritis: 30–50%
  - In patients with SLE: 8–30%

ETIOLOGY

Pathogenesis is largely unknown but thought to be multifactorial. Most models incorporate environmental, immune-mediated and genetic factors. Overview is as follows:

- Glandular cells are activated by environmental factors like a virus.
- Salivary gland epithelium and lacrimal glands become infiltrated with lymphocytes in a periductal or periacinar distribution.
- Cytokines produced by the lymphocytes recruit other immune cells, but may also lead to decreased production of fluid secretion themselves.
- In genetically susceptible individuals, auto-antibodies and immune complexes are formed.
- Auto-antibodies and lymphocytic infiltration of extra-glandular tissues are likely responsible for the extra-glandular manifestations of the disease.

ASSOCIATED CONDITIONS

- Secondary Sjögren's syndrome is usually associated with rheumatologic diseases including:

  - Rheumatoid arthritis
  - Systemic lupus erythematosus
  - Systemic sclerosis
  - Less commonly: Polymyositis, dermatomyositis, relapsing polychondritis, fibromyalgia
- Sicca symptoms can also be found in association with other non-rheumatologic disorders
  - Approximately 10% of the patients with autoimmune thyroid disorder also have Sjögren's syndrome.
  - Hypothyroidism
  - Multiple sclerosis
  - Alzheimer's disease

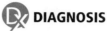 **DIAGNOSIS**

SIGNS AND SYMPTOMS

- Signs and symptoms can be divided into those consistent with sicca syndrome (glandular manifestations) and extra-glandular manifestations.
- Sicca syndrome is the presenting complaint in 85% of the patients with Sjögren's syndrome.
- Extra-glandular manifestations, present in 10–15% of those with primary disease, include the following:
  - General: Fever, fatigue, adenopathy
  - Skin-purpura, vasculitis, vitiligo, xerosis, alopecia, cutaneous lymphomas
  - Pulmonary-interstitial pneumonitis, tracheobronchial sicca
  - GI: Esophageal dysmotility, gastritis, primary biliary cirrhosis, celiac sprue
  - Cardiac-pericarditis, pulmonary HTN
  - Renal: Interstitial nephritis common
  - Musculoskeletal: Arthritis, arthralgia, myalgia
  - Neurologic: Neuropathies, mainly sensory
  - Psychiatric: Depression, anxiety

History

- Dry eyes or kerato-conjunctivitis sicca (KCS)
  - Patients complain of dry, burning or itchy eyes
  - May report "foreign body" sensation
  - Dry eye symptoms are frequently worsened by environmental irritants such as
    - Air conditioning or wind
    - Smoke
    - Low humidity
  - Dry eyes may not be noted until coincident dehydrating condition or illness develops or new medication with anticholinergic side effects started
- Dry mouth or xerostomia
  - Complain of "cotton-mouth," dysphagia
  - Need to drink extra fluids, even at night or may come to office with a bottle of water and sip from it during examination ("water bottle sign")
  - Notice altered taste, tongue, and mouth burning
  - Complain of swollen glands
  - History of multiple dental caries or oral thrush
- Extra-glandular symptoms correlate with the manifestations previously listed

Physical Exam

- On ocular exam may see
  - Corneal abrasions or ulcers
  - Evidence of ocular infection

- Oral examination may show
  - Dry, fissured tongue or buccal mucosa
  - Diminished or absent salivary pool
  - Enlargement of salivary glands and/or sialoliths
  - Parotid gland swelling (bilateral) may be noted
    - Common in primary Sjögren's syndrome
    - Unusual in secondary Sjögren's syndrome

TESTS
Lab
- Elevated ESR
- ANA positive in 65% of patients
- RF positive in 90% of patients
- Anti-SSA (anti-Ro)
  - Not specific for Sjögren's syndrome
  - Present in 70–80% of primary but <10% of secondary Sjögren's syndrome patients
- Anti-SSB (anti-La)
  - Higher specificity than SSA
  - Present in 50–75% of primary but <5% of secondary Sjögren's syndrome patients
- Can also see anemia of chronic disease
- Polyclonal hypergammaglobulinemia

Imaging
- Parotid sialography may show anatomic abnormalities of salivary ducts
- A salivary gland scintigraphy can be used to give information on glandular uptake, resting function, and discharge.

Diagnostic Procedures/Surgery
- To diagnose KCS:
  - Schirmer's test
    - Performed by placing small strip of filter paper under lower eyelid and measure degree of wetting for 5 minutes
      - <10 mm in 5 minutes is abnormal
      - <5 mm in 5 minutes is consistent with diagnosis of KCS
  - Rose-bengal test
    - Ocular staining with rose bengal 1% solution used to detect areas of abnormal epithelium
    - Von Bijsterveld scoring system is used
    - A score of ≥4 is positive test
- To diagnose xerostomia:
  - Sialometry is used to demonstrate objective evidence of salivary gland dysfunction
    - Patient expectorates all saliva into preweighed cup for 15 minutes
    - Significant flow rate: <0.1 mL per minute
  - Need to repeat test more than once due to variation in saliva flow
- Minor salivary gland biopsy:
  - This is the "gold standard" for diagnosis.
  - Positive result is focal lymphocytic sialadenitis
    - A focus score of >1 per 4 mm^2 is diagnostic.

Pathologic Findings
- The salivary gland biopsy shows lymphoepithlial infiltration of the exocrine areas of the gland.
  - Composed mainly of CD4 T cells
  - Evidence of destruction of glandular tissue
- Adjacent areas may appear normal.
- Diagnostic criteria as proposed by collaborative European-North American study group
  - Presence of 4 of 6 criteria, (including histopathologic feature or auto-antibodies) has sensitivity of 93.5% and specificity of 94% for Sjögren's syndrome

- Ocular symptoms: Dry eyes, foreign body sensation, frequent use of ocular lubricants
- Oral symptoms: Dry mouth, swollen salivary glands, liquids required to swallow food
- Ocular signs: Positive Schirmer's or rose bengal test
- Histopathologic feature: Focal lymphocytic sialadenitis as indicated by focus score >1 per 4 mm^2 of minor salivary gland biopsy
- Salivary gland involvement: Positive result of salivary scintigraphy, parotid sialography or unstimulated salivary flow test
- Auto-antibodies: At least 1 positive result, RF, ANA, anti-SSA or anti-SSB
  - Exclusion criteria: Head and neck irradiation, lymphoma, AIDS, hepatitis C, sarcoidosis, use of anticholinergic drugs, graft-versus-host disease

DIFFERENTIAL DIAGNOSIS
- Rheumatologic disorders
  - Rheumatoid arthritis
  - Systemic lupus erythematosus
  - Polymyalgia rheumatica
- Infectious processes
  - Mumps
  - Hepatitis C
  - HIV
- Infiltrative processes
  - Amyloidosis
  - Sarcoidosis
- Parotid tumors, although more likely unilateral
- Medications, notably tricyclic antidepressants
- History of irradiation
- Multiple sclerosis
- Immune complex disease
- Graft versus host disease

 ## TREATMENT

GENERAL MEASURES
Sicca symptoms are treated with lubrication and avoidance of the aggregating factors.
- Eye symptoms:
  - Artificial tears
  - Wear glasses outdoors
  - Avoid drying medications, hair dryers
- Oral symptoms:
  - Saliva substitutes
  - Use of sugar-free hard candies or gum to stimulate saliva flow
  - Good dental hygiene, fluoride toothpaste
  - Avoid alcohol, smoking
- Use of humidifiers may decrease symptoms

 ## MEDICATION (DRUGS)

First Line
In patients with residual salivary gland function, a secretagogue (cholinergic agonist) can be used.
- Pilocarpine hydrochloride (Salagen)
  - Dose: Start with 5 mg PO at night and increase weekly up to 5 mg or more q.i.d. (max dose 30 mg/day)
  - May take up to 3 months to reach full effect

- Side effects: Diaphoresis, urinary frequency
- May also alleviate other sicca syndromes
- Cevimeline hydrochloride (Evoxac)
  - Available if patient not tolerate or achieve response with pilocarpine
  - Max dose: 30 mg PO t.i.d.
- NSAIDs and salicylates
  - First-line treatment for myalgias, arthralgias
  - May not be well tolerated due to decreased salivary flow and esophageal motility
  - Topical or rectal suppository formulation
- Hydroxychloroquine sulfate
  - Dose: 200 mg b.i.d.
  - Useful for myalgias, arthralgias, adenopathy, fatigue, and salivary gland swelling
  - Not shown to increase tear flow

Second Line
- Methotrexate
  - Dose: 7.5–25 mg PO per week
  - Can be given by IM or SC injection
  - Used if refractory to hydroxychloroquine
- Corticosteroids
  - Used to treat refractory cases
  - Most helpful for vasculitis, pneumonitis, neuropathy, nephritis
  - No effect on sicca symptoms
  - High doses (1 mg/kg/day) used in life-threatening cases
  - Usual side effects are more pronounced in patients with Sjögren's syndrome especially periodontal disease, oral candidiasis
- Cyclophosphamide
  - For life threatening disease
  - Dose: IV pulse therapy 0.5–1 g/m^2/day
  - Used with caution due to high incidence of lymphoma in Sjögren's syndrome
- Other
  - Azathioprine: (1 to 2 mg/kg/day) or Leflunomide may be useful in selected patients
  - TNF, etanercept not shown to be beneficial
  - Interferon currently being studied in trials

SURGERY
Punctal occlusion may help with tear retention and improve tear flow.

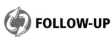 **FOLLOW-UP**

Issues for Referral
- Ophthalmic consultation
- Frequent dental check-ups
- Frequent rheumatologic follow-up

PROGNOSIS
- Sicca symptoms require diligent care of eyes and dentition
- Most patients do well

COMPLICATIONS
Risk of lymphoma in Sjögren's syndrome is 40 times that of general population
- B-cell neoplasm most common
- Some reports of virus associated lymphomas
- MALT lymphomas, both pulmonary and gastric, may develop in Sjögren's syndrome patients

Pregnancy Considerations
- Increased incidence of congenital heart block if mother positive for Anti-SSA or Anti-SSB
- If there is evidence of fetal heart block, oral dexamethasone can be given to try to prevent permanent damage to the fetal cardiac conduction system.

REFERENCES
1. Asmussen KH, Bowman SJ. Outcome measures in Sjögren's syndrome. *Rheumatol.* 2001;40:1085–1088.
2. Cush JJ, Kavanaugh A, Stein MC. *Rheumatology, Diagnosis & Therapeutics*. Philadelphia: Lippincott; 2005.
3. Dawson LJ, Smith PM, Moots RJ, et al. Sjögren's syndrome—time for a new approach. *Rheumatol.* 2000;39:234–237.
4. Derk CT, Vivino FB. A primary care approach to Sjögren's syndrome. *Postgrad Med.* 2004;116:49–56.
5. Fox RI. Sjögren's syndrome. *Lancet.* 2005;366:321–331.

 MISCELLANEOUS

Perioperative considerations
- Routine use of humidified oxygen
- Artificial tears and ocular lubricants to avoid corneal abrasions

CODES
ICD9-CM
710.2 Sjögren's Syndrome

KEY WORDS
- Dry Eyes
- Dry Mouth
- Autoimmune Disease
- Salivary Gland Enlargement
- Lymphoma

SKIN CANCERS, COMMON

Mohsin K. Malik, MD
Lynn E. Iler, MD

KEY CLINICAL POINTS

- Sun exposure is the major risk factor for the development of skin cancer, but skin cancer can occur on any skin surface
- 3 main types
  - Basal cell carcinoma
    - High incidence in the U.S. population
    - Rarely metastasizes but local invasion can cause significant tissue destruction Squamous cell carcinoma
    - Incidence and risk in between basal cell carcinoma and melanoma
  - Melanoma
    - Least common of 3 types of skin cancer
    - Early detection and treatment is key to long-term survival
    - Invasive melanoma has poor prognosis
- Surgical excision is the treatment of choice

 BASICS

DESCRIPTION

The 3 most common skin cancers are important causes of morbidity and mortality in the U.S.

- Basal and squamous cell carcinoma are non-melanoma skin cancers derived from keratinocytes
  - Basal cell carcinoma classically presents as a pearly papule or nodule on head and neck
  - Squamous cell carcinoma classically presents as a rough, hyperkeratotic papule or nodule on chronically sun-exposed skin
- Melanoma is a skin cancer derived from melanocytes that is relatively common in the U.S., and classically presents as a new or changing pigmented lesion.
- All 3 cancers have subtypes that vary in clinical and pathological presentations

GENERAL PREVENTION

Sun protection is the major form of prevention. Methods include:

- Limit sun exposure between 10 a.m. and 4 p.m. when intensity is the greatest
- Stay in the shade when outdoors
- Cover exposed skin with a wide-brimmed hat, long sleeves, pants, and sunglasses
- Use a sunscreen with SPF 15 or greater and re-apply frequently

EPIDEMIOLOGY

About 1 in 71 lifetime risk for developing melanoma, even higher for non-melanoma skin cancer

Incidence

- About 900,000 new basal cell carcinomas in the overall United States population, accounting for about 1/4 of all diagnosed cancers
- About 200,000 new squamous cell carcinomas overall in the United States
- In the United States, 26,000 new cases of melanoma in women yearly
  - Incidence is increasing faster than for any other cancer
  - 6th most common cancer in women by incidence (excluding combined nonmelanoma skin cancers)

RISK FACTORS

- Sun exposure is the major risk factor for all 3 types of skin cancers.
- Additional risk factors for melanoma include:
  - History of sunburns
  - Personal or family history of melanoma
  - Specific phenotypic features including
    - Fair skin
    - Tendency to sun burn
    - Blonde or red hair
    - Blue or green eyes
  - High number of typical nevi
  - Atypical nevi
- Additional risk factors for squamous cell carcinoma include:
  - Scars or burns
  - Ionizing radiation
  - Exposure to arsenic or aromatic hydrocarbons

ETIOLOGY

Environmental and genetic factors contribute to the development of skin cancer, but ultraviolet radiation (sun exposure) is the most important etiological agent.

ASSOCIATED CONDITIONS

Several conditions predispose to the development of skin cancers

- Basal cell:
  - Chronic immunosuppression
  - Xeroderma pigmentosum
  - Basal cell nevus syndrome
- Squamous cell:
  - Chronic immunosuppression
  - Xeroderma pigmentosum
  - Human papilloma virus: Anogenital squamous cell carcinoma
  - Actinic keratoses: Can be clinically indistinguishable from early squamous cell carcinoma. About 60% of squamous cell carcinoma arises from actinic keratoses, but individual actinic keratosis has low risk of progression to cancer
- Melanoma:
  - Chronic immunosuppression
  - Xeroderma pigmentosum
  - Familial atypical multiple mole and melanoma syndrome (dysplastic nevus syndrome)

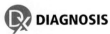 **DIAGNOSIS**

SIGNS AND SYMPTOMS

History

Any of the following should alert the physician to a possible skin cancer:

- A new skin lesion
- A skin lesion that is changing in size, shape, or color
- A sore that does not heal
- Personal or family history of skin cancer
- History of sunburns or radiation

Physical Exam

- Basal cell carcinoma
  - Commonly presents on chronically sun-exposed skin, and characteristically presents as a pearly papule or nodule
  - Rolled borders may be present

- Telangiectasias may be present
- Lymph nodes should be examined in a patient with skin cancer or a history of skin cancer
- Squamous cell carcinoma
  - Commonly presents on chronically sun-exposed skin, especially the face, pinnae, backs of the hands, forearms, and lower legs
  - Generally presents as a hyperkeratotic papule, nodule, or plaque, with or without erythema
  - May develop crust or ulceration
  - Less frequently can develop into a cutaneous horn
- Melanoma
  - Commonly presents on the legs and backs of women, but can occur on any skin or mucosal surface including the scalp, nails, mouth, and labia
  - Any new or changing pigmented lesion in an adult should be examined
  - May be raised or flat with the surface of the skin
  - Generally presents as a new or changing lesion with one or more of the "ABCDs"
    - Asymmetry
    - Border irregularity
    - Color variegation (more than one color)
    - Diameter >6 mm

TESTS
Lab
Baseline and yearly chest x-ray and LDH in patients with an invasive melanoma

Diagnostic Procedures/Surgery
Biopsy provides histological diagnosis of clinically suspected skin cancers
- Nonmelanoma skin cancers
  - Shave or punch biopsy may be performed depending on anatomic site and size
  - Shave biopsy:
    - May miss deeper histological features
    - May be more easily performed and with more control using a sterile razor blade held in the hand and bent in a curve
- Melanoma
  - Punch biopsy should be performed on suspected melanoma
    - May be excisional or incisional based on clinical suspicion, location, and size of lesion

ALERT
- A shave biopsy is never indication in a lesion suspected to be melanoma.
- Once a shave biopsy has been performed on a melanoma, depth of invasion cannot be measured.
- If available, a dermatoscope can aid in the examination of pigmented lesions.

Pathologic Findings
- Basal cell carcinoma
  - Atypical basophilic basaloid cells extending into the dermis, typically with peripheral palisading
- Squamous cell carcinoma
  - Atypical squamous cells that extend from the epidermis into the dermis
- Melanoma
  - Asymmetric proliferation of cytologically atypical single and nested melanocytes throughout the epidermis with or without dermal invasion

DIFFERENTIAL DIAGNOSIS
- Pigmented lesions:
  - Nevus
  - Atypical nevus
  - Seborrheic keratosis
- Nonpigmented lesions:
  - Actinic keratosis
  - Dermatofibroma

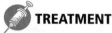 **TREATMENT**

GENERAL MEASURES
- Surgical excision and Mohs micrographic surgery are important modalities in treating basal and squamous cell carcinoma. Other forms of local destruction can also be used depending upon depth of the tumor.
- Surgical excision is the treatment of choice for melanoma.
  - Invasive melanomas with aggressive histological features might benefit from a sentinel lymph node biopsy
  - In asymptomatic patients with melanoma thickness <4 mm and without evidence of metastasis, routine lab studies or imaging have limited value

SPECIAL THERAPY
Radiotherapy
Less commonly used for nonmelanoma skin cancer than other modalities
- Can be used for select basal and squamous cell carcinoma which are low-risk and small in size
- Also useful as adjuvant therapy in some invasive cancers

 MEDICATION (DRUGS)

- Topical therapy for basal and squamous cell carcinoma
  - 5-Flurouracil 5% cream:
    - Greatest utility in treating actinic keratoses, but has been used for primary, superficial, low-risk basal and squamous cell carcinoma
    - Irritation, inflammatory response, and discomfort at application sites can be severe and cause discontinuation
  - Imiquimod 5% cream:
    - Effective treatment for actinic keratoses and primary, low-risk superficial basal cell carcinoma
- Systemic therapy for melanoma
  - High-dose interferon alpha provides benefit in surgically resected, lymph-node positive melanoma
  - Dacarbazine, temozolomide, and other cytotoxic agents provide limited benefit in metastatic disease

SURGERY
- Surgical excision is most common treatment method, and has advantage of providing histological examination of tumor margins
  - Basal cell carcinoma: 3–5 mm margin of resection
  - Squamous cell carcinoma: 4–6 mm margin of resection
  - Melanoma
    - In situ: 5 mm margin of resection
    - <2 mm depth of invasion: 10 mm margin of resection
    - ≥2 mm depth of invasion: 20 mm margin of resection
    - Lymph node dissection if clinical evidence of lymph node involvement
  - Further treatment indicated if tumor extends to deep or lateral margins on histological examination

- Most surgical excisions can be done on an outpatient basis with primary closure, but flaps or grafts may be required for large excisions or excisions where cosmetic outcome is a concern
- Electrodessication and curettage (ED&C)
  - Appropriate for low-risk, superficial basal or squamous cell carcinoma
  - Relatively low-risk and well tolerated procedure, but does not provide tissue for histological examination
- Cryotherapy
  - Liquid nitrogen applied by spray or probe causes local tissue destruction
  - Generally used for treatment of actinic keratoses, but can be used for low-risk basal or squamous cell carcinoma
- Mohs micrographic surgery
  - A procedure where tumor is excised, tissue is examined on frozen section, and further tissue is excised if tumor extends to surgical margins. Appropriate for low-risk, superficial basal or squamous cell carcinoma
  - Provides more favorable outcome for high-risk basal and squamous cell carcinoma compared to simple surgical excision

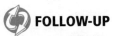 **FOLLOW-UP**

Issues for Referral
Basal and squamous cell carcinoma should be referred for Mohs surgery in cases of high-risk features including:
- Recurrence
- High-risk location such as eyelid, ears, nose, lips
- Tumor size >20 mm (or >5–10 mm for basal cell in high-risk locations)
- Morpheaform, infiltrative, or other aggressive histological features of basal cell carcinoma
- Perineural involvement

PROGNOSIS
- Melanoma
  - For localized disease (stage I and II), the most important prognosticators are tumor thickness and ulceration
  - For advanced disease, important prognosticators are the number of metastatic nodes (stage III) and sites of metastases (stage IV)
  - Selected ten year survival:
    - Stage IA ($\leq$1 mm, no ulceration): 88%
    - Stage IIA (1.01–2 mm, ulceration): 64%
    - Stage IIC (>4 mm, ulceration): 32%
    - Stage III (nodal involvement): 18–63%
    - Stage IV (metastases): 6–16%

- Basal and squamous cell carcinoma
  - 90–95% cure rate overall with surgical resection
  - >97% cure rate overall with Mohs micrographic surgery
  - Cure rates somewhat lower with other modalities
  - Recurrences tend to occur in the first 3 years

COMPLICATIONS
- Patients who have had a skin cancer are at increased risk for a subsequent skin cancer
- Local recurrences can occur with all skin cancer

PATIENT MONITORING
Patients with a history of skin cancer need to be followed closely.
- For tumors excised with negative margins, semiannual follow-up for the first two years and then annual follow-up is a reasonable strategy for routine surveillance
- Any changes in the excised skin cancer, or any new lesions suspicious for skin cancer, should be evaluated immediately

REFERENCES

1. Albert MR, Weinstock MA. Keratinocyte carcinoma. *CA Cancer J Clin*. 2003;53:292–302.
2. Balch CM, Soong SJ, Gershenwald JE, et al. Prognostic factors analysis of 17,600 melanoma patients: Validation of the American Joint Committee on Cancer melanoma staging system. *J Clin Oncol*. 2001;19:3622–3634.
3. Bataille V, Bishop JA, Sasieni P, et al. Risk of cutaneous melanoma in relation to the numbers, types and sites of naevi: A case-control study. *Br J Cancer*. 1996;73:1605–1611.
4. Elwood JM, Jopson J. Melanoma and sun exposure: An overview of published studies. *Int J Cancer*. 1997;73:198–203.
5. Sober AJ, Chuang TY, Duvic M, et al. Guidelines of care for primary cutaneous melanoma. *J Am Acad Dermatol*. 2001;45:579–586.
6. Thissen MR, Neumann MH, Schouten LJ. A systematic review of treatment modalities for primary basal cell carcinomas. *Arch Dermatol*. 1999;135:1177–1183.

CODES
ICD9-CM
- 173 Basal or squamous cell carcinoma
- 172 Malignant melanoma of skin

KEY WORDS

- Skin Cancer
- Basal Cell Carcinoma
- Squamous Cell Carcinoma
- Melanoma
- Mohs

SUBSTANCE ABUSE
Jody A. Underwood, MD

KEY CLINICAL POINTS

- Substance abuse/dependence develops more rapidly in women than men.
- Substance abuse/dependence complicates pregnancy and increases the risk of abnormalities in the newborn.
- Treatment should include cormorbid conditions and involve family members.

 BASICS

DESCRIPTION

- Dependence: Repeated substance use, with or without physical dependence.
- Abuse: Substance use that deviates from accepted medical or social norms.
- Intoxication: Substance use that causes a reversible syndrome effecting mental functions.
- Withdrawal: A syndrome that occurs after stopping or reducing the amount of a substance previously used.
- Tolerance: Original dose of a substance produces a decreased effect or larger doses must be taken to obtain same effect observed with original dose.
- Types of substances:
  - CNS depressants: Alcohol, barbiturates, benzodiazepines, inhalants, and opioids
  - CNS stimulants: Amphetamines, caffeine, cocaine, and nicotine
  - Hallucinogens: Cannabis, LSD, mescaline, psilocybin, and ecstasy (MDMA)

GENERAL PREVENTION

Counseling along with education:

Educate about the use of addictive prescription medications

EPIDEMIOLOGY

- According to the National Comorbidity Survey (NCS) approximately 6% of American women between the ages of 15 and 54 have a lifetime diagnosis of drug use disorders
  - Male > Female (1.6:1)
- The prevalence of prescription drug use, abuse, and dependence is higher for women than for men (i.e., pain relievers, tranquilizers, stimulants, sedatives).
- Women develop substance abuse and dependence patterns more rapidly than men.
- Women abuse hallucinogens and opioids less than men, but use cocaine and amphetamines equally.
- Women are more likely to smoke or use cocaine intranasally than intravenously.

RISK FACTORS

Risk factors for substance use:

- Family history of drug abuse
- Personality disorders
- Depression
- Involvement with a drug-dependent partner

Genetics

The genetic influence for drug use, abuse, or dependence is greater for men than for women (33% versus 11%).

PATHOPHYSIOLOGY

Substances stimulate the limbic system:

Nucleus accumbens and ventral tegmental area most affected

ASSOCIATED CONDITIONS

- Women who abuse substances are more likely than men to have comorbid or primary psychiatric diagnoses:
  - Mood disorders
  - Anxiety disorders
  - Eating disorders
  - Pathological gambling
- Women who smoke cannabis report panic attacks more frequently than men.

Pregnancy Considerations

- Cocaine use is associated with increased rates of obstetric and postpartum complications
  - Meconium staining
  - Premature rupture of membranes
  - Prematurity and reduced birth weight and height
  - Abruptio placentae
  - Attention deficits, impulsivity, and hyperactivity in offspring
- Opioid use:
  - During pregnancy, stabilize with the lowest effective dose of methadone or buprenorphine rather than detoxify.
  - Buprenorphine is associated with reduced neonatal withdrawal because of low placental transference of drug.
- Opioid withdrawal syndrome in newborns:
  - Seizures, sleep abnormalities, feeding difficulties, and weight loss
  - Treatment: Opioids, sedatives, clonidine, and benzodiazepines
- Tobacco smoking:
  - Increased risk of premature delivery is related to its stimulating effects on oxytocin.
  - Increases the risk of fetal growth retardation, sudden infant death syndrome, low birth weight and height, and hypertension.

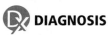 **DIAGNOSIS**

See Description

SIGNS AND SYMPTOMS

Female substance users:

- May have physical symptoms (see physical exam)
  - Miosis: Opioids
  - Mydriasis, pressured speech: Stimulants
  - Slurred speech, slowed motor response, gait disturbance: Depressants
  - Altered mental status: All substances
- May have the same severity of symptoms of problematic substance use (alcohol and opioids) as men, yet seek treatment sooner.
- May have a greater subjective response to cocaine than men.

History

Obtain information about past and present use:

- Type of substances used
- Quantity and frequency of use
- Age when substance use began
- Amount of money and time spent on obtaining substances—screen for illegal activities such as prostitution, assault, and theft to pay for substances
- History of prior substance abuse treatment or psychiatric treatment
- Withdrawal: Presence of delirium tremens or withdrawal seizures

ALERT

Because detecting and evaluating substance-abusing patients is difficult:

- Obtain information from other sources (i.e., family members, coworkers)
- Remember that patients often underestimate the amount of substance used.

Physical Exam

- Perform an extensive psychiatric and medical assessment
- Physical symptoms of substance use:
  - Subcutaneous or IV users:
    - Scars
    - Abscesses, infections
    - Heart murmur (bacterial endocarditis)
    - RUQ tenderness (hepatitis)
    - Thrombophlebitis
    - Signs of tetanus
  - Intranasal use (cocaine, heroin):
    - Deviated or perforated nasal septum
    - Nasal bleeding
    - Tetanus
  - Smokers of crack, marijuana or other drugs and inhalant abusers:
    - Bronchitis
    - Asthma
    - Chronic respiratory conditions

TESTS

Lab

- Toxicology: Urine/blood tests: Usually positive for up to 2 days after use of most substances, and up to 30 days for cannabis.
- Pregnancy test: Defines treatment options
- Prolactin level:
  - Cocaine can induce hyperprolactinemia that may cause several changes in the menstrual cycle.
  - Cannabis can produce significant, transient decreases in plasma level of prolactin and luteinizing hormone during the luteal phase.
  - Nicotine can inhibit the release of prolactin and luteinizing hormone.

DIFFERENTIAL DIAGNOSIS

- Hyperthyroidism
- Psychosis
- Delirium
- Anxiety
- Depression

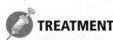 ## TREATMENT

INITIAL STABILIZATION

- Observe for possible overdose and polysubstance intoxication
- Evaluate for medical conditions
- Provide supportive treatment

Discontinue the use of substances as quickly as possible:

- Detoxification (outpatient, partial hospital, or inpatient)
  - Use medications to treat physiologically dependent patients (patient who use alcohol, sedatives, or opioids)
  - Treat with phenobarbital, benzodiazepines (lorazepam or chlordiazepoxide), methadone, or buprenorphine
- Mutual help groups:
  - AA (alcoholics anonymous)
  - NA (narcotics anonymous)
  - Women only groups

- Involve family/source of social support at every stage of treatment. Mutual help groups:
  - Al-Anon
  - Alateen
  - Narc-Anon

GENERAL MEASURES

Treatments that may reduce the likelihood that the patient will return to substance abuse:

- Treat comorbid depressive and anxiety disorders.
- Involve the family/social support.
- Encourage treatment for patient's partner if he or she abuses substances also.
- Treat comorbid physical conditions.
- Be mindful of a woman's menstrual cycle when counseling about smoking cessation as quitting during premenstrual symptoms may be more difficult.

Complementary and Alternative Medicine

- Yoga
- Deep relaxation
- Exercise
- Acupuncture

 ## MEDICATION (DRUGS)

- Opioid dependent patients who have failed abstinence-based treatments:
  - Consider maintenance with an opioid agonist: Methadone or buprenorphine
  - Consider naltrexone: Opioid antagonist that blocks the effect of opioids
- Pharmacologic treatment for nicotine dependence:
  - Nicotine replacement
  - Bupropion: Contraindicated in women with an eating disorder

 ## FOLLOW-UP

- Referrals to mutual help groups
- Group and individual therapy
- Continued involvement of the family
- Medication maintenance, if indicated
- Continue to screen for comorbid psychiatric disorders

PROGNOSIS

- Relapse is common
- Educate patient that long-term sobriety may require multiple attempts

COMPLICATIONS

- Substance abuse:
  - Is involved in most cases of domestic violence
  - Affects domestic partners, children and the elderly
  - Is a major cause of motor vehicle injuries and fatalities
- IVDU:
  - HIV
  - Hepatitis B and C
  - Syphilis and other sexually transmitted diseases
- Tobacco use:
  - Increased risk for impaired immune response, cardiovascular disease, and cancer of the lung and bladder
  - Increased rates of breast, ovarian, and cervical cancers
  - Lung cancer mortality rates surpass breast cancer as the most frequent cause of death

PATIENT MONITORING
Provide frequent motivation checks

REFERENCES

1. American Psychiatric Association. *Diagnostic and Statistical Manual of Mental Disorders*. 4th ed. Washington, DC: American Psychiatric Association; 2000.
2. Burt BK, Hendrick VC. *Clinical Manual of Women's Mental Health*. Washington, DC: American Psychiatric Publishing, Inc; 2005.
3. Sadock B, Sadock V. *Kaplan & Sadock's Pocket Handbook of Clinical Psychiatry*. 4th ed. Philadelphia: Lippincott Williams & Wilkins; 2005.
4. Yager J, Anderson A, Devlin M, et al. Practice guidelines for the treatment of patients with substance use disorders: Alcohol, cocaine, opioids. In: *Practice Guidelines for the Treatment of Psychiatric Disorders*. 2nd ed. Washington, DC: American Psychological Association; 2002:249–324.
5. Zilberman M, Blume S. Substance abuse and abuse in women. In: Romans S, Seeman M, ed. *Women's Mental Health A Life Cycle Approach*. Philadelphia: Lippincott Williams & Wilkins; 2006:179–190.

CODES
ICD9-CM
- 304.00 Opioid dependence
- 305.50 Opioid abuse
- 304.40 Amphetamine dependence
- 305.70 Amphetamine abuse
- 304.20 Cocaine dependence
- 305.60 Cocaine abuse
- 304.10 Sedative, hypnotic or anxiolytic dependence
- 305.40 Sedative, hypnotic or anxiolytic abuse
- 304.30 Cannabis dependence
- 305.20 Cannabis abuse
- 304.50 Hallucinogen dependence
- 305.30 Hallucinogen abuse
- 305.1 Nicotine dependence
- 304.80 Polysubstance dependence (excludes opioids)

KEY WORDS
- Substance Dependence
- Substance Abuse
- Drug Use

SYSTEMIC LUPUS ERYTHEMATOSUS

Lori Lieberman-Maran, MD

KEY CLINICAL POINTS

- Systemic Lupus Erythematosus (SLE) is an autoimmune disease commonly affecting women of childbearing years.
- Variable clinical symptoms from mild (rash and arthritis) to severe organ-threatening disease
- Treatment:
  - Ranges from treatment with NSAIDs to potent immunosuppressive medications
  - Guided by degree of severity of symptoms and organ system involvement

 BASICS

DESCRIPTION

- SLE is a chronic inflammatory autoimmune disease with multiorgan involvement
- Characterized by excessive autoantibody production, immune complex formation, and tissue injury

EPIDEMIOLOGY

- Peak incidence occurs in women between the ages of 15–45, but can occur at any age.
- Female to male ratio:
  - Ratio 10:1 between the age of 15–45
  - Ratio 2:1 during childhood or post-menopause
- More common in African-Americans, Afro-Caribbeans, and Hispanic Americans

Incidence

In the United States, 2–8 cases per 100,000 person years

Prevalence

- Approximately 40–50 cases per 100,000 in the general population
- One of the most common autoimmune diseases in women during childbearing years

RISK FACTORS

There are no known risk factors in SLE, but there are triggers to the immune system that may initiate the cellular response in SLE:
- Ultraviolet light
- Drugs
- Viruses

Genetics

- Does not follow typical inheritance pattern, but there is about a 10% chance that any given patient with SLE will have another family member with SLE
- Concordance rate of identical twin is 24% compared to fraternal twins of 2–3%
- Associated with HLA-DR2 and DR3

PATHOPHYSIOLOGY

- Complex autoimmune disease involving the interaction of both T cells and B cells primarily producing pathogenic autoantibodies
- Autoantibody production is driven by polyclonal B cell activation and autoantigen-driven immune stimulation
- Autoantibodies mediate tissue injury by immune complex deposition

ETIOLOGY

- Unknown etiology
- Genetic susceptibility and environmental factors both contribute to its pathogenesis

ASSOCIATED CONDITIONS

SLE may occur with other autoimmune diseases such as:
- Hemolytic anemia
- Thyroiditis
- Idiopathic thrombocytopenia purpura
- Fibromyalgia can occur in 1/3 of the patients with SLE

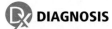 **DIAGNOSIS**

SIGNS AND SYMPTOMS

Classification of SLE includes the presence of at least 4 out of the 11 criteria:
- Malar rash
- Discoid rash
- Photosensitivity
- Oral ulcers
- Arthritis (nonerosive)
- Serositis
  - Pleuritis
  - Pericarditis
- Renal involvement
  - Persistent proteinuria >0.5 g/day or 3+
  - Presence of cellular casts
- CNS involvement
  - Seizures
  - Psychosis
- Hematologic abnormalities
  - Hemolytic anemia
  - Leukopenia
  - Thrombocytopenia
- Immunologic markers
  - Antibodies to native DNA, Smith antigen
  - Anticardiolipin IgG, IgM, lupus anticoagulant
  - False positive serologic test for syphilis
- Anti-nuclear antibody (ANA)

History

- Constitutional complaints are common presenting features of SLE:
  - Malaise, fatigue, fever, and weight loss
- Diverse clinical presentations depending on organ system involved:
  - Rash, joint pain, myalgias, Raynaud's, seizure, headache, pleuritic chest pain, oral ulcers, photosensitivity, or alopecia

Physical Exam

Can have a variety of physical findings depending on organ system involved such as:
- Arthritis: Usually symmetric involving small joints in hands, wrists, and knees
- Rash
- Oral ulcers
- Alopecia

TESTS

Lab

- Hematologic abnormalities:
  - Leukopenia
  - Anemia
  - Thrombocytopenia

- Renal abnormalities:
  - Elevated creatinine
  - Proteinuria
  - Active urinary sediment
- Hypocomplementemia (C3, 4)
- Autoantibodies:
  - ANA: Positive in virtually all patients with SLE (98%), but lack specificity
  - Antibodies to double stranded DNA
    - Present in 60–90% of patients with SLE
    - Specificity of 95%
    - Presence of these antibodies may be associated with development of nephritis
  - Anti-Smith antibodies
    - Present in 10–30% of patients with SLE
    - Specificity of 75–100%
  - Antiphospholipid antibodies
    - Present in 30–50% of patients with SLE

Imaging
Imaging is not needed for diagnosis but may be helpful depending on the clinical situation:
- Plain radiograph of involved joints
- Chest radiograph
- Echocardiography
- Magnetic resonance imaging

Diagnostic Procedures/Surgery
Biopsy of an involved organ (kidney or skin) may be necessary for diagnostic purposes and to help guide treatment decisions

Pathologic Findings
- Inflammation, blood vessel abnormalities (vasculopathy or vasculitis), and immune-complex deposition.
- WHO Classification of Lupus Nephritis:
  - Class I: Normal glomeruli
  - Class II: Mesangial nephritis
  - Class III: Focal proliferative glomerulonephritis
  - Class IV: Diffuse proliferative glomerulonephritis
  - Class V: Membranous glomerulonephritis
  - Class VI: Chronic sclerosing glomerulonephritis

DIFFERENTIAL DIAGNOSIS
Extremely broad differential diagnosis for SLE since it has a wide variety of clinical presentations. Some categories to consider include:
- Infection
- Malignancy
- Endocrinopathy
  - Hypothyroidism
- Rheumatic disease
  - Systemic vasculitis
  - Rheumatoid arthritis
  - Polymyositis
  - Still's disease
  - Fibromyalgia
- Medication side effects
  - Carbamazepine, hydralazine, isoniazid, methyldopa, minocycline, phenytoin, procainamide, sulfasalazine, quinidine, ethosuximide, chlorpromazine, and penicillamine
  - There have been several case reports that the newer biologic agents (TNF alpha antagonists) can cause drug induced lupus including etanercept and infliximab

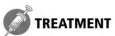 ## TREATMENT

INITIAL STABILIZATION
Patients with SLE generally require medications to control their symptoms as well as lifestyle modifications to prevent flares.

SPECIAL THERAPY
All patients with SLE should be counseled on proper use of sunscreens and avoidance of ultraviolet light since this is known to trigger flares.

 ## MEDICATION (DRUGS)

- Nonsteroidal anti-inflammatory drugs (NSAIDs):
  - Used to treat arthritis and soft tissue complaints and mild serositis
  - Caution in patients with renal insufficiency
- Corticosteroids:
  - Typically prescribed orally in low, medium (0.5 mg/kg) or high doses (1 mg/kg) depending on the manifestation
  - Pulse steroids (IV methylprednisolone 1 gm for 3 consecutive days) used to treat severe organ-threatening features of disease
- Anti-malarials:
  - Used to treat constitutional symptoms, musculoskeletal complaints, skin rashes, and pleuritic chest pain
  - Hydroxychloroquine 400 mg/day
    - Most commonly prescribed antimalarial
  - Generally well tolerated
  - Annual ophthalmologic exam is recommended as can cause ocular toxicity
- Immunosuppressive medications:
  - Azathioprine: 1.5–2.5 mg/kg/day
    - Used as steroid sparing agent and as maintenance therapy for nephritis
    - Can cause bone marrow suppression and hepatotoxicity
  - Cyclophosphamide
    - Used to treat nephritis and in some cases of CNS lupus
    - Associated with several adverse side effects including bladder toxicity, ovarian failure, bone marrow suppression, and increased risk of infection
  - Mycophenolate mofetil: 1–3 gm/day
    - New evidence supports use as induction and maintenance therapy for nephritis
    - Generally well tolerated; few adverse effects including leukopenia, nausea, and diarrhea

Pregnancy Considerations
- SLE is not associated with infertility unless patient treated with cyclophosphamide which can lead to premature ovarian failure
- Pregnancy should be planned for a time when disease (especially renal) is relatively well controlled
- Maternal morbidity includes flares (especially renal), preeclampsia, preterm labor, and thrombosis (primarily in those with antiphospholipid antibodies)
- Fetal morbidity includes fetal loss, preterm birth, intrauterine growth retardation, and neonatal lupus
- Medications should be adjusted during pregnancy to avoid risk to the fetus:
  - Must consider the risks and benefits of medications in pregnant patients with SLE
  - The safety of hydroxychloroquine is unknown, but has been used safely in pregnancy.

- Prednisone is relatively safe at low doses, but potential risks include gestational diabetes, preeclampsia, and cleft palate.
- Azathioprine does have a small risk of harm to the fetus but is used cautiously in certain patients.

SURGERY
Renal transplantation is an alternative for lupus patients who develop renal failure.

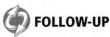 **FOLLOW-UP**

Issues for Referral
- A rheumatologist should follow patients with SLE closely.
- Consider referral to nephrologist, dermatologist, and/or neurologist.

PROGNOSIS
- There is a 3-fold to 5-fold increased mortality compared with the general population.
- The 10-year survival rate approaches 90% and the 20-year survival rate approaches 70%.
- Early deaths are generally due to active disease, especially renal or CNS; later deaths result from complications of SLE or treatment.
- Most crucial predictor of mortality is renal disease; the second is CNS disease.
- Patients of African or Hispanic descent appear to have greater mortality rates.

COMPLICATIONS
Complications and mortality result directly from disease activity or treatment toxicity and include:
- Cardiovascular (CV) disease
  - Premature atherosclerosis is now recognized as a serious concern in patients with SLE.
  - There is a 10-fold to 50-fold increase in CV disease compared to age matched controls.
- Infection
- Renal failure
- Cerebrovascular events
- Osteonecrosis

PATIENT MONITORING
- Patients with SLE should be carefully followed to monitor disease activity.

- Routine laboratory tests include:
  - CBC
  - ESR
  - Urinalysis and serum creatinine
  - DsDNA levels
  - Complement levels (C3, C4)
- Clinical indices used to assess disease activity in research studies include:
  - Systemic lupus erythematosus disease activity index (SLEDAI)
  - Systemic lupus activity measure (SLAM)
  - British isles lupus assessment group (BILAG)

REFERENCES

1. Bjornadal L, Yin L, Granath F, et al. Cardiovascular disease a hazard despite improved prognosis in patients with systemic lupus erythematosus: Results form a Swedish population based study 1964–95. *J Rheumatology*. 2004;31:713–719.
2. Boumpas D, Austin H, Fessler B, et al. Systemic lupus erythematosus: Emerging concepts-part 1: Renal, neuropsychiatric, cardiovascular, pulmonary, and hematologic disease. *Ann Intern Med*. 1995;122:940–950.
3. Boumpas D, Fessler B, Austin H, et al. Systemic lupus erythematosus: Emerging concepts-part 2: Dermatologic and joint disease, the antiphospholipid syndrome, pregnancy and hormonal therapy, morbidity and mortality, and pathogenesis. *Ann Intern Med*. 1995;123:42–53.
4. Ginzler E, Dooley M, Aranow C, et al. Mycophenolate mofetil or intravenous cyclophosphamide for lupus nephritis. *N Engl J Med*. 2005;353:2219–2228.
5. Hochberg M, Silman A, Smolen J, et al., eds. *Rheumatology*. 3rd ed. Edinburgh: Mosby; 2003.

CODES
ICD9-CM
710.0 Systemic lupus erythematosus

KEY WORDS
- Autoimmune Disease
- SLE
- Nephritis

TEMPORALMANDIBULAR JOINT SYNDROME

Jamie K. Kemp, MD
Kelly A. McGarry, MD

KEY CLINICAL POINTS

- Temporomandibular joint (TMJ) syndrome is second only to headache as a cause of head and facial pain.
- Symptoms can be exacerbated by:
  - Stressful life events
  - Conditions such as teeth grinding (bruxism), jaw clenching, and dental malocclusion
    - Referral to dentist for bite place appliance can improve symptoms
- NSAIDs with jaw exercises are first line therapy

 ## BASICS

DESCRIPTION

- TMJ syndrome is a group of symptoms that includes:
  - Pain in the temporomandibular joint
  - Headache
  - Other facial pain, and
  - Dysfunction of the temporomandibular joint
- There may be associated clicking or crepitus
- It may be due to problems within the joint itself or to dysfunction of the muscles or connective tissues of the area around the joint.

EPIDEMIOLOGY

- It has been estimated that 10% of the male population and 20% of the female population has at some point had symptoms consistent with TMJ dysfunction.
- TMJ syndrome is seen disproportionately in women between 20 and 50 years of age.
- It is second only to headache as a cause of head and facial pain.

RISK FACTORS

- Emotional stress and anxiety tend to exacerbate the symptoms.
- Rheumatoid arthritis, and less commonly, osteoarthritis, can affect the temporomandibular joint.

PATHOPHYSIOLOGY

- The temporomandibular joint is a synovial joint with a fibrocartilage meniscus serving as the articulating surface.
- Connective tissues and the muscles of mastication surround the joint.
- Presumably, dysfunction of any part of the temporomandibular region can cause pain.

ETIOLOGY

It is not clear exactly what causes the symptoms of TMJ syndrome, but there are associated conditions that can exacerbate pain:

- Jaw clenching or tooth grinding (bruxism)
- Dental malocclusion
- Malalignment of the jaws
- TMJ articular disc disease
- Anxiety, depression, and stress

ASSOCIATED CONDITIONS

- Anxiety and depression
- Fibromyalgia
- Increased cervical lordosis
- Bruxism

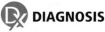 ## DIAGNOSIS

TMJ is diagnosed almost exclusively in the outpatient setting.

SIGNS AND SYMPTOMS

- Most patients complain of unilateral pain and stiffness in the jaw or the side of the face.
- The pain is described as a dull ache that may radiate to the ear, jaw, or neck.
- Symptoms usually become more apparent with chewing.
- Some patients may complain of an audible clicking with opening of the jaw.
- There may be locking of the jaw or limited opening of the jaw.

History

- The symptoms of TMJ tend to wax and wane, and there are commonly symptom-free periods.
- There is often a precedent stressful life event before an episode of symptoms.

Physical Exam

- There may be facial asymmetry; the muscles of the affected side may be atrophied or hypertrophied.
- Crepitus may be noted with opening and closing of the jaw.
- Palpation of the muscles around the TMJ may reveal marked tenderness.
- Palpation of TMJ may reveal tenderness:
  - Joint should be palpated both laterally and posteriorly in open and closed positions
  - Lateral: Place fingers at depression below zygomatic arch, 1–2 cm anterior to tragus
  - Posterior: Place fingers behind tragus at each external acoustic meatus and pull forward while patient opens and closes mouth
- The clinician should also examine the ears, cervical spine, and teeth to evaluate for possible other causes of pain.

TESTS

The diagnosis is usually made on the basis of symptoms and exam findings.

Lab

- Only rarely are lab tests indicated.
- If there are associated symptoms or findings that suggest another connective tissue disease, such as lupus or rheumatoid arthritis, then laboratory testing should be ordered accordingly.

Imaging

MRI:

- Imaging procedure of choice, but should be reserved for severe or complex cases.
- Most common MRI findings include derangements of the articular disc and degenerative bony changes.
- MRI findings do not always correlate with symptoms or their severity and should be interpreted in light of the history and physical.

Diagnostic Procedures/Surgery

Joint arthrography is rarely performed and has largely been replaced by MRI.

DIFFERENTIAL DIAGNOSIS

Less common but potentially serious causes of facial and head pain should be considered:

- Rheumatoid arthritis
- Tumors of the bone and connective tissue, including tumors that metastasize to bone
- Dental disease
- Temporal arteritis
- Trigeminal neuralgia

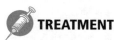 **TREATMENT**

GENERAL MEASURES

The most important step in treatment of TMJ disorder is to identify factors that exacerbate symptoms and to attempt to treat these individual entities.

SPECIAL THERAPY

Patients with significant bruxism jaw clenching, or malocclusion should be fitted for a bite plate appliance by a dentist to lessen these exacerbating factors.

Physical Therapy

- Jaw exercises and physical therapy have been shown to be helpful in patients with TMJ syndrome.
- However, patients must be referred to a therapist who has training in oral rehabilitation.
- Low-level laser therapy:
  - Although some early reports demonstrated pain relief, a recent study showed no significant difference in pain relief between the treatment and placebo groups although both groups reported some improvement.
  - Can be done through referral to PT

Complementary and Alternative Medicine

Acupuncture and biofeedback have both been shown to reduce symptom frequency and severity in patients with temporomandibular joint dysfunction.

 MEDICATION (DRUGS)

First Line

- NSAIDs, when used in conjunction with jaw exercises, are first line therapy for TMJ dysfunction.
- Tricyclic antidepressants and muscle relaxants at bedtime are also helpful, especially in patients with early morning symptoms.
  - Amitriptyline: 25 mg PO at hour of sleep
    - Improvement in 75% of outpatients in one small study
  - Cyclobenzaprine: 10–30 mg PO at hour of sleep
    - May need to increase dose over first 2 weeks as tolerated
    - May take 7–10 days to achieve improvement

Second Line

- If there is evidence of arthritis of the temporomandibular joint, a corticosteroid injection into the joint may be helpful, but should be performed by a practitioner with expertise in this procedure.
- Botulinum: A toxin injection is quickly becoming an accepted treatment of TMJ pain, but should only be performed by a practitioner with expertise.

SURGERY

Patients with significant joint derangement or who fail medical therapy may be referred for arthroscopic surgery, including meniscectomy and disc repair.

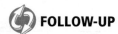 **FOLLOW-UP**

Issues for Referral

- Patients with jaw clenching, grinding, or bruxism should be referred to a dentist for bite plate appliance fitting.
- Patients with severe complaints that do not respond to conservative therapy may warrant referral to an oral/maxillofacial surgeon or an endodontist.

PROGNOSIS

- Patients with TMJ syndrome generally have waxing and waning symptoms.
- Many patients will experience relief with conservative therapy, although few patients will experience permanent relief from their symptoms.

COMPLICATIONS

If not monitored, TMJ syndrome can turn into a chronic pain disorder.

REFERENCES

1. Arthritis and Allied Conditions. 15th ed. Philadelphia: Lippincott Williams and Wilkins; 2005.
2. Bonica's Management of Pain. 3rd ed. Philadelphia: Lippincott, Williams, and Wilkins; 2001.
3. DeAbreu VR, Campari CM, DeFatima Zanirato Lizarelli R, et al. Low-intensity laser therapy in the treatment of temporomandibular disorders: A double-blind study. J Oral Rehabil. 2005;32:800.
4. Mishra KD, Gatchel RJ, Gardea MA. The relative efficacy of 3 cognitive-behavioral treatment approaches to temporomandibular disorders. J Behav Med. 2000;23:293.
5. Nicolakis P, Erdogmus B, Kopf A, et al. Effectiveness of exercise therapy in patients with internal derangement of the temporomandibular joint. J Oral Rehabil. 2001;28:1158.
6. Rizzatti-Barbosa CM, Nogueira MT, de Andrade ED, et al. Clinical evaluation of amitriptyline for the control of chronic pain caused by temporomandibular joint disorders. Cranio. 2003;21:221–225.
7. Yuasa H, Hidemichi Y, Kenichi K, et al. Randomized clinical trial of primary treatment for temporomandibular joint disk displacement without reduction and without osseous changes: A combination of NSAIDs and mouth-opening exercise versus no treatment. Oral Surg Oral Med Oral Pathol Oral Radiol Endo. 2001;91:671.

CODES

ICD9-CM

- 524.60 TMJ disorders
- 524.62 Arthralgia of the TMJ
- 524.64 TMJ sounds on opening and/or closing of the jaw

KEY WORDS

- Headache
- Jaw Pain
- Face Pain
- Jaw Clicking
- Jaw Locking

TOBACCO USE

Michelle A. Stozek Anvar, MD

KEY CLINICAL POINTS

- Smoking cessation should always be a major health care goal as quitting can have a significant impact on disease.
- Relapse rates are high for smokers who quit during pregnancy.

 BASICS

DESCRIPTION
Smoking, especially cigarettes, is a major health concern and requires regular screening and counseling.

GENERAL PREVENTION
Physician intervention for smoking cessation has shown to have a positive impact in cessation rates.

EPIDEMIOLOGY
Per the CDC in 2003:
- Adults that smoke tobacco: 21%
  - Women: 19.2%
  - Men: 24.1%
- High school students that smoke: 22%
- Middle school students that smoke: 8%
- Data vary for pregnant women but from 11–22% of pregnant women smoke and in some parts of the United States rates may be even higher.

ASSOCIATED CONDITIONS
- Cardiac:
  - Smoking is associated with approximately a 6-fold increase in myocardial infarction compared to women who have never smoked.
  - There is a decrease in myocardial events after quitting in both patients with and without prior cardiovascular events.
- Pulmonary:
  - Smoking cessation reduces the rates of decline in FEV1.
  - Many smokers have a decrease in cough and sputum production in the 1st smoke-free year.
- Malignancy:
  - Lung cancer is now one of the leading causes of cancer related death in women.
  - Almost twice as many women in the United States will die of lung cancer in 2005 than from breast cancer.
  - Tobacco use is also associated with many other malignancies (head and neck, esophageal, bladder, cervical, and pancreatic)
- Fertility:
  - Smoking >10 cigarettes per day has been associated with impaired fertility.
  - In addition, studies suggest that smoking can lead to premature aging of the ovary.
- Osteoporosis:
  - Tobacco use is a major risk factor for loss of bone density.

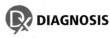 **DIAGNOSIS**

History
- Screening for smoking should be done regularly. The "5 A's" are designed to help evaluate smokers:
  - Ask: Systematically identify all tobacco users at every visit
  - Advise: Strongly urge all tobacco users to quit
  - Assess: Determine willingness to make a quit attempt
  - Assist: Aid the patient in quitting
  - Arrange: Arrange follow-up

Physical Exam
- Physical exam may be normal
- If pulmonary obstruction occurs, may find:
  - Prolonged expiration and wheezes on forced exhalation
  - Hyperinflation
  - Increased anteroposterior diameter of chest
  - Decreased breath sounds
  - Heart sounds often become distant
  - Coarse crackles at lung bases
- Concern for malignancy:
  - Weight loss
  - Hemoptysis
  - Lymphadenopathy

TESTS
Pulmonary function tests:
- To detect lung disease that may be attributable to cigarette use
- May be useful to show patients documented evidence of the negative consequences of smoking when lung disease is detected
- Abnormal PFTs may provide motivation to quit

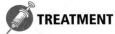 **TREATMENT**

GENERAL MEASURES
- After screening for smoking, the patient's readiness to quit should be assessed. They may fall into the following categories:
  - Precontemplative: Patient is not ready or interested in quitting
  - Contemplative: Patient is considering quitting in the future
  - Determination: Patient is actively planning to quit or has started to try
  - Action: Patient is actively trying to quit or quit less than 6 months ago
  - Maintenance: Patient quit more than 6 months ago
- Behavioral changes
  - Providing even brief advice about quitting smoking increases the likelihood that a smoker will successfully quit and remain a nonsmoker in the future.
- Suggested interventions:
  - Quit date: Choose a day in the future to quit
  - Prepare for quit date
    - Identify triggers and develop alternate plan
    - Avoid situations and places that triggered smoking in the past
    - Inform friends and family of plan for their support and assistance
    - Be aware of nicotine withdrawal and how it can be treated
  - Patient education regarding potential weight gain
  - Exercise and healthy diet should be discussed
- Counseling;
  - Cognitive
    - The goal of cognitive therapy is to reframe the way a patient thinks about smoking.
    - Smokers are taught techniques of distraction, positivism, relaxation, and mental imagery.
    - Offered encouragement and motivation

- Behavioral
  - Behavioral therapy teaches patient to avoid stimuli that trigger smoking, such as stress, alcohol, and associating with other smokers.
  - Other interventions include altering the usual smoking routine, preparing for cigarette cravings, and addressing withdrawal.
  - Intensive counseling
    - Can be associated with a 22% rate of quitting
    - Limited counseling (<3 minutes) is associated with a 13% quit rate.
- See Substance Abuse chapter

SPECIAL THERAPY
Complementary and Alternative Medicine
- Acupuncture: A 2002 Cochran review of 22 studies comparing acupuncture to sham acupuncture showed no difference in quit rates.
- Hypnotherapy has not been shown to reliably affect rates of quitting.
- Telephone quit lines: Many states have numbers when patients can easily access advice and treatment programs for quitting.

MEDICATION (DRUGS)

- Buprorion: An antidepressant with action on norepinephrine and dopamine is approved for use in smoking cessation:
  - 150 mg dose once daily for 3 days then 150 mg b.i.d. for 7–12 weeks
  - Doses should be at least 8 hours apart
  - Avoid dosing at bedtime as may cause insomnia
  - Quit date should be 1–2 weeks after starting medication.
  - Class B in pregnancy
  - Contraindicated in patients with a seizure disorder or eating disorder
  - Can be used in combination with nicotine
- Other SSRIs have not been shown to have the same effect.
- Clonidine and nortyptilline may be as effective as bupropion.
- Nicotine replacement:
  - Decreases the symptoms of nicotine withdrawal (insomnia, irritability, anxiety, dysphoria, and increased appetite with weight gain)
  - There are a variety of forms available: Patch, gum, inhaler, and nasal spray.
  - Dose is dependent on amount of nicotine used previously.
  - Nicotine replacement decreases the symptoms of nicotine withdrawal.
  - It has been shown to be safe even in patients with cardiovascular disease.
  - Class D in pregnancy

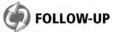

FOLLOW-UP

PATIENT MONITORING
Follow-up for continued patient screening and support should be provided.

Pregnancy Considerations
See Pregnancy, Substance Abuse chapter

REFERENCES

1. Abbot NC, Stead LF, White AR, et al. Hypnotherapy for smoking cessation. *Cochrane Database System Rev*. 1998;2:CD001008.
2. Bernstein IM, Mongeon JA, Badger GJ, et al. Maternal smoking and its association with birth weight. *Obstet Gynecol*. 2005;106:986–991.
3. Ford C, Zlabek JA. Nicotine replacement therapy and cardiovascular disease. *Mayo Clinic Proceedings*. 2005;80:652–656.
4. Hughes JR, Stead LF, Lancaster T. Antidepressants for smoking cessation. *Cochrane Database System Rev*. 2004;4:CD000031.
5. Joseph AM, Norman SM, Ferry LH, et al. The safety of transdermal nicotine as an aid to smoking cessation in patients with cardiac disease. *N Engl J Med*. 1996;335:1792.
6. Lancaster T, Stead LF. Physician advice for smoking cessation. *Cochrane Database System Rev*. 2004;4:CD000165.
7. Schroeder SA. What to do with a patient who smokes. *JAMA*. 2005;294:482–487.
8. White AR, Rampes H, Ernst E. Acupuncture for smoking cessation. *Cochrane Database System Rev*. 2002;2:CD000009.

MISCELLANEOUS

Quick Reference Guide for Clinicians located at: http://www.surgeongeneral.gov/tobacco/tobaqrg.htm#Contents

KEY WORDS
- Tobacco Cessation
- Smoking Cessation

TRICHOMONAS VAGINALIS

Iris L. Tong, MD

KEY CLINICAL POINTS

- *Trichomonas vaginalis (T. Vaginalis)* infection is one of the most common sexually transmitted infections (STI).
- It is associated with increased rates of:
  - HIV transmission
  - Complications in pregnancy
  - Infertility
  - Cervical Intraepithelial Neoplasia (CIN)
- HIV and STD screening should be performed on all patients with *T. vaginalis* infection.

 BASICS

DESCRIPTION

- Trichomoniasis is the 3rd leading cause of vaginitis in women, after bacterial vaginosis and yeast vaginitis.
- *Trichomonas vaginalis* is the causative organism:
  - Protozoan
  - Motile organism with 4 flagella
  - Transmitted via sexual contact
- *Trichomonas* infection is the most common STD aside from human papilloma virus (HPV):
  - More common than Chlamydia trachomatis or Neisseria gonorrhea
  - May receive less attention because it is not a reportable disease

GENERAL PREVENTION

Safe sex practices will decrease transmission of *T. vaginalis*.

EPIDEMIOLOGY

Incidence
- Approximately 120 million women worldwide become infected each year.
- There are an estimated 5 million new cases per year in the United States.

Prevalence
- Affects 180 million women worldwide
- Accounts for up to 25% of vaginal infections in women
- Among young adults in the United States, higher prevalence among African American women

RISK FACTORS
- Unprotected intercourse
- Multiple sexual partners
- Intrauterine device (IUD)
- Tobacco use
- Other STIs

ETIOLOGY
- Transmission of *Trichomonas vaginalis* via sexual contact
- *Trichomonas* can be transmitted via man-to-woman and woman-to-woman contact.
- Incubation period of 5–10 days in general, but can range from 1–28 days.

ASSOCIATED CONDITIONS
Patients with trichomoniasis may be at risk for other STIs.

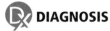 DIAGNOSIS

SIGNS AND SYMPTOMS
Up to 50% of women are asymptomatic.

History
- Unprotected sexual intercourse
- Copious, foul-smelling vaginal discharge
  - Color of discharge ranging from white to yellow-green
- Pruritus
- Vaginal irritation
- Dysuria
- Dyspareunia
- Abdominal pain in 10%

Physical Exam
- Vulvar and vaginal erythema
- Frothy white or green discharge
- "Strawberry" cervix
  - Erythematous cervix with punctuate hemorrhages
- Absent or mild cervical motion tenderness
- Mild lower abdominal discomfort
- Focal tenderness/masses usually absent

ALERT
Elevated vaginal pH and increased number of WBCs on wet prep are consistent with diagnosis of trichomonosis.

Lab
- Vaginal pH >4.5 (normal = 4.5)
- Light microscopy (see below):
  - 45–60% sensitivity
  - >95% specificity when motile trichomonads visualized
- DNA probe:
  - 92% sensitivity, 98–99% specificity
  - Commercially available probe which simultaneously detects the presence of *Candida* species, *Gardnerella vaginalis*, and *T. vaginalis* from a single vaginal swab
  - Results within hours
  - Must be performed by laboratory
- Pap smear:
  - Trichomonads often found incidentally on routine Pap smear
  - Sensitivity ranges from 24–67%, specificity up to 99.9% in some studies
- Urinalysis:
  - Trichomonads often found incidentally on urinalysis
- Culture:
  - Modified Diamond's medium is gold standard
    - 98% sensitivity, 100% specificity
    - Diagnosis within 2–7 days
    - Some systems designed for specimen collection and culture in provider's office
    - Culture generally not used because of length of time for diagnosis and lack of availability of culture medium
- Polymerase chain reaction (PCR):
  - 84% sensitivity, 94% specificity
  - Emerging as a very accurate diagnostic method
  - Only available in research settings

- Immunochromatography:
  - New, rapid test using detection of Trichomonas antigen
  - Diagnosis within 10 minutes
  - Sensitivity and specificity ~95%
  - Performed in provider office
- STI screening:
  - HIV
  - Chlamydia
  - Gonorrhea
  - Syphilis
  - Hepatitis B and C

ALERT

- Samples for pH, microscopy, DNA probe, and culture should be obtained from the posterior fornix or vaginal wall.
- Obtaining a sample from cervical os may reveal normal cervical mucous.

Diagnostic Procedures/Surgery

Light microscopy:

- Presence of motile organisms and increased number of white blood cells (WBCs)
  - WBCs and *T. vaginalis* are similar in size and shape, but only trichomonads are motile
- Wet preparation slide
  - Place thin layer of discharge on glass slide
  - Add one drop of normal saline to slide
- Organisms not visualized by light microscopy in up to 50% of women with culture-confirmed infection
- Likelihood of visualizing organisms may be increased by
  - Adding normal saline immediately to slide
  - Warming slide
  - Decreasing intensity of substage lighting on microscope
  - Viewing slides immediately after collection
    - Increasing time interval between collection and examination decreases visualization of motile trichomonads
    - In a study of 65 slide preparations, 20% initially positive for motile trichomonads became negative within 10 minutes
- Negative result does not rule out infection

DIFFERENTIAL DIAGNOSIS

- Bacterial vaginosis
- Vulvovaginal candidiasis
- Atrophic vaginitis
- Cervicitis

TREATMENT

GENERAL MEASURES

- Abstain from sexual intercourse until both partners treated
- Encourage safe sex practices

MEDICATION (DRUGS)

First Line

Metronidazole: 2 g PO × 1 dose

Second Line

Metronidazole: 500mg PO b.i.d. × 7 days

- Cure rate of single-dose or 7-day regimen is >90%
- Common side effects: Nausea, vomiting, metallic taste, and gastrointestinal upset
- Patients should be cautioned to avoid alcohol

ALERT

- Partners should also be treated
- Patients should avoid sexual intercourse until both partners are treated successfully

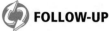

FOLLOW-UP

DISPOSITION

Cure rate with Metronidazole: 90%

Admission Criteria

Treatment is primarily outpatient

Issues for Referral

Consider referral to obstetrician/gynecologist or infectious disease specialist if symptoms persist after treatment.

COMPLICATIONS

- Antibiotic resistance:
  - Resistance rate according to Center for Disease Control (CDC): 2.5–5%
  - Regimens for resistance organisms:
    - 1st failure:
      - Retreat with Metronidazole 500 mg b.i.d. × 7 days
    - 2nd failure:
      - Metronidazole: 2 g PO every day × 3–5 days or
      - Tinidazole: 500 mg PO q.i.d. with 500 mg intravaginally b.i.d. × 14 days or
      - Paromomycin: 5 g intravaginally every day for 14 days
  - If above regimens are not effective, the CDC is available for consultation (www.cdc.gov/std)
- Recurrence:
  - Rate of recurrence can be decreased by
    - Treating sexual partner
    - Advising patients to avoid sexual intercourse until both partners are treated successfully.
    - Participating in safe sexual practices
- Complications in pregnancy (see below)
  - Increased risk of transmission of HIV
  - Increases susceptibility of uninfected individuals
  - Increases infectivity of infected individuals
- Infertility:
  - Women with prior *Trichomonas* infection are at increased risk of tubal infertility
    - Risk of infertility may increase with number episodes of trichomoniasis
    - May be secondary to concomitant *Chlamydia* or *Gonorrhea* infection
  - *Trichomonas* may alter sperm motility and viability in men
- Pelvic inflammatory disease (PID)
  - Higher rate of PID among women with *Trichomonas* infection than uninfected women
  - Among women colonized with *Chlamydia*, higher rate of symptomatic disease in those who were also infected with *Trichomonas*
- CIN:
  - *Trichomonas* infection has been associated with higher risks of subsequent CIN
  - Unclear if *Trichomonas* alone or the coinfection of *Trichomonas* and *HPV* contributes to the development of CIN
- Post-operative Infection:
  - Women with trichomonosis more likely to develop vaginal cuff cellulitis or abscess

Pregnancy Considerations

- *Trichomonas* infection is associated with:
  - Premature ruptures of membranes

– Preterm labor
– Low birth weight
- There is a possible risk of teratogenicity with the use of metronidazole in the first trimester
- The CDC recommends treating symptomatic pregnant women with a single 2 g dose of metronidazole, but does not recommend treating asymptomatic pregnant women:
  – Treatment of asymptomatic infection has not been shown to prevent associated risks in pregnancy
  – A recent meta-analysis of 14 studies revealed that treatment of trichomoniasis during pregnancy did not decrease the incidence of preterm birth

PATIENT MONITORING

Patients with trichomoniasis should be screened for STIs including HIV.

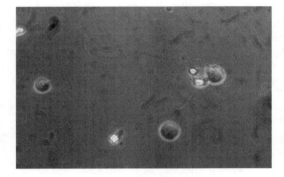

Figure 1 Trichomonads are similar in size to and difficult to distinguish from WBCs unless they are motile.

REFERENCES

1. Egan ME, Lipsky MS. Diagnosis of vaginitis. *Am Fam Physician*. 2000;62:1095.
2. Forna F, Gulmezoglu AM. Interventions for treating trichomoniasis in women. *Cochrane Database Syst Rev*. 2000;3:CD000218.
3. Kingston MA, Bansal D, Carlin EM. Shelf-life of trichomonas. *Int J STD AIDS*. 2003;14:28–29.
4. Owen MK, Clenney TL. Management of vaginitis. *Am Fam Physician*. 2004;70:2125–2132.
5. Soper D. Trichomoniasis: Under control or undercontrolled? *Am J Obstet Gynecol*. 2004;190:281–290.
6. Wendel KA, Erbelding EJ, Gaydos CA, et al. Trichomonas vaginalis polymerase chain reaction compared with standard diagnostic and therapeutic protocols for detection and treatment of vaginal trichomoniasis. *Clin Infect Dis*. 2002;35:576–580.

ADDITIONAL READING

Sobel JD, Nyirjesy P, Brown W, et al. Tinidazole therapy for metronidazole-resistant vaginal trichomoniasis. *Clin Infect Dis*. 2001;33:1341–1346.
Miller WC, Swygard H, Hobbs MM, et al. The prevalence of trichomoniasis in young adults in the United States. *Sex Transm Dis*. 2005;32:593–598.

CODES

ICD9-CM
131.01 Trichomonal vulvovaginitis
616.1 Vaginitis and vulvovaginitis
623.5 Vaginal discharge NOS

KEY WORDS

- Vaginal Discharge
- Vaginal Itching
- *Trichomonas Vaginalis*
- Sexually Transmitted Disease

T

UNINTENDED PREGNANCY

Eleanor Bimla Schwarz, MD, MS

KEY CLINICAL POINTS

Unintended pregnancy is common and preventable

DESCRIPTION
70% of women of reproductive age are sexually active and do not want to become pregnant, but could become pregnant if they or their partners do not use contraception or if their method fails.

GENERAL PREVENTION
- Choosing a contraceptive:
  - Consider efficacy, ease of use, visibility to partner, duration of efficacy, return to fertility on discontinuation, non-contraceptive health benefits, potential contraindications, and acceptability of side effect profile.
  - All forms of contraception safe during lactation:
    - Estrogen containing contraceptives may transiently decrease milk supply.
    - Intrauterine device (IUD) or depot medroxy-progesterone acetate (DMPA) are options.
    - Women breastfeeding infant <6 months (*without* formula supplementation) and without return of menses may rely on lactational amenorrhea as contraception.
- Efficacy:
- % with unintended pregnancy within 1st year of use

	Typical Use	Perfect Use	Continued use at 1 year
Levonorgestrel IUD (Mirena)	0.1	0.1	81
Vasectomy	0.15	0.1	100
Tubal ligation	0.5	0.5	100
Copper T IUD (ParaGard)	0.8	0.6	78
DMPA	3	0.3	56
Contraceptive ring	8	0.3	68
Contraceptive patch	8	0.3	68
Contraceptive pills	8	0.3	68
Male condom	15	2	53
Female condom	21	5	49
Diaphragm	16	6	57
Cervical cap	16–32	9–26	46–57
Sponge	16–32	9–20	46–57
Withdrawal	27	4	43
No method	85	85	

  - Studies have yet to demonstrate superiority to pills despite better compliance with ring/patch.
  - Progestin-only pills must be taken at same time every day. Delays of 1 hour result in significant loss of efficacy.
- Duration of efficacy:
  - Contraceptives labeled "D" and "X" by FDA not indicated during pregnancy but do NOT induce birth defects if used while pregnant.
- Initiating a contraceptive:
  - Starting a method day patient is seen by MD (rather than waiting for first Sunday of menses) increases rates of continuation without increasing side effects.
  - A backup method is required for 7 days after initiation of all hormonal methods.

	Labelled	Evidence
Levonorgestrel IUD (Mirena)	5 years	7 years
Copper IUD (ParaGard)	10 years	12 years
DMPA	12 weeks	13 weeks
Contraceptive ring	3 weeks	4 weeks
Contraceptive patch	1 week	1 week
Contraceptive pills	Daily	Daily
Male/female condom, sponge	Single use	Single use
Vasectomy	Indefinite	Indefinite
Tubal ligation	Indefinite	Indefinite
Diaphragm/cervical cap	Indefinite	Indefinite

  - Initial side effects tend to wane after first 3 months.
  - Continuous use of appropriate forms of contraception is safe and decreases rates of unintended pregnancy.
  - Withdrawal bleeding decreases irregular spotting but not necessary for health reasons.
    - Oral contraceptives limiting menses to 4 ×/year available (Seasonale, Seasonique).
  - IUD insertion is simple and quickly learned.
- Managing side effects:
  - Breakthrough bleeding: Can be caused by poor compliance with medication. Can manage by:
    - Increasing estrogen dose
    - Changing progestin
    - If above ineffective, induce withdrawal bleed with progesterone
  - Nausea: Decrease estrogen
  - Breast tenderness: Decrease estrogen or change progestin
  - Acne: Use a combined hormonal contraceptive or try changing progestin
  - Headaches: Common:
    - No evidence that combined hormonal contraception causes headaches.
    - If associated with hormone withdrawal, consider continuous use of hormones
    - If a woman develops headache with aura, estrogen should be stopped
  - Weight gain: No evidence that combined hormonal contraception causes weight gain
    - Increase exercise, decrease caloric intake
    - Consider changing progestin
  - Decreased libido: Change progestin
  - Return to fertility after discontinuing method:
    - Immediate: Pills, patch, ring, and IUD
    - Delayed: DMPA (by 9–10 months)
  - Irregular bleeding commonly caused by DMPA, progestin only pills, and levonorgestrel IUD
- Non-contraceptive benefit of various methods:
  - Decreased risk of ovarian/endometrial cancer:
    - Methods which suppress ovulation: DMPA and hormonal methods (pills, patch, or ring), but not levonorgestrel or copper IUD.
  - Decreasing blood loss/dysmenorrhea: Hormonal methods (pills, patch, or ring), DMPA, and levonorgestrel IUDs.
  - Protect against symptomatic PID: Barrier methods, hormonal contraception (pills, patch, or ring), DMPA, and levonorgestrel IUD.

– Acne reduction
  • Hormonal methods (pills, patch, or ring)
– Reduction of sickle cell crises: DMPA
– Possible reduction in seizures: DMPA
• Emergency contraception:
  – More effective the sooner it is used
  – Regimens:
    • Plan B pills: Most effective regimen
    • Levonorgestrel: 0.75 mg q12h × 2 doses
      o Both pills can be taken at once and provide efficacy up to 5 days after contraceptive emergency
      o Few side effects: 10% with nausea
      o Approximately 75% decrease in risk of pregnancy
      o Very safe; available over the counter to women >18 years
      o No contraindications to use at any age
      o Does not induce miscarriage/birth defects
      o Recommend patients keep supply at home
      o Advance provision reduces access barriers, increases timely use, and does not increase sexual risk-taking
    • Copper T IUDs inserted up to 7 days after contraceptive emergency also effective.

EPIDEMIOLOGY
Prevalence
• Approximately 49% of pregnancies among American women are unintended; half of these are terminated.
• Induced abortion is one of the most commonly performed medical procedures.
  – In 2002, 1.29 million abortions performed in the United States.
  – Each year in the United States, 1 in 50 women ages 15–44 have an abortion.
  – Approximately 35% of the women in the United States have had abortion by age 45.
• All forms of contraception are cost-effective.
• In countries where abortion is illegal and unsafe, unintended pregnancy continues to cause significant morbidity and mortality, as it did in the United States prior to Roe v. Wade.

ASSOCIATED CONDITIONS
• Sexually transmitted infections (STI):
  – Chlamydia (can be asymptomatic), gonorrhea, HIV, trichomonas, syphilis, and hepatitis B and C.
  – Condom use should be recommended.
• Rape and intimate partner violence

SCREENING
History
• Contraindications to estrogen containing contraceptives include:
  – Smoking after age 35
  – Multiple risk factors for CAD
  – History of clot or vascular disease
  – Migraine with aura
  – History of breast cancer
  – Cirrhosis or active hepatitis
• Medications which increase hepatic metabolism and decrease efficacy of hormonal methods: Anti-convulsants, St. John's wort, rifampin, and griseofulvin.
  – Most antibiotics do not impact efficacy
• Contraindications to IUD insertion:
  – Current STI or STI within last 3 months
    • Increased risk of pelvic infection within first 20 days after insertion
    • After initial period, infection risk is similar to that for general population

– Nulliparity NOT contraindication to use of IUD
• Contraindications to DMPA:
  – Blood pressure >160/100
  – Current or past breast cancer
  – Current DVT/PE
• Relative contraindications to DMPA:
  – Major depression
  – Significant concern of weight gain
  – Concern about bone mineral density (BMD):
    • Decreases about 3% per year for the first 2 years of use and then stabilizes
    • Upon cessation, BMD returns to normal

Physical Exam
• Rule out hypertension (>160/100) before initiating hormonal contraception.
• There is no need to do a Pap, pelvic, or breast exam before starting a contraceptive method.
• Weight >90 kg/200 lbs decreases (but does not eliminate) efficacy of the patch and pills.

TESTS
Lab
• Check urine hCG before initiating a method
• High sensitivity urine pregnancy tests are positive 1 week after conception (20 mIU/mL hCG)
• "Missed period" ≅2 weeks after conception
• Home pregnancy tests are high sensitivity tests

 TREATMENT

• Adoption:
  – 1% of women with unintended pregnancies plan for adoption
  – Referral resources are available at: http://naic.acf.hhs.gov/
• Abortion:
  – Medication or aspiration abortion has no adverse effect on women's future fertility, mental health, or risk of breast cancer.
  – Case-fatality rate for legal abortion is <1 death per 100,000 procedures.
  – 1 in 15,000 women who carry a pregnancy to term die from complications of childbirth.
  – The earlier a pregnancy is terminated the safer the procedure is:
    • In the United States, 87% of the counties have no abortion provider.
    • Approximately 34% of American women of reproductive age live in these counties.
  – The U.S. has 4 times as many centers which seek to deter women from having abortions as clinics which provide abortion
  – Reliable information about clinics providing abortion services is available at:
    • http://www.plannedparenthood.org or
    • http://www.prochoice.org.
  – Pre-abortion screening includes:
    • Rule out ectopic pregnancy
    • Determine gestational age
    • Rh status
    • Hematocrit
    • Chlamydia status
  – Monitor women on anticoagulation carefully
  – Women with abnormal heart valves do not require antibiotic prophylaxis

- Medication abortion:
  - Can be induced up to 9 weeks from last menstrual period using:
    - Mifepristone 200 mg PO and
    - Misoprostol 800 mg PO or intravaginal
  - Mifepristone:
    - Not available in pharmacies
    - Clinicians must sign provider agreement in order to prescribe mifepristone.
    - In certain states, advanced practice clinicians may also provide mifepristone.
    - Information on how to do this is available at http://www.earlyoptionpill.com/.
  - Vaginal bleeding expected for 8–17 days.
  - Side effects include:
    - Cramping/pelvic pain:
      o Treat with ibuprofen 800 mg t.i.d.
      o Approximately 10–30% of women also require narcotics to control the 1st day of cramping
    - GI symptoms (due to misoprostol): Nausea 30%, vomiting 20%, and diarrhea 20–50%
    - Fever/chills in first 24 hours: 15–60%
  - Provision of mifepristone requires a plan to treat potential complications:
    - Incomplete abortion
      o Vacuum aspiration is needed by 1–3%
    - Major hemorrhage
      o Transfusion needed by 1 in 500 women
  - No requirement to have signed agreement from colleagues to provide aspiration or transfusion services.
  - Fatal *Clostridium sordellii* infection:
    - Affected 1 in 100,000 women in California
    - Ongoing investigation of these cases by CDC
    - Presenting symptoms: Pelvic pain and malaise, without fever
  - Contraindications include:
    - Coagulopathy
    - Systemic corticosteroid use or adrenal failure
    - Suspected ectopic pregnancy
    - Inherited porphyrias
  - Remove IUDs before mifepristone use
  - Regimens using methotrexate and misoprostol alone are less effective and associated with more side effects.
- Aspiration abortion:
  - Can be performed until viability (24 weeks from last menstrual period) under Roe v. Wade.
  - Large majority (88%) performed before 12 weeks
  - The duration of the procedure is about 5 minutes.
  - Including counseling and follow-up observation, total visit time approximately 4 hours.
  - Some states require multiple visits or waiting period before obtaining abortion services.
  - Safest to perform aspiration procedure without general anesthesia as anesthesia significantly greater risk than procedure itself.
  - Most women have adequate pain control from paracervical block, ibuprofen 800 mg, PRN acetaminophen with hydrocodone/diazepam.
  - After 12 weeks, misoprostol and/or osmotic cervical dilators are used to help dilate cervix:
    - Women must make 2 visits to a clinic, even in states without mandated waiting periods.
    - Cervical dilation is initiated on 1st visit, and uterus is emptied on second visit.
  - The day after an aspiration procedure, women can resume their usual activities:
    - Generally no need for pain medication

- No fever
  - Women traditionally advised to avoid sex and tampons until bleeding stops (about 2 weeks).
    - May decrease post-abortal infection
    - No formal evidence to support this practice
  - If a woman has excessive pain, bleeding, or fever after an abortion, consider:
    - Retained tissue (treated by repeat aspiration)
    - Infection (treat with antibiotics)
    - Perforation (a very rare complication, may rarely require surgical repair)

 FOLLOW-UP

- Women should be seen 2 weeks after medication abortion to ensure completion of abortion.
- Many women are excellent candidates for IUD:
  - Can be placed immediately following an aspiration abortion (on the same day), or
  - After a medication abortion has been completed (at a follow up visit)

REFERENCES

1. Mosher WD, Martinez GM, Chandra A, et al. Use of contraception and use of family planning services in the United States: 1982–2002. *Advance Data from Vital and Health Statistics*; 2004;350:1–36.
2. Westhoff C, Morroni C, Kerns J, et al. Bleeding patterns after immediate vs. conventional oral contraceptive initiation: A randomized, controlled trial. *Fertil Steril*. 2003;79:322–329.
3. Loder E, Buse D, Golub J. Headache as a side effect of oral contraceptives: A systematic review. *Am J Obstet Gynecol*. 2005;193:636–649.
4. Henshaw SK. Unintended pregnancy in the United States. *Fam Plann Perspect*. 1998;30:24–29.
5. Finer LB, Henshaw SK. Estimates of United States abortion incidence in 2001 and 2002. The Alan Guttmacher Institute. Available at: http://www.guttmacher.org/pubs/2005/05/18/ab_incidence.pdf.
6. Jones RK, Darroch JE, Henshaw SK. Patterns in the socioeconomic characteristics of women obtaining abortions in 2000–2001. *Perspect Sex Reprod Health*. 2002;34:226–235.
7. State Facts About Abortion: Texas. The Alan Guttmacher Institute. Available at: http://www.guttmacher.org/pubs/sfaa/texas.html, accessed October 18, 2005.
8. Sonnenberg FA, Burkman RT, Hagerty CG, et al. Costs and net health effects of contraceptive methods. *Contraception*. 2004;69:447–459.
9. World Health Organization. *Medical Eligibility Criteria for Contraceptive Use*. 3rd ed. Geneva: WHO, 2004.
- USEFUL WEBSITES
  - www.managingcontraception.org
  - www.agi-usa.org
  - www.contraceptiononline.org
  - www.arhp.org

KEY WORDS

- Termination of Pregnancy
- Abortion
- Contraception
- Birth Control
- Oral Contraceptive Pills

URINARY INCONTINENCE

Vivian W. Sung, MD, MPH

KEY CLINICAL POINTS

- Urinary incontinence is a common, treatable disorder.
- Only 13% of women with incontinence will actively seek help.
- There are many minimally invasive options for treating urinary incontinence.
- Incontinence is often associated with pelvic organ prolapse.

 ## BASICS

DESCRIPTION

- Urinary incontinence is defined as any involuntary leakage of urine that is unacceptable to the patient.
- Urinary incontinence is rarely life threatening, but may result in insecurity, embarrassment, depression, social disengagement, and/or psychological and functional decline.
- In 1995, annual direct cost in United States was approximately $16.3 billion:
  - Approximately 1–3% of costs for diagnosis and treatment
  - Up to 70% of costs were for routine care including laundry and protective garments
- Most common types of urinary incontinence:
  - Stress incontinence:
    - Urethra fails to maintain watertight seal
    - Results in leakage with increases in intraabdominal pressure
  - Urge incontinence:
    - Episodes of large volume loss secondary to uninhibited detrusor contractions
    - Disruption of coordinated components of bladder filling and emptying
  - Mixed incontinence:
    - Combination of stress and urge incontinence
    - Approximately 30% of women presenting with incontinence will have mixed components
  - Urinary retention:
    - Inability to empty bladder completely with voiding
    - Can result in "overflow" incontinence
  - Functional incontinence:
    - Occurs when patient with intact lower urinary tract unable/unwilling to reach toilet to void
    - Visual impairment, limited manual dexterity, and limited mobility

EPIDEMIOLOGY

Incidence

- Limited information available on incidence of incontinence, given the long latency period.
- In women 60 years and over, incidence estimated at 20% per year.

Prevalence

- Rates vary due to different definitions of incontinence in surveys and literature.
- Among adult women in the community, prevalence ranges from 9–69%.
- In nursing homes, prevalence >50%.

RISK FACTORS

- Female sex
- Pregnancy/childbirth
  - Of pregnant women, 50% report incontinence, but the majority will resolve after delivery.
- Parity is risk factor in younger women but is weakly associated in older women
- Age: Peak in prevalence from 40–60 years
- Menopause
- Obesity
- Smoking
- Chronic increase in intra-abdominal pressure
  - Chronic cough, asthma
- Other medical comorbidities

PATHOPHYSIOLOGY

Weakening or injury of pelvic supportive structures (connective tissue, pelvic floor muscles, and nerves)

ETIOLOGY

- Stress incontinence
  - Urethral hypermobility
    - Loss of muscular and/or fascial supports compromise ability of urethra to maintain watertight seal with increases in intra-abdominal pressure
  - Intrinsic sphincter deficiency
    - Intrinsic muscular tone is weakened
    - Reduces resting urethral tone and resistance to increases in intra-abdominal pressure
- Urge incontinence
  - Muscular
    - Myogenic changes in detrusor muscle may lead to overactivity/underactivity of bladder
  - Neurologic
    - Postoperative effects
    - Aging
    - Spinal cord disease
    - Multiple sclerosis
    - Diabetes
    - Parkinsonism
    - Cerebrovascular accident
- Urinary retention
  - Outflow obstruction
    - Failure of urethra or pelvic floor to relax during voiding
    - Pelvic organ prolapse
    - Neoplasms
    - Prior anti-incontinence procedures
  - Hypotonic bladder
    - Detrusor unable to generate enough pressure to overcome urethral resistance
    - Autonomic, peripheral neuropathy
    - Pharmacologic (anticholinergics, calcium channel blockers, adrenergic agonists)
    - Radiation fibrosis
- Transient causes: Delirium, infection, pharmacologic (antihypertensives, antidepressants, hypnotics), endocrine (diabetes, hypercalcemia), stool impaction

ASSOCIATED CONDITIONS

- Pelvic organ prolapse frequently
- Fecal incontinence commonly (69%)
- Depression

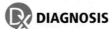 ## DIAGNOSIS

SIGNS AND SYMPTOMS

Symptoms may progress and regress
- Leakage of urine

- Pad use
- Need to change clothes after accidents
- Uncontrollable large volume accidents (urge incontinence)
- "Key in door" urge incontinence: Severe urge or leakage upon arriving home
- Limitations in usual activities
  - Restrictions in physical activities to avoid embarrassing accidents
- Social disengagement
  - Avoids social functions or going out of the house to avoid embarrassing accidents
- Sexual dysfunction
  - Avoids sexual relations due to leakage or fear of leakage during intercourse
  - Avoids sexual relations due to altered body image and embarrassment

History
- Symptom type
  - Stress incontinence: Leakage with coughing, sneezing, laughing, exercise, or exertion
  - Urge incontinence: Uncontrollable urinary urge, large volume accidents, urinary frequency, nocturia
  - Urinary retention: Incomplete emptying, double voiding, voiding difficulty
- Severity of symptoms
  - Duration of symptoms
  - Frequency and amount of leakage
  - Pad use
- Exacerbating factors
  - Medications (diuretics, alpha-blockers, etc.)
- Coexisting pelvic floor disorders
  - Sensation of bulge or pressure in vagina
  - Urinary tract infections
  - Defecatory dysfunction
  - Fecal incontinence
- Impact on quality of life
  - Actual versus desired activity level
  - Psychosocial impact
- Fluid and caffeine intake
- Prior therapies and effectiveness (physical therapy, Kegel exercises, medications, surgery)

Physical Exam
- Pelvic examination
  - Assess pelvic organ support
  - Assess neurologic function
  - Assess pelvic muscle strength
- Cough stress test: Objective demonstration of stress incontinence

TESTS
- Urodynamic testing if significant prolapse to rule out associated stress incontinence
  - Indications:
    - Diagnosis unclear based on initial history and physical
    - Symptoms not consistent with exam findings
    - Patient not improved with initial treatment
    - Prior anti-incontinence surgery
    - Clinical trials where urodynamics testing results serve as outcomes
  - Some advocate urodynamics testing if surgical intervention is planned
- Post void residual to rule out retention

Lab
Urinalysis and culture to rule out infection
Other Tests
- Voiding diary
- Cystometrogram
- Cystoscopy and renal ultrasound or CT scan in patients with recurrent urinary tract infections

DIFFERENTIAL DIAGNOSIS
See Etiology section

TREATMENT

GENERAL MEASURES
- The goal of treatment is to achieve a cure or minimize the impact of the condition.
- Treatment strategy should consider the severity of symptoms, degree of bother, associated pelvic floor conditions, prior surgery, and patient's willingness to accept risks and success rates of different interventions.
- It is important to remember that many women may report satisfaction even if incontinence is not completely resolved.
- Observation is appropriate in patients with symptoms not severe enough to start intervention.

Diet
- Stress incontinence
  - Weight loss
  - Smoking cessation
- Urge incontinence
  - Decrease caffeine and fluid intake
  - Smoking cessation

Physical Therapy
- Stress incontinence
  - Pelvic floor rehabilitation, Kegel exercises, and physical therapy
    - Pelvic floor training shown to be better than no treatment or placebo, but difficult to compare studies due to methodology
    - Regimen: 3–4 sets of 10 squeezes × 3–4 months
    - Side effects are rare and reversible
    - Requires diligent performance by patients
    - Many patients perform incorrectly and thus may benefit from physical therapy
    - Long-term success unclear
- Urge incontinence
  - Pelvic floor rehabilitation and physical therapy

SPECIAL THERAPY
- Stress Incontinence: Continence pessary
- Urge Incontinence: Bladder retraining
  - May be used in cognitively intact patients
  - Patient voids every 2 hours, regardless of urge
  - Relaxation techniques to suppress urgency to prolong interval between voids
  - If patient gets urge during 2-hour time period, should NOT run to the bathroom
    - Patient to concentrate on suppressing urge
    - Can use Kegel squeeze to suppress urge
  - Once urge is suppressed, patient should WALK slowly to restroom
  - When accident-free for 2 days, can increase time interval between voids by 30–60 minutes
  - Continue until patient voiding every 3–4 hours without incontinence

MEDICATIONS (DRUGS)

- Stress Incontinence: Pharmacotherapy limited
  - Tricyclic antidepressants: Imipramine
    - Efficacy ~60% based on small studies
    - Starting dose = 10 mg every day
    - Can increase to 75 mg every day
  - Duloxetine (currently investigational)
- Urge incontinence
  - Anti-cholinergics: Efficacy around 60%
    - Do not use in women with narrow angle glaucoma
    - Start at lower dose and titrate based on response after 3–4 weeks of therapy
    - Similar efficacy among different medications
  - Tolterodine (Detrol):
    - Immediate release (IR) 1–2 mg b.i.d. or extended release (ER) 2–4 mg every day
    - Standard starting dose = ER 4 mg every day
  - Oxybutynin (Ditropan):
    - IR 2.5–5 mg b.i.d. or ER 5–30 mg
    - Standard starting dose = ER 5–10 mg every day
  - Trospium (Sanctura): 20 mg b.i.d.
  - Solifenacin (Vesicare): 5–10 mg every day
  - Darifenacin (Enablex): 7.5–15 mg every day
    - Side effects: Dry mouth (most common), constipation, and CNS (anxiety, confusion)

SURGERY

- Stress incontinence
  - Urethral bulking agents (collagen, carbon-coated zirconium oxide beads, and ethylene vinyl alcohol):
    - Outpatient or office procedure
    - Performed with cystoscopy
    - Improves urethral coaptation
    - Success rates: 13–78%
    - Collagen degrades over time, therefore concern regarding long-term success
    - Overall very low risk and may be offered to women with multiple comorbidities
    - For collagen, prior skin testing required
  - Midurethral slings:
    - Permanent, synthetic sling
    - Outpatient procedure or overnight stay
    - Minimally invasive
    - Local or minimal regional anesthesia
    - Low complication rates (urinary retention 2%; sling erosion <1%; de novo urinary urgency 5%)
    - Success rates: 84–87% at 2–5 years
  - Traditional bladder neck slings:
    - Various sling materials available
    - More dissection than midurethral slings
    - Hospital stay: 1–2 days
    - Success rate: 83% at 2 years
  - Retropubic colposuspension:
    - Sutures placed to stabilize bladder neck
    - Abdominal or laparoscopic approach
    - 1–2 days hospital stay
    - Success rate: 84% at 2 years
- Urge incontinence
  - Sacral neuromodulation

 FOLLOW-UP

Issues for Referral
- Failed conservative or medical management
- Prior gynecologic/urologic surgery
- Recurrent urinary tract infections
- Associated severe pelvic organ prolapse

REFERENCES
1. Brown JS, Grady D, Ouslander JG, et al. Prevalence of urinary incontinence and associated risk factors in postmenopausal women. *Obstet Gynecol*. 1999;94:66–70.
2. Hannestad YS, Rortveit G, Sandvik H, et al. A community-based epidemiologic survey of female urinary incontinence: The Norwegian EPICONT study. *J Clin Epidemiol*. 2000;53:1150–1156.
3. Nygaard IE, Heit M. Stress urinary incontinence. *Obstet Gynecol*. 2004;104:607–620.
4. Ouslander JG. Management of overactive bladder. *N Engl J Med*. 2004;350:786–799.
5. Rogers RG, Kammerer-Doak D, Coates KW, et al. A new instrument to measure sexual function in women with urinary incontinence or pelvic organ prolapse. *Am J Obstet Gynecol*. 2001;184:552–558.

ADDITIONAL READING
Walters MD, Karram MM, eds. *Urogynecology and Reconstructive Pelvic Surgery*. 2nd ed. St. Louis: Mosby, Inc.; 1999.
Bent AE, Ostergard DR, Cundiff GW, et al., eds. *Urogynecology and Pelvic Floor Dysfunction*. 5th ed. Philadelphia: Lippincott Williams & Wilkins; 2003.

CODES
ICD9-CM
- 625.6 Stress urinary incontinence
- 788.31 Urge incontinence
- 788.38 Overflow incontinence
- 788.33 Mixed incontinence
- 788.41 Urinary frequency
- 788.63 Urinary urgency
- 788.2 Urinary retention, unspecified
- 788.21 Incomplete bladder emptying
- 788.34 Incontinence without awareness
- 596.51 Overactive bladder

KEY WORDS
- Urinary Incontinence
- Pelvic Floor Disorders
- Urinary Retention
- Pelvic Organ Prolapse

URINARY TRACT INFECTION

Jennifer Jeremiah, MD

KEY CLINICAL POINTS

- Symptomatic UTI in healthy women can be treated empirically
- In general, short course 3-day therapy is as effective as 7-day therapy in uncomplicated UTI
- Antibiotic choice should be based on regional resistance to *E. coli*

 BASICS

DESCRIPTION

Urinary tract infections (UTI) represent the most common bacterial infection in pregnant and nonpregnant women
- Infections may be symptomatic or asymptomatic
  - Symptoms include dysuria, frequency, urgency, hematuria, and/or suprapubic pain
  - Fever >38°C, flank pain, nausea or vomiting suggest upper tract infection and require more aggressive evaluation and treatment
- Infections may be complicated or noncomplicated
  - Uncomplicated UTI occurs in patients with normal genitourinary tract, without recent instrumentation and with symptoms in the lower urinary tract
  - Complicated UTIs are associated with the following and increase likelihood of treatment failure
    - Abnormalities of the urinary tract
    - Existence of foreign body (i.e., indwelling catheter, stone)
    - Infection with resistant pathogens
    - Patient characteristics including advanced age, diabetes, menopause, spinal cord injury, multiple sclerosis, immunosuppression or immunodeficiency, and recent antibiotic use

EPIDEMIOLOGY
- More than 1/2 of all women will have a symptomatic UTI in their lifetime.
- Approximately 2–14% of pregnant women will also have asymptomatic bacteruria during pregnancy.
- *Escherichia coli* is the most common pathogen accounting for 75–95% of infections.
- *Staphylococcus saprophyticus* is second accounting for 2–20%.
- Other less common pathogens include the enterobacteriaceae, *klebsiella*, *proteus*, and *enterococcus faecalis*.
- Pyuria and symptoms of UTI without positive standard urine culture may suggest infection with *Chlamydia trachomatis*.
- Accompanying vaginal discharge may also suggest infection with *Neisseria gonorrhea* or *Trichomonas vaginalis*.

RISK FACTORS
Sexual intercourse is one of the most important risk factors for uncomplicated UTI. Other risk factors include:
- Instrumentation
- Anatomic predisposition
- Poor patient compliance
- Infrequent voiding
- Diaphragm and tampon use

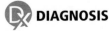 **DIAGNOSIS**

- The diagnosis of UTI relies on clinical symptoms and urinalysis with or without urine culture.

- In a healthy woman with classic symptoms and absence of vaginal discharge, the likelihood of infection is >90% and empiric treatment should be considered.

History
- Lower tract infection:
  - Dysuria
  - Urgency
  - Suprapubic pain
- Upper tract infection or pyelonephritis:
  - Abrupt onset of fever and chills
  - Nausea and vomiting
  - Back pain

Physical Exam
- Lower tract infection:
  - Physical exam may be normal
- Upper tract infection or pyelonephritis:
  - Fever
  - Unilateral or bilateral flank pain
  - Tenderness over costovertebral angles

Lab
- Dipstick urinalysis positive for leukocyte esterase and/or nitrates is 75% sensitive and 82% specific for UTI
- Microscopic hematuria may be present in 40–60% of patients
- Urine culture:
  - Midstream pyuria on unspun urine with 100,000 colony forming units (CFU) per ml is diagnostic
  - Should be considered for patients who fail initial treatment or will likely have atypical or resistant organisms
  - Lower colony counts should be considered positive in women with symptoms

DIFFERENTIAL DIAGNOSIS
- Interstitial cystitis
- Vaginitis
- Urethritis
- Sexually transmitted disease

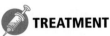 **TREATMENT**

Treatment should alleviate symptoms and prevent complications.
- Antibiotic choice
  - In areas where resistance of *E. coli* to trimethoprim-sulfamethoxazole (TMP-SMX) is <20%, TMP-SMX is recommended
  - Fluoroquinolones like ciprofloxacin should be used in regions with higher resistance
- Length of treatment for uncomplicated UTI
  - Short course (3-day) therapy
    - As effective as longer courses in uncomplicated UTI
    - Increases patient compliance
    - Decreases drug complication
    - Reduces costs
    - May decrease resistance
  - Both TMP-SMX and fluoroquinolones may be given for short course treatment
- Length of treatment for complicated UTI
  - Oral fluoroquinolones like ciprofloxacin for 7–14 days offers reasonable cure
  - Parenteral therapy should be considered for complicated UTI with drug-resistant pathogens or poor tolerance of oral medications

- Asymptomatic Infections should be treated in the setting of:
  - Mechanical abnormalities
  - Parenchymal renal disease
  - Diabetes mellitus
  - Pregnancy
  - Immunocompromised states

Pregnancy Considerations

- Physiologic changes in pregnancy increase risk of UTI
- Asymptomatic infection if left untreated may predispose to complications including:
  - Pyelonephritis
  - Preterm delivery
  - Low birth weight infants
- Insufficient data still exists to support short course therapy in pregnancy although has been employed with success.
  - Effective antibiotic choices may include: Cephalexin, nitrofurantoin, amoxicillin, and ampicillin.

Diet

Cranberry has been studied for treatment and prevention of UTI.

- It is thought to prevent bacterial adherence to host cell surface membranes.
- Currently there is no clear evidence for use in treatment of UTI.
- Studies may suggest a role in prophylaxis.
- It appears to be a safe, well-tolerated herbal supplement without significant drug interactions.

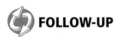 FOLLOW-UP

DISPOSITION

Patients who fail to respond to antibiotics to which the pathogen should be susceptible within 24–48 hours should be considered for repeat urine culture and imaging studies to rule out urinary tract pathology.

REFERENCES

1. David RD, DeBlieux PM, Press R. Rational antibiotic treatment of outpatient genitourinary infections in a changing environment. *Am J Med*. 2005;118:7S–13S.
2. Evidence-Based Clinical Practice. 3-day course of antibiotics as effective as 7-day course for older women with urinary tract infection. *Evidence-based Healthcare Public Health*. 2004; 8:314–315.
3. Lynch DM. Cranberry for prevention of urinary tract infection. *Am Fam Physician*. 2004;70:2175–2177.
4. Mehnert-Kay SA. Diagnosis and management of uncomplicated urinary tract infections. *Am Fam Physician*. 2005;72:451–456.
5. Mittal P, Wing DA. Urinary tract infections in pregnancy. *Clin Perinatol*. 2005;32:749–764.
6. Sheffield JS, Cunnigham FG. Urinary tract infection in women. *Obstet Gynecol*. 2005;106:1085–1092.

CODES

ICD9-CM

- 599.0 UTI
- 595.0 Acute cystitis

KEY WORDS

- Dysuria
- Cystitis
- Pyelonephritis

U

UTERINE FIBROIDS

Mary H. Hohenhaus, MD

KEY CLINICAL POINTS

- Common in reproductive age women
- Most are asymptomatic, but can cause significant morbidity
- Too few well-designed studies to compare treatments
  - Individualize treatment based on woman's age, anticipated timing of menopause, symptom severity, size and number of myomas, other medical conditions, and a discussion of her preferences and desire for pregnancy

 BASICS

DESCRIPTION

- Uterine myomas are benign smooth muscle cell tumors, also called fibroids and leiomyomas
- Described by location, although most myomas involve more than one layer of the uterus
  - Subserosal: Projects into the pelvis, causing irregular uterine contour; may be pedunculated
  - Intramural: Within uterine wall
  - Submucosal: Projects into the uterine cavity
  - May arise from cervix or broad ligament
- Range from microscopic to easily palpable, size described in gestational weeks
- May be single or multiple
- Most common solid pelvic tumor in women, most common indication for hysterectomy

GENERAL PREVENTION

- Oral contraceptives may prevent myomas by suppressing cyclic variation of hormones
- Although diets high in green vegetables have been associated with a lower relative risk, no evidence that dietary intervention prevents myomas

EPIDEMIOLOGY

- True incidence and prevalence are unknown because myomas are usually asymptomatic
- Typically become symptomatic in women between the ages of 30–40
- Black women are 2–3 times more likely to develop myomas than white women
- Black women tend to be younger at both time of diagnosis and hysterectomy, have higher uterine weights, and are more likely to be anemic

Incidence

Estimated at 12.8/1000 women aged 25–44

Prevalence

- Clinically apparent in approximately 20–40% of reproductive age women.
- May exceed 75% in surgical pathology series

RISK FACTORS

- Nulliparity
- Oral contraceptive use before age 16
- Black race

Genetics

- Family and twin studies suggest a genetic predisposition
- Associated with 2 hereditary syndromes:
  - Reed's syndrome: Uterine and subcutaneous myomas
  - Bannayan-Zoana syndrome: Uterine myomas, lipomas, and hemangiomas

PATHOPHYSIOLOGY

- Abnormal uterine bleeding
  - Increased vascularity and venous congestion
  - Increased surface area of uterine cavity
- Compression of pelvic structures
- Acute pelvic pain
  - Torsion of pedunculated myoma
  - Protrusion of submucosal myoma through cervix
  - Infarction as myoma outgrows blood supply
- Impaired fertility
  - Distortion of uterine cavity may interfere with sperm transport or implantation

ETIOLOGY

- 2-step process:
  - Transformation of normal smooth muscle cell to cell with high density of receptors that respond to cyclic hormone variation
  - Clonal proliferation of abnormal muscle cells
- Likely involves multiple growth factors
- Perimenopausal growth related to high estrogen levels during anovulatory cycles

ASSOCIATED CONDITIONS

- Iron-deficiency anemia
- Endometritis
- Adenomyosis
- Impaired fertility

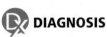 **DIAGNOSIS**

PRE-HOSPITAL

May be found incidentally on bimanual examination of the uterus or on pelvic imaging ordered for unrelated symptoms

SIGNS AND SYMPTOMS

- Pelvic/reproductive
  - Heavy, prolonged, painful menses (submucosal myomas)
    - May be associated with fatigue, pallor, shortness of breath, palpitations
  - Pelvic pressure or fullness
  - Acute pelvic pain
- Gastrointestinal
  - Increased abdominal girth
  - Constipation, tenesmus (posterior myomas)
- Urinary
  - Frequency, urgency (anterior myomas)

History

- Menstrual, sexual, obstetrical histories
- Quantify blood loss during menses

Physical Exam

- Enlarged, firm, irregular uterus
- Peritoneal signs (infarcted myoma)
- Conjunctival pallor, tachycardia

TESTS

Lab

- β-hCG
- Complete blood count
- Iron, total iron-binding capacity, ferritin
- Type and crossmatch before surgery

Imaging
- Abdominal plain films may show concentric calcifications
- Transvaginal ultrasound to confirm diagnosis, evaluate for ovarian neoplasm
- Renal ultrasonography to evaluate for urinary obstruction
- Magnetic resonance imaging to visualize individual myomas, distinguish between benign myomas and malignant sarcomas, detect adenomyosis
- Hysterosalpingography to define extent of submucous myomas before surgery or to evaluate uterine cavity and patency of fallopian tubes

Diagnostic Procedures/Surgery
Endometrial biopsy to evaluate abnormal bleeding

Pathologic Findings
- Multinodular uterine tumor
- Smooth muscle fibers organized in bundles, surrounded by fibrous tissue

DIFFERENTIAL DIAGNOSIS
- Abnormal uterine bleeding
  - Anovulation
  - Endometrial hyperplasia or malignancy
- Pelvic pain
  - Endometriosis
  - Adenomyosis
  - Ectopic pregnancy
  - Torsion or rupture of ovarian cyst
  - Pelvic inflammatory disease
- Pelvic mass
  - Pregnancy
  - Adenomyosis, uterine polyp
  - Ovarian malignancy
  - Leiomyosarcoma

TREATMENT

PRE-HOSPITAL
- No data to support treatment in asymptomatic women; watchful waiting is appropriate
- Drug therapy may control symptoms, reduce myoma size, and help correct anemia before surgery, but does not appear to improve surgical outcomes
- Consider autologous blood donation before surgery

INITIAL STABILIZATION
- Control severe bleeding and pain
- Treat iron-deficiency anemia

MEDICATION (DRUGS)

- Can reduce myoma size and uterine volume as well as bleeding
- May be sufficient for women nearing menopause
- Side effects and expense limit long-term use
- None shown to improve fertility
- Myomas regain pretreatment size within months after drug is stopped
- Oral contraceptives may prevent but will not treat established myomas
- Gonadotropin-releasing hormone (GnRH) agonists
  - Cause hypoestrogenic state
    - Leuprolide: 3.75 mg IM monthly or 11.25 mg IM depot every 3 months

- Nafarelin: 400 mcg intranasally b.i.d. (alternate nostrils)
- Goserelin: 3.6 mg implant SC every 28 days
  - Reduce uterine size by up to 65% and induce amenorrhea in most women
  - Associated with hot flushes, vaginal dryness, mood swings, and bone loss, although addition of hormone replacement therapy (HRT) may reduce side effects
  - Not well studied beyond 6 months of use
- Danazol, an androgenic steroid, and progestins may be useful for inducing amenorrhea, but are not approved for treatment of myomas in the US
- Mifepristone, selective estrogen response modifiers, and interferon alfa may have benefit, but their use is largely investigational

SURGERY
- Indications for surgery
  - Contraindication to or intolerance of drug therapy
  - Failure of medical management to control abnormal bleeding or anemia
  - Concern for malignancy
  - Mass effect causing pain, pressure, or urinary or gastrointestinal tract symptoms
  - Distortion of uterine cavity causing infertility or repeated pregnancy loss
- Carries risk of infection, bleeding, damage to adjacent organs, adhesion formation

ALERT
Rapid growth (increase in uterine size by 6 weeks in 1 year) in a nonpregnant woman or growth in a menopausal woman suggests malignancy and should prompt surgical removal.
- Hysterectomy
  - Definitive treatment as it eliminates symptoms and the development of new myomas
  - Indicated for extensive disease, suspected malignancy, and myomas in association with other pelvic abnormalities
  - Associated with significant improvement in symptoms and quality of life
  - Appropriate only for women who do not desire future pregnancy
- Abdominal myomectomy
  - Removal of myomas via laparotomy while preserving uterus
  - Indicated for multiple myomas or uterus >16 weeks in size
  - Preferred in women desiring future pregnancy as risk of uterine rupture is extremely low
  - Removal of multiple myomas may involve more time and greater blood loss than hysterectomy
- Laparoscopic myomectomy
  - Removal of myomas via laparoscope while preserving uterus
  - Indicated for 1 or 2 easily accessible myomas <8 cm in diameter and uterine size <16 weeks
  - Risk of uterine rupture is controversial
- Hysteroscopic myomectomy
  - Removal of submucosal myomas via operative endoscope introduced through the cervix
  - May be performed as same-day surgery with local anesthesia and sedation
  - More effective when combined with endometrial ablation, but ablation precludes future pregnancy
- Myolysis
  - Coagulation of myoma via laparoscopy
  - May carry increased risk of adhesions and uterine rupture

U

- Uterine artery embolization
  - Procedure under fluoroscopic guidance in which gel, beads, or coils are introduced through a catheter in the common femoral artery to the uterine artery
  - Disrupts blood supply to myoma causing degeneration
  - Minimally invasive procedure under conscious sedation, rapid recovery compared with hysterectomy
  - Usually requires overnight hospitalization for pain control
  - Resolution of bleeding symptoms in up to 90% reported at 6 months, but not well studied
  - Associated with significant pain and fever; sepsis and death have been reported
  - Disruption of blood supply to ovaries and endometrium causing permanent amenorrhea reported in up to 3% of women under 40
  - Long-term effect on fertility and pregnancy outcomes not known

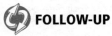 **FOLLOW-UP**

Issues for Referral
- Refer to fertility specialist to evaluate for other causes of infertility
- Refer to urology for management of ureteral obstruction

Pregnancy Considerations
- Large myomas may be associated with pain and premature labor
- Rapid growth may occur in response to estrogen, increased blood flow, or edema
- Risk of abruption increases if the placenta overlies a myoma
- Considerations after myomectomy
  - Adhesions may impair fertility
  - Postpone pregnancy at least 6 months
  - Cesarean delivery may be preferable

PROGNOSIS
- Most symptomatic women require surgery
- May recur after myomectomy
  - Risk increases with number of myomas
  - Up to 50% recurrence at 5 years
  - Up to 25% require second surgery
- Regress during menopause
- HRT may stimulate growth

COMPLICATIONS
- Secondary infection of degenerating myoma
- Osteoporosis secondary to GnRH agonist

- Cytogenetic studies suggest leiomyosarcomas develop from separate pathway, but malignant transformation of myomas has been described

PATIENT MONITORING
- Asymptomatic myomas may be followed by exam or ultrasound every 3 months to determine growth pattern, then every 6 months if stable
  - Examine at same time in cycle to limit effects of hormonal stimulation on tumor size
- Watchful waiting may be appropriate for large, asymptomatic myomas in women approaching menopause if malignancy has been excluded
- Annual bone mineral density studies if GnRH agonist is continued >6 months; consider calcium and bisphosphonate therapy

REFERENCES
1. ACOG Committee on Gynecologic Practice. Uterine artery embolization. *Obstet Gynecol*. 2004;103:403–404.
2. Myers ER, Barbar MD, Gustilo-Ashby T, et al. Management of uterine leiomyomata: What do we really know? *Obstet Gynecol*. 2002;100:8–17.
3. Olive DL, Lindheim SR, Pritts EA. Non-surgical management of leiomyoma: Impact on fertility. *Curr Opinion Obstet Gynecol*. 2004;16:239–243.
4. Stewart EJ. Uterine fibroids. *Lancet*. 2001;357:293–298.
5. Wallach EE, Vlahos NF. Uterine myomas: An overview of development, clinical features, and management. *Obstet Gynecol*. 2004;104:393–406.

CODES
ICD9-CM
- 218.0 Submucous leiomyoma of uterus
- 218.1 Intramural leiomyoma of uterus
- 218.2 Subserous leiomyoma of uterus
- 218.9 Leiomyoma of uterus, unspecified

KEY WORDS

- Dysmenorrhea
- Fibroid
- Hysterectomy
- Leiomyoma
- Menorrhagia
- Myoma
- Myomectomy

VENOUS THROMBOEMBOLISM

Benjamin L. Sapers, MD

KEY CLINICAL POINTS

- Venous thromboembolism (VTE) is a common and, if untreated, highly lethal disease. Keeping a low threshold of suspicion for this condition is always a good idea.
- Pregnancy and the use of OCPs increase the risk of VTE significantly.

 BASICS

DESCRIPTION
Deep venous thrombosis (DVT) is a fibrin clot most commonly found in the deep veins of the lower extremities. Pulmonary embolism (PE) occurs when such clots migrate to the pulmonary venous circulation. VTE may describe either or both of these conditions.

GENERAL PREVENTION
Patients who have had surgery and/or prolonged hospitalizations have a heightened risk for VTE.

- Subcutaneous heparin, low-dose coumadin, LMWHs, and intermittent sequential compression devices (SCDs) with thromboembolism-deterrent stockings (TEDS) decrease the risk of VTE.
- LMWHs probably are the most effective when the risk of VTE is high (e.g., immediately after orthopedic surgery).
- Early mobilization of patients after surgery and during hospitalization minimizes VTE risk.

EPIDEMIOLOGY
Incidence
- Approximately 1.9/1000 in people age >45
- For each 10 year increase in age, the incidence doubles.
- Women over the age of 75 have an incidence of 2.7/1000.
- The risk of VTE among women taking combined estrogen-progesterone oral contraceptive pills (OCP) is 3 times that of controls. The risk among pregnant women is 3–4 times that of women on OCP.

RISK FACTORS
Virchow's Triad: Venous stasis, hypercoagulability, and/or vessel wall injury

- General risks
  - Age >40, history or family history of DVT, pregnancy or recent post-partum, OCP use, obesity, inflammatory bowel disease, nephrotic syndrome, hypertension, congestive heart failure, stroke, pneumonia, cancer, tobacco use, recent surgery (requiring >30 minutes of anesthesia within 1 month), prolonged air travel (more than 3100 miles), trauma and/or fracture (specifically of tibial, femoral or pelvic), shock, diabetic ketoacidosis.
- Blood dyscrasias
  - Major risk: Antiphospholipid antibodies, antithrombin III, protein C or S deficiency, homozygosity for factor V Leiden mutation, prothrombin G20210A mutation.
  - Minor risk: Heterozygosity for factor V Leiden or prothrombin G20210A mutations, hyperhomocysteinemia, myeloproliferative disorders, high factor VIII levels
  - In pregnancy, protein S and homocysteine (if taking folate supplements) levels may be decreased and factor VIII levels increased

PATHOPHYSIOLOGY
- Acute PE causes increased pulmonary vascular resistance due to:
  - Physical obstruction of blood flow
  - Hypoxia-induced vasoconstriction from released humoral factors (serotonin, thrombin, histamine).
- Resultant increase in pulmonary artery pressure leads to increased right ventricular (RV) afterload which in more severe cases may cause RV dilation and failure.

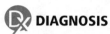 **DIAGNOSIS**

SIGNS AND SYMPTOMS
- Pulmonary Embolism: Dyspnea, chest pain (pleuritic or non), low grade fever, hemoptysis, syncope, tachypnea, tachycardia, and hypotension
  - Approximately >80% of PEs are associated with DVTs and some of these may be asymptomatic
- DVT: Pain, swelling, skin discoloration, and low grade fever
  - Approximately >20% of symptomatic DVTs associated with asymptomatic PE

Physical Exam
- Often unrevealing
- Most common findings include tachycardia and hypoxia
- Right heart strain (jugular venous distention, new tricuspid regurgitation murmur, accentuated P2, RV heave) and hypotension may be present

TESTS
Lab
- CBC to detect blood dyscrasias and obtain baseline platelet count prior to heparin use.
- PT/PTT for baseline prior to anticoagulation.
- EKG to rule out other causes and to evaluate for right heart strain.
- Arterial blood gas (ABG)
  - Should be used only if further evaluation of respiratory status is necessary
  - A normal A-a gradient can be seen in up to 20% of patients with PE
  - With low pre-test probability, normal A-a gradient may help rule out PE
- CXR (<0.001 rads exposure) to evaluate for alternative diagnoses and to compare with V/Q scan if done. Probably unnecessary if CT Angiogram is ordered.
- Troponin I–if elevated may support diagnosis of myocardial infarct but as it and BNP can be elevated with PE, it has been suggested as a marker for severity of PE.
- Serum D-dimer
  - Negative predictive value is up to 99%, but positive predictive value is only 30%.
  - Accuracy varies according to assay type, enzyme-linked immunoadsorbent assays have highest sensitivities.
  - Decreased specificity in pregnant women, but sensitivity remains high.

Pregnancy Considerations
A total gestational radiation exposure of <0.5 rad is recommended for pregnant women. Exposures of up to 5 rad have not been associated with significant fetal injury in the majority of studies.

Diagnostic Procedures

Assess the pretest probability for VTE.

- Pretest Probability for VTE assessment tool
  - PE more likely than competing diagnoses = 3 points
  - Swelling or pain on palpation of legs = 3 points
  - HR >100 = 1.5 points
  - Previous DVT and/or PE = 1.5 points
  - Immobilization >3 days or surgery within last month = 1.5 points
  - Hemoptysis = 1 point
  - Malignancy, active or treated within the last 6 months = 1 point
    - <2 points = low pretest probability
    - 2–6 points = intermediate probability
    - >6 points = high probability
- Low pre-test probability
  - Check D-dimer
  - If (–), no further testing
- Intermediate or high pre-test probability
  - Lung imaging for possible PE
  - Lower extremity US if possible DVT

Imaging

- Lower extremity ultrasound (US):
  - Because calf veins are not well visualized with traditional US technique, US should be repeated on day 7 to rule out clot propagation. As pregnant women may have more prompt propagation; an additional sonogram should be done on day 2 or 3.
  - Full leg ultrasound + D-dimer as accurate as serial ultrasounds in recent studies.
  - Serial negative leg ultrasounds do not abrogate need for lung imaging when the pre-test probability is moderate or high.
  - While pedal edema is most pronounced in third trimester, the risk of VTE is nearly uniform throughout gestation.
- V/Q Scan:
  - A normal V/Q scan effectively rules out pulmonary embolism.
  - Ventilation is 0.01–0.02 rads exposure; perfusion is 0.01–0.03
  - Does not require IV contrast
  - Approximately 50–70% of test results are nondiagnostic (20% in pregnant women as they tend to be younger and have fewer comorbidities)
  - Safest option in pregnant women.
    - Low- and intermediate-probability tests should be followed by leg US.
    - If negative, serial ultrasounds (+/– D-dimer) or pulmonary angiogram (PA gram) should be performed.
- CT angiogram:
  - The test of choice to rule out PE
  - Accuracy may be comparable to PA gram.
  - When V/Q scan and CTA had discordant results, CTA demonstrated correct diagnosis 92% of the time
  - IV contrast load and radiation exposure (0.2–0.3 rads) equivalent to that of PA gram
  - May rule in alternative diagnosis
  - May help diagnose right heart strain
- Pulmonary angiogram
  - Gold standard
  - Complication rate in 4 studies investigating PE
    - Rate of death was 0.0–0.5%
    - Major complication rate ≤3% (severe contrast reaction, renal failure, and cardiac arrest)

DIFFERENTIAL DIAGNOSIS

- PE: Pneumonia, asthma, COPD exacerbation, myocardial infarction, pulmonary edema, anxiety, aortic dissection, pericardial tamponade, lung cancer, pulmonary HTN, rib fracture, pneumothorax, costochondritis, and/or musculoskeletal pain
- DVT: Cellulitis, superficial thrombophlebitis, calf muscle strain or tear, popliteal cyst, venous insufficiency, knee or ankle pathology, asymmetric cardiac edema, drug induced edema, lymphedema, and/or lipedema

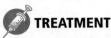 **TREATMENT**

INITIAL STABILIZATION

Patients may be hypotensive and hypoxic with severe PE. Fluid resuscitation and pressors should be initiated when necessary.

GENERAL MEASURES

Both PE and VTE can be painful.

- NSAIDs should be used with caution as may exacerbate bleeding risk.
- Acetaminophen in high doses has been associated with an elevation in INR with coumadin.
- Judicious use of opioids may be required for symptomatic management.

Activity

No compelling evidence that early ambulation promotes DVT propagation. Some guidelines recommend that normal ambulation can begin on day 2 of treatment with LMWH.

Special Therapy

Graduated compression stockings with DVT may decrease risk of chronic venous disease of involved leg.

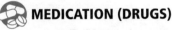 **MEDICATION (DRUGS)**

- Heparins (Low Molecular Weight Heparins [LMWH] and Unfractionated Heparin [UFH])
  - Current standard of care for acute DVT/PE including during pregnancy
  - LMWH
    - Starting dose is 1 mg/kg SC b.i.d.
    - Has been associated with fewer deaths and major bleeds than UFH
  - UFH
    - Higher risk of heparin-induced thrombocytopenia and osteoporosis with long-term use than LMWH
    - Still has a role in patients with
      - ○ Weight >100 kg
      - ○ Condition which may require rapid reversal of anticoagulation
      - ○ Renal insufficiency
    - Dosed by weight and monitored by PTT
  - Neither UFH nor LWMH cross the placenta nor are they secreted into breast milk.
- Coumadin
  - Generally started once therapeutic LWMH (or UFH) at doses of 2.5–10 mg/day depending on patient's age and comorbidities
  - LMWH is continued until the INR is 2–3 for 2 consecutive days.
  - Chronic use of LMWH may be preferred in cancer related VTE.
  - Anticoagulation is continued for a total of 3–6 months when VTE is thought to be provoked and at least 6 months when not.

– In most cases, a second unprovoked episode of VTE should be treated with a lifetime of anticoagulation
– Probably safe in first 6 weeks of gestation but increased risk of bone, facial and central nervous system abnormalities if used later. Since it does cross the placenta, can lead to neonatal bleeding on delivery.
- Thrombolytics
  – Indications
    - Massive pulmonary embolus
    - Cardiogenic shock
    - Evidence of right heart strain by Echo
  – Thrombolytic therapy has not been shown to decrease mortality, although may decrease the sequela of chronic pulmonary HTN
  – Surgical or catheter embolectomy may be attempted in patients who are otherwise at high risk for bleeding.
- Inferior vena cava filter (IVCF)
  – May be temporary or permanent
  – Indications:
    - Patients with known DVT when a clear contraindication to anticoagulation exists
    - Adjunctive therapy for significant proximal propagation of DVT in a patient on appropriate anticoagulation
  – IVCFs may themselves become nidus for clot
    - Risk of PE decreases acutely with known DVT but this benefit is lost within 2 years
    - Associated with increased risk of chronic venous disease and recurrent DVTs within 2 years of placement

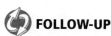

FOLLOW-UP

DISPOSITION
- Patients with PE can be discharged safely if hemodynamically stable and therapeutic on coumadin (INR = 2–3)
- Clinically stable patients with acute DVT and with good social support can be managed as outpatients on LWMH and coumadin.

PROGNOSIS
- Good prognosis for VTE with timely treatment
- For unprovoked VTE events, recurrence rate off anticoagulants is high and optimal length of treatment is 6 months

PATIENT MONITORING
- Close monitoring as outpatients to detect recurrence and to maintain a therapeutic INR

- If INR is therapeutic on 2 consecutive measurements, interval between blood checks can be increased, but never to more than 1 month.
- Patients should be aware that many foods and medications can alter INR.
  – Should report any new medications including over-the-counter and herbals
  – May benefit from nutrition consult and handouts on high Vitamin K foods

REFERENCES

1. Bates SM, Ginsberg JS. How we manage venous thromboembolism during pregnancy. *Blood*. 2002;100:3470–3478.
2. Goldhaber SZ, Elliott CG. Acute pulmonary embolism: Part I epidemiology, pathophysiology, and diagnosis. *Circ*. 2003;108:2726–2729.
3. Goldhaber SZ, Elliott CG. Acute pulmonary embolism: Part II risk stratification, treatment, and prevention. *Circ*. 2003;108:2832–2838.
4. Kanne JP, Lalani TA. Role of computed tomography and magnetic resonance imaging for deep venous thrombosis and pulmonary embolism. *Circ*. 2004;109:I15–I21.
5. Kearon C, Ginsberg JS, Kovacs MJ, et al. Comparison of low-intensity warfarin therapy with conventional-intensity warfarin therapy for long-term prevention of recurrent venous thromboembolism. *NEJM*. 2003;349:631–639.
6. Quiroz R, Kucher N, Zou KH, et al. Clinical validity of a negative computed tomography scan in patients with suspected pulmonary embolism: A systematic review. *JAMA*. 2005;293:2012–2017.

CODES
ICD9-CM
- 415.1 Pulmonary embolism and infarction
- 673 Obstetrical pulmonary embolism
- 453.40 Venous embolism and thrombosis of unspecified deep vessels of lower extremity

KEY WORDS

- Venous Thromboembolism
- Pulmonary Embolism
- Deep Venous Thrombosis

V

VULVAR LICHEN SCLEROSIS

Mohsin K. Malik, MD
Lynn E. Iler, MD

KEY CLINICAL POINTS

- Lichen sclerosis is a chronic, inflammatory and scarring skin disease of unknown cause:
  - Pruritus is major symptom
  - Scarring of the labia can lead to significant pain and functional impairment
  - Can resemble sexual abuse
- Ultrapotent topical steroids are effective, first-line therapy
- Up to 5% lifetime risk of developing squamous cell carcinoma of the vulva

 BASICS

DESCRIPTION
- Lichen sclerosis is a chronic inflammatory and scarring disease of the skin.
- Starts as hypopigmented, atrophic plaques around the vagina and anus and later progresses to scarring
- Long-standing disease can lead to narrowing of the introitus, absorption of labia minora, and scarring of the clitoral hood.

EPIDEMIOLOGY
- Good epidemiological data is lacking.
- More common on vulva than penis, female to male ratio between 6:1 and 10:1.
- More common in older women.
- More commonly reported in whites.

Incidence
- Peak incidence in 6th decade (about 14/100,000)
- Second, smaller peak in incidence in prepubertal girls

ETIOLOGY
- Cause remains unknown
- Autoimmune mechanism implicated
  - Lichen sclerosis clusters with autoimmune disease, 41% of women have autoantibodies.
  - Some histological similarities with autoimmune diseases affecting the skin, including scleroderma and systemic lupus erythematosus.
- Infectious etiology has also been implicated
  - *Borrelia burgdorferi*, the most likely pathogenic agent
  - However, women in the United States do not have evidence of increased exposure.
- Exacerbation of lesions with local trauma (Koebnerization)
  - Lichen sclerosis may first become apparent after itching and subsequent scratching from candidiasis, vaginitis, or other local process.
  - Scratching exacerbates the pruritis of lichen sclerosis, creating an itch-scratch cycle.

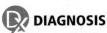 DIAGNOSIS

SIGNS AND SYMPTOMS
- May begin asymptomatically
- Vulvar or perineal symptoms include:
  - Pruritus (mild to severe)
  - Pain/burning/soreness
  - Dysuria
  - Dryness/dyspareunia (adults)
  - Vaginal discharge
  - Genital/anal bleeding
  - Labial stenosis/fusion (late sequelae)
  - Constipation (generally in children)
  - Girls are more likely than women to report urinary or bowel symptoms
- Lichen sclerosis can clinically resemble sexual abuse.
  - The 2 diagnoses are not mutually exclusive.
  - In one series, sexual abuse was suspected in 3/4 of girls eventually diagnosed with lichen sclerosis only.

Physical Exam
Diagnosis can often be made on clinical grounds, especially in children.
- Early disease may have only hypopigmentation or changes of skin texture
- Often intensely pruritic
- Findings include
  - Atrophic plaques in "figure-8" or "hourglass" distribution around the vulva and anus
  - Hypo/hyperpigmentation
  - Wrinkled texture of skin (subtle)
  - Excoriation, cracks, fissures, erosion, telangiectasias, bullae
  - Vulvar scarring (labial adhesion/fusion/stenosis)
  - Secondary infection
  - Non-genital involvement (oral, back/shoulders) is uncommon

TESTS
Lab
Despite reports of autoantibodies in patients with lichen sclerosis, a workup for autoimmune disease is generally not warranted.

Diagnostic Procedures/Surgery
Punch biopsy for evaluation of suspicious areas.

Pathologic Findings
Histological examination is often required to establish the diagnosis.

Changes include thinning of the epidermis, degeneration of basal layer, inflammatory cells in the upper dermis, and homogenization of papillary dermis

DIFFERENTIAL DIAGNOSIS
- Atopic dermatitis (eczema)
- Post-inflammatory hypo/hyperpigmentation
- Lichen simplex chronicus
- Candidal vulvovaginitis
- Bacterial vaginosis
- Lichen planus
- Scleroderma
- Vitiligo
- Sexual abuse

 MEDICATION (DRUGS)

First Line
- Ultrapotent topical steroids are first-line therapy
  - Options include:
    - Clobetasol propionate 0.05% ointment (Temovate 0.05% ointment)

- Halobetasol propionate 0.05% ointment (Ultravate 0.05% ointment)
- Cream, gel, or liquid versions of these steroids are not ultrapotent and are not appropriate first-line therapy
- Apply b.i.d. for 3 months
- Taper based on response
- A 30 g tube lasts about 3 months
- Maintenance therapy is generally required
  - No optimal protocol
  - Moderate to ultrapotent topical steroids applied 2–3 times weekly generally prevent recurrence
- Rare side effects of topical steroids include local skin atrophy and adrenal suppression

Second Line
- Other medical treatments include retinoids (oral or topical) and topical androgens, progesterones, or estrogens, but these are not as effective.
- Antihistamines (hydroxyzine) may be required in women with severe pruritus, or who exacerbate lesions by scratching.

SURGERY
- Surgery may be required to repair functional impairment caused by scarring.
- Indications include:
  - Narrowed introitus
  - Fused labia
  - Buried clitoris
- Vulvectomy does not provide surgical cure for lichen sclerosis because of the high post-operative recurrence rate.

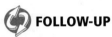 FOLLOW-UP

Issues for Referral
To dermatologist to confirm diagnosis and biopsy any changed areas.

PROGNOSIS
- Ultrapotent topical corticosteroids are effective treatment:
  - Relief of symptoms in most patients
  - Complete resolution of disease in about 25%
  - Symptoms generally improve in days
  - Skin changes improve over months
  - May prevent scarring if used early
  - Treatment can reverse some of the histological changes but not scarring
- Small subset of girls have resolution of disease at menarche

COMPLICATIONS
Up to 5% long-term risk of developing squamous cell carcinoma of the vulva.
- Not known if treatment reduces risk for malignancy
- Usually occurs in older patients but has been reported in women as young as 18

PATIENT MONITORING
Long-term surveillance for malignancy with semiannual to annual exam is warranted given increased risk of squamous cell carcinoma.

REFERENCES

1. Cooper SM, Gao XH, Powell JJ, et al. Does treatment of vulvar lichen sclerosus influence its prognosis? *Arch Dermatol*. 2004;140:702–706.
2. Dalziel KL, Wojnarowska F. Long-term control of vulval lichen sclerosus after treatment with a potent topical steroid cream. *J Reprod Med*. 1993;38:25–27.
3. Fujiwara H, Fujiwara K, Hashimoto K, et al. Detection of Borrelia burgdorferi DNA (B garinii or B afzelii) in morphea and lichen sclerosus et atrophicus tissues of German and Japanese but not of US patients. *Arch Dermatol*. 1997;133:41–44.
4. Meffert JJ, Davis BM, Grimwood RE. Lichen sclerosus. *J Am Acad Dermatol*. 1995;32:393–416.
5. Meyrick RH, Ridley CM, McGibbon DH, et al. Lichen sclerosus et atrophicus and autoimmunity-a study of 350 women. *Br J Dermatol*. 1988;118:41–46.
6. Powell JJ, Wojnarowska F. Lichen sclerosus. *Lancet*. 1999;353:1777–1783.
7. Scurry JP, Vanin K. Vulvar squamous cell carcinoma and lichen sclerosus. *Australas J Dermatol*. Jun 1997;38(Suppl 1): S20–S25.

CODES
ICD9-CM
701.0

KEY WORDS
- Lichen Sclerosis
- Dyspareunia
- Squamous Cell Carcinoma
- Koebnerization

V

VULVAR MASS

Kelly Bossenbroek, MD
Melissa Nothnagle, MD

KEY CLINICAL POINTS

- Vulvar mass has a broad differential diagnosis, the most worrisome being cancer.
- Any lesion that is increasing in size or has an unusual appearance should be biopsied.
- Patients should be referred to a surgeon for any diagnostic biopsy that cannot safely be done in the office.
- Risk factors for vulvar cancer include smoking, human papilloma virus (HPV) infection, HIV infection, and advanced age.

 BASICS

DESCRIPTION

A wide variety of pathologic processes can present as a vulvar mass. These can be classified as benign, pre-cancerous, or malignant, although many of these entities are points on a spectrum of disease. For example lichen sclerosus can lead to vulvar epithelial neoplasia (VIN), which can progress to squamous cell carcinoma.

- Benign disease:
  - Benign tumors can be cystic (mucous cyst, Bartholin's cyst), anatomic (hernia), or solid (fibroma, lipoma).
  - Infections and abscesses also can present as a mass.
- Premalignant disease:
  - The undifferentiated type of VIN is associated with HPV infection (especially subtypes 16 and 18) and often affects younger women.
  - The differentiated type of VIN is often keratinizing and is associated with lichen sclerosis but not with HPV infection.
- Malignant disease:
  - The most common form of vulvar cancer is squamous cell carcinoma.

GENERAL PREVENTION

- VIN and squamous cell carcinoma are associated with HPV infection. Preventing HPV infection by postponing the age of first intercourse and limiting the number of sexual partners may help prevent these diseases.
- Smoking cessation
- Regular gynecological exams including visual inspection of the external genitalia to diagnose and treat early premalignant disease.

EPIDEMIOLOGY

Vulvar cancer is most common in women between the ages of 65 and 75. However, 15% of newly diagnosed patients are under the age of 40.

Incidence

- According to the American Cancer Society, approximately 4,000 vulvar cancers will be diagnosed in the United States in 2005.
- Among elderly women the annual incidence is 20 per 100,000.

Prevalence

Vulvar cancer accounts for 0.6% of all cancers in women.

RISK FACTORS

- HPV infection
- HIV infection
- Advanced age
- Smoking

PATHOPHYSIOLOGY

- The pathologic processes underlying vulvar diseases are variable.
- The exact mechanism of HPV-associated malignant transformation is not completely elucidated, but may be due to cell cycle augmentation by HPV-encoded proteins.

ETIOLOGY

- HPV infection is associated with VIN, a premalignant finding which can progress to squamous cell carcinoma.
- Vulvar cancer in older women is associated with chronic inflammation (often reported by the patient as chronic itching) leading to squamous cell hyperplasia, which may progress to VIN and squamous cell carcinoma.

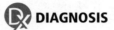 DIAGNOSIS

SIGNS AND SYMPTOMS

Malignant diseases:

- VIN
  - Long history of vulvar pruritus (most common symptom of VIN)
  - Affected area is often thicker and lighter in color than the surrounding skin
- Invasive vulvar cancer:
  - Vulvar lump or mass (most common sign)
  - Vulvar bleeding, discharge, or pain
  - Dysuria

History

- Importantly, women with vulvar cancer present to their physician an average of 6 months after symptoms develop. Women should be asked routinely about vulvar itching and discomfort.
- Patients with vulvar disorders often complain of chronic pruritus, pain, burning, irritation, or a palpable mass.

Physical Exam

- Vulvar cancer usually presents as a raised lesion which may be ulcerated or condylomatous.
- Most squamous cell carcinomas occur on the labia majora and are unifocal.
- Mucous cysts are found on the labia minora or at the introitus.
- Bartholin's cysts are found in the labia minora at 4 and 8 o'clock. Usually they are pea-sized, but can be quite large when inflamed or infected.
- Skene's duct cysts are located adjacent to the urethral meatus.

TESTS

Imaging

Imaging is generally not useful in identifying or diagnosing tumors of the vulva. However, MRI or CT scan can be used to detect regional lymph node metastasis.

Diagnostic Procedures/Surgery

- Any suspicious lesion on the vulva should be biopsied using excisional or punch biopsy, which can be done under local anesthesia in the primary care office. Large or highly suspicious lesions may be referred to a gynecologist for biopsy.
- Benign tumors such as fibromas, lipomas, or hidradenomas should be excised if they are painful, bleeding, rapidly growing, or cosmetically bothersome.
- Asymptomatic sebaceous cysts can be left untreated. Incision and drainage is indicated for infected cysts.

- A firm nodule on the labia minora can be mistaken for a Bartholin's cyst when it is actually Bartholin's gland carcinoma. Due to the increased risk of this type of carcinoma in women over 40 years old, masses should be biopsied in women of this age group.
- Bartholin's gland abscesses can be treated by placement of a Word catheter or by marsupialization.

Pathologic Findings
- Histologically, squamous cell carcinoma is the most common type of vulvar cancer. However, melanoma, basal cell carcinoma, verrucous carcinoma, Paget's disease, and other types of cancers also occur on the vulva.

DIFFERENTIAL DIAGNOSIS
- Benign disease:
  - Fibroma (most common benign solid tumor of the vulva)
  - Lipoma
  - Hidradenoma
  - Sebaceous cyst
  - Epidermoid cyst
  - Pilonidal cyst
  - Condyloma acuminatum
  - Bartholin's gland cyst or abscess
  - Fistula or abscess due to Crohn's disease
- Malignant and premalignant disease:
  - VIN I, II, III (pre-cancerous lesions)
  - Squamous cell carcinoma (most common malignancy of the vulva)
  - Melanoma
  - Bartholin's gland carcinoma
  - Basal cell carcinoma
  - Sarcoma
  - Lymphoma
  - Endodermal sinus tumor
  - Merkel cell carcinoma

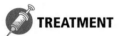 **TREATMENT**

SURGERY
Surgical excision is the treatment of choice for patients with vulvar cancer.
- The goal of surgery is to remove the primary lesion with a 1 cm margin as well as any associated lymph nodes.
- Vulvar cancers are also staged surgically.
- Repeat excision is the best treatment for local recurrence.

Pregnancy Considerations
Excision of asymptomatic benign lesions should be delayed until after delivery due to increased risk of bleeding. However, diagnostic biopsy and excision for potential malignancy should not be postponed.

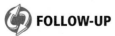 **FOLLOW-UP**

PROGNOSIS
5-year survival rate for vulvar cancer is 70%.

Early detection and treatment improves survival.

PATIENT MONITORING
Patients with a history of vulvar cancer should be monitored closely for disease recurrence at the excision site as well as metastasis to the inguinal lymph nodes.

Examine patients for new masses, skin breakdown and/or ulceration.

REFERENCES

1. American Cancer Society. What are the key statistics for vulvar cancer? Available at: http://www.cancer.org.
2. Blumstein HA. Bartholin gland diseases. *Emedicine*, May 24, 2004.
3. Canavan T, Cohen D. Vulvar cancer. *Am Fam Physic*. 2002;66:1269–1274.
4. Eilber KS, Raz S. Benign cystic lesions of the vagina: A literature review. *J Urology*. 2003;170:717–722.
5. Feller ER, Ribaudo S, Jackson ND. Gynecologic aspects of Crohn's disease. *Am Fam Physic*. 2001;64:1725–1728.
6. Larrabee R, Kylander DJ. Benign vulvar disorders. Identifying features, practical management of nonneoplastic conditions and tumors. *Postgrad Med*. 2001;109:151–164.
7. Naumann RW. Surgical treatment of vulvar cancer. *Emedicine*, Nov 11, 2004.
8. The 2004 ASCO annual meeting proceedings (post-meeting edition). *J Clin Oncol*. 2004;22:5028.

ADDITIONAL READING
Tavassoli FA, Devilee P, eds. World Health Organization Classification of Tumours. Pathology and Genetics of Tumours of the Breast and Female Genital Organs. Lyon: IARC Press; 2003.
Sinard JH. Outlines in Pathology. Philadelphia: WB Saunders; 1996.

CODES
ICD9-CM
- 079.4 HPV infection
- 184.4 Malignant neoplasm of vulva
- 214.9 Lipoma any site
- 233.3 Carcinoma in situ
- 229.9 Benign lesion
- 616.1 Vaginitis/Vulvitis
- 616.2 Bartholin's gland cyst
- 616.3 Bartholin's gland abscess
- 624.1 Atrophy of vulva
- 698.9 Pruritus
- 705.83 Hidradenitis suppurativa
- 706.2 Sebaceous cyst

CPT
- 56405 Vulvar abscess – incision and drainage
- 56420 Bartholin's Gland abscess – incision and drainage
- 56440 Marsupialization
- 56501-56515 Destruction of vulvar lesion
- 56605-56606 Perineal biopsy
- 56740 Bartholin's Gland excision

KEY WORDS
- HPV Infection
- Squamous Cell Carcinoma
- Chronic Pruritus
- Vulvar Mass
- Vulvar Cancer

V

VULVODYNIA

Lori A. Boardman, MD, ScM

KEY CLINICAL POINTS

- Vulvodynia is a chronic pain syndrome and is not psychological in origin.
- Approximately 40% of women with vulvodynia do not seek treatment; 60% of those who seek treatment see 3 or more physicians prior to diagnosis.
- Current treatment options are largely empirical and rarely evidence-based:
  - No single treatment effective in all women
  - Improvement may take weeks to months

 ## BASICS

DESCRIPTION
- Characterized by chronic vulvar burning, irritation or rawness in the absence of skin disease or infection.
- Tend to fall into 2 different groups based on location of pain, although overlap possible:
  - Generalized vulvodynia describes involvement of entire vulva by persistent, chronic pain that is burning, stinging or irritating
  - Localized vulvodynia specifies involvement of a portion of vulva, such as the vestibule (vulvar vestibulitis) or clitoris
  - In both instances, pain may be provoked (e.g., intercourse, tampon insertion) or spontaneous or mixed

EPIDEMIOLOGY
- 3/4 of women with vulvodynia have pain on contact, with the remaining 25% experiencing spontaneous burning or knife-like pain.
- Cumulative incidence similar in African American and white women.
- Hispanic women may be more likely to experience chronic vulvar pain compared to African American or white women.
- Chronic vulvar pain on contact decreases with increasing age.

Prevalence
Recent population-based evidence indicates:
- Approximately 16% of the United States population report histories of chronic vulvar burning or pain on contact lasting 3 months or longer.
- Approximately 7% currently experiencing such discomfort

RISK FACTORS
Proposed triggers historically include but are not limited to:
- Recurrent vaginal infections (most commonly, yeast and bacterial vaginosis)
- Use of oral contraceptives
- Destructive treatments (e.g., trichloroacetic acid) or irritants (e.g., topical medications)
- Repetitive physical or sexual abuse, most often by primary family member (associated with vulvodynia in recent population-based study)

Genetics
Specific genetic variants (or polymorphisms) appear to be associated with risk of vestibulitis:
- Homozygosity for allele 2 of interleukin-1 receptor antagonist
- At least 1 of 6 melanocortin-1 receptor polymorphisms
  - If both present, additive risk for vestibulitis

ETIOLOGY
- Multifactorial process involved in development of vulvodynia
- End result: Neuropathic pain (most frequently, burning)

ASSOCIATED CONDITIONS
Higher incidence of:
- Interstitial cystitis
- Irritable bowel syndrome
- Fibromyalgia

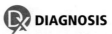 ## DIAGNOSIS

SIGNS AND SYMPTOMS
- Symptoms include vulvar burning, stinging, irritation, or rawness.
- Itching may be present, but should not predominate.
- Clinical signs limited to possible vestibular erythema in those with vestibulitis.

History
- Exact symptoms as well as location and duration of pain
- Previous diagnoses and treatments
- Use of skin irritants

Physical Exam
- If cutaneous or mucosal disease present, evaluate (including possible biopsy) and treat first
- If no visible disease, perform cotton swab test (see below)
- If tender or patient describes burning with touch, perform fungal culture
- If culture negative, institute general measure and treatment

TESTS
- Cotton swab test:
  - Using moistened Q-Tip, palpate vestibule (area just outside hymen) at 2, 4, 6, 8, and 10 o'clock
  - Patient quantifies pain as absent, mild, moderate or severe
- Wet mount and KOH preparations, vaginal pH
- Vaginal fungal culture
- Vulvar biopsy of suspicious areas

Pathologic Findings
Biopsy is not indicated in absence of clinical findings

DIFFERENTIAL DIAGNOSIS
- Cyclic vulvovaginitis
- Atypical candidiasis (non-albicans species)
- Vulvar dermatoses (e.g.,allergic or contact dermatitis, lichen sclerosus, lichen simplex chronicus)

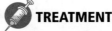 ## TREATMENT

GENERAL MEASURES
- Cotton underwear during day and none at night
- Avoid irritants (perfumes, shampoos)
- Cleanse with water and pat dry
- If needed, emollients without preservatives

Diet
Use of low-oxalate diet with calcium citrate supplementation controversial and evidence to support treatment disputed.

Biofeedback and Physical Therapy
- Used for both localized and generalized pain
- Particularly helpful if vaginismus present
- Includes internal and external soft tissue mobilization and myofascial release, trigger-point pressure, electrical stimulation; pelvic floor retraining, biofeedback
- Success rates (variably measured from pain decrease to return to intercourse) range from 35–79%

Complementary and Alternative Medicine
Reports indicate frequent use of complementary health methods and products by patients with vulvar pain
- Dietary alterations most common method
- Nutritional and herbal supplements most common product
- Acupuncture beneficial in one small study

 ## MEDICATION (DRUGS)

Multiple treatments often used with no clear superiority demonstrated; randomized trials rare
- Topical:
  - A 5% lidocaine ointment most commonly prescribed
    - Approximately 76% of women with vestibulitis able to have intercourse following 6–8 weeks nightly therapy (compared to 36% at baseline)
  - A 0.025% capsaicin cream
    - Significant decreases in pain and increases in ability to have intercourse seen following 12 weeks daily therapy among vestibulitis patients
  - Others: gabapentin cream (requires compounding pharmacy), amitriptyline cream
- Injectable:
  - Triamcinolone acetonide 1% and bupivacaine
  - Submucosal methylprednisolone and lidocaine
    - Approximately 68% of a small population of vestibulitis patients with favorable response following weekly injections over 3 weeks
  - Interferon α
    - Long-term improvement variable
    - Side effects include fever, malaise, myalgia
- Oral:
  - Tricyclic antidepressants
    - Use lower doses in elderly, do not stop abruptly in any patient
    - Avoid use in presence of cardiac abnormalities or in those using MAOIs
  - Gabapentin and carbamazepine
  - Full pain response for all oral medications not evident for 3–4 weeks
  - Slowly increase doses of all medications to allow development of tolerance to side effects

SURGERY
- Surgery not indicated in women with generalized vulvodynia
- Vestibulectomy reserved for women with long-standing vestibulitis recalcitrant to other therapies
  - Success rates vary widely and are lower in those with primary vestibulitis (always had pain with insertion) and those with interstitital cystitis
  - Complications: Blood loss, wound infection or separation, granulation tissue, and continued pain

 ## FOLLOW-UP

PROGNOSIS
- Even with appropriate therapy, rapid resolution unusual
- Realistic goals crucial
  - Expected level of improvement (in pain, sexual function) may change during therapy and will vary from patient to patient
- Early counseling for women with sexual pain (including sex therapy, couples counseling, and/or psychotherapy) crucial

REFERENCES

1. Haefner H, Collins M, Davis G, et al. The vulvodynia guide. *J Reprod Med*. 2005;9:40–51.
2. Harlow B, Stewart E. A population-based assessment of chronic unexplained vulvar pain: Have we underestimated the prevalence of vulvodynia? *J Am Med Womens Assoc*. 2003;58:82–88.
3. Moyal-Barracco M, Lynch P. 2003 ISSVD terminology and classification of vulvodynia: A historical perspective. *J Reprod Med*. 2004;49:772–777.
4. National Institute of Child Health and Human Development. Vulvodynia: Toward Understanding a Pain Syndrome (04-5462). Washington, DC: United States Government Printing Office; 2004.

ADDITIONAL READING

Stewart E, Spencer P. *The V Book: A Doctor's Guide to Complete Vulvovaginal Health*. New York: Bantam Publishers; 2002.

CODES
ICD9-CM
- 625.9 Vulvodynia
- 616.10 Vulvar vestibulitis

KEY WORDS

- Vulvar Pain
- Vestibulitis
- Dyspareunia

INDEX

Page numbers followed by *f* indicate figures; page numbers followed by *t* indicate tabular material.

Index

Mirtazapine, 26, 83
Miscarriage, 8–9, 100, 258, 260, 269–273
Misoprostol, 9, 273, 328
Missed abortion, 8–9, 271–273
Mitotane, 80
Mitoxantrone (Novantrone), 176
Mittelschmerz, 174
Mixed incontinence, 329–331
MMI. *See* Methimazole
MMSE. *See* Mini-mental status test
Modafinil, 177, 188
MODY. *See* Maturity-onset diabetes of young
Mofetil, 38
Mohs micrographic surgery, for skin cancer, 310–312
Moist skin, 150, 241
Monoamine oxidase inhibitors (MAOIs), 26, 83, 97, 300
Mononucleosis, 114–116
Monospot, 114
Mood changes, 14*t*, 129, 186–187
Mood disorder, 82, 123
Mood stabilizers, 184, 221
Mood swings, 59, 91, 281
Morbid obesity, 183–185
Morning headache, 187
Morning stiffness, 123, 292
Morning tiredness, 187
Morphea, 295–297
Morphine, 224, 237
Motor response, slowed, 313
Mouth, dryness of, 307–309
MPC. *See* Mucopurulent cervicitis
MS. *See* Multiple sclerosis
MTX. *See* Methotrexate
Mucocutaneous lesions, 304
Mucopurulent cervicitis (MPC), 204–205
Mucopurulent discharge, 204
Mucosal bleeding, 5–7
Mucus
  dry oral, 238, 262
  passage of, 164
Multiple sclerosis (MS), 175–177
Muscle cramps, 244
Muscle inflammation, 85
Muscle mass, increase of, 138
Muscle tension, 25
Muscle twitches, 261
Muscle wasting, 133, 136, 150, 238
Muscle weakness, 79, 85, 150, 238
Musculoskeletal pain, 122–123, 281
Myalgias, 59, 122–123, 153, 296, 307, 316
Mycobacterium tuberculosis, 267–269
Mycophenolate, 38
Mycophenolate mofetil, 86, 317
Mycoplasma hominis, 39
Mydriasis, 313
Myelin sheath, autoimmune disease attack on, 175
Myobloc. *See* Botulinum toxin
Myocardial Infarction, 75–77
Myolysis, for uterine fibroids, 335
Myomas, 334–336
Myomectomy, for uterine fibroids, 335
Myopathy, 150

Mysoline, 113
Myxedema, 244–246
Myxedema coma, 153–154

Nabothian cysts, 178–179
Nadolol, 130
Nafarelin, 33, 109, 335
NAFLD. *See* Nonalcoholic fatty liver disease
Nails, brittle, 153
Naladixic acid, 286
Naltrexone, 14–15, 314
Namenda. *See* Memantine
Naratriptan (Amerge), 130
Narcolepsy, 161–163
Narcotics, 237
Nasal congestion, 264
NASH. *See* nonalcoholic steatohepatitis
Nateglinide, 89
Nausea, 14*t*, 25, 59, 93, 129, 133, 192, 194, 196, 204, 226, 233, 235, 238, 247, 255, 262, 277, 332
Nausea and vomiting in pregnancy (NVP), 238–240
Neck
  pain in, 75, 104, 150
  stiffness in, 236, 286
Neck vein distention, 71
Nedocromil, 30*t*
Neisseria gonorrhoeae, 42, 203–207, 300, 304, 332–333
Nelfinavir, 143
Nelson syndrome, 80
Neonatal Graves' disease, 241–243
Neonatal TB, 269
Nephritis, 307
  Lupus, 316–318
Nephropathy, 90
Nerve compression, 198
Neural tube defects, 258, 260
Neurocognitive deficits, 186
Neuroleptics, 20, 221
Neuropathy, 90, 129, 136
Neuropsychological impairment, 246
Nevirapine, 143
Newborn care, by women with seizure disorders, 259
NHPCC. *See* Hereditary nonpolyposis colorectal cancer
Niacin, 146
Niaspan, 146
Nicotine, 261, 290, 313–315, 322
Nicotinic acid, 146
Nifedipine, 230, 253, 290–291, 296
Night sweats, 59, 142, 171, 268
Nimodipine, 131
Nipple
  discharge from, 48–49, 120
  inversion of, 44
  pain in, 51, 169–170
Nipple confusion, 51
Nipple stimulation, 124
Nitrates, 76
Nitrofuradantoin, 36
Nitrofurantoin, 278, 279, 333
Nitroglycerin, 291
Nitroglycerine, 64, 253
Nitroprusside, 253

NMDA-receptor antagonist, 20, 102
Nocturia, 187
Nodules, 10, 49–50, 292, 310–311
Nonalcoholic fatty liver disease (NAFLD), 180–182
Nonalcoholic fatty liver with cryptogenic cirrhosis, 180–182
Nonalcoholic steatohepatitis (NASH), 180–182
Nonimmune fetalis hydrops, 200–202
Nonrestorative sleep, 161, 187
Nonsteroidal anti-inflammatory drugs (NSAIDs), 6, 8, 49, 62, 78, 93–94, 109, 120, 123, 127, 130, 158–159, 174, 190, 198, 200–202, 236–237, 251, 265, 281, 293, 309, 316–317, 320, 338
Norgestimate, 218
Nortriptyline, 83, 131, 221, 236
Nortyptilline, 322
Novantrone. *See* Mitoxantrone
NSAIDs. *See* Nonsteroidal anti-inflammatory drugs
Numbing, against past trauma, 298
Nuvaring, 94
NVP. *See* Nausea and vomiting in pregnancy

Obesity, 10, 22–23, 75–77, 155, 180–182, 183–188, 217–218, 235, 284*t*, 286–288
Obsessive compulsive disorder (OCD), 25–27, 96–97
Obstructive sleep apnea syndrome (OSAS), 161–163, 186–188
Obstructive sleep apnea-hypopnea syndrome (OSAHS), 186
OC. *See* Oral contraceptives
OCD. *See* Obsessive compulsive disorder
OCPs. *See* Oral contraceptives
Octreotide, 64
Odynophagia, 142
Ofloxacin, 205
Olanzapine (Zyprexa), 20
Oligomenorrhea, 5, 155, 217–219
Oligo-ovulation, 217
Olsalazine, 159
Omalizumab, 29
Omega-3 fatty acids, 221
Ondanzetron, 239
Onycholysis, 150
Ophthalmopathy, 150
Opiates, 69, 124, 190
Opioids, 14–15, 123, 130, 261–262, 338
  abuse of, 313–315
Opium, 118
Optic neuritis, 175–177
Oral contraceptive pills (OCPs). *See* Oral contraceptives
Oral contraceptives (OC), 6, 11, 47, 120, 126, 131, 138–139, 158, 167, 172, 174, 192, 194, 218, 234, 281, 286, 301, 326, 334–335, 337–339, 344–345
Oral hairy leukoplakia, 114–116
Oral laceration, 111

Index